Landmark Papers in Cardiovascular Medicine

Landmark Papers in . . . series

Landmark Papers in Cardiovascular Medicine

Edited by

Dr Aung Myat BSc(Hons) MB BS MRCP

Specialist Registrar in Cardiology and
BHF Clinical Research Training Fellow
West Midlands Deanery and
BHF Centre of Research Excellence
The Rayne Institute, St Thomas' Hospital,
King's College London, UK

Professor Anthony H. Gershlick BSc(Hons) MB BS MD FRCP

Professor of Interventional Cardiology
University of Leicester, UK

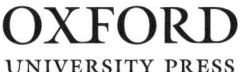

OXFORD
UNIVERSITY PRESS

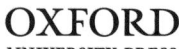

OXFORD
UNIVERSITY PRESS

Great Clarendon Street, Oxford, OX2 6DP,
United Kingdom

Oxford University Press is a department of the University of Oxford.
It furthers the University's objective of excellence in research, scholarship,
and education by publishing worldwide. Oxford is a registered trade mark of
Oxford University Press in the UK and in certain other countries

© Oxford University Press 2012

The moral rights of the author[s] have been asserted

First Edition published in 2012

Impression: 1

All rights reserved. No part of this publication may be reproduced, stored in
a retrieval system, or transmitted, in any form or by any means, without the
prior permission in writing of Oxford University Press, or as expressly permitted
by law, by licence or under terms agreed with the appropriate reprographics
rights organization. Enquiries concerning reproduction outside the scope of the
above should be sent to the Rights Department, Oxford University Press, at the
address above

You must not circulate this work in any other form
and you must impose this same condition on any acquirer

British Library Cataloguing in Publication Data
Data available

Library of Congress Cataloging in Publication Data
Library of Congress Control Number: 2012940771

ISBN 978–0–19–959476–4

Printed and bound by
CPI Group (UK) Ltd, Croydon, CR0 4YY

Oxford University Press makes no representation, express or implied, that the
drug dosages in this book are correct. Readers must therefore always check
the product information and clinical procedures with the most up-to-date
published product information and data sheets provided by the manufacturers
and the most recent codes of conduct and safety regulations. The authors and
the publishers do not accept responsibility or legal liability for any errors in the
text or for the misuse or misapplication of material in this work. Except where
otherwise stated, drug dosages and recommendations are for the non-pregnant
adult who is not breast-feeding

Links to third party websites are provided by Oxford in good faith and
for information only. Oxford disclaims any responsibility for the materials
contained in any third party website referenced in this work.

Foreword

Landmark Papers in Cardiovascular Medicine by Dr Aung Myat and Professor Tony Gershlick represents an outstanding collection of articles and associated commentary. This book is part of the prestigious Oxford University Press series. Distinguished authors from around the globe have been assembled and have successfully identified key papers from the past four decades—papers that have informed clinical practice, shaped professional society guidelines, and spawned further research.

The editors start off their book with a section on coronary heart disease, and then cover electrophysiology, heart failure, hypertension, valvular heart disease, and cardiac imaging—the major disciplines within cardiology. Within each of these sections, authors present the seminal papers in the field. Beyond providing mere summaries of these papers, the authors provide contextual background, as well as a critique of the strengths and weaknesses of the papers. They also provide expert perspective on the impact the papers have had on the field, as well as key learning points, and additional references for those who want to pursue a specific topic in greater detail. Essentially, the book summarizes the major papers that would have been covered in an academic journal club conducted over the past forty years, with the added benefit of assessing what is truly important and durable through the lens of time.

This book will be of great interest to those who practice or study cardiovascular medicine. For the physician in training, this book provides the perfect preparation to quote the relevant medical literature on rounds and appear erudite (and, in fact, be erudite). I hope you find the book as stimulating, educational, and exciting as I did.

Deepak L. Bhatt, MD, MPH, FACC, FAHA, FSCAI, FESC
Professor of Medicine, Harvard Medical School
Chief of Cardiology, VA Boston Healthcare System
Director, Integrated Interventional Cardiovascular Program,
Brigham and Women's Hospital & VA Boston Healthcare System
Senior Investigator, TIMI Study Group
Boston, United States

Preface

'Why' is always the question. Compiling a book entitled *'Landmark Papers in Cardiovascular Medicine'* is no small undertaking. As with all such projects, it requires the assistance and dedication of busy authors to produce high quality manuscripts against a backdrop of over-ambitious editors and publisher-driven deadlines. In this instance the effort required has been that much greater since, for each chosen discipline of cardiovascular medicine, all of the papers published over the past 40 years were to be considered for inclusion in the appropriate chapter, reviewed where indicated, read forensically, then analysed, and a decision taken to select (or not) the source for inclusion. If chosen, the papers had to be summarized, and then came the difficult bit—considering their contemporary relevance and adjudicating on their importance, and indicating the reasons why.

In completing this book we were privileged to draw upon the ability, enthusiasm, and drive of junior colleagues who prepared the first summary drafts for each chapter. Their contribution should not be underestimated and their efforts bode well for their futures and for that of their chosen disciplines. We were also extremely fortunate to be able to muster the support of the cognoscenti: senior researchers who have published extensively in the field. These senior authors know and have used these data (and those not selected) over many years, building on all publications to generate new hypotheses and incrementally advanced research studies. They were handed the difficult and unenviable job of finally selecting the papers to be included, reviewing the junior doctors' summary reviews, modifying and fine tuning the arguments where needed, and then writing the all-important commentaries at the beginning and end of each chapter. Clearly, the selection of a source as a 'Landmark Paper' is a decision based on individual professional experience and some, may be many, will not agree with the choices. There cannot be, however, a right or wrong choice, merely the opinion of experienced senior researchers in the field. Unexpressed reader criticism, debate, and controversy over the choices they have made may stimulate others to choose their own personal list. The reader should not get confused by the differing order of the papers. We gave the authors free rein on how they wished to present their chapters—some chose a chronological order, others hierarchical, others interweaving papers to tell an important historical story. The variance prevents conformity and makes the overall text more interesting. We are lucky that all contributions are of the highest quality.

So 'why'? Most importantly we feel that to have available an analytical understanding of what went before will always foster robust thinking and hopefully evolve novel concepts and research data of equally high quality. Contemporary research doesn't just appear out of thin air. Instead the evidence base that constitutes any discipline is the bedrock for understanding the strengths and weaknesses of the medicine we practice. We hope and believe that such a book will educate beyond the boundaries of the papers presented, inspire, and encourage readers to generate future robust data in order to support current and future clinical practice. Moreover many training schemes worldwide have entry, mid, or exit exams—it is all here, between these covers.

We hope this tome achieves its aims. If even one reader is inspired sufficiently by what went before to begin to build new data and understandings for the future, then our combined efforts have been worthwhile.

Tony Gershlick and Aung Myat

Acknowledgements

First and foremost we owe a huge debt of gratitude to our panel of expert authors. It is they that have selected the landmark papers we have included in this text. It is their choices that will no doubt court some degree of controversy despite the justification and detailed analysis. By virtue of their position, scientific track records, and their standing in the wider cardiovascular community, these esteemed experts are hugely busy people. We therefore thank each and every one of them wholeheartedly for believing in the project and their willingness to devote their valuable time to its success.

Second, we thank our junior colleagues for their energy and enthusiasm for the project. They have worked tirelessly and challenged themselves without reproach to extract every nuance from each of the papers they have summarized. We have been exacting in what we required from the landmark paper appraisals and we have been hugely impressed at what we have received.

Third, we must pay tribute to our colleagues at Oxford University Press, namely Helen Liepman, Elizabeth Chadwick, Imogen Lowe, Susan Crowhurst, and Charles Haynes for their trust, guidance, and ultimately patience, for a manuscript which has taken the best part of two years to compile. Thanks too to Priya Sagayaraj at Cenveo Publisher Services.

And last, but by no means least, we thank, unreservedly, our families, friends and colleagues for their unerring support and understanding.

Aung Myat and Tony Gershlick

I also acknowledge financial support from the Department of Health via the National Institute for Health Research (NIHR) comprehensive Biomedical Research Centre award to Guy's and St Thomas' NHS Foundation Trust in partnership with King's College London and King's College Hospital NHS Foundation Trust, alongside a British Heart Foundation Clinical Research Training Fellowship.

And finally I would like to take this opportunity to thank, wholeheartedly, my mentors: Professors Redwood, Marber, and Gershlick, for their belief, guidance and unequivocal support.

Aung Myat

Contents

Part V **Valvular heart disease**

Part VI **Cardiac imaging**

Part VII

Part VIII

Part IX

Contributors

Dr Dawn Adamson
Consultant Cardiologist
University Hospitals of Coventry and Warwickshire
NHS Trust
Coventry, UK
No conflicts of interest to declare

Dr Amit P. Amin MD MSc
Assistant Professor
Division of Cardiology, Department of Medicine
Washington University School of Medicine,
St. Louis, Missouri, USA
No conflicts of interest to declare

Dr Suzanne Arnold MD
Fellow, Cardiovascular Diseases
Saint Luke's Mid America Heart Institute and the
University of Missouri-Kansas City,
Kansas City, Missouri, USA
No conflicts of interest to declare

Dr Kaleab Asrress
Specialist Registrar in Cardiology
BHF Clinical Research Fellow
The Rayne Institute
St Thomas' Hospital
London, UK
No conflicts of interest to declare

Dr Natalia Briceno BSc MB BS MRCP
ST3 Cardiology
Kent, Surrey and Sussex Deanery, UK
No conflicts of interest to declare

Dr Donna M. Buchanan PhD
Researcher/Outcomes Manager, Saint Luke's Mid
America Heart Institute and
Teaching Assistant Professor, University of
Missouri-Kansas City School of Medicine,
Kansas, Missouri, USA
No conflicts of interest to declare

Dr Paul Chan MD
Associate Professor of Internal Medicine
Mid America Heart Institute and the University of
Missouri-Kansas City,
Kansas City, Missouri, USA
No conflicts of interest to declare

Dr Gerry Coghlan MD FRCP
Consultant Cardiologist & Pulmonary
Hypertension Lead, London, UK
Royal Free London NHS Trust
No conflicts of interest to declare

Dr David J. Cohen MD MSc
Missouri Endowed Chair in Cardiovascular Research
University of Missouri-Kansas City School of Medicine,
Kansas City, Missouri, USA
Dr Cohen has received Research Grant Support from
Medtronic, Boston Scientific, Abbott Vascular, Eli Lilly,
Eisai Pharmaceuticals, Astra-Zeneca, Biomet, and
Edwards Lifesciences and consulting income from
Medtronic, Abbott Vascular, and Eli Lilly

Professor John GF Cleland
Professor of Cardiology
Hull York Medical School (at University of Hull)
Castle Hill Hospital
Kingston-upon-Hull
East Riding of Yorkshire,
Yorkshire, UK
No conflicts of interest to declare

Professor Nick Curzen BM(Hons) PhD FRCP
Consultant Cardiologist and Professor of
Interventional Cardiology
University Hospital Southampton NHS
Foundation Trust,
Southampton, UK
No conflicts of interest to declare

Dr William R Davies
Cardiology Specialist Registrar
Papworth Hospital NHS Foundation Trust,
Cambridgeshire, UK
No conflicts of interest to declare

Dr Kalpa De Silva
Specialist Registrar and Research Fellow
in Cardiology
St. Thomas' Hospital
King's College London, UK
No conflicts of interest to declare

Professor Michael Frenneaux
Regius Professor of Medicine
School of Medicine & Dentistry
University of Aberdeen,
Aberdeen, UK
Professor Frenneaux is inventor of method of use patents for Perhexiline in heart muscle diseases. He sits on a clinical units adjudication committee for the SIGNIFY trial, which is sponsored by Servier. He has received speaker fees from A.Menarini. He sits on an advisory panel for Cephalon Inc.

Dr John Fryearson
Cardiology Registrar
Severn Deanery, Bristol, UK
No conflicts of interest to declare

Professor Bernard J Gersh
Professor of Medicine, Mayo Clinic College of Medicine,
Consultant in Cardiovascular Diseases, Mayo Clinic, Arizona, USA
Declarations:
Ortho-McNeil Janssen Scientific Affairs – Member of the Executive Committee for the ORBIT-AF Registry
Amorcyte Inc. – Member of a DSMB
Abbott Laboratories – Member of a DSMB
GE Healthcare – General Consulting
St Jude Medical Inc. – Member of a DSMB
Medispec Limited – Member of a DSMB
Merck & Co Inc. – Participation in the DEFINE Study
Boston-Scientific – Member of a DSMB
Baxter Healthcare Corporation – Member of a DSMB

Dr Kaushik Guha MBBS BSc (Hons) MRCP
Clinical Cardiology Fellow
Royal Brompton Hospital
National Heart & Lung Institute, Imperial College, London, UK
No conflicts of interest to declare

Dr Paul A. Gurbel M.D.
Director, Sinai Center for Thrombosis Research
Sinai Hospital of Baltimore
Associate Professor of Medicine
Johns Hopkins University School of Medicine, Baltimore, Maryland, USA
Dr Gurbel reported serving as a consultant for Daiichi Sankyo, Lilly, Pozen, Novartis, Bayer, AstraZeneca, Accumetrics, Nanosphere, Sanofi-Aventis, Boehringer Ingelheim, Merck, Medtronic, Iverson Genetics, CSL, and Haemonetics; receiving grants or grants pending from the National Institutes of Health, Daiichi Sankyo, Lilly, Pozen, CSL, AstraZeneca, Sanofi-Aventis,
Haemoscope, Medtronic, Harvard Clinical Research Institute, and Duke Clinical Research Institute; receiving payment for lectures, including service on speakers' bureaus from Lilly, Daiichi Sankyo, Nanosphere, Sanofi Aventis, Merck, and Iverson Genetics; receiving payment for development of educational presentations from Schering-Plough, the Discovery Channel, and Pri-Med; and holding patents in the area of personalized antiplatelet therapy and interventional cardiology.

Dr James Harrison MA MRCP
BHF Clinical Research Fellow in Cardiac Electrophysiology
Divisions of Imaging Sciences & Biomedical Engineering & Cardiovascular Medicine
King's College London
St. Thomas' Hospital
London, UK
No conflicts of interest to declare

Dr Robert A Henderson DM FRCP FESC
Consultant Cardiologist
Trent Cardiac Centre
Nottingham University Hospitals NHS Trust, Nottingham, UK
No conflicts of interest to declare

Dr S Iyengar
Specialist Registrar in Radiology and Cardiac Imaging Fellow
Peninsula Radiology Academy and Peninsula Medical School
Plymouth, UK
No conflicts of interest to declare

Dr Hasan Jilalhawi
Cedars-Sinai Medical Center, Los Angeles, USA
Dr Jilalhawi is a consultant to Edwards Lifesciences, St Jude Medical and Venus Medtech.

Dr Roy Jogiya
SpR Cardiology
London Deanery, London, UK
No conflicts of interest to declare

Dr Dean J. Kereiakes MD FACC FSCAI
Medical Director, The Christ Hospital Heart and Vascular Center/The Lindner Research Center
Professor of Clinical Medicine, Ohio State University, Columbus, Ohio, USA
Dr Kereiakes has received grant and/or research support from Daiichi Sanyko, Inc. and consulting fees from Daiichi Sankyo/Eli Lilly & Co. and Medpace

Dr Jamal N Khan
Clinical Research Fellow in Cardiovascular
Sciences
Glenfield Hospital, Leicester, UK
No conflicts of interest to declare

Dr Mikhail Kosiborod MD FACC FAHA
Associate Professor
St. Luke's Mid America Heart Institute
University of Missouri-Kansas City,
Kansas City, Missouri, USA
Dr Kosiborod reports receiving research grants from the
American Heart Association and Medtronic Diabetes
and has been a Consultant/Advisory Board member for
Medtronic Diabetes, Genentech, Sanofi-Aventis, Gilead,
Kowa Pharmaceuticals, and Boehringer-Ingelheim.

Dr Tushar Kotecha
ST3 Cardiology
London Deanery, London, UK
No conflicts of interest to declare

Dr Pier Lambiase PhD FRCP
Senior Lecturer & Honorary Consultant Cardiologist
Cardiology Department
Heart Hospital, University College London,
London, UK
No conflicts of interest to declare

Dr Francisco Leyva
Consultant Cardiologist
Queen Elizabeth Hospital, University Hospitals
Birmingham NHS Trust
Reader in Cardiology, University of Birmingham,
Birmingham, UK
Dr Leyva has been a consultant to and has received
speaker honoraria and research support from Medtronic
Inc., St Jude Medical, Sorin and Boston Scientific.

Dr Boon Lim
Specialist Registrar in Cardiac Electrophysiology
Heart Hospital, University College London,
London, UK
No conflicts of interest to declare

Dr Nick Linton MEng MRCP
MRC Clinical Research Fellow in Cardiac
Electrophysiology
Divisions of Imaging Sciences & Biomedical
Engineering & Cardiovascular Medicine
King's College London
St. Thomas' Hospital
London, UK
No conflicts of interest to declare

Professor Gregory YH Lip MD, FRCP (London, Edinburgh, Glasgow), DFM, FACC, FESC
Professor of Cardiovascular Medicine
University of Birmingham Centre for Cardiovascular
Sciences
Birmingham City Hospital, Birmingham, UK
Professor Lip has served as a consultant to
Bayer, Astellas, Merck, Sanofi, BMS/Pfizer,
Daiichi-Sankyo, Biotronik, Portola and Boehringer
Ingelheim and has been on the speakers' bureau
for Bayer, BMS/Pfizer, Boehringer Ingelheim, and
Sanofi Aventis.

Professor Theresa A McDonagh MBBS BSc MRCP MD FESC
Consultant Cardiologist and Professor of Clinical
Cardiology
King's College Hospital
Denmark Hill
London, UK
No conflicts of interest to declare

Dr Nestor Mercado MD PhD FESC
Interventional Cardiology Fellow
Swedish Heart and Vascular Institute, Seattle,
Washington, USA
No conflicts of interest to declare

Professor Mark J Monaghan PhD FRCP (Hon) FACC FESC
Director of Non-Invasive Cardiology
King's College Hospital
Denmark Hill, London, UK
No conflicts of interest to declare

Dr William Moody
British Heart Foundation Clinical Research Fellow and
SpR Cardiology
Queen Elizabeth Hospital, University Hospital
Birmingham NHS Foundation Trust and
School of Clinical and Experimental Medicine,
College of Medical and Dental Sciences, University
of Birmingham,
Birmingham, UK
No conflicts of interest to declare

Dr Mani Motwani
Cardiovascular Research Fellow,
University of Leeds, Leeds, UK
No conflicts of interest to declare

Dr Larry Mulligan PhD FAHA
Senior Principal Scientist and Technical Fellow
Medtronic Inc.,
Hertfordshire, UK
No conflicts of interest to declare

Dr Aung Myat BSc(Hons) MBBS MRCP
Specialist Registrar in Cardiology and BHF
Clinical Research Training Fellow
West Midlands Deanery and
BHF Centre of Research Excellence,
The Rayne Institute, St Thomas' Hospital,
King's College, London, UK
No conflicts of interest to declare.

Dr Julian O M Ormerod
SpR Cardiology
Department of Cardiovascular Medicine
Birmingham University,
Birmingham, UK
No conflicts of interest to declare

Dr Mark O'Neill DPhil FRCP FHRS
Consultant Cardiologist & Reader in Clinical Cardiac
Electrophysiology
Divisions of Imaging Sciences & Biomedical
Engineering & Cardiovascular Medicine
King's College London
St. Thomas' Hospital
London, UK
No conflicts of interest to declare

Dr Alexander R. Opotowsky MD MPH
Boston Adult Congenital Heart Service
Children's Hospital Boston
Brigham and Women's Hospital
Harvard Medical School,
Boston, Massachusetts, USA
No conflicts of interest to declare

Dr Jayan Parameshwar
Consultant Cardiologist
Transplant Unit
Papworth Hospital NHS Foundation Trust,
Cambridgeshire, UK
No conflicts of interest to declare

Dr Tania Pawade
SpR Cardiology
West Midlands Deanery,
Birmingham, UK
No conflicts of interest to declare

Dr Divaka Perera
Senior Lecturer and Consultant Cardiologist
St. Thomas' Hospital
King's College London, UK
No conflicts of interest to declare

Professor Nicholas Peters
Professor of Cardiology and Head of Cardiac
Electrophysiology, Imperial College London, and
Consultant Cardiologist at Imperial College Healthcare
NHS Trust, London, UK
No conflicts of interest to declare

Dr Ricardo Petraco
Specialist Registrar in Cardiology and Clinical
Research Fellow
Imperial College London,
London, UK
No conflicts of interest to declare

Dr Sven Plein
British Heart Foundation Senior Clinical
Research Fellow
Multidisciplinary Cardiovascular Research Centre &
Leeds Institute of Genetics, Health and Therapeutics,
University of Leeds, Leeds, UK
Dr Plein has received research grant support from
Philips Healthcare.

Dr Bernard Prendergast
Consultant Cardiologist
Oxford University Hospitals NHS Trust,
Oxford, UK
No conflicts of interest to declare

Professor C A Roobottom
Professor of Radiology & Peninsula Radiology
Academy Head
Derriford Hospital & Peninsula Medical School
Plymouth, UK
No conflicts of interest to declare

Dr Adam Salisbury MD
Fellow, Cardiovascular Diseases
Saint Luke's Mid America Heart Institute and the
University of Missouri-Kansas City,
Kansas City, Missouri, USA
No conflicts of interest to declare

Dr Nalyaka Sambu
Specialist Registrar in Cardiology
Wessex Cardiothoracic Unit, University Hospital
Southampton NHS Foundation Trust,
Southampton, UK
No conflicts of interest to declare

Dr Joerg Seeburger MD PhD
Consultant Cardiac Surgery
Department of Cardiac Surgery, Heart Centre Leipzig,
Leipzig, Germany
No conflicts of interest to declare

Dr Fu Siong Ng
Clinical Lecturer in Cardiology
National Heart & Lung Institute
Imperial College London,
London, UK
No conflicts of interest to declare

Dr Kim Smolderen
Assistant Professor
Saint Luke's Mid America Heart Institute
AHA/Spina Outcomes Research Center, Kansas City,
Missouri and
Department of Medical Psychology and
Neuropsychology,
Tilburg University, The Netherlands
No conflicts of interest to declare

Professor John Spertus MD MPH FACC FAHA
Daniel Lauer/Missouri Endowed Chair
Tenured Professor of Medicine, UMKC
Saint Luke's Mid America Heart Institute/UMKC
University of Missouri-Kansas City,
Kansas City, Missouri, USA
No conflicts of interest to declare

Dr Ray W. Squires PhD
Professor of Medicine
Program Director, Cardiovascular Health &
Rehabilitation
Mayo Clinic
Rochester, Minnesota, USA
No conflicts of interest to declare

Dr Christopher D Steadman MB ChB MRCP
Specialist Registrar in Cardiology
Queen Elizabeth Hospital, Birmingham, UK
No conflicts of interest to declare

Dr Luke D. Tapp BSc MB BS MRCP
Research Fellow, University of Birmingham Centre
for Cardiovascular Sciences, City Hospital
Birmingham and Honorary Research Associate,
School of Clinical and Experimental Medicine,
University of Birmingham, Birmingham, UK
No conflicts of interest to declare

Dr Udaya S. Tantry Ph.D.
Lab Director

Sinai Center for Thrombosis Research
Sinai Hospital of Baltimore,
Baltimore, Maryland, USA
Dr Tantry reported receiving travel support and
fees for lectures from Accumetrics.

Dr Randal J. Thomas MD MS
Director, Cardiovascular Health Clinic
Mayo Clinic
Rochester, Minnesota, USA
No conflicts of interest to declare

Dr Christopher Valerio
Clinical Research Fellow in Pulmonary Hypertension
Royal Free London NHS Trust, London, UK
No conflicts of interest to declare

Dr Richard W Varcoe
Locum Consultant Cardiologist
Trent Cardiac Centre
Nottingham University Hospitals NHS Trust,
Nottingham, UK
No conflicts of interest to declare

Dr Lakshmi Venkitachalam MD
Assistant Professor
Dept. of Biomedical and Health Informatics,
University of Missouri-Kansas City School of Medicine,
Kansas City, Missouri, USA
No conflicts of interest to declare

Dr Adie Viljoen
Consultant Metabolic Physician
Dept. Metabolic Medicine/Chemical Pathology
Lister Hospital, London, UK
Dr Viljoen has been involved in research studies and/or
received lecture honoraria and consultancy/advisory
fees in the last 3 years from: Abbott, Astra Zeneca, Eli
Lilly, Merck Sharp Dohme, Novo Nordisk, Pfizer, Roche,
Sanofi Aventis, Takeda.

Professor Gary Webb MD
Director, Adolescent and Adult Congenital Heart
Program
Cincinnati Children's Hospital Heart Institute
Cincinnati, Ohio, USA
No conflicts of interest to declare

Dr Anthony Wierzbicki
Dept. Metabolic Medicine/Chemical Pathology
Guy's & St. Thomas' Hospitals NHS Foundation Trust,
London, UK
No conflicts of interest to declare

Professor Friedrich Wilhelm Mohr MD PhD
Medical Director Heart Centre and Chief of Staff
Department of Cardiac Surgery, Heart Centre Leipzig,
Leipzig, Germany
No conflicts of interest to declare

Professor Bryan Williams MD FRCP FESC FAHA
Professor of Medicine
Institute of Cardiovascular Sciences
University College London,
London, UK
No conflicts of interest to declare

Dr Matthew Wright PhD MRCP
Consultant Cardiologist/Electrophysiologist
Divisions of Imaging Sciences & Biomedical
Engineering & Cardiovascular Medicine

King's College London
St. Thomas' Hospital
London, UK
No conflicts of interest to declare

Professor Anji Yetman MD
Professor, Pediatrics
Director, Marfan Cardiology Clinic
Director, Adult Congenital Heart Disease Program
University of Utah, Utah, USA
No conflicts of interest to declare

List of abbreviations

AAS	acute aortic syndrome
ACC	American College of Cardiology
ACCORD	action to control risk in diabetes
ACE	angiotensin converting enzyme
ACEi	angiotensin converting enzyme inhibitors
ACS	acute coronary syndrome
ADONIS	American-Australian-African trial with dronedarone in atrial fibrillation or flutter patients for the maintenance of sinus rhythm
ADP	adenosine diphosphate
AEC	automatic exposure control
AERP	atrial effective refractory periods
AF	atrial fibrillation
AFASAK	aspirin vs. warfarin standard dose
AFCAPS/TexCAPS	air force/Texas coronary atherosclerosis prevention study
AFCL	atrial fibrillation cycle length
AFFIRM	atrial fibrillation follow-up investigation of rhythm management study
AFI	atrial fibrillation investigators
AFl	atrial flutter
AH	atrial-His
AHA	American Heart Association
A-HEFT	African-American heart failure trial
AIM-HIGH	active intervention in metabolism of low HDL/high triglycerides and impact on global health outcomes
ALIVE	amiodarone as compared with lidocaine for shock-resistant ventricular fibrillation
ALLHAT	antihypertensive and lipid-lowering treatment to prevent heart attack trial
AMI	acute myocardial infarction
AMI	acute myocardial infarction
ANOVA	analysis of variance
ARB	angiotensin receptor blocker
ARBITER	arterial biology for the investigation of the treatment effects of reducing cholesterol
ARREST	amiodarone for resuscitation after out-of-hospital cardiac arrest due to ventricular fibrillation
ARTS	arterial revascularization therapies study
ARVC	arrhythmogenic right ventricular cardiomyopathy
AS	aortic stenosis
ASA	acetylsalicylic acid
ASCOT	Anglo-Scandinavian coronary outcomes study
ASD	atrial septal defect
ASPIRE	action on secondary prevention through intervention to reduce events
AT	atrial tachycardia
ATHENA	a placebo-controlled, double-blind, parallel arm trial to assess the efficacy of dronedarone 400 mg bid for the prevention of cardiovascular hospitalization or death from any cause in patients with atrial fibrillation/ atrial flutter
ATLAS	assessment of treatment with lisinopril and survival
ATP	adeonsine tri-phosphate
ATP-II	adult treatment panel report-II
AUC	area under ROC curve
AURORA	study to evaluate the use of rosuvastatin in subjects on regular hemodialysis: an assessment of survival and cardiovascular events
AV	aortic valve
AVA	aortic valve area
AVERT	atorvastatin versus revascularization treatments trial
AVID	antiarrhythmics versus implantable defibrillators
AVNRT	atrioventricular nodal re-entry tachycardia
AVR	aortic valve replacement
AVSD	atrioventricular septal defect
BAFTA	Birmingham atrial fibrillation treatment of the aged study
BARI	bypass angioplasty revascularization investigation
BBC ONE	British bifurcation coronary study
BENESTENT	Belgium Netherlands STENT arterial revascularization therapies study
BHF	British Heart Foundation
β-MHC	β-myosin heavy chain
BMI	body mass index

BMPR2	bone morphogenetic protein receptor 2
BMS	bare metal stenting
BNP	B-type natriuretic peptides
BP	blood pressure
BREATHE-2	bosentan randomized trial of endothelin antagonist therapy for PAH
BV	biventricular
CABG	coronary artery bypass grafting
CABRI	coronary artery bypass revascularization investigation
CAC	coronary artery calcium
CAD	coronary artery disease
CAFA	atrial fibrillation anticoagulation study
CAFE	conduit artery function evaluation
CAMIAT	Canadian amiodarone myocardial infarction trial investigators
CAPS	cardiac arrhythmia pilot study
CARDia	coronary artery revascularization in diabetes trial
CARDS	collaborative atorvastatin diabetes study
CARE-HF	cardiac resynchronization-heart failure
CARISMA	cardiac arrhythmias and risk stratification after acute myocardial infarction
CARPREG	cardiac disease in pregnancy
CASS	coronary artery surgery study
CAST	cardiac arrhythmia suppression trial
CBF	collateral blood flow
CCB	calcium channel blockers
CCS	Canadian Cardiovascular Society
CCS	clinical composite score
CCS	cardiovascular society angina grading
CCT	cardiac computed tomography
CCT	cholesterol treatment trialists' collaboration
ccTGA	congenitally-corrected TGA
CTD-PAH	connective tissue disease-associated pulmonary arterial hypertension
CE-MARC	clinical evaluation of magnetic resonance imaging in coronary heart disease
CETP	cholesterol ester transfer protein
CFI	collateral flow index
CFR	coronary flow reserve
CHAD	CVD–heart attack–diabetes
CHAMP	cardiovascular hospitalization atherosclerosis management programme

CHARM	candesartan in heart failure assessment of reduction in mortality and morbidity
CHD	coronary heart disease
CHEER	chest pain evaluation in the emergency room
CHF	congestive heart failure
CHO	Chinese hamster ovary
CHRISTMAS	carvidelol hibernating reversible ischaemia trial: marker of success
CIBIS	the cardiac insufficiency bisoprolol study
CK	creatine kinase
CL	cycle length
CMR	cardiac magnetic resonance
COMET	carvedilol or metoprolol European trial
COMPANION	comparison of medical therapy, pacing and defibrillation in heart failure
CONSENSUS	cooperative north Scandinavian enalapril survival study
COPD	chronic obstructive pulmonary disease
COPERNICUS	carvedilol prospective randomized cumulative survival
CORONA	controlled rosuvastatin in the multinational trial in heart failure
COURAGE	clinical outcomes utilizing revascularization and aggressive drug evaluation
CPVT	catecholaminergic polymorphic ventricular tachycardia
CR	cardiac rehabilitation
CRCARE	cardiac rehabilitation care continuity through automatic referral evaluation
CRP	C-reactive protein
CRT	cardiac resynchronization therapy
CRT-D	CRT with a defibrillator
CRT-P	CRT without a defibrillator
CS	coronary sinus
CSX	cardiac syndrome X
CT	computed tomography
CTCA	computed tomography coronary angiography
CTEPH	chronic thrombo-embolic pulmonary hypertension
CTI	cavotricuspid isthmus
CURE	clopidogrel in unstable angina to prevent recurrent events
CVA	cerebrovascular accident
CVD	cardiovascular disease

CW	continuous-wave
Cx43	connexin43
CXA	coronary angiography
D2B	door-to-balloon
DAIS	diabetes atherosclerosis intervention study
DAL-OUTCOMES	efficacy and safety of dalcetrapib in patients with recent acute coronary syndrome
DANAMI	danish trial in acute myocardial infarction
DAPT	dual antiplatelet therapy study
DART	diet and re-infarction trial
DASI	Duke activity status index
DC	direct current
DCM	dilated cardiomyopathy
DEFER	multi-centre randomized study to compare deferral vs. performance of PCI of non-ischaemic-producing stenoses
DES	drug eluting stenting
DETECT	early, simple and reliable DETECTion of pulmonary arterial hypertension (PAH) in systemic sclerosis (SSc)
DHA	docosahexaenoic acid
DHF	dyssnchronous heart failure
DIAMOND	Danish investigations of arrhythmia and mortality on dofetilide
DIONYSOS	short-term, randomized, double-blind, parallel-group study to evaluate the efficacy and safety of dronedarone versus amiodarone in patients with persistent atrial fibrillation
DLP	dose length product
DOSE	diuretic optimization strategies evaluation
DSE	dobutamine stress echocardiography
DSM	diagnostic and statistical manual
DSMB	data and safety monitoring board
DT	deceleration time
d-TGA	d-transposition of the great arteries
EBCT	electron-beam computed tomography
ECG	electrocardiogram
ECMO	extracorporeal membrane oxygenation
ECTCM	ECG-controlled tube current modulation
ED	effective dose
ED	emergency department
EDIC	echo-dobutamine international cooperative
EF	ejection fraction

EFFECT	enhanced feedback for effective cardiac treatment
EMIAT	european myocardial infarct amiodarone trial
EMPHASIS-HF	eplerenone in mild patients hospitalization and survival study in heart failure
EP	electrophysiology
EPA	eicosapentaenoic acid
EPIC	echo-persantine international cooperative
ERACI	argentine randomized trial of coronary angioplasty with stenting versus coronary bypass surgery in patients with multivessel disease
ERO	effective regurgitant orifice
ESC	European Society of Cardiology
ESR	erythrocyte sedimentation rate
ETT	exercise tolerance test
EURIDIS	European trial in atrial fibrillation or flutter patients receiving dronedarone for the maintenance of sinus rhythm
EUROASPIRE	European action on secondary prevention through intervention to reduce events
FAME II	fractional flow reserve versus angiography for multi-vessel evaluation II
FFR	fractional flow reserve
FHS	Framingham heart study
FISH	fluorescence in situ hybridization
FREEDOM	future revascularization evaluation in patients with diabetes mellitus: optimal management of multi-vessel disease
FRISC II	the Framingham and Fast revascularization during instability in coronary artery disease (FRISC) II trial
FRS	Framingham risk score
GISSI-2	second gruppo italiano por lo studio della streptochinasi nell'infarto miocardic
GISSI-P	gruppo italiano per lo studio della sopravvivenza nell'infarto miocardico (prevenzione)
GPCR	G-protein coupled receptor
GUSTO	global utilization of streptokinase and t-PA for occluded coronary arteries
GWAS	genome-wide association study
HAS-BLED	hypertension, abnormal renal/liver function, stroke, bleeding history or predisposition, labile INR, elderly, drugs/alcohol concomitantly score
HCM	hypertrophic cardiomyopathy

HDL-C	high-density lipoprotein cholesterol		JUPITER	justification for the use of statins in prevention: an intervention trial evaluating rosuvastatin
HEAAL	heart failure end point evaluation of angiotensin II antagonists losartan trial		LA	left atrial
HeFNEF	heart failure with normal ejection fraction		LAA	left atrial appendage
HEMOR$_2$RHAGES	hepatic or renal disease, ethanol abuse, malignancy, older age (>75 years), rebleeding, reduced platelet count or function, hypertension (uncontrolled), anemia, genetic factors, excessive fall risk, and stroke		LAD	left anterior descending
			LAR	lifetime attributable risk
			LBBB	left bundle branch block
			LDL-C	low-density lipoprotein cholesterol
			LGE-CMR	late gadolinium-enhanced CMR
			LIFE	losartan intervention for endpoint reduction in hypertension
HF	heart failure		LM	left main coronary disease
HFpEF	heart failure with preserved ejection fraction		LMWH	low molecular weight heparin
HHV 6	human herpes virus type 6		LTA	light transmittance agregometry
HLHS	hypoplastic left heart syndrome		LV	left ventricle
HOPE	heart outcomes prevention evaluation		LVAD	left ventricular assist device
HOT CAFE	how to treat chronic atrial fibrillation		LVAS	left ventricular assist system
HPR	high on-treatment platelet reactivity		LVEDVI	left ventricle end-diastolic volume index
HPS	heart protection study		LVEF	left ventricular ejection fraction
HPS-2/THRIVE	heart protection study-2/treatment of HDL to reduce the incidence of vascular events		LVESD	left ventricular end-systolic diameter
			LVESV	left ventricular end systolic volume
			LVESVI	left ventricular end systolic volume index
HR	hazard ratio		LVOT	left ventricular outflow tract
Hyd-Iso	hydralazine and isosorbide dinitrate		LVSD	left ventricular systolic dysfunction
HYVET	hypertension in the very elderly trial		MA	maximal amplitude
IC	intracoronary		MACCE	major adverse cardiac and cerebrovascular events
ICA	invasive coronary angiography		MACE	major adverse cardiac events
ICD	implantable cardioverter defibrillator		MADIT-CRT	multicentre automatic defibrillator implantation trial with cardiac resynchronization therapy
IHD	ischaemic heart disease			
ILLUMINATE	investigation of lipid level management to understand its impact in atherosclerotic events		MADIT-II	multicentre automatic defibrillator implantation trial II
			MASS	medicine, angioplasty, or surgery study
IMA	internal mammary artery		MATE	medicine versus angiography in thrombolytic exclusion
IMPROVE-IT	improved reduction of outcomes: vytorin efficacy international trial			
			MBG	myocardial blush grade
INR	international normalized ratio		MDCT	multidetector CT
I-PRESERVE	irbesartan in patients with heart failure and preserved ejection fraction		MERIT-HF	metoprolol CR/XL randomized intervention trial in congestive heart failure
IRA	infarct-related artery			
ISIS-1	first International Study of Infarct Survival		MI	myocardial infarction
ISIS-2	second international study of infarct survival		MIAMI	metoprolol in acute myocardial infarction
IV	instrumental variable		MIBI	methoxyisobutylisonitrile
IVC	inferior vena cava		MINAP	myocardial infarction national audit project
JELIS	Japan EPA lipid intervention study			
JNC-V	joint national committee-V			
J-RHYTHM	Japanese rhythm management trial for atrial fibrillation study			

MIRACLE	multicenter insync randomized clinical evaluation	PASP	pulmonary artery systolic pressure
M-LVDP	mean left ventricular diastolic pressure	PBMV	percutaneous balloon mitral valvotomy
MONICA	multinational monitoring of cardiovascular disease project	PCI	percutaneous coronary intervention
		pCMBS	p-chloromercuriphenylsulphonic acid
mPAP	mean pulmonary artery pressure	PCR	polymerase chain reaction
MPI	myocardial perfusion index	PCWP	pulmonary capillary wedge pressure
MPRI	myocardial-perfusion reserve index	PEP-CHF	perindopril in elderly people with chronic heart failure
MR	mitral regurgitation	PET	positron emission tomography
MRA	magnetic resonance angiography	PHV	percutaneous heart valve
MRA	minimalo-corticoid antagonist	POBA	plain old balloon angioplasty
MRC	Medical Research Council	PPAR	peroxisomal proliferator activating receptor
MRI	magnetic resonance imaging		
MR-IMPACT	magnetic resonance imaging for myocardial perfusion assessment in coronary artery disease trial	PPH	primary pulmonary hypertension
		PPHN	persistent pulmonary hypertension of the newborn
MR-INFORM	MR perfusion imaging to guide management of patients with stable coronary artery disease	PPV	positive predictive value
		PPVI	percutaneous pulmonary valve implant
		PROBE	prospective, randomised, open-label, blinded-end point
MRS	magnetic resonance spectroscopy		
MS	mitral stenosis	PROCAM	prospective cardiovascular münster study
MUGA	multi-gated acquisition scan		
MVA	mitral valve area	PROSPECT	predictors of response to CRT
MVR	mitral valve replacement	PROSPER	prospective study of pravastatin in the elderly at risk
NCEP	national cholesterol education program		
NHANES	national health and nutrition survey	PROTECTION I	prospective multicenter study on radiation dose estimates of cardiac CT angiography in daily practice I
NHLBI	National Heart, Lung, and Blood Institute		
NHP	Nottingham Health Profile		
NICE	National Institute for Health and Clinical Excellence	PROVE-IT-TIMI 22	pravastatin or atorvastatin evaluation and infection therapy–thrombolysis in myocardial infarction 22
NNT	number-needed-to-treat		
NPV	negative predictive value	PST	post-systolic thickening
NRAF	National Registry of Atrial Fibrillation	PUFA	polyunsaturated fatty acid
NSTEMI	non-ST elevation infarction	PV	pulmonary vein
NSVT	non-sustained ventricular tachycardia	PVd	pulmonary vein diastolic
NYHA	New York Heart Association	PVI	pulmonary vein isolation
OAC	oral anticoagulation	PVR	pulmonary vascular resistance
OD	optical density	PVs	pulmonary vein systolic
OMT	optimal medical therapy	PW	pulsed-wave
ONTARGET	ongoing telmisartan alone and in combination with ramipril global endpoint trial	QALY	quality adjusted life year
		QCA	quantitative coronary angiography
		QI	quality improvement
ORT	orthodromic reciprocating tachycardia	QoF	quality outcomes framework
PA	pulmonary artery	RAA	renin-angiotensin-aldosterone
PACES	patient-centred episode system	RALES	randomized aldactone evaluation study
PAH	pulmonary arterial hypertension	RAP	right atrial pressure
PAPI	pharmacogenomics of antiplatelet intervention	RAS	renin-angiotensin-aldosterone system

RAVEL	randomized study with the sirolimus-eluting velocity balloon-expandable stent in the treatment of patients with de novo native coronary artery lesions
RCA	right coronary artery
RCT	randomized conrolled trial
RE-LY	randomized evaluation of long term anticoagulant therapy
RELY-ABLE	long-term multi-centre extension of dabigatran treatment in patients with atrial fibrillation who completed RE-LY trial
RethinQ	cardiac-resynchronization therapy in heart failure with narrow QRS complexes
REVERSAL	reversal of atherosclerosis with aggressive lipid lowering
REVERSE	resynchronization reverses remodeling in systolic left ventricular dysfunction RF radiofrequency
RIPCORD	routine pressure wire assessment influence management strategy at coronary angiography for diagnosis of chest pain
RITA-2	second randomized intervention treatment of angina trial
ROC	receiver operating characteristic
ROMICAT	rule out myocardial infarction using computer assisted tomography
RSMR	risk-standardized mortality rate
RT	real-time
RV	right ventricle
RVOT	right ventricular outflow tract
RVSP	right ventricular systolic pressure
RWMA	regional wall motion abnormalities
SADS	sudden adult death syndrome
SALTIRE	scottish aortic stenosis and lipid lowering trial, impact on regression
SAQ	Seattle angina questionnaire
SCD	sudden cardiac death
SEAS	simvastatin and ezetimibe in aortic stenosis
SHARP	study of heart and renal protection
SHIFT	systolic heart failure treatment with ifinhibitor ivabradine trial
SHOCK	should we emergently revascularize occluded coronaries for cardiogenic shock trial
SIHD	stable ischaemic heart disease
SK	streptokinase
SMASH-VT	substrate mapping and ablation in sinus rhythm to halt ventricular tachycardia

SNP	single nucleotide polymorphism
SOC	standard-of-care
SOLVD	studies of left ventricular dysfunction
SoS	stent or surgery trial
SPAF	stroke prevention and atrial fibrillation
SPECT	single positron emission tomography
SR	sinus rhythm
SR	strain rate
ST	stent thrombosis
STEMI	ST-elevation myocardial infarction
STICH	surgical treatment for ischemic heart failure
SVC	superior vena cava
SVT	supraventricular tachycardia
SWISSI II	Swiss interventional study on silent ischemia type II
SWORD	Survival with oral d-sotalol
SYNTAX	synergy between PCI with taxus and cardiac surgery trial
T2DM	type 2 diabetes mellitus
TACTICS-TIMI 18	treat angina with aggrastat and determine cost of therapy with an invasive or conservative strategy-thrombolysis in myocardial infarction 18
TAPAS	thrombus aspiration during percutaneous coronary intervention in acute myocardial infarction study
TAVI	transcatheter aortic valve implantation
TC	total cholesterol
TDI	tissue Doppler imaging
TEG	thromboelastography
TGA	the great arteries
TIA	transient ischaemic attack
TIME	trial of invasive versus medical therapy in elderly
TIMI	thrombolysis in myocardial infarction
TLR	target lesion revascularization
TMS	transmurality scoring
TNF	tumour-necrosis factor
TOE	trans-oesophageal echocardiography
ToF	tetralogy of Fallot
t-PA	tissue plasminogen activator
TTE	transthoracic echocardiography
TUNEL	terminal deoxynucleotidyl transferase dutp nick end labelling
TVR	target vessel revascularization
TXA2	thromboxane A2

UA	unstable angina		VF	ventricular fibrillation
UFH	unfractionated heparin		V-HeFT	vasodilator-heart failure trials
UKPDS	United Kingdom prospective diabetes study		VSD	ventricular septal defect
VA	ventriculoarterial		VT	ventricular tachycardia
VA	veterans affairs		WASH	warfarin/aspirin study in heart failure
VA-HIT	veterans administration HDL intervention trial		WATCH	warfarin and antiplatelet therapy in chronic heart failure
VALHeFT	valsartan heart failure trial investigators		WHO	World Health Organization
VALIANT	valsartan in acute myocardial infarction		WMSI	wall-motion score index
VANQWISH	veterans affairs non-Q-wave infarction strategies in-hospital		WOSCOPS	west of Scotland coronary prevention study
VINO	value of first day angiography/angioplasty In evolving Non-ST segment elevation myocardial infarction, an open multicenter randomized trial		XMR	X-ray radiography and magnetic resonance
			YLS	years of life saved

Part I

Coronary heart disease

Chapter 1

Epidemiology, outcomes, and quality of care

Dr Kim Smolderen, Dr Amit Amin, Dr Suzanne Arnold, Dr Donna Buchanan, Dr Paul Chan, Dr David Cohen, Dr Mikhail Kosiborod, Dr Nestor Mercado, Dr Adam Salisbury, Dr Lakshmi Venkitachalam, and Professor John Spertus

Introduction

Epidemiology is the study of large populations of patients aimed at documenting incidence and prevalence of disease, with a goal to also define the causes of disease. Dating back to Hippocrates, who systematically sought to understand the cause of disease, the field has grown increasingly sophisticated in its methods and insights. While seminal epidemiologists like John Snow—who identified the cause of a cholera epidemic in England in 1854—helped found the field, the landmark Framingham study helped to shape the field in cardiology by providing some of the most powerful insights into the risk factors for cardiovascular disease. In fact, it remains an important source

of information as the programme is still active today and is continually expanding its analyses of genetic, biomarker, and physiological determinants of heart disease. The methods of the field have matured substantially throughout the years and now incorporate a myriad of novel risk factors, including genetics and environmental exposures, as a means of identifying the causes of disease.

Although epidemiology has a centuries-old tradition of providing insights into the causes and prognosis of disease, outcomes research is a much younger discipline, coming into its own over just the past decade. It is emerging as an increasingly important discipline, as medicine struggles to incorporate new technologies in an era of decreasing financial resources for healthcare systems. In fact, the increased funding for comparative effectiveness research in the United States underscores the demand for outcomes research, a field of scientific inquiry that examines the results of healthcare interventions and policy. It is not defined by any particular method, but rather, it leverages multiple methodologies, including epidemiology, health services research, economics and decision analysis, qualitative research, and advanced statistical methodologies and study designs[1,2]. What principally defines the field of outcomes research is its focus on the end results of healthcare and its disciplined efforts to define the patient characteristics, processes of care, and the infrastructure in which care is delivered that are associated with those outcomes. Of course, the relevant outcomes extend beyond mortality and disease progression to include patients' health status (symptoms, function, and quality of life) and the costs of care.

Since Paul Ellwood's Shattuck Lecture about outcomes management in 1988[3], the long-term goal of outcomes research has been to gather empirical data from ongoing patient care, and use this to determine how medical care is affecting patients' outcomes to better inform the medical fraternity and patients alike about how they are likely to fare if they undergo alternative treatment options. Often using observational data, outcomes researchers have sought to describe the comparative effectiveness of different therapies. This concept has been extended in recent years to the systematic quantification of healthcare quality as a means for improving care. Research studies now commonly explore the application of evidence-based guidelines, pursue qualitative studies of higher and lower performing healthcare systems, and methodologically inquire about the processes of medical decision making. These insights can then be translated into novel tools to improve the safety, timeliness, equity, efficiency, evidence-base, and patient-centeredness of healthcare[4].

The fields of both epidemiology and outcomes research have benefited enormously over the past few decades from improved computing power, better analytic methods, the availability of large datasets, and the study of clinical behaviour. In this chapter, we highlight a small, somewhat subjective, sample of the seminal articles that have laid the foundation for the current state of the art of these scientific disciplines. We sought to capture a broad spectrum of representative articles that reflect 'growth areas' of the field. Landmark articles are, generally, those that have spawned numerous investigators to further understand the determinants of patients' outcomes and how care is currently delivered so that these outcomes can be improved. We not only relied upon the collective experience of the authors, but also surveyed a number of our colleagues in epidemiology and outcomes research to solicit their input. Paring down the numerous excellent suggestions was a challenge and the selected articles are intended to encourage the reader to further explore these disciplines, which will ultimately lead to improvements in the delivery of healthcare and patients' outcomes.

An assessment of clinically useful measures of the consequences of treatment

Laupacis A, Sackett DL, Roberts RS. *N Engl J Med* 1988; 318: 1728–33.

Background

Randomized controlled trials are considered the gold standard for establishing clinical efficacy. However, translating these results to clinical care can be difficult. This challenge is further compounded by the fact that the results of clinical trials are often expressed in different terms, such as the absolute difference in outcomes between the groups, the relative risk (the ratio) of having an outcome with one treatment versus another, and the relative risk reduction (1 minus the relative risk). All three of these representations of the data may be confusing for physicians to explain to patients. Also, since trials have different patient populations and different durations of follow-up, it can be difficult for clinicians to compare and contrast the results of different studies.

Article summary

This article is a well-articulated thought piece that explains the alternative methods for summarizing the results of a clinical trial. The authors advocate for a novel metric, the number-needed-to-treat (NNT), which is calculated as 1/absolute risk reduction. The clinical interpretation of this number is simple: how many patients need to be treated for the period of time studied for 1 not to have the outcome. The authors extend this concept to also express the number who would experience harm from the new treatment and to normalize the results for different periods of observation in different trials. They eloquently enumerate the challenges of this metric and also emphasize how it can be useful in prioritizing treatments for an individual patient. The use of this measure should facilitate more transparent sharing of evidence from clinical trials with patients so that they can better understand the benefits of treatment.

Strengths and limitations

While framing the results of a single clinical trial using the NNT is easy and straightforward, integrating multiple studies, even of the same treatment, is difficult. While meta-analyses can be helpful in getting a more robust estimate of treatment benefit, these are rarely available. Importantly, this concept underscores the relationship between patients' baseline risk and the benefit they may receive from treatment. If the relative risk reduction is constant, then the greater a patient's risk for an outcome, the greater the expected absolute risk reduction and the lower the NNT. This concept—the heterogeneity of patient benefit—forms the foundational rationale for clinical decision making and has been used to highlight the 'risk-treatment' paradox in cardiovascular disease and the need for strategies to target those with the greatest potential for benefit from treatment. Another important challenge of using the NNT is that it fails to incorporate the uncertainty of estimates in a clinical trial and confidence intervals need to be generated, although they seldom are.

Impact on the field

This article is one of the seminal conceptual contributions to the field of evidence-based medicine and the

translation of evidence into practice. Many clinical trials now report their results in terms of NNT and it has been extended from dichotomous outcomes (such as mortality and rehospitalizations) to quality of life, such that they can be categorized into outcomes of clinically meaningful benefit. It also remains one of the most straightforward ways to communicate the benefits of therapy to patients, although substantial improvements in such communication remain a pressing challenge for the profession.

Learning points

♦ Creating simple, intuitive methods for summarizing the results of clinical trials so that they can be more readily applied to clinical practice is challenging.

♦ The number-needed-to-treat (NNT) is the reciprocal of the absolute risk reduction and indicates how many patients would need to be treated with a new therapy for one to avoid an adverse outcome.

Further reading

- Guyatt GH, Sackett DL, Cook DJ. Users' guides to the medical literature. II. How to use an article about therapy or prevention. A. Are the results of the study valid? Evidence-Based Medicine Working Group. *JAMA* 1993; 270: 2598–601.
- Guyatt GH, Sackett DL, Cook DJ. Users' guides to the medical literature. II. How to use an article about therapy or prevention. B. What were the results and will they help me in caring for my patients? Evidence-Based Medicine Working Group. *JAMA* 1994; 271: 59–63.
- Kent DM, Rothwell PM, Ioannidis JP, Altman DG, Hayward RA. Assessing and reporting heterogeneity in treatment effects in clinical trials: a proposal. *Trials* 2010; 11: 85.

Smoke-free legislation and hospitalizations for acute coronary syndrome

Pell JP, Haw S, Cobbe S, Newby DE, Pell AC, Fischbacher C, McConnachie A, Pringle S, Murdoch D, Dunn F, Oldroyd K, Macintyre P, O'Rourke B, Borland W. *N Engl J Med.* 2008; 359(5): 482–491.

Background

Since the 1964 report by Surgeon General Luther Terry and subsequent epidemiological studies, there has been growing public awareness of the association between

smoking and heart disease. Numerous educational or taxation programmes have since been developed worldwide to curb the use of tobacco. More recently, studies have reported worse outcomes among people exposed to second-hand smoke. As a result, bans on tobacco use in public places have been implemented in several countries to address the risk of passive smoke exposure among non-smokers. However, prior studies of passive exposure to second-hand smoke have been limited by retrospective data collection, small sample sizes, and lack of information on patients' smoking status and exposure to second-hand smoke. This article, published by Pell *et al.*, reports on rates of acute coronary syndrome (ACS) prior to and after implementation of the 'Smoking, Health and Social Care Act' in Scotland in 2005, with a focus on the legislation's impact on non-smokers. In anticipation of this legislation, the authors coordinated their research efforts around this act and prospectively collected patient data with adequate controls.

Article summary

The authors prospectively compared the number of admissions for ACS before and after the implementation of the smoking ban legislation. They enrolled all ACS patients that were admitted to nine hospitals—hospitals whose catchment areas accounted for 63% of all ACS admissions in Scotland—during the previous ten months (June 2005–March 2006) and after the smoking ban (June 2006–March 2007). The researchers defined an ACS admission as one with a detectable level of cardiac troponin after an emergency admission for chest pain. Apart from the routine troponin measurements that were performed in all admitted patients with chest pain, serum cotinine levels, and a self-reported smoking history were obtained. Patients were classified as smokers, never smokers, or former smokers. In addition, the authors ensured the robustness of their findings with historical and geographical controls. They compared rates of ACS prior to implementation of the smoking ban in Scotland (historical control) and contemporaneously with England (geographic control), which had not implemented a smoking ban. Overall, the researchers documented a 17% reduction in hospital admissions for ACS after the enactment of the smoke-free legislation, compared to a 3% mean annual reduction in the historical control and 4% in the geographic control. The number of prevented admissions involving non-smokers accounted for the majority (67%) of the decrease in ACS events. This was confirmed by a reduction in serum cotinine levels in the non-smokers.

Strengths and limitations

In this study, the authors provide an example of a well-designed epidemiologic study. Data were prospectively

collected and the disease state of interest, ACS, was defined using a commonly accepted and standardized definition. The authors ensured that their results were not due to temporal trends through the use of both a historical control (pre- vs. post-implementation) and a geographic control (contemporaneous population not exposed to the intervention). Finally, the authors confirmed self-reported rates of smoking exposure (primary and secondary) with physiologic measurements of cotinine levels. In summary, their study design is viewed as a model for establishing strong associations in population studies. There were, however, several potential limitations in this study. Serum cotinine levels were used instead of saliva specimens to measure patients' exposure to smoke, which likely resulted in an underestimation of cotinine levels. And although the study suggests that the reduction in ACS may have been greater among women than among men, and among older individuals, these findings will need further replication and may not be extrapolated to other populations, as culture and climate differences may produce demographic differences in smoking patterns.

Impact on the field

This paper was the first to thoroughly document the impact of implementing a smoking ban in public areas on public health. Through its methodological rigour, it defined a strong epidemiologic association, backed by biochemical markers, between exposure to second-hand smoke and cardiac events in non-smokers. This study nicely demonstrated how legislation could be used as a tool to protect individuals from the harmful effects of smoking. Because of the strength of this study's findings, other cities and countries have adopted smoking bans and tobacco manufacturers are less likely to mount legislative challenges based upon questionable health benefits alone.

Learning points

- This study was the first to prospectively and thoroughly document the impact of legislation banning smoking in public places on ACS events among non-smokers exposed to second-hand smoke.
- It provides a good example of using epidemiology to support public policy initiatives.

Further reading

- Deyton L, Sharfstein J, Hamburg M. Tobacco product regulation—a public health approach. *N Eng J Med* 2010; 362(19): 1753–6.

- Schroeder SA, Warner KE. Don't forget tobacco. *N Eng J Med* 2010; 363(3): 201–4.

Prediction of coronary heart disease using risk factor categories

Wilson PWF, D'Agostino RB, Levy D, Belanger AM, Silbershatz H, Kannel WB. *Circulation* 1998; 97: 1837–47.

Background

Coronary heart disease (CHD) remains the leading cause of death in the United States, with one in three adults expected to develop the disease during their lifetime. Given the magnitude of the problem, it is not surprising that the scientific community has invested enormous efforts and resources in developing accurate and easy-to-use tools to predict the risk of CHD, an important foundation for developing rational prevention strategies.

Cardiovascular risk assessment and prevention have been the cornerstones for many large-scale epidemiological studies, including the Framingham Heart Study (FHS), one of the earliest and best-known population-based studies of men and women free from overt CHD. Established in 1960, this study provided important insights into the epidemiology of CHD and helped identify actionable risk factors that were subsequently incorporated into primary prevention guidelines. The article under review is a landmark example of how critical information from population-based research can be successfully translated to a simple, yet powerful, algorithm for clinical practice.

Article summary

With the explicit objective of incorporating multivariable estimates of risk, as advocated by the Joint National Committee-V (JNC-V) and the National Cholesterol Education Program (NCEP) Adult Treatment Panel report-II (ATP-II), Wilson and colleagues examined data from a population-based sample of 2489 men and 2856 women, 30–74 years old, and free from overt CHD at baseline in the FHS. Detailed information on demographics, medical history, and laboratory data were ascertained at baseline and participants were followed for over 12 years for the development of CHD (angina pectoris, recognized and unrecognized myocardial infarction, coronary insufficiency and CHD death). 'Hard' CHD events included total CHD without angina pectoris. Information on events was obtained from study clinic visits and review of medical records from physicians' offices and hospitalizations.

The predominant risk factors of interest were blood pressure (BP), total cholesterol (TC), low-density lipoprotein cholesterol (LDL-C), and high-density lipoprotein cholesterol (HDL-C). Age-adjusted linear or logistic regression models were used, as appropriate, to examine the relationship between these risk factors with the development of CHD. Cox proportional hazards regression models were used to estimate the relative risk of 12-year CHD outcomes across risk factor categories and were then adapted to provide ten-year incidence estimates. To simplify implementation, sex-specific score sheets were developed to calculate ten-year absolute risks for total CHD, hard CHD (total CHD without angina pectoris), and low-risk total CHD for persons of the same age and sex.

During follow-up, a total of 383 men and 227 women developed CHD, which was significantly associated with categories of BP, smoking, diabetes, TC, LDL-C, and HDL-C (p = 0.001 for all). In multivariable models, the attributable risk percentage for BP level that exceeded high normal (≥130/85) was 28% in men and 29% in women. The corresponding estimate for elevated TC (≥200 mg/dL) was 27% and 34%, respectively. The discriminatory ability of prediction models, quantified using c-statistics, was similar for models with categorical and continuous forms of risk factors. Using the beta-coefficients from the Cox proportional hazards models, sex-specific score sheets were developed to predict CHD according to the distribution of important risk factors. As an example of use of these score sheets, a 55-year-old man with a TC of 250 mg/dL, HDL-C of 39 mg/dL, and blood pressure of 146/88 who is diabetic and a non-smoker has an estimated absolute 10-year CHD risk of 31% with a relative risk of 1.9 as compared with a 55-year old man with average risk factor levels.

Strengths and limitations

The Framingham Heart Study is one of the earliest population-based, prospective studies to conduct a thorough examination of the epidemiology of CHD in a large sample of men and women with long-term follow-up. The present study builds on previous work from the FHS to efficiently incorporate risk factors into simple risk prediction tools, thus meeting a well articulated need by the JNC and NCEP panels. Importantly, this approach integrates information from multiple risk factors to provide an estimate of both absolute and relative CHD risk in middle-aged adults free from overt CHD and has been successfully incorporated into clinical practice. Some limitations of the study are as follows. First, the study cohort was predominantly middle-class Caucasian subjects with an average age of ~50 years, potentially limiting its accuracy in younger individuals and other racial/ethnic cohorts. Second, the model provides estimates of intermediate-term (ten-year), but not long-term (lifetime), risk of CHD, thus limiting the extent of risk prediction in young subjects with low short-term but high lifetime risk for CHD. Third, the CHD model does not incorporate other important cardiac risk factors such as family history or physical activity and was constructed prior to identification of novel markers of inflammation (e.g. C-reactive protein), subclinical atherosclerosis (coronary calcification), or socioeconomic status. These limitations notwithstanding, the FHS provides a unique, practical system for estimating global CHD risk.

Impact on the field

Assessment of risk status is especially crucial in primary prevention efforts, as it determines the choice and intensity of treatment strategies in patients without manifest disease. This disease prediction algorithm has enabled much more practical implementation of primary prevention guidelines. This also highlights the importance of moving beyond the 'one risk factor at a time' approach by simultaneously considering multiple risk factors in estimating equations. The clinical importance of this tool is further underscored by the inclusion of this scoring system as a means to assess ten-year CHD risk in the 2001 NCEP ATP III guidelines. Overall, this landmark publication, in particular, and the Framingham Study, in general, have defined and shaped the practice of preventive cardiology in the United States.

Learning points

- Higher levels of blood pressure are associated with higher levels of age, body mass index, diabetes, and total cholesterol (TC) in the overall cohort, with sex-specific associations seen in LDL cholesterol (LDL-C) and HDL cholesterol (HDL-C).
- In multivariable models that included age, smoking status, and diabetes, the risk of CHD was significantly higher for (1) hypertension stages I–IV (vs. normal BP of <130/85 mmHg), (2) TC categories of 200–239 and ≥240 mg/dL (vs. <200 mg/dL), and (3) HDL-C levels <35 and ≥60 mg/dL (vs. 35–59 mg/dL) in men and women. In models that replaced TC with LDL-C categories, the risk of CHD was greater with LDL-C ≥160 mg/dL (vs. <130 mg/dL) and magnitude similar to TC categories.

Further reading

- Ridker PM, Buring JE, Rifai N, Cook N. Development and Validation of Improved Algorithms for the Assessment of Global Cardiovascular Risk in Women: The Reynolds Risk Score. *JAMA* 2007; 297: 611–9.

Effect of variability in the interpretation of coronary angiograms on the appropriateness of use of coronary revascularization procedures

Leape LL, Park RE, Bashore TM, Harrison JK, Davidson CJ, Brook RH. *Am Heart J* 2000; 139: 106–13.

Background

Previous clinical trials comparing coronary artery bypass grafting (CABG) with medical therapy had found that patients with left main or three-vessel coronary artery disease benefit from CABG. In contrast, there was no benefit of CABG in the lower-risk groups, such as those with one-vessel disease, who are often more appropriately treated medically or by percutaneous coronary intervention (PCI). These findings were reflected in the American College of Cardiology/American Heart

Association (ACC/AHA) Clinical Practice Guidelines by Eagle *et al.*, which strongly endorsed CABG for left main disease and recommended against its use in the setting of one or two-vessel coronary disease not involving the proximal left coronary artery (*Circulation* 1999; 100(13): 1464–80). Like CABG, the decision to recommend PCI also hinges strongly upon the accurate assessment of coronary stenoses. New York State, in the US, had developed public reporting of physician performance and had been particularly aggressive in applying standards of appropriateness, based upon work by the RAND Corporation. While previous studies had suggested variability in interpretation of coronary angiograms, no study had yet linked this variation to patients' clinical care and medical decision making.

Article summary

Leape *et al.* obtained a sample of 308 angiograms from 15 New York hospitals that were randomly sampled from several strata to represent a diverse group of institutions. Angiograms were randomly selected within three groups: overall group, those with three-vessel disease who underwent CABG, and those with one-vessel disease who underwent PCI. Films were blindly reviewed by a panel of expert angiographers at the Core Angiographic Laboratory at Duke University and were graded on technical quality, presence/location/severity of coronary stenoses, and appropriateness for PCI or CABG. A consensus was reached and compared with the original cardiologists' interpretations to assess variation.

The expert panel found technical deficiencies in over half of cases, most often due to inadequate separation or opacification of vessels. In fact, 12 were of such poor quality that the panel stated that no accurate interpretation could be made. Core lab readings tended to show less significant disease (no stenosis in 16% of vessels previously read as showing significant disease), less severity of stenosis (43% lower, 6% higher), and lower extent of disease (23% less, 6% more) than the original clinical interpretations. The impact of these variations on the potential appropriateness of revascularization was substantial. Among 83 patients who had undergone CABG for three-vessel disease that were rated 'necessary' or 'appropriate' by the New York cardiologists, 14 (17%) were reclassified as inappropriate or uncertain for CABG by the Duke panel. Of the single-vessel disease patients who had undergone PTCA, 10% of those rated necessary or appropriate by New York cardiologists' readings were classified as inappropriate or uncertain when Duke panel readings were used. The finding that some patients had undergone

invasive treatments, including CABG, for no significant CAD raised significant concerns for the field.

Strengths and limitations

As early as 1975, Detre *et al.* demonstrated substantial inter- and intra-observer variation in angiogram interpretation (*Circulation* 1975; 52: 979–86), and despite substantial technical advances in image quality and operator experience, this variation has persisted to the extent that erroneous interpretation was evident in ~30% of cases. What distinguishes Leape's study is that they then linked this variation to the clinical decision to undergo CABG and PCI. The findings of this study suggested that a significant number of patients were undergoing a major operation that was potentially unnecessary, based on erroneous data. The inadequacies of single-observer interpretation of angiograms are obvious, particularly when these are used for decisions as important as whether or not to recommend CABG or PCI. Despite these data, there are currently no mandates for more than one operator to interpret an angiogram prior to proceeding with coronary revascularization.

Impact on the field

The Institute of Medicine estimates that tens of thousands of Americans die each year from errors in their care, and hundreds of thousands suffer or barely escape non-fatal injuries that a truly high-quality care system could prevent. Patient safety issues include not only errors such as administering the wrong drug or dosage to a patient, but also encompass aspects of misdiagnosing the presence or severity of disease and making critical treatment decisions as a result of these misinterpretations. The first step in improving safety is to learn about the causes of error and to use this knowledge to design systems of care that prevent errors. Although angiograms were known to have variations in interpretation, Leape's study extended this finding to demonstrate that this variation resulted in inappropriate treatments for some patients. While this study should have led to a dramatic redesign of healthcare, potentially to include mandatory 'catheterization conferences' to review cases with colleagues prior to treatment, this has not happened.

Learning points

- This study described marked technical deficiencies in the quality of angiography in routine clinical practice.

◆ When interpreted by an expert panel, there was substantial variation in the interpretation of coronary angiograms, with panel readings tending to show less significant disease, less severity of stenoses, and a reduced extent of disease. The effect led to an overestimation of treatment appropriateness for CABG by 17% and for PCI by 10%.

◆ Although prior work had also shown large inter- and intra-observer variability in angiogram interpretation, Leape *et al.* were the first to link this variation to medical decision making, suggesting that many patients are undergoing major procedures based upon erroneous data.

◆ This study highlighted the need to extend patient safety evaluations to interpretation of diagnostic tests such as angiograms, particularly when the interpretation of these tests results in major treatment decisions that could have critical consequences for the patient.

Further reading

● Detre KM, Wright E, Murphy ML, Takaro T. Observer agreement in evaluating coronary angiograms. *Circulation.* 1975, 52(6): 979–86. Evaluated 22 physicians' interpretations of 13 coronary angiograms on two separate occasions and found substantial inter- and intra-observer variation in interpretation. This finding was replicated in multiple studies over the following 20 years.

● Eagle KA, Guyton RA, Davidoff R, Ewy GA, Fonger J, Gardner TJ, Gott JP, Herrmann HC, Marlow RA, Nugent W, O'Connor GT, Orszulak TA, Rieselbach RE, Winters WL, Yusuf S, Gibbons RJ, Alpert JS, Garson A Jr, Gregoratos G, Russell RO, Ryan TJ, Smith SC Jr. ACC/AHA guidelines for coronary artery bypass graft surgery: executive summary and recommendations: A report of the American College of Cardiology/American Heart Association Task Force on Practice Guidelines (Committee to revise the 1991 guidelines for coronary artery bypass graft surgery). *Circulation* 1999; 100(13): 1464–80.

● Patel MR, Dehmer GJ, Hirshfeld JW, Smith PK, Spertus JA. ACCF/SCAI/STS/AATS/AHA/ASNC 2009 Appropriateness Criteria for Coronary Revascularization: a report by the American College of Cardiology Foundation of Appropriateness Criteria Task Force, Society for Cardiovascular Angiography and Interventions, Society of Thoracic Surgeons, American Association for Thoracic Surgery, American Heart Association, and the American Society of Nuclear Cardiology Endorsed by the American Society of Echocardiography, the Heart Failure Society of America, and the Society of Cardiovascular Computed Tomography. *J Am Coll Cardiol* 2009; 53(6): n530–53.

Effect of coronary artery bypass graft surgery on survival: overview of ten-year results from randomized trials by the Coronary Artery Bypass Graft Surgery Trialists' Collaboration

Yusuf S, Zucker D, Passamani E, Peduzzi P, Takaro T, Fisher LD, Kennedy JW, Davis K, Killip T, Norris R, Morris C, Mathur V, Varnauskas E, Chalmers TC. *Lancet* 1994; 344: 563–70.

Background

During the 25 years since coronary artery bypass graft (CABG) surgery was introduced, it was clear that the operation relieved angina and probably improved quality of life. However, the effect of CABG on long-term prognosis, particularly within clinical subsets, had been more difficult to establish.

Article summary

Yusuf *et al.* compared the effect of CABG with medical therapy on long-term survival in patients with stable coronary artery disease (CAD) using an individual patient-level data meta-analysis. The investigators included patients with stable CAD (stable angina not severe enough to necessitate surgery on grounds of symptoms alone) from clinical trials who were randomly assigned CABG surgery or medical treatment. The primary aims were to compare the effects of a strategy of routine CABG surgery with one of initial medical therapy on mortality at five, seven, and ten years among all patients. The major secondary aims were to assess the interaction between the extent of coronary artery disease, the degree of LV dysfunction, and patients' risks for mortality with CABG surgery. In the study, 1324 patients were assigned to CABG surgery and 1325 to medical management between 1972 and 1984. The proportion of patients in the medical treatment group who had undergone CABG surgery was 25% at five years, 33% at seven years, and 41%

at ten years, whereas 93.7% of patients assigned to the surgery group underwent CABG surgery. The CABG group had significantly lower mortality than the medical treatment group at five years (10.2% vs. 15.8%; OR 0.61 [95% CI 0.48–0.77], p <0.001), seven years (15.8% vs. 21.7%; OR 0.68 [0.56–0.83], p <0.001), and ten years (26.4% vs. 30.5%; OR 0.83 [0.70–0.98]; p = 0.03). The risk reduction correlated with the severity of angiographic coronary disease, with the greatest relative risk reduction apparent among patients with left main disease and lesser benefit among patients with two or three-vessel disease (relative to one-vessel disease as the reference group). Although relative risk reductions in subgroups defined by other baseline characteristics were similar, the absolute benefits of CABG surgery were most pronounced in patients in the highest risk categories. This effect was most evident when several prognostically important clinical and angiographic risk factors were combined to stratify patients according to their overall risk of long-term mortality. For example, over ten years, estimated life expectancy gains were minimal in the low-risk group, 5.0 months in the intermediate-risk group, and 8.8 months in the high-risk group (p for trend = 0.003).

Strengths and limitations

The main strength of this study was the integration of patient-level data from multiple clinical trials to better define the mortality benefits of CABG and to understand the association of patient characteristics with these benefits. Using data from randomized clinical trials as the basis for the analysis is also a key advantage that enabled the authors to limit the impact of selection bias and confounding on their results.

While this was a state-of-the-art analysis, there are nonetheless several limitations in applying this analysis of CABG vs. medical treatment to contemporary care, both inherent in the study itself and in its application to current care. With regards to limitations due to the study design, only patients who met the inclusion and exclusion criteria of the original studies were included. The generalizability of these findings to the broader population to whom the results are applied is unknown. In addition, there are several limitations to applying these findings to contemporary care. First of all, during the timeframe of the original randomized trials that were pooled for this study, CABG surgery was performed before the widespread use of internal mammary artery (IMA) grafts which have better long-term patency rates than saphenous vein grafts and have subsequently been linked to improved long-term survival. In addition, the patient population for this meta-analysis excluded patients aged >65 years and included only 3% women, whereas contemporary CABG is performed commonly in both of these groups. Finally, medical therapy has improved substantially since the timeframe of this study. In particular, antiplatelet agents were used in only 20% of patients, lipid lowering agents were not widely used, and statins were not available. Although beta blockers were available when these studies were done, their full benefit had not been documented. Were these trials replicated today, it is likely that most patients would receive many of these effective therapies. Whether these changes would mitigate the survival advantage of CABG is unknown.

Impact on the field

Current guideline indications for CABG surgery in stable coronary artery disease are based on this meta-analysis. As such, CABG is indicated for patients with significant left main CAD, one or two-vessel coronary artery disease, and patients with underlying LV dysfunction. In addition, CABG is recommended for patients at high risk of mortality. In fact, the case for a survival advantage from CABG in left main coronary disease, despite the aforementioned limitations, is so great that contemporary clinical trials comparing coronary revascularization with medical therapy still exclude these patients from randomization.

This is a landmark paper for several reasons. First of all, it is one of the first large-scale pooled analyses of patient-level data from randomized clinical trials and demonstrates the benefit of such meta-analyses to reveal important subgroup effects that were not apparent in the original trials. Moreover, this study demonstrates the principle that targeting therapies to the highest risk populations leads to greater absolute benefits—thus optimizing the cost-effectiveness of the intervention. The results of this study form the basis for many of our contemporary guidelines and appropriateness measures with regard to patient selection for coronary artery bypass surgery.

Learning points

- Coronary artery bypass surgery surgery is effective for symptom improvement but does not reduce the incidence of non-fatal myocardial infarction.
- A strategy of initial CABG surgery is associated with lower mortality than one of medical management, with delayed surgery if necessary, especially in high-risk and medium-risk patients with stable CAD.

Further reading

- Boden WE. Chapter 25: Medical management of stable coronary artery disease. In: Yusuf S, Cairns JA, Camm AJ, Fallen EA, Gersh BJ, eds *Evidence Based Cardiology*. 3rd edn. Oxford: Wiley-Blackwell, 2010.
- Brown ML, Sundt TM. Chapter 27: Surgical coronary artery revascularization. In: Yusuf S, Cairns JA, Camm AJ, Fallen EA, Gersh BJ, eds *Evidence Based Cardiology*. 3rd edn. Oxford: Wiley-Blackwell, 2010.

These two chapters are excellent contemporary overviews of the medical and surgical management of patients with stable coronary artery disease.

Risk-treatment mismatch in the pharmacotherapy of heart failure

Lee DS, Tu JV, Juurlink DN, Alter DA, Ko DT, Austin PC, Chong A, Stukel TA, Levy D, Laupacis A. *JAMA* 2005; 294(10): 1240–7.

Background

A key principle that guides the application of medical treatments is that patients who are at the greatest risk for poor outcomes are likely to derive the most benefit from an intervention. This concept, that absolute risk reduction is proportional to patients' underlying risk, has been reflected in numerous studies of cardiovascular interventions. As early as the late 1990s, however, a surprising pattern had begun emerging in the literature. In practice, a wide variety of cardiovascular interventions ranging from thrombolytic therapy, statins, heart failure treatments, and, more recently, the use of bleeding avoidance therapies at the time of percutaneous coronary intervention were actually provided less frequently to the patients at highest risk and with the greatest potential to benefit. Some have attributed this apparent 'risk-treatment paradox' to a greater burden of contraindications to therapy among those who are at the greatest risk for poor outcomes, while others felt it reflected a reluctance on the part of physicians to provide therapies to patients who are 'too old' or 'too sick', despite strong evidence that the absolute risk reduction might be greatest in these patients. Lee and colleagues examined provision of evidence-based treatments in a large cohort of patients admitted with congestive heart failure to see if this risk-treatment mismatch was apparent in heart failure management and to understand whether contraindications to therapy, or other life-limiting comorbidities, might explain any mismatch between risk, benefit, and treatment.

Article summary

The authors leveraged a cohort of patients aged 79 or younger, hospitalized with systolic heart failure at 103 hospitals in Ontario, Canada, between 1999 and 2001. Patients were stratified into low, average, and high risk of one-year mortality using a validated risk prediction score.

Prescription rates for angiotensin converting enzyme (ACE) inhibitors, angiotensin receptor blockers (ARBs), and beta blockers were assessed at discharge, and in the first 90 days after discharge among patients aged 65 and older for whom prescription drug benefit records were available. The authors specified several analyses to better understand how comorbidities, complications, hospital, and physician characteristics might influence heart failure medication prescriptions. For instance, sensitivity analyses included limiting the population to patients without life-limiting, non-cardiac comorbidities and studying prescription rates in subsets of patients without renal insufficiency (for ACE inhibitors and ARBs), patients without chronic lung disease or bradycardia (for beta blockers) and in patients without hypotension.

Low-risk patients were most likely to receive each of these medications, both at discharge and in follow-up, with progressively lower rates of drug use in those with average or high risk. This pattern was apparent in those without life-limiting, non-cardiac comorbidities, after excluding patients with hypotension and specific contraindications to each therapy. Adjusting for age, sex, physician specialty, and age and hospital type, this pattern persisted, suggesting the widespread pervasiveness of this practice.

Strengths and limitations

The major strength of this study was the detailed examination of the role of potential contraindications to therapy on prescribing patterns for these critical evidence-based treatments. Finding persistent risk-treatment mismatch in several sensitivity analyses suggests that patient contraindications and physician specialty do not explain the risk-treatment paradox. This study focused on in-patients in Ontario, but there is little reason to suspect that these findings are not generalizable to other health-care systems.

Impact on the field

Although this study was not the first to bring attention to the risk-treatment paradox, it was instrumental in demonstrating that this paradox is not simply due to the greater rate of contraindications to therapy in higher-risk patients. This is a landmark paper because of the steps taken by the authors to understand whether the relationship between provision of therapy and underlying risk persisted after accounting for several actual or perceived contraindications to treatment. These data strongly suggest that ineligibility for therapy alone does not explain the risk-treatment paradox. Since these lifesaving therapies can lead to the greatest absolute reduction in adverse outcomes among the highest risk patients, this study highlights a major opportunity for quality improvement. These findings support the growing focus on assessment of performance measures to ensure that evidence-based interventions are applied uniformly in clinical practice.

Learning points

- Absolute risk reduction from an intervention is proportional to patients underlying risk, yet many cardiovascular therapies, in real world practice, are withheld from those at highest risk who have the most potential to benefit and are preferentially used in those with the least potential to benefit.
- Even after accounting for contraindications for therapy, this risk-treatment paradox persisted for key evidence-based heart failure treatments, highlighting a key opportunity for quality improvement. This pattern had been previously demonstrated in therapies used in the management of CHD.

Further reading

- Krumholz HM, Murillo JE, Chen J, et al. Thrombolytic therapy for eligible elderly patients with acute myocardial infarction. *JAMA*. 1997; 277(21): 1683–8. Older patients were less likely to receive thrombolytics, despite evidence suggesting greater benefit in elderly patients.
- Ko DT, Mamdani M, Alter DA. Lipid-lowering therapy with statins in high-risk elderly patients: the treatment-risk paradox. *JAMA*. 2004; 291(15): 1864–70. Study reporting an inverse relationship between baseline risk of death and probability of receiving statins among elderly patients with cardiovascular disease or with diabetes.

Depression following myocardial infarction: impact on six-month survival

Frasure-Smith N, Lesperance F, Talajic M. *JAMA* 1993; 270(15): 1819–25.

Background

In 1628, William Harvey noted that: 'For every affection of the mind that is attended either with pain or pleasure, hope or fear, is the cause of an agitation whose influence extends to the heart.' Yet as cardiology developed a keener appreciation for biological and physiological mechanisms of disease, the importance of patients' psychological status on their disease and outcomes was diminished. Nevertheless, the importance of a mind-body connection in cardiac disease was repeatedly emphasized by some of history's greatest physicians, such as Sir William Osler, who articulated the perceived association between behavioural patterns and the subsequent development of cardiac disease. In the mid 1960s, cardiologists Friedman and Rosenman, who studied middle-aged men, introduced the concept of the type A behaviour pattern—a constellation of behaviours including a constant sense of time urgency, hostility, and competitive 'drive'—that appeared to be associated with cardiovascular disease. Unfortunately, the work on the type A behaviour in cardiac disease was considered by the clinical and research community to be inconclusive and disagreement on the assessment and management of the behaviour pattern further diminished enthusiasm for the concept of the mind-body connection. However, the seminal work by Frasure-Smith et al., demonstrating an important association between depression following acute myocardial infarction (AMI) and outcomes, re-opened this important area of research in cardiac disease.

Article summary

The authors studied the association between a Diagnostic and Statistical Manual of Mental Disorders (DSM)-III-R diagnosis of major depression in AMI patients and the subsequent six-month cardiac mortality in a prospective, observational, follow-up study. A total of 222 patients

(78% males) were enrolled from a cardiac unit in an academic hospital in Montreal, Quebec. Patients were interviewed between 5 and 15 days following their AMI, using a diagnostic interview to establish a DSM diagnosis of major depression. The primary outcome was survival status at six months, for which the authors obtained information from patients' medical records, interviews with family members or other witnesses, and death certificates. Deaths were adjudicated by a team of independent cardiologists. A major disorder of depression was diagnosed in 16% of patients at the time of the interview. A total of 12 patients died at six-month follow-up, of which 50% were depressed at inclusion. The mortality in depressed patients was significantly higher than in non-depressed AMI patients (17% vs. 3%; adjusted HR for Killip class and prior AMI = 4.29, 95% CI 3.14–5.44, p = 0.013).

Strengths and limitations

The work by Frasure-Smith *et al.* was the first to prospectively evaluate the link between depression, as established by a psychiatric diagnostic interview, and AMI prognosis. Whereas prior research only included male patients, this study was also the first to include both men and women. Importantly, the authors explicitly considered clinical markers of post-AMI mortality, including Killip class, frequency of premature ventricular contractions, and ejection fraction, and found depression to not only be independently associated with mortality, but also to be more strongly associated with survival than any of these traditional markers of poor prognosis. Despite the great impact of this seminal work, it is important to recognize that this early work had significant limitations—including limited power, a high participation-refusal rate of approximately 30%, being a single-centre study, short follow-up, and the fact that the duration criterion of two weeks underlying a DSM diagnosis of major depression was not used.

Impact on the field

The publication of this work reawakened researchers to the prognostic importance of patients' psychosocial status on clinical outcomes after AMI. It spurred substantially more research in this area. The work by Frasure-Smith *et al.* was replicated multiple times afterwards, using larger samples allowing for more rigorous adjustment for confounding factors, and using not only a formal DSM diagnosis of depression, but also self-report questionnaires questioning patients about symptoms of depression and linking these with subsequent adverse outcomes among a variety of cardiac conditions. Through the extension of this work on depression and cardiac

disease, a 'manageable' explanation of the mind-body link in cardiac disease was thought to be offered, and subsequently introduced a series of treatment modalities that have been developed in psychiatry for the management of the cardiac patient with depression. Two well-known intervention trials—one focusing on Sertraline treatment and the other on cognitive behavioural therapy—were not, however, able to demonstrate a survival benefit for depressed cardiac patients undergoing these treatments for their depression. These negative findings and more recent evidence from the Heart and Soul Study have underscored the importance of behavioural and lifestyle factors (e.g. physical inactivity) in explaining the association between depression and adverse outcomes in cardiac disease and expanded our understanding of the importance of adequate management of comorbid depression in cardiac patients. Challenges for the future include designing and integrating actionable and sustainable protocols to improve recognition of depression in cardiac disease, allowing depressed patients to get appropriate treatment for their depressive symptoms and examining ways to leverage depressive symptoms as a means for further cardiovascular risk-stratification so that more aggressive cardiac treatment may be considered for those at higher risk for subsequent mortality.

Learning points

- This study was the first to prospectively document the association between a diagnosis of major depression and AMI prognosis—in both men and women—and created new interest in this area of research.
- This study stimulated a large body of research to further replicate their findings, and ongoing efforts to further clarify the mechanisms underlying the association between depression and cardiac disease. While current efforts to address depression have failed to improve cardiovascular outcomes—although depressive symptoms have been reduced—novel treatment strategies, such as collaborative care, are beginning to show promise in improving the prognosis of depressed patients with significant cardiovascular disease.

Further reading

- Glassman AH, O'Connor CM, Califf RM, *et al.* Sertraline treatment of major depression in patients with acute MI or unstable angina. *JAMA* 2002; 288(6): 701–9.

- Berkman LF, Blumenthal J, Burg M, *et al.* Effects of treating depression and low perceived social support on clinical events after myocardial infarction: the Enhancing Recovery in Coronary Heart Disease Patients (ENRICHD) Randomized Trial. *JAMA* 2003; 289(23): 3106–16.

- Whooley MA, de Jonge P, Vittinghoff E, *et al.* Depressive symptoms, health behaviors, and risk of cardiovascular events in patients with coronary heart disease. *JAMA*. 2008; 300(20): 2379–88.

Effect of PCI on quality of life in patients with stable coronary artery disease

William S. Weintraub, M.D., John A. Spertus, M.D., M.P.H., Paul Kolm, Ph.D., David J. Maron, M.D., Zefeng Zhang, M.D., Ph.D., Claudine Jurkovitz, M.D., M.P.H., Wei Zhang, M.S., Pamela M. Hartigan, Ph.D., Cheryl Lewis, R.N., Emir Veledar, Ph.D., Jim Bowen, B.S., Sandra B. Dunbar, D.S.N., Christi Deaton, Ph.D.,Stanley Kaufman, M.D., Robert A. O'Rourke, M.D., Ron Goeree, M.S., Paul G. Barnett, Ph.D., Koon K. Teo, M.D., and William E. Boden, M.D., for the COURAGE Trial Research Group. *N Eng J Med* 2008; 359: 677–87.

Background

Since its dissemination in the 1980s, percutaneous coronary intervention (PCI) has grown rapidly, to the point that it is performed >600,000/year in the United States alone. Although PCI reduces mortality in the setting of primary reperfusion for an ST-elevation myocardial infarction (STEMI), no mortality benefit has been demonstrated in patients with chronic stable ischaemic heart disease (SIHD). Accordingly, the primary benefit of PCI in patients with SIHD is relief of angina and improved quality of life. However, patients' health status (their symptoms, function, and quality of life) also improves with medical therapy, raising a key question—how effective is a strategy of optimal medical therapy (OMT) in comparison to PCI and medical therapy in the treatment of chronic stable angina? This was addressed in the Clinical Outcomes Utilizing Revascularization and Aggressive Drug Evaluation (COURAGE) trial, which randomized patients with stable obstructive coronary disease to a strategy of PCI plus OMT versus medical therapy alone. The primary results of that study showed no differences, for a mean of 4.5 years, in the rates of death and non-fatal MI. Yet COURAGE substantially elevated the field of clinical research in SIHD by prospectively designing a thorough assessment of patients' general and disease-specific health status. While some previous randomized studies had examined health status outcomes, they had been limited by the use of generic instruments, coarse assessments of angina, and limited follow-up of patients' health status.

Article summary

The COURAGE trial enrolled SIHD patients with ≥70% proximal stenosis of at least one coronary artery with inducible ischaemia or at least one coronary stenosis ≥80% with classic anginal symptoms and excluded patients with recent revascularization, ejection fraction <30% or refractory heart failure, contraindications to PCI, ongoing CCS class IV angina, and significant left main disease. Patients in both arms received aggressive, evidence-based, risk factor modification and anti-anginal therapy which was titrated regularly according to study protocol. Patient-centred health status outcomes were collected using both the disease-specific Seattle Angina Questionnaire (SAQ) and the generic RAND-36 to quantify health status. Over a follow-up of at least 30 months, patients had serial assessments of their health status prior to randomization and at one, three, six, and twelve months, followed by yearly assessments over the course of follow-up.

At baseline, the majority of patients reported anginal symptoms, with only about one-fifth being asymptomatic. Seattle Angina Questionnaire scores in each of the five domains improved significantly in both groups during the follow-up period. Early health status gains were greater in patients randomized to PCI, but patients who were treated medically experienced substantial and sustained improvements in angina frequency, angina stability, and quality of life, which was evident as early as the first month of follow-up. In fact, the difference between PCI + OMT and OMT alone at six months was only about 25% of the difference in the change experienced by OMT patients from baseline to six months. The early advantage with PCI faded with time, such that no significant health status differences were apparent between the groups at the 36-month follow-up. In terms of number needed to treat, the data indicated that 17 patients would need to be

treated with PCI + OMT for one patient to have significantly greater relief of angina than OMT alone, while 12.5
and 11 would need PCI + OMT for one patient to have
significant benefit in quality of life and physical function,
respectively. Another important insight from this study
was that baseline angina frequency was a critical determinant of health status improvement after PCI. After
dividing patients into tertiles of baseline angina severity,
PCI offered the greatest benefit to those with the most
severe baseline angina, reflecting the principle that the
sickest patients are most likely to benefit from treatment.

Strengths and limitations

First, rather than a direct comparison of PCI to medical
therapy, this was a strategy trial comparing upfront PCI
versus medical therapy. The use of a strategy trial, that
allowed crossovers from OMT alone to PCI in those with
refractory symptoms, is much more reflective of usual
clinical practice. Second, the quality of life data were carefully collected at frequent intervals using both disease-
specific and generic instruments, allowing careful
comparison of health status improvements over time,
using valid, reliable, and responsive tools. This was the
first trial of PCI vs. medical therapy to capture such
detailed health status data, including more detailed
assessments of angina than prior studies, which focused
on assessments of CCS class from the providers', rather
than the patients', perspectives. Among the limitations of
this study are the low enrolment of women (15%) and
minorities (14%), reflecting the large number of Veterans' Affairs sites, which may influence the generalizability of these findings. There were also missing health status
data at each follow-up, ranging from 15% to over 30%.
These data, however, were addressed using state-of-the-art
multiple imputation strategies. The results are encouraging in that careful medical therapy can result in marked
improvements in health status, with PCI to be safely
deferred, pending an assessment of patients' initial
response to OMT alone.

Impact on the field

This report from a pivotal, randomized clinical trial
represents an important extension of the primary outcome by providing a detailed description and comparison of health status outcomes, which can often be more
important to patients than survival and MI. The role of
early PCI in the management of stable CAD was further
clarified by finding that the most symptomatic patients
stood to benefit most from early PCI, which yielded
immediate and large improvements in health status.

We consider it a landmark paper because it highlights the
importance of considering all relevant outcomes in trials,
including health status. The COURAGE trial leveraged a
strong focus on disease-specific, patient-centred outcomes, which is particularly appropriate for chronic diseases, such as SIHD, for which the primary benefit of
treatment is controlling symptoms and improving quality
of life.

The inclusion of patient-centered outcomes, quantified by the SAQ, highlighted two of the COURAGE
study's key findings: (1) that medical therapy provides
sustained improvement in health status of similar magnitude to PCI in follow-up and (2) that baseline burden of
symptoms is a major determinant of benefit from PCI.
These findings were provided by the intentional inclusion of a disease-specific measure for CAD, which provided more dramatic and clinically interpretable insights
than a generic measure.

Learning points

- This study provided key insights, suggesting
  that an initial strategy of PCI is associated with
  greater early health status benefits compared
  with medical therapy, but that medical therapy
  leads to substantially improved health status and
  similar health status outcomes to those patients
  who initially received PCI by the third year of
  follow-up.
- Strategy trials such as COURAGE, which allow
  crossover from medical therapy alone to PCI
  in those with refractory symptoms, yield more
  generalizable data since they are more reflective of
  routine clinical practice.
- Patient-centred outcomes such as health status
  are of critical importance in studying the impact
  of interventions, and inclusion of disease-specific
  instruments allows more accurate assessment of
  the impact of treatments on patients' symptoms,
  function, and quality of life.

Further reading

- Boden WE, O'Rourke RA, Teo KK, *et al.* Optimal medical
  therapy with or without PCI for stable coronary disease.
  NEJM. 2007, 356 (15):1503–1516. Initial COURAGE publication, which provided the key insight that a strategy of initial PCI was not associated with a lower risk of the primary
  end point of death or non-fatal myocardial infarction in
  comparison with optimal medical therapy.

- Pocock SJ, Henderson RA, Clayton T, Lyman GH, Chamberlain DA. Quality of life after coronary angioplasty or continued medical treatment for angina: three-year follow-up in the RITA-2 trial. Randomized Intervention Treatment of Angina. *J Am Coll Cardiol* 2000; 35 (4): 907–914. The RITA-2 trial compared the strategy of initial PCI to medical therapy, and included long-term follow-up of health status outcomes. However, it was limited by its use of only disease-specific health status instruments, which are less sensitive to clinical change than disease specific instruments
- Strauss WE, Fortin T, Hartigan P, Folland ED, Parisi AF. A comparison of quality of life scores in patients with angina pectoris after angioplasty compared with after medical therapy. Outcomes of a randomized clinical trial. Veterans Affairs Study of Angioplasty Compared to Medical Therapy Investigators. *Circulation*. 1995; 92(7): 1710–19. The Veterans Affairs Study of Angioplasty Compared to Medical Therapy (ACME Trial), which randomized patients with single-vessel CAD to PCI or medical therapy, was the first to use validated instruments to compare the health status benefits of these competing treatments in stable CAD. The study was limited by its brief duration of follow-up, inclusion of only patients with single vessel CAD and its use of only generic health status instruments.

Strategies for reducing the door-to-balloon time in acute myocardial infarction

Bradley EH, Herrin J, Wang Y, Barton BA, Webster TR, Mattera JA, Roumanis SA, Curtis JP, Nallamothu BK, Magid DJ, McNamara RL, Parkosewich J, Loeb JM, Krumholz HM. *N Eng J Med* 2006; 355: 2308–20.

Background

Because delays in door-to-balloon (D2B) times for ST-elevation myocardial infarction (STEMI) are associated with lower survival, the ACC/AHA STEMI guidelines in 2004 recommended a D2B time of <90 minutes as a core quality measure for the management of STEMIs. However, the steps needed to achieve recommended D2B times were poorly defined, and progress in shortening D2B times was slow. In this setting, this study evaluated the effect of 28 hospital-based strategies to reduce D2B times across 365 hospitals that were elicited from qualitative research methods.

Article summary

This study used novel mixed (both qualitative and quantitative) methods to examine the impact of hospital strategies on D2B time. Hospitals were asked to provide information in a survey on 28 proposed strategies to reduce D2B time. The effect of these strategies on D2B time was then evaluated using hierarchical multivariable models, with each site characterized as a random effect. To facilitate the interpretation of the effect of each strategy on D2B time, all independent variables were centred on their means.

The majority of hospitals (>50%) had median D2B times that exceeded the 90-minute benchmark (mean [±SD] of the hospital median D2B time: 100.4 ± 23.5 minutes). Six strategies were identified in risk-adjusted

models to be associated with faster D2B times: (1) having emergency medicine physicians activate the catheterization laboratory (mean reduction in D2B time, -8.2, 95% CI [-14.3,-2.0] minutes); (2) having a single call to a central page operator activate the laboratory (-13.8, 95% CI [-21.2,-6.4] minutes); (3) having the emergency department activate the catheterization laboratory while the patient is en route to the hospital (-15.4, 95% CI [-24.2, -6.6] minutes); (4) expecting staff to arrive in the catheterization laboratory within 20 minutes after being paged compared to >30 minutes (-19.3, 95% CI [-6.0,-32.7] minutes); (5) having an attending cardiologist always on site (-14.6, 95% CI [-25.7,-3.6] minutes); and (6) having staff in the emergency department and the catheterization laboratory use real-time data feedback (-8.6, 95% CI [-13.6,-3.6] minutes). These strategies, however, were present only in a minority of hospitals and therefore the study highlighted the potential for improved implementation of these strategies in shortening D2B times.

Strengths and limitations

This was the first study to systematically identify which hospital strategies could be employed to improve D2B times for patients presenting with a STEMI. Many of the strategies were not being commonly used in US hospitals and yet could be implemented with existing resources. Since its publication, most hospitals in the US have implemented these strategies, and D2B times have dramatically decreased, with median hospital D2B times for most hospitals now <90 minutes. The authors' use of novel methodologies, including qualitative interviews to determine which strategies were associated with improved quality of care, provides a methodological paradigm for future hospital quality improvement initiatives. There were also several potential limitations. Due to the cross-sectional survey design, causality could not be established. It is possible that some of the recommended strategies were surrogates for unmeasured hospital care processes that lead to shorter D2B times. The survey data were reported by a single respondent at the hospital, and the reported policies and practices were not independently confirmed. Finally, this study does not apply to patients who were transferred from other hospitals.

Impact on the field

Until the mid-2000s there existed a large degree of variation in D2B times and consequently suboptimal outcomes in STEMI patients. This was the first study, which demonstrated why D2B times in real-world clinical practice were so variable, and what could be done to address this deficiency. It was instrumental in bridging the gap between clinical trials and practice and led to a national D2B initiative that translated the study's results to the routine care of STEMI patients. It thus epitomizes a paradigm of generating novel insights into practice and translating them to routine clinical care.

Learning points

♦ While the benchmark for a timely primary PCI is a D2B time of less than 90 minutes, achieving this goal was difficult for most hospitals.

♦ This study, using novel mixed methods, was the first to systematically evaluate and identify hospital-based strategies that could shorten D2B times.
♦ This study laid the foundation for a national movement to reduce D2B times and provided a methodological paradigm for future quality improvement initiatives.

Further reading

● Bradley EH, Nallamothu BK, Herrin J, et al. National efforts to improve door-to-balloon time results from the Door-to-Balloon Alliance. J Am Coll Cardiol. 2009; 54(25): 2423–9.
● Krumholz HM, Bradley EH, Nallamothu BK, et al. A campaign to improve the timeliness of primary percutaneous coronary intervention: Door-to-Balloon: An Alliance for Quality. JACC Cardiovasc Interv. 2008; 1(1): 97–104.
● Krumholz HM, Wang Y, Chen J, et al. Reduction in acute myocardial infarction mortality in the United States: risk-standardized mortality rates from 1995–2006. JAMA 2009; 302(7): 767–73.
● Nallamothu BK, Bates ER, Herrin J, Wang Y, Bradley EH, Krumholz HM; NRMI Investigators. Times to treatment in transfer patients undergoing primary percutaneous coronary intervention in the United States: National Registry of Myocardial Infarction (NRMI)-3/4 analysis. Circulation 2005; 111(6): 761–7.
● Nallamothu BK, Krumholz HM, Ko DT, et al. Development of systems of care for ST-elevation myocardial infarction patients: gaps, barriers, and implications. Circulation 2007; 116(2): e68–72.
● Pinto DS, Kirtane AJ, Nallamothu BK, et al. Hospital delays in reperfusion for ST-elevation myocardial infarction: Implications when selecting a reperfusion strategy. Circulation 2006; 114(19): 2019–25.

Cost effectiveness of thrombolytic therapy with tissue plasminogen activator as compared with streptokinase for acute myocardial infarction

Mark DB, Hlatky MA, Califf RM, Naylor CD, Lee KL, Armstrong PW, Barbash G, White H, Simoons ML, Nelson CL. N Engl J Med 1995; 332(21): 1418–24.

Background

The success of primary reperfusion for STEMI with streptokinase (SK) led to efforts to develop more effective, fibrin-specific thrombolytics. The first second-generation thrombolytic was tissue plasminogen activator (t-PA). However, two large, international, randomized

clinical trials of t-PA vs. SK—GISSI-3 and ISIS-2—did not show any reduction in mortality with t-PA as compared with SK. It was in this setting that a very large 'megatrial', the Global Utilization of Streptokinase and Tissue Plasminogen Activator for Occluded Coronary Arteries (GUSTO) was conducted to compare t-PA vs. SK for the treatment of patients with STEMI. Of note, in GUSTO, the t-PA dose used was the relatively novel 'accelerated' dose in which the full infusion was given over 1.5 hours (with two-thirds in the first 30 minutes) as compared with the traditional three-hour infusion that had been tested in previous trials.

In addition to evaluating clinical end points, a novel aspect of this trial was the inclusion of a pre-specified economic analysis, embedded within the trial, to evaluate the cost-effectiveness of t-PA as compared with SK. The goal of this analysis was to evaluate whether the observed survival benefits of t-PA were worth the much higher up-front cost of the drug. As such, this was one of the first cost-effectiveness studies in the cardiovascular literature to be based directly on empirical data from a clinical trial.

Article summary

The economic study was performed concurrently within the GUSTO clinical trial. The authors used a modified societal perspective to identify relevant costs, although indirect costs (e.g. time lost from work) and non-medical costs were not included. Effectiveness was measured in terms of life expectancy. Specifically, survival to one year was assessed via the follow-up data available from the trial. After one year, the authors assumed that the hazard of death did not depend on the thrombolytic agent (i.e. the survival curves of SK and t-PA were parallel), and they used the Duke Databank (n = 4379) to estimate survival from year 1 to year 14. Beyond year 14, to estimate the tail of the survival curve, they used a mathematical function (the Gompertz function) that approximates survival. Thus, they used advanced modelling techniques to estimate long-term survival. Both survival and costs were discounted at an annual rate of 5%. The end point was the incremental cost-effectiveness ratio for t-PA vs. SK, expressed in terms of cost per life year gained. In addition to the base-case analysis, the authors also conducted several sensitivity analyses to assess the impact of various parameters on the cost-effectiveness ratio.

The estimated cumulative medical costs (hospital costs plus physicians' fees) at one year, exclusive of the cost of the thrombolytic agent, averaged $24,575 for patients treated with SK and $24,990 for patients treated with t-PA—a difference of $415. When the drug costs for the thrombolytic agent were added, the incremental, undiscounted costs for each patient who received t-PA were $2845. The projected life expectancy for the GUSTO population was 15.41 years for patients treated with t-PA vs. 15.27 years for patients treated with SK—an undiscounted increase in life expectancy for the t-PA group of 0.14 year per patient (i.e. 14 additional years of life per 100 patients treated with t-PA). The cost-effectiveness ratio for the use of t-PA instead of streptokinase was $32,678 per year of life saved, a favourable ratio as compared with the accepted benchmark, at that time, of $50,000/LY gained.

Strengths and limitations

The economic study was prospectively designed at the inception of the main clinical trial, which sought to enrol all eligible patients and did not alter routine clinical care beyond administering the fibrinolytic agent. This article, published in 1995, was the first trial-based, prospective cost-effectiveness study that set a new standard for the integration of cost-effectiveness analyses into future randomized trials. The collection of data to estimate the costs of treating the patients randomly assigned to the various groups was part of the original study design. Therefore, these researchers could analyse both detailed clinical information and prospectively collected economic data on an unusually large number of patients. This study was thus instrumental in bridging the gap between the clinical and economic aspects of randomized trials. Although the methods and interpretation of this study have been subject to criticism, a more definitive trial comparing these strategies was not performed after this mega-trial, and the Food and Drug Administration approved claims of superiority for t-PA by its manufacturer. Soon after publication of these studies, use of t-PA increased and it became the standard-of-care in the US, prior to the era of primary angioplasty.

Learning points

- The GUSTO investigators were the first to design a cost-effectiveness study to be prospectively implemented alongside a clinical trial.
- This study established how a more expensive treatment for acute MI can still be cost-effective from a societal perspective.
- This study set the foundation, and provided a model for, conducting future cost-effectiveness studies, such as those incorporated into the Bypass Angioplasty Revascularization Investigation (BARI) and COURAGE trials.
- The GUSTO trial found that the rapid ('accelerated') administration of t-PA reduced overall mortality by 15% (relative risk reduction) and 1% absolute risk reduction, as compared with streptokinase.

> ◆ The cost-effectiveness ratio for accelerated t-PA vs.
> streptokinase was $32,678 per year of life saved—a
> value that compared favourably with many other
> commonly accepted medical interventions.

Further reading

- Holmes DR Jr, Califf RM, Topol EJ. Lessons we have learned from the GUSTO trial. Global Utilization of Streptokinase and Tissue Plasminogen Activator for Occluded Arteries. *J Am Coll Cardiol* 1995; 25(7 Suppl): 10S–17S.
- Krumholz HM, Pasternak RC, Weinstein MC, *et al.* Cost effectiveness of thrombolytic therapy with streptokinase in elderly patients with suspected acute myocardial infarction. *N Engl J Med* 1992; 327(1): 7–13.
- Maggioni AP, Franzosi MG, Santoro E, White H, Van de Werf F, Tognoni G. The risk of stroke in patients with acute myocardial infarction after thrombolytic and antithrombotic treatment. Gruppo Italiano per lo Studio della Sopravvivenza nell'Infarto Miocardico II (GISSI-2), and The International Study Group. *N Engl J Med* 1992; 327(1): 1–6.
- Mark DB. Clinical and economic lessons from studies of coronary thrombolysis. *J Vasc Interv Radiol* 1995; 6(6 Pt 2 Suppl): 94S–101S.
- Mark DB. Economics and Quality of Life After Acute Myocardial Infarction: Insights from GUSTO-I. *J Thromb Thrombolysis* 1996; 3(2): 151–5.

Does more intensive treatment of acute myocardial infarction in the elderly reduce mortality? Analysis using instrumental variables

McClellan M, McNeil BJ, Newhouse JP. *JAMA* 1994; 272: 859–66.

Background

A critical challenge for outcomes research is to evaluate the outcomes for alternative treatment strategies. While this is straightforward in randomized clinical trials (RCTs), it is much more challenging in observational studies where treatment is selected by the physician, and not randomly allocated. While RCTs are considered the gold standard for providing unbiased estimates of treatment effect, they are often impractical to address the vast majority of clinical questions. Consequently, investigators have increasingly sought to leverage clinical registries and administrative databases for comparative effectiveness research. However, it is well recognized that these non-randomized, observational studies are highly prone to selection biases and risk-adjustment using conventional analytical techniques is often inadequate for accounting for unmeasured sources of variation in treatment selection.

Article summary

By applying a novel econometric technique—the instrumental variable (IV) approach—to understand the incremental survival benefit of varying treatment intensities, the article by McClellan *et al.* marks an important methodological advancement in the field of outcomes research. In this study, the authors linked claims and administrative data from the Health Care Financing Administration (Medicare) to examine the association between the intensity of using invasive procedures (cardiac catheterization, percutaneous transluminal coronary angioplasty, coronary artery bypass graft surgery) and mortality following AMI. From an initial cohort of 218,427 Medicare beneficiaries 64 years or older who experienced an AMI in 1987, patients missing information on ZIP code (1.2%), admitted initially to a hospital more than 100 miles from residence (4.9%) or those living in Alaska (0.04%) were excluded. Then, the use of invasive procedures during the 90 days after the initial admission was identified and vital status of patients ascertained at varying time intervals. Estimates of mortality difference between treatment groups were obtained using both the conventional analysis of variance (ANOVA) method and the IV approach. For the IV analysis, the authors used the differential distances from patients' residences to the nearest hospitals with particular characteristics (availability of catheterization or revascularization facilities, volume of AMIs treated in the elderly) as the instrument, something associated with treatment, but otherwise not expected to be associated with survival.

Among 205,021 Medicare beneficiaries admitted with AMI in 1987, 46,760 (23%) patients underwent catheterization within 90 days, of whom approximately half underwent subsequent revascularization. Patients who received invasive procedures had much lower mortality at all time intervals ranging from one day after admission to >4 years. Since these patients were also younger and had fewer comorbid conditions, it is likely that they differed from those patients who did not receive invasive procedures for a variety of important, but unmeasured, clinical characteristics (e.g. disease severity, AMI location). Although adjustment for observed differences in baseline characteristics using ANOVA attenuated the unadjusted treatment effect, use of invasive procedures was still associated with an implausible 28.1% lower mortality at four years after hospitalization.

In contrast, comparisons of patient groups that differed only in differential distances from hospitals with invasive capabilities demonstrated a much lower marginal benefit of invasive treatment on mortality at 1–4 years after AMI. Despite the similarity in observed health characteristics, patients living closer to a catheterization hospital were significantly more likely to receive invasive procedures. The difference in mortality rates between the two groups at 90 days, however, was only 0.4 absolute percentage-points (58.1% vs. 58.5%) at four years. Thus, the IV analysis suggests that use of cardiac catheterization yields only a 0.6 percentage-point relative risk reduction in four-year mortality—at least in patients who are 'marginal' from the standpoint of the instrument. Similar results were observed in patients who were admitted to high versus low volume hospitals.

The authors conclude that in elderly Medicare beneficiaries with AMI: (1) the use of cardiac catheterization and revascularization is independent of observed health characteristics but is performed less frequently in patients living in rural areas, women, and black people, and (2) the use of invasive procedures affords only a marginal, and possibly no clinically-important, survival benefit after AMI.

Strengths and limitations

This study was among the first to utilize the large administrative Medicare database to understand the degree to which the availability of technological capabilities may influence treatment decisions and outcomes in AMI. Importantly, this study was also the first to introduce and apply a novel econometric approach, instrumental variable analysis, to account for important selection biases.

Critics of observational studies have traditionally cited issues of unmeasured confounding and selection bias to question the validity of conclusions derived from observational studies. Adequate adjustment for confounding is especially challenging in registries and administrative databases as exposure is determined by a complex interplay between patient and provider factors. Prior to the study by McClellan *et al.*, investigators relied primarily on conventional multivariable adjustment to account for differences in patient characteristics between

treatment groups. The usefulness of these methods, however, depends on richness and clinical detail of the available data, which is often not very detailed in administrative datasets. Moreover, even detailed clinical datasets may not identify all potential confounders. Developing alternative approaches for risk adjustment is therefore critical for establishing the validity of comparative effectiveness research based on observational data. By explicitly demonstrating and accounting for the impact of patient selection on mortality in the elderly receiving varying intensities of invasive procedures after AMI, this article by McClellan and colleagues represents a critical methodological advancement in outcomes research involving non-randomized studies. Although the results apply only to 'marginal' patients, those that are really eligible for either treatment and whose treatment selection is determined primarily by the instrument, and would not be applicable to those with clinical characteristics mandated for one approach or the other, it remains the most powerful technique for minimizing the biases in non-random treatment allocation.

Learning points

- ◆ Elderly Medicare beneficiaries with AMI who underwent invasive procedures (cardiac catheterization and revascularization) were younger, had less comorbidity, and were more likely to be admitted to hospitals with cardiac catheterization facilities or high AMI volumes.
- ◆ Proximity to hospital types (with or without catheterization facility, high vs. low AMI volume) was a strong independent determinant of treatment intensity after an AMI and was uncorrelated with observed patient characteristics status.
- ◆ Incremental use of invasive procedures across varying treatment intensities was associated with minimal survival benefit in the 'marginal' elderly patients, that is, those patients who underwent procedures mainly because they lived near a high intensity hospital. Most of the benefit was observed on day 1 before use of invasive procedures and is thus more likely attributable to strategies other than the procedures.
- ◆ Instrumental variable (IV) analysis provides a powerful analytical approach to derive less biased estimates of treatment effect in the presence of unmeasured confounding in non-randomized studies.

Further reading

• Stukel TA, Fisher ES, Wennberg DE, Alter DA, Gottlieb DJ, Vermeulen MJ. Analysis of observational studies in the presence of treatment selection bias: effects of invasive cardiac management on AMI survival using propensity score and instrumental variable methods. *JAMA* 2007; 297(3): 278–85. This study provides a more contemporary analysis of the impact of treatment intensity following AMI in elderly Medicare beneficiaries enrolled in 1994–95 and followed for a longer time period of seven years and compares the sensitivity of results to the type of analytical technique used— multivariable regression, propensity scores, IV analysis.

Racial inequalities in the use of procedures for patients with ischaemic heart disease in Massachusetts

Wenneker MB, Epstein AM. *JAMA* 1989; 261: 253–7.

Background

Eliminating disparities in care and outcome on the basis of race and gender is a major goal of a high-quality healthcare system and is codified by the Institute of Medicine's commitment to equity. Prior studies had suggested that black people are treated with fewer cardiac procedures than white people. However, these studies had been single-centre studies or population-based analyses that lacked sufficient multivariable adjustment.

Article summary

Wenneker and Epstein sought to determine whether differences in treatment between black and white patients were attributable to race after adjusting for important clinical and socioeconomic confounders. They evaluated administrative data from the Massachusetts Health Data Consortium on patients discharged from Massachusetts hospitals in 1985. Patients whose principal diagnosis was a disease of the circulatory system or chest pain (i.e. myocardial infarction, unstable angina, etc.) or who underwent coronary angiography, coronary artery bypass graft surgery (CABG), or coronary angioplasty were included for analysis.

The authors first calculated age and sex-adjusted utilization rates based on the Massachusetts population. They found that procedural utilization did not differ by race for patients admitted for chest pain or circulatory disorders. However, white patients were more than twice as likely to undergo angioplasty or CABG. Next, the authors performed a hospital-based analysis to examine for racial differences among patients admitted for chest pain and related syndromes, to account for the fact that black and white patients may have differential rates of admission for cardiac problems. They found substantial differences by race for use of coronary angiography and revascularization: as compared with black patients, white patients were 1.3 times more likely to undergo angiography (95% CI 1.1,1.6, p <0.01), 1.9 times more likely to undergo CABG (95% CI 1.3,2.7, p <0.001), and 1.7 times more likely to undergo angioplasty (95% CI 0.9,3.1, p <0.08). These racial differences persisted after adjustment for demographics, comorbidities, and median zip code income.

Strengths and limitations

There are certain limitations to this study that should be acknowledged, although it should also be recognized that statistical techniques that are so readily employed today were not available at the time this was published. Although this study used a large administrative database, it was limited to Massachusetts residents (only 3% were black) and hospitals, a region of the US known to practice more evidence-based care. Thus, the treatment patterns and patient populations at these hospitals may not reflect those in other parts of the country. The researchers were also limited in the number of confounders for which they were able to adjust. Certain comorbidities, such as diabetes and kidney disease, were not captured in this database, are more prevalent in black patients, and may have impacted treatment decisions. Finally, more sophisticated techniques that are commonly used today, such as propensity score matching and hierarchical modelling, may have provided less biased estimates of racial differences.

Despite its limitations, this was a seminal study in identifying variations in care that differ by race—a field of inquiry that has greatly expanded after the publication of this work and continues to be an area of active investigation. Although this study was not the first to suggest that there was a difference by race in the use of cardiac procedures, it was the first to use a large multi-site database and multivariable adjustment to account for potential confounders. For example, the authors adjusted for insurance status and median zip code income to demonstrate that differences by race were not simply attributable to racial differences in access to care or neighbourhood income. Moreover, they compared utilization rates among black and white patients who were hospitalized with eligible cardiac conditions to control for potential differences in hospitalization rates for cardiac conditions between blacks and whites. Collectively, their systematic approach has become a paradigm for subsequent studies of racial differences.

Impact on the field

Healthcare systems throughout the world have struggled to address disparities in care. In the US, rectifying racial disparities is a national priority and is one of the primary goals of the US Department of Health and Human Services' Healthy People 2010 agenda and of the Institute of Medicine, which includes 'equity' as one of six key domains of healthcare quality. While documenting that the variation in care was a necessary first step in understanding whether true disparities in care were occurring, it was important to document whether adverse consequences occur as a result of differential treatment. Wenneker and Epstein were very careful to note that they could not conclude, based on their study findings, that black patients were undertreated or harmed by undergoing fewer procedures, as a higher procedure rate among white patients may simply reflect procedural overuse in white patients rather than underuse in black patients. However, this paper highlighted the need to better understand the reasons for variations in treatment which may occur in specific patient subgroups and whether these differences may affect patient outcomes. Since this report, numerous investigators have continued to document racial differences in the use of invasive cardiac procedures, even after controlling for clinical characteristics, mechanisms of reimbursement, organization of healthcare

services, and availability of technology at individual hospitals. In addition to stimulating multiple studies that have attempted to dissect the complex relationships between race, treatment, and outcomes, Wenneker and Epstein's article also provided a framework for future inquiries to examine potential disparities in care by sex, age, income, and other subgroups.

Learning points

- Black patients who are hospitalized for serious cardiac conditions were less likely than white patients to undergo coronary angiography, angioplasty, or CABG.
- Wenneker and Epstein were the first to document these differences using a large multi-site database and to use multivariable adjustment to control for important potential confounders of the complex relationship between race and treatment.
- This study established the analytic framework for multiple subsequent studies that have further documented variations in cardiac treatments based on race, socioeconomic status, age, and sex.

Further reading

- Chen J, Rathore SS, Radford MJ, Wang Y, Krumholz HM. Racial differences in the use of cardiac catheterization after acute myocardial infarction. *N Engl J Med* 2001; 344: 1443–9.
- Peterson ED, Wright SM, Daley J, Thibault GE. Racial variation in cardiac procedure use and survival following acute myocardial infarction in the Department of Veterans Affairs. *JAMA* 1994; 271: 1175–80.
- Spertus JA, Jones JG, Masoudi FA, Rumsfeld JS, Krumholz HM. Factors Associated With Racial Differences in Myocardial Infarction Outcomes. *Ann Intern Med* 2009; 150: 314–24.

Reduction in acute myocardial infarction mortality in the United States: risk-standardized mortality rates 1995–2006

Krumholz HM, Wang Y, Chen J, Drye EE, Spertus JA, Ross JS, Curtis JP, Nallamothu BK, Lichtman JH, Havranek EP, Masoudi FA, Radford MJ, Han LF, Rapp MT, Straube BM, Normand S-LT. *JAMA* 2009; 302: 767–73.

Background

Acute myocardial infarction (AMI) has been at the forefront of quality initiatives, with numerous reports examining the patterns of, and disparities in the use of, recommended care. Early reports examining the quality of care in AMI documented significant underuse of potentially lifesaving therapies in the setting of an MI and highlighted an important opportunity to improve the application of evidenced-based care in routine clinical practice. Since then, both public and private agencies have augmented the focus on quality care by targeting specific aspects of care, including time to reperfusion and use of evidence-based medicines, which have been codified into performance measures for both quality improvement and accountability[1, 2]. Although the creation of performance measures and their subsequent public reporting would be expected to improve outcomes, the temporal change in mortality after AMI, and its variability across hospitals, had not been examined in the modern era.

Article summary

In this observational study of Medicare beneficiaries discharged with AMI, Krumholz and colleagues sought to delineate changes in outcomes, and the variability in survival, across a decade of performance measurement. They analysed 3,195,672 discharges in 2,755,370 patients discharged from non-federal acute care hospitals in the United States between 1 January 1995, and 31 December 2006 and estimated hospital-level, 30-day risk-standardized mortality rates (RSMRs). Patients included were 65 years or older (mean, 78 years) who had at least a 12-month history of fee-for-service enrolment prior to the index hospitalization. Patients discharged alive within one day of an admission (not against medical advice) and those transferred from one acute care hospital to another without a principal discharge diagnosis of AMI at both hospitals, were excluded. A 'control' cohort of non-AMI hospitalizations among patients 65 years or older who were discharged from acute care hospitals and who did not have a principal diagnosis of AMI was also created to contrast results from the AMI cohort.

The primary end point was 30-day all-cause mortality and the primary hospital end point was 30-day all-cause RSMR. Secondary outcomes included in-hospital mortality, length of stay, and discharge disposition. Information on age, sex, 2 AMI location variables, 8 cardiovascular history variables, and 15 other variables that identify additional coexisting illnesses were derived from in-patient and outpatient administrative claims. Using a previously validated risk model[3] standardized hospital-specific estimates and quantitative summaries of between-hospital variation after adjusting for case mix were computed.

Compared to those discharged in 1995, the characteristics of patients discharged in 2006 were reflective of older patients with more comorbid conditions and prior coronary revascularization. In spite of these temporal changes, the 30-day mortality rate decreased from 18.9% in 1995 to 16.1% in 2006, and in-hospital mortality decreased from 14.6% to 10.1%, with a parallel reduction in the mean length of stay from 7.9 (SD, 6.3) days to 7.0 (SD, 6.0) days. At the patient level, the odds of dying within 30 days of admission if treated at a hospital 1 SD above the national average relative to that if treated at a hospital 1 SD below the national average were 1.63 (95% CI: 1.60, 1.65) in 1995 and 1.56 (95% CI: 1.53, 1.60) in 2006. Hospital-specific RSMRs decreased from 18.8% in 1995 to 15.8% in 2006 (odds ratio [95% CI]: 0.76 [0.75, 0.77]), suggesting an absolute risk reduction of 3%, meaning that for every 33 AMIs in 2006, one more patient would be alive 30 days later than similar patients cared for in 1995. Furthermore, all indices of between-hospital heterogeneity decreased from 1995 to 2006: coefficient of variation from 11.2% to 10.8%, the inter-quartile range from 2.8% to 2.1%, and the between-hospital variance from 4.4% to 2.9%, suggesting much more consistent outcomes across hospitals. In contrast, no significant trends were observed for other non-AMI conditions, where a focus on performance measurement and improvement had not occurred.

Strengths and limitations

This study was conducted using the large, national Medicare database and relied upon a more standardized follow-up period of 30 days rather than the more inconsistent and invalid use of in-hospital events. Yet the data was derived from administrative claims and, as such, lacked important information on process measures and medications, such that attribution to the full range of performance measures could not be confirmed. Thus, a limitation of the analysis is its inability to delineate the specific mechanism of improved outcomes, potentially including improved use of evidence-based pharmacotherapy, reperfusion techniques, or quality improvement initiatives and public reporting. The time period of the analysis also coincides with the widespread use of troponin testing and it is unclear how this may have influenced the pattern of hospital mortality. Nevertheless, documenting the substantial reduction in RSMRs and decreased variability across hospitals signifies substantial improvements in outcomes and improved consistency across centres that had not been observed in other conditions.

Impact on the field

Medicine is facing an unprecedented demand for performance measurement and accountability for healthcare quality. Evidence is needed to show that initial efforts are associated with benefits that warrant the cost and effort needed to support this trend. This study by Krumholz *et al.* serves to illuminate the potential of healthcare providers to achieve appreciable improvement in cardiovascular outcomes. First, on average, 1 more patient of every 33 admitted in 2006, as compared with 1995, is now alive 30 days after their event. Second, this improved quality of care is now provided more homogenously across hospitals throughout the country. These developments underscore the value of systematic and collaborative efforts to target and achieve improvements in outcomes. Furthermore, this study has opened avenues for further research, such as identifying the specific cause(s) for improvement and promoting the use of best practices, exploring the extent of improvement in under-served and high-risk patient subgroups (women, minorities) and examining factors that may explain the residual variation between hospitals when caring for AMI patients.

Learning points

♦ Compared to 1995, Medicare enrollees discharged with AMI a decade later are older, with a

greater number of them reporting concomitant comorbidities and prior revascularization.

♦ Yet, at the patient level, the odds of dying within 30 days of admission if treated at a hospital 1 SD above the national average relative to that if treated at a hospital 1 SD below the national average were 1.63 (95% CI: 1.60, 1.65) in 1995 and 1.56 (95% CI: 1.53, 1.60) in 2006.

♦ At the hospital level, risk-standardized mortality rates showed an absolute reduction of 3% with a concomitant reduction in between-hospital variation, reflecting a more homogenous provision of improved care across the country.

Further reading

● Krumholz HM, Merrill AR, Schone EM, *et al.* Patterns of hospital performance in acute myocardial infarction and heart failure 30-day mortality and readmission. *Circ Cardiovasc Qual Outcomes.* 2009, 2(5): 407–13. With national hospital quality profiling efforts extending from measuring processes of care to the assessment of short-term outcomes, this study provides an important contribution by highlighting the variation in 30-day mortality and readmission rates by region and hospital characteristics for two critical conditions in contemporary practice.

Effectiveness of public report cards for improving the quality of cardiac care: the EFFECT study: a randomized trial

Tu JV, Donovan LR, Lee DS, Wang JT, Austin PC, Alter DA, Ko DT. *JAMA* 2009; 302(21): 2330–7.

Background

Public reporting of hospital performance is an increasingly common, albeit controversial, strategy to improve quality of care. However, no large randomized trial had previously been conducted to evaluate the effectiveness of public reporting on improving quality of care.

Researchers at the Institute for Clinical Evaluative Sciences in Canada explored the impact of public reporting on performance of hospitals treating patients with acute myocardial infarction (AMI) and congestive heart failure (CHF). Evidence-based guidelines are well established for these heart conditions, but the guidelines are not always followed as part of routine clinical care, thus providing an opportunity to close the gap between optimal and actual clinical practice.

Article summary

In the Enhanced Feedback for Effective Cardiac Treatment (EFFECT) trial, Tu *et al.* hypothesized that public release of hospital report cards would improve the quality of cardiac care provided. The trial involved 86 hospital corporations in Ontario, Canada, where no prior public reporting initiatives were in place. At each hospital, a target sample of 125 charts for AMI and/or CHF patients (total n = 15,997 patients) was abstracted by an experienced cardiology research nurse. A population-based cluster randomized trial design was used. Hospitals were randomized to early (January 2004) or delayed (September 2005) feedback of a public report card regarding their hospital's baseline performance (April 1999 to March 2001) on a set of 12 AMI and 6 CHF national process-of-care quality indicators. The performance reports for the early feedback hospitals were publicly released at a press conference, on the Web, and received extensive media (television, radio, and newspaper) coverage. There was no press release or media coverage when the delayed feedback hospitals received their performance reports. Follow-up data (April 2004 to March 2005) was collected to assess changes in outcomes. The co-primary outcome measures were changes between baseline and follow-up for AMI and CHF composite, quality care, indicator scores. Secondary outcome measures included individual quality indicators comprising the composite scores, hospital report card impact survey regarding quality improvement (QI) initiatives launched in response to the early feedback report cards, and hospitals' all-cause mortality rates.

Results showed most process-of-care indicators improved at a similar rate over time in both groups of hospitals. The public release of hospital report cards was not associated with significantly greater improvement in the overall composite AMI and CHF quality indicators at the early feedback hospitals as compared with the delayed feedback hospitals. However, for individual indicators, significantly greater improvement was seen in the early vs. delayed feedback hospitals for the percentage of AMI patients receiving fibrinolytic therapy prior to transfer to a coronary care or intensive care unit and for the percentage of CHF patients receiving an ACE inhibitor or an ARB for left ventricular dysfunction. Also, in response to the publicly released early feedback report card, early feedback hospitals were significantly more likely to engage in QI initiatives as compared with the delayed feedback hospitals. For example, within the early feedback group, ten hospitals changed their policies to allow emergency department physicians to administer fibrinolytics without specialist consultation, five hospitals opened up CHF clinics, and there was an increase in the use of ACE inhibitors and ARBs for patients with left ventricular dysfunction. Most importantly, the mean 30-day AMI mortality rates were significantly lower for the early feedback hospitals compared to the delayed feedback hospitals, especially for patients presenting with STEMI. Although the CHF mortality rates were not significantly different across hospital feedback groups, the mean one-year CHF mortality rates were significantly lower among CHF patients with left ventricular dysfunction at the early feedback hospitals.

Strengths and limitations

The primary strength of this study is that it is the first to use the rigorous randomized clinical trial methodology to evaluate whether public report cards improve quality of care. Although improvement was seen in early feedback hospitals for many secondary outcomes, study limitations could have made it difficult to detect differences in the primary outcomes of composite AMI and CHF quality indicators.

Specifically, it was not possible to blind the delayed feedback group to the media coverage of the early feedback group. The fact that several delayed feedback hospitals also started QI initiatives in response to the early feedback report card may have diminished group differences in the study outcomes. A trial that used more frequent and timely feedback of publicly released report cards on a regular basis could have been more effective. In response to public reporting of performance, the QI projects undertaken varied in nature, timing, and focus. Using multidisciplinary QI teams at each hospital to implement a consistent system-wide initiative might have improved quality of care across hospitals. The relatively short, one-year, follow-up period may not have been long enough to see the full potential impact of quality improvement initiatives. Also, results of this trial conducted in the Canadian publically funded healthcare system may not generalize to other healthcare models such as the 'market-driven' system in the United States.

Impact on the field

Policy mandates are increasing the public reporting of hospital quality and this study is the first to subject public accountability to the rigorous standards of a randomized trial. This study was recognized as the '2010 Article of the Year' by the Canadian Institutes of Health Research for its contribution to the advancement of health services research and clear impact on healthcare policy in Canada. The methods and results of the EFFECT trial provide a model to other health care systems on how to improve the quality of care and may lead the way for public reporting as a cost-effective strategy to encourage the translation of evidence-based guidelines into improved clinical practice. The rigour of this study provides justification to international trends to transparently measure and report hospitals' quality of care.

Learning points

- This randomized trial provides rigorous data showing the benefits of the public release of hospital report cards on improvement in quality of cardiac care.

◆ Despite negative findings for the co-primary outcomes of AMI and CHF composite quality care indicator scores, the study found that publicly released report cards stimulated local, hospital-specific QI initiatives and practice changes that may have had a cumulative effect leading to better outcomes, such as improved survival after AMI.

Further reading

● O'Connor GT, Plume SK, Olmstead EM, *et al.* A regional intervention to improve the hospital mortality associated with coronary artery bypass graft surgery. The Northern New England Cardiovascular Disease Study Group. *JAMA* 1996; 275(11): 841–6.

Use of medical resources and quality of life after acute myocardial infarction in Canada and the United States

Mark DB, Naylor CD, Hlatky MA, Califf RM, Topol EJ, Granger CB, Knight JD, Nelson CL, Lee KL, Clapp-Channing NE, Sutherland W, Pilote L, Armstrong PW. *N Engl J Med* 1994; 331: 1130–5.

Background

Hospitals, regions, and countries often adopt standards of clinical practice that may differ widely. In the setting of acute myocardial infarction (AMI), the US tends to apply invasive risk stratification and revascularization aggressively, while Canada, at least in the 1990s, did not. Exploiting national variations in care can provide an important opportunity to examine differences in practice patterns on clinical outcomes, including quality of life.

Article summary

To compare the use of medical resources and quality of life outcomes among patients in the US and Canada during the year after acute myocardial infarction (AMI), an analysis of North American patients who were enrolled in the Global Utilization of Streptokinase and t-PA for Occluded Coronary Arteries (GUSTO) trial was used to examine the outcomes of different patterns of post-AMI management. From the overall study population of 41,021 patients, the economic and quality of life substudy included 2600 US patients and 400 Canadian patients—approximately 1/8 of the overall population from these two countries.

The primary outcomes of interest were utilization of medical resources and health-related quality of life during the year after AMI. Data on the utilization of medical resources was collected on all study participants from the time of study enrolment to one-year follow-up. At each follow-up interview, patients were asked about medical care during the interval, including hospitalizations, cardiac catheterization, coronary angioplasty, coronary bypass surgery, nursing home placement, and outpatient

visits to 11 different types of practitioners or care facilities. Quality of life was measured with a battery of generic instruments. Functional status was assessed using the Duke Activity Status Index, the Katz Activities of Daily Living Scale, and a single four-level question about the effects of the patient's health on overall functioning. Angina and dyspnoea were assessed using the Rose questionnaires. Perceptions of general health were assessed on a scale ranging from excellent to poor that was taken from the National Health Interview Survey as well as a 0–100 rating scale. General psychological well-being was evaluated with a ten-item scale created for this study from published instruments, as well as the Carroll Depression Scale. In addition to a baseline assessment (which was performed during the initial hospitalization), follow-up assessments of health-related quality of life were performed by structured telephone interviews at 30 days, 6 months, and 1 year after enrolment.

During the initial hospitalization, length of stay was ~1 day longer for the Canadian patients as compared with the US patients, but they had a much lower rate of cardiac catheterization (25% vs. 72%, p <0.001), coronary angioplasty (11% vs. 29%, p <0.001), and coronary bypass surgery (3% vs. 14%, p <0.001). By one year, 24% of the Canadian and 53% of the US patients had undergone angioplasty or bypass surgery (p <0.001). The Canadians had more visits to physicians during the follow-up year (p <0.001), but fewer visits to specialists (p <0.001). There were no significant difference in one-year mortality or 30-day functional status between the Canadian and US patients. In contrast, one-year functional status improved to a greater extent, as measured by the Duke Activity

Status Index (DASI) (30 vs. 35, p <0.001), among the US patients compared with the Canadian patients. While there was no difference in general health perceptions (p = 0.39), US patients were less likely to report chest pain or dyspoea at one year than their Canadian counterparts (34% vs. 21% and 45% vs. 29%, respectively; p <0.001). In conclusion, the Canadian patients, who were managed less aggressively than US patients, had more cardiac symptoms and worse functional status one year after AMI than the US patients.

Strengths and limitations

This is one of the first studies to examine the relationship between intensity of healthcare services (mainly coronary revascularization procedures) and a broad range of patient-centered outcomes after AMI. By taking advantage of a 'natural experiment' in healthcare delivery between the US and Canadian systems, the authors were able to demonstrate that despite a lack of survival benefit, the greater intensity of revascularization procedures performed in the US was associated with modest benefits in patients' health status at one year. Whether these benefits are worth the additional cost remains an open question.

There are several important limitations to this study. The rates of invasive cardiac procedures for Canada in the GUSTO trial were higher than typical of the country overall, potentially leading to an underestimation of the reported differences in quality of life, chest pain, and shortness of breath. The authors suggest that physicians that participated in the trial were more aggressive and probably more technologically oriented than the overall population of physicians caring for AMI patients in Canada.

Patients' functional status was measured with generic (not disease-specific measures, as used in COURAGE, above) instruments and the assessment of angina was performed with a diagnostic questionnaire, rather than one designed to quantify frequency or severity.

However, the consistency of the results obtained with a wide array of standard instruments, rather than relying on a single instrument, supports the general conclusions of this study.

Impact on the field

This study was one of the first to exploit variations in care across countries to examine the association of different practice patterns with clinical and health status outcomes. It is considered a classic example of exploiting a clinical trial to provide insights into the association of non-randomized aspects of care on outcomes.

Learning points

- ◆ Acute myocardial infarction patients in the US are more likely to undergo revascularization procedures than Canadian patients.
- ◆ The difference in the use of revascularization procedures between the US and Canada is associated with increased functional capacity and global health scores in patients in the US compared to Canada.

Further reading

- McNeil BJ. Shattuck Lecture—Hidden barriers to improvement in the quality of care. *N Engl J Med* 2001; 345: 1621–6. General overview on the hidden barriers that promote differences in patterns of practice, use of procedures, technology, and quality of care across the US.
- Peterson ED, Califf RM. Chapter 45. Quality of Care and Medical Errors in Cardiovascular Disease. In: Topol EJ. *Textbook of Cardiovascular Medicine*. 3rd edn. Lippincott William & Wilkins, 2006. Contemporary review on the current quality indicators for cardiovascular care and procedures.

Conclusion

The field of epidemiology and outcomes research is rapidly evolving. Dedicated to generating insights that improve the clinical care for patients, the field relies on a wide variety of research techniques. As exemplified by the selected articles, qualitative research methods, administrative data, and clinical trials are analysed using advanced statistical methods to remove potential biases

and target disparities, alternative processes of care and improved survival and health status (symptoms, function, and quality of life) outcomes. Patient, process of care, and treatment variables are studied to illuminate their relationship to outcomes and to target novel interventions to optimize outcomes. As exemplified by the improvements in AMI survival, these research efforts offer the opportunity to improve the care and treatment of patients with cardiovascular disease.

References

1. Krumholz HM. Outcomes research: generating evidence for best practice and policies. *Circulation* 2008;118: 309–18.

2. Krumholz HM, Peterson ED, Ayanian JZ, *et al.* Report of the National Heart, Lung, and Blood Institute working group on outcomes research in cardiovascular disease. *Circulation* 2005; 111: 3158–66.

3. Ellwood PM. Shattuck lecture—outcomes management. A technology of patient experience. *N Engl J Med.* 1988; 318(23):1549–56.

4. Institute of Medicine. *Crossing the Quality Chasm: A New Health System for the Twenty-first Century.* Washington: National Academy Press; 2001.

Chapter 2

Lipids and cardiovascular disease

Dr Adie Viljoen and Dr Anthony Wierzbicki

Introduction

Atherosclerotic plaques were noted to contain waxy deposits (cholesterol) by Fallopius in 1575 and in 1914 Anitschkow showed that cholesterol feeding led to atherosclerosis in a rabbit. The results of early lipid-lowering trials such as the Coronary Drug Project (clofibrate; niacin; d-thyroxine and oestrogen), World Health Organization Clofibrate Trial, Lipid Research Clinics (cholestyramine), and Programme on Surgical Correction of Hyperlipidaemia (ileal bypass surgery) were unclear, with some therapies showing no benefit (d-thyroxine and oestrogen) and the rest giving reductions in cardiovascular disease (CVD) events but not total mortality within the trial period. In some cases, for instance with clofibrate, mortality increased. Later trials (e.g. Helsinki Heart Study) failed to clarify the situation. A cholesterol controversy arose stating that cholesterol reduction might reduce CVD but increase other causes of mortality. The identity of the LDL-receptor was clarified and a class of drugs designed to block the rate-limiting step in cholesterol synthesis (2-hydroxy-methyl-glutaryl (HMG)-CoA reductase inhibitors) and increase LDL clearance was discovered. It remained to determine what their effects were in clinical practice.

A landmark paper in this field should fundamentally influence medical practice by setting a new paradigm for diagnosis, treatment, or by defining audit standards for the effectiveness of diagnosis or treatment so that improvements in care can be introduced and managed equitably.

Further reading

- Brown MS, Dana SE, Goldstein JL. Regulation of 3-hydroxy-3-methylglutaryl coenzyme A reductase activity in cultured human fibroblasts. Comparison of cells from a normal subject and from a patient with homozygous familial hypercholesterolemia. *J Biol Chem* 1974 Feb 10; 249(3): 789–96.
- Endo A. A gift from nature: the birth of the statins. *Nat Med* 2008 Oct; 14(10): 1050–2.
- Finking G, Hanke H. Nikolaj Nikolajewitsch Anitschkow (1885–1964) established the cholesterol-fed rabbit as a model for atherosclerosis research. *Atherosclerosis* 1997 Nov; 135(1): 1–7.

- Oliver MF. Doubts about preventing coronary heart disease. *BMJ* 1992; 304: 393–4.
- Steinberg D. The pathogenesis of atherosclerosis. An interpretive history of the cholesterol controversy, part IV: the 1984 coronary primary prevention trial ends it—almost. *J Lipid Res* 2006 Jan; 47(1): 1–14.

Scandinavian Simvastatin Survival Study (4S)

The Scandinavian Simvastatin Survival Study Group. Randomised trial of cholesterol lowering in 4444 patients with coronary heart disease: the Scandinavian Simvastatin Survival Study (4S). *Lancet* 1994; 344: 1383–9.

Background

At the time when the Scandinavian Simvastatin Survival Study (4S) was formulated the Expert Panels in Europe and the United States had started recommending the lowering of cholesterol (specifically LDL-C)—especially in patients with known coronary heart disease (CHD). No previous trial had been able to convincingly show that lowering cholesterol prolongs life.

Methods and results

The trial randomized 4444 patients with angina pectoris or previous myocardial infarction (MI) and cholesterol 5.5–8.0 mmol/L to simvastatin 20–40 mg or placebo. Simvastatin reduced LDL-C by 35% and mortality (256 [12%] vs. 182 [8%] deaths) by 30% (95% CI 0.58–0.85, p = 0.0003) after 5.4 years. In the open-label follow-up a 15% (3–26) reduction in mortality (414 vs. 468 deaths) was seen over 10.4 years driven by a 24 (10–36)% reduction in CHD mortality (238 vs. 300 deaths; p = 0.0018). No difference was noted in mortality from and incidence of cancer.

Strengths and limitations

The 4S trial showed the survival benefit of statins in patients with CHD. It was performed in a high-risk group with high initial cholesterol levels. No previous unifactorial lipid-lowering trial had demonstrated total or even CHD mortality during the planned follow-up period, though both niacin and ileal bypass had shown long-term post-trial benefits. Further, but underpowered, subgroup analyses of 4S showed benefits in diabetes, women, and older individuals.

Conclusions

This was the first trial to show that treatment of a secondary prevention population with a statin results in a 30% decrease in mortality and in cardiovascular events in all major subgroups.

Learning points

- In a high-risk secondary prevention population statin therapy reduces total mortality.
- In this population statins reduce all types of CVD events, hospital admissions, and are cost saving.
- Statins are safe as no increase is seen in non-CVD mortality and no significant side-effects are seen.
- Long-term follow-up of the 4S population shows no increase in rates of cancer with statin therapy.

Further reading

- Consensus conference. Lowering blood cholesterol to prevent heart disease. *JAMA* 1985; 253: 2080–6.
- European Atherosclerosis Society. Strategies for the prevention of coronary heart disease: a policy statement of the European Atherosclerosis Society. *Eur Heart J* 1987; 8: 77–88.
- Miettinen TA, Pyörälä K, Olsson AG, *et al.* Cholesterol-lowering therapy in women and elderly patients with myocardial infarction or angina pectoris: findings from the Scandinavian Simvastatin Survival Study (4S). *Circulation* 1997; 96: 4124–5.
- Strandberg TE, Pyörälä K, Cook TJ, *et al.* Mortality and incidence of cancer during 10-year follow-up of the Scandinavian Simvastatin Survival Study (4S). *Lancet* 2004; 364: 771–7.

The West of Scotland Coronary Prevention Study (WOSCOPS)

Shepherd J, Cobbe SM, Ford I, Isles CG, Lorimer AR, MacFarlane PW, McKillop JH, Packard CJ. Prevention of coronary heart disease with pravastatin in men with hypercholesterolemia. *N Engl J Med* 1995; 333: 1301–7.

Background

Primary prevention is the long-term goal in lipid-lowering therapy, as up to 33% of patients who experience their first event die almost immediately. The problem with primary prevention trials is to find a high-risk population with a high prevalence of the desired CVD risk factor to which the trial therapy is directed. The West of Scotland population has one of the highest rates of CVD in the UK.

Methods and results

The West of Scotland Coronary Prevention Study (WOSCOPS) compared pravastatin 40 mg to placebo in 6595 middle-aged men without a history of MI with a mean total cholesterol of 272 mg/dL (7.0 mmol/L). Pravastatin reduced LDL-C by 26% and CHD events by 31% (17–43) (p <0.001) after 4.9 years. The WOSCOPS showed a 22% reduction in mortality (p = 0.051). In the ten-year, post-trial follow-up CHD death was reduced by 17% (8.6% vs.10.3%; p = 0.02); and by 24% over the entire period (11.8% vs. 15.5%; p <0.001). There was no increase in non-cardiovascular deaths or cancer.

Strengths and limitations

This study was the first to clearly demonstrate the unequivocal benefit of statin therapy in a primary prevention setting and almost achieved a benefit on total mortality. A few patients with CHD did enter the WOSCOPS trial and it was argued that these accounted for all the benefit. However, the treatment effect was similar in all subgroups within the study. Post-hoc analyses suggested that the benefits in WOSCOPS were more than expected for LDL-C reduction alone, giving rise to the idea of the potential pleiotropic actions of statins. Women were excluded from WOSCOPS.

Conclusion

This was the first lipid trial to show that statin therapy reduces CHD events in a high-risk male primary prevention population and almost confirmed a reduction in total mortality.

Learning points

- ◆ Statin therapy reduces CHD events in a male primary prevention population.
- ◆ Continued follow-up of the WOSCOPS study population showed a continuing reduction in CVD morbidity and mortality with no increase in rates of cancer.

Further reading

- Ford I, Murray H, Packard CJ, Shepherd J, Macfarlane PW, Cobbe SM. Long-term follow-up of the West of Scotland Coronary Prevention Study. *N Engl J Med* 2007; 357: 1477–1486.
- Frick MH, Elo O, Haapa K, *et al*. Helsinki Heart Study: primary-prevention trial with gemfibrozil in middle-aged men with dyslipidemia: safety of treatment, changes in risk factors, and incidence of coronary heart disease. *N Engl J Med* 1987; 317: 1237–45.
- The Lipid Research Clinics Coronary Primary Prevention Trial results. I. Reduction in incidence of coronary heart disease. *JAMA* 1984; 251: 351–64.

Heart Protection Study (HPS)

Heart Protection Study Collaborative Group. MRC/BHF Heart Protection Study of cholesterol lowering with simvastatin in 20,536 high-risk individuals: a randomised placebo-controlled trial. *Lancet* 2002; 360: 7–22.

Background

Limited evidence existed on the effects of statins in some high-risk groups, in particular those with diabetes, females, or the elderly; and those with below average LDL-C concentrations. Epidemiological studies had suggested benefits of anti-oxidant vitamins but no trial had yet assessed their benefits on cardiovascular outcomes. The HPS study investigated the role of statins and anti-oxidants in a large diverse high-risk population.

Methods and results

A group of 20,536 adults (aged 40–80 years) with CHD, other occlusive arterial disease, or diabetes were randomized in a 2 x 2 design to 40 mg simvastatin, antioxidant vitamins, or placebo. No effect was seen with vitamins after five years. All-cause mortality was reduced by 11% (1328 [12.9%] vs. 1507 [14.7%]; p = 0.0003) with simvastatin. The proportional reduction in event rates was similar in every subcategory including stroke, peripheral artery disease, diabetes; male or female, age >70 years; and patients with LDL-C <3.0 mmol/L (116 mg/dL), or total cholesterol <5.0 mmol/L (193 mg/dL).

Strengths and limitations

It was the first study to provide direct robust evidence on the benefits of statins in all groups. This trial provided extensive data on safety. To date, it is the largest trial of statin lipid-lowering treatment. It included more subjects with diabetes (5963) and patients >65 years (1069) than other lipid trials targeted specifically at these two patient cohorts (i.e. Collaborative AtoRvastatin Diabetes Study (CARDS) and the Prospective Study of Pravastatin in the Elderly at Risk (PROSPER)).

However, there were a number of limitations. The HPS was one of the first studies to use an active drug run-in phase. Despite recruiting mostly statin experienced patients, 30% of patients discontinued therapy. During the trial all secondary prevention patients, including those with diabetes, had to be started on lipid–lowering treatment following the results of other trials. This increased the placebo group drop-in rate to 14% by the end of the trial. This effect is likely to have reduced the efficacy of the statin intervention, which has been

estimated at a 33% reduction in events per 1 mmol/L LDL-C as opposed to the 24% found in the intention-to-treat analysis. The HPS has also been used as evidence for the use of statins in type 1 diabetes but numbers were very small.

Conclusion

The trial showed that simvastatin therapy produces a consistent 25% reduction in CVD events in all patient groups, including a large sub-group with diabetes.

Learning points

+ The HPS study showed that simvastatin therapy resulted in a consistent reduction in CVD events in all groups recruited to the trial.
+ Statin therapy reduced CVD events in a population with diabetes.
+ Statin therapy produced a consistent 25% relative risk reduction even at low initial levels of LDL-C.

Further reading

- Collins R, Armitage J, Parish S, Sleight P, Peto R. MRC/BHF Heart Protection Study of cholesterol-lowering with simvastatin in 5963 people with diabetes: a randomised placebo-controlled trial. *Lancet* 2003; 361(9374): 2005–16.
- MRC/BHF Heart Protection Study Investigators. MRC/BHF Heart Protection Study of cholesterol-lowering therapy and of antioxidant vitamin supplementation in a wide range of patients at increased risk of coronary heart disease death: early safety and efficacy experience. *Eur Heart J* 1999; 20(10): 725–41.
- MRC/BHF Heart Protection Study Investigators. MRC/BHF Heart Protection Study of antioxidant vitamin supplementation in 20,536 high-risk individuals: a randomised placebo-controlled trial. *Lancet* 2002; 360(9326): 23–33.

Pravastatin or atorvastatin evaluation and infection therapy—thrombolysis in myocardial infarction 22 (PROVE IT–TIMI 22)

Cannon CP, Braunwald E, McCabe CH, Rader DJ, Rouleau JL, Belder R. Intensive versus moderate lipid lowering with statins after acute coronary syndromes. *N Engl J Med* 2004; 350(15): 1495–504.

Background

It was not clear whether lowering lipid levels further would increase the clinical benefit or whether statin

therapy would be beneficial in acute coronary syndromes (ACS). Much was made of the pleiotropic effects of statins as opposed to the LDL-C lowering effects (see WOSCOPS) and given the different dose response curves for reductions in markers of inflammation (e.g. C-reactive protein; CRP) and LDL-C it was hypothesized that more aggressive lipid-lowering therapy would not deliver increased benefits in a high-risk group of patients with inflammation. The observation that *Chlamydia pneumoniae* was associated with atherosclerotic plaques suggested that a possible benefit could be gained from gatifloxacin antibiotic therapy, although results from this part of the trial were not reported in this paper.

Methods and results

The Pravastatin or atorvastatin evaluation and infection therapy–thrombolysis in myocardial infarction 22 (PROVE-IT-TIMI 22) study randomized, in a 2 x 2 design, 4162 patients admitted with ACS in the preceding ten days to 40 mg pravastatin or 80 mg atorvastatin and a ten-day course of gatifloxacin or placebo, every month of the trial. The primary end point was CVD events. The antibiotic arm showed no benefits. In the statin arm the pravastatin arm achieved a median LDL-C level of 95 mg/dL (2.46 mmol/L) and atorvastatin 62 mg/dL (1.60 mmol/L). A 16% (5–26) reduction in CVD events in favour of atorvastatin was seen at two years (p = 0.005).

Strengths and limitations

This landmark study comparing two statins did not meet the pre-specified criterion for equivalence (<15% difference) but showed superiority of more intensive treatment.

The effects were proportional to LDL-C reduction, but the differences in dose-response to outcome plots continued the debate about whether it was the LDL-C lowering or anti-inflammatory effects of statins that were most relevant (see Figure 2.1). The PROVE-IT study confirmed the results of the Reversal of Atherosclerosis with Aggressive Lipid Lowering (REVERSAL) study which measured atheroma volume by intravascular ultrasound and the Arterial Biology for the Investigation of the Treatment Effects of Reducing Cholesterol (ARBITER) study using carotid intima media thickness which had shown that atorvastatin 80 mg was superior to pravastatin 40 mg.

Conclusion

The PROVE-IT trial provided the first evidence that more aggressive lipid-lowering therapy was associated with greater benefit in patients presenting with ACS.

Learning points

- Statins are effective in reducing CHD events in patients with ACS.
- More aggressive statin therapy is more effective than standard therapy in reducing CVD events.
- Statins have different dose-efficacy relationships for LDL-C reduction and reduction of CRP. The greatest effect in PROVE-IT was found in patients with greater LDL-C and higher CRP levels.

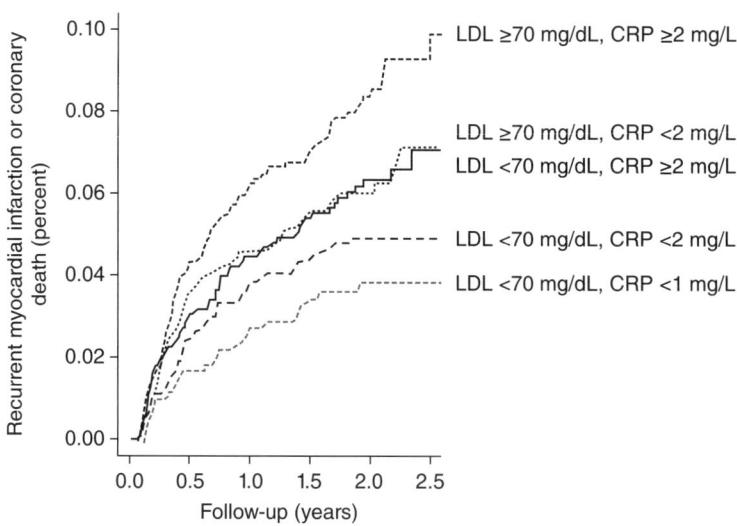

Figure 2.1 Clinical relevance of achieved LDL and achieved CRP following treatment with statin.

Adapted from Ridker PM, *et al*. C-Reactive Protein Levels and Outcomes after Statin Therapy. *New Engl J Med* 2005; 352: 20–28, with permission.

Further reading

- Bonetti PO, Lerman LO, Napoli C, Lerman A. Statin effects beyond lipid lowering—are they clinically relevant? *Eur Heart J* 2003; 24: 225–48.
- Nissen SE, Tuzcu EM, Schoenhagen P, *et al.* for the REVERSAL Investigators. Effect of Intensive Compared With Moderate Lipid-Lowering Therapy on Progression of Coronary Atherosclerosis. *JAMA* 2004; 291: 1071–80.
- Taylor AJ, Kent SM, Flaherty PJ, Coyle LC, Markwood TT, Vernalis MN. ARBITER: Arterial Biology for the Investigation of the Treatment Effects of Reducing Cholesterol: a randomised trial comparing the effects of atorvastatin and pravastatin on carotid intima medial thickness. *Circulation* 2002; 106: 2055–60.

Justification for the Use of statins in Prevention: an Intervention Trial Evaluating Rosuvastatin (JUPITER)

Ridker PM, Danielson E, Fonseca FA, Genest J, Gotto AM Jr, Kastelein JJ, Koenig W, Libby P, Lorenzatti AJ, MacFadyen JG, Nordestgaard BG, Shepherd J, Willerson JT; Glynn RJ; JUPITER Study Group. Rosuvastatin to prevent vascular events in men and women with elevated C-reactive protein. *N Engl J Med* 2008; 359(21): 2195–207.

Background

The use of statins in primary prevention was encouraged in guidelines, but the exact CVD risk cutoffs for treatment and the LDL-C target were still unclear. Analysis of CRP in the 5742 participants of the primary prevention Air Force/Texas Coronary Atherosclerosis Prevention Study (AFCAPS/TexCAPS) had shown that lovastatin reduced CHD events in patients with high LDL-C, but also in patients with high CRP. Statin therapy showed little benefit in the group with low LDL-C and low CRP. Thus, CRP screening might provide a method to improve the targeting of statin therapy.

Methods and results

The Justification for the Use of statins in Prevention: an Intervention Trial Evaluating Rosuvastatin (JUPITER) trial assigned 17,802 patients with LDL-C <130 mg/dL (3.4 mmol/L) and CRP >2.0 mg/L to rosuvastatin 20 mg or placebo. The primary end point was CVD events. Rosuvastatin reduced LDL-C by 50% and CRP by 37%. The trial was stopped early after 1.9 years. The number of CVD events were reduced by 44 (31–54)% by rosuvastatin (142 vs. 251 events; p <0.00001). The MI rate was reduced by 54 (30–70)%, stroke by 48 (31–66)%, intervention or ACS by 47 (30–60)%, total CVD events by 47 (31–60)% (all p <0.00001) and mortality by 20 (3–33)% (p = 0.02). All subgroups showed consistent effects. No increase in myopathy was seen but the statin arm did have a higher incidence of physician-reported diabetes and a small rise in HbA_{1c}. Further analyses showed rosuvastatin reduced events in women, the elderly, patients with impaired renal function, and also venous thromboembolism.

Strengths and limitations

This trial is a landmark study as it included large numbers of women and the elderly. It confirmed the clinical relevance of the inflammation in atherosclerosis and extended the benefits of statin treatment to a low-risk population. Trials that are stopped early tend to show disproportionate benefits of intervention. In the field of lipid-lowering such criticisms have applied to the Collaborative Atorvastatin Diabetes Study (CARDS), Anglo-Scandinavian Coronary Outcomes Study (ASCOT), and JUPITER studies. Additional controversy has been added by the magnitude of the effects; the relatively low event and fatality rates; the applicability of CRP to routine clinical practice; and questioning whether the trial really recruited a 'low risk' population, as the calculated Framingham ten–year cardiovascular disease risk (used for treatment stratification in the UK) was ~18% though coronary heart disease risk (used for treatment stratification in the USA) was <20%.

Conclusion

This trial showed that statin therapy in patients with moderate CHD risk additionally stratified by having high levels of the inflammation-associated CVD risk factor CRP produces significant rapid benefits.

Further reading

● Libby P. Inflammation and atherosclerosis events. *Nature* 2002; 420: 868–74.

● de Lorgeril M, Salen P, Abramson J, *et al*. Cholesterol lowering, cardiovascular diseases, and the rosuvastatin-JUPITER controversy: a critical reappraisal. *Arch Intern Med* 2010; 170(12): 1032–6.
● Montori VM, Devereaux PJ, Adhikari NK, *et al*. Randomised trials stopped early for benefit: a systematic review. *JAMA* 2005; 294(17): 2203–9.
● Ridker PM, Rifai N, Clearfield M, *et al*. Measurement of C-reactive protein for the targeting of statin therapy in the primary prevention of acute coronary events. Air Force/Texas Coronary Atherosclerosis Prevention Study Investigators. *N Engl J Med* 2001; 344: 1959–1965.
● Ridker PM. Rosuvastatin in the primary prevention of cardiovascular disease among patients with low levels of low density lipoprotein cholesterol and elevated high-sensitivity C-reactive protein: rationale and design of the JUPITER trial. *Circulation* 2003; 108: 2292–7.

Cholesterol treatment trialists' collaboration

Baigent C, Keech A, Kearney PM, Blackwell L, Buck G, Pollicino C. Efficacy and safety of cholesterol-lowering treatment: prospective meta-analysis of data from 90,056 participants in 14 randomised trials of statins. *Lancet* 2005 Oct 8; 366(9493): 1267–78.

Cholesterol Treatment Trialists' (CTT) Collaboration. Efficacy and safety of more intensive lowering of LDL cholesterol: a meta-analysis of data from 170,000 participants in 26 randomised trials. *Lancet* 2010; 376(9753): 1670–81.

Background

The early meta-analyses of lipid lowering therapy (1996) showed benefits with statins and maybe a small effect of omega-3 fatty acids. The availability of a large number of statin trials that were mostly, but not all, positive allowed a comprehensive meta-analysis to be performed of their efficacy and safety. This data was especially relevant for groups which were relatively under-represented in the trials, such as women, the elderly, primary prevention, patients with strokes, diabetes, or other non-coronary disease.

Methods and results

The first analysis (2005) comprised a prospective meta-analysis of data from 90056 patients from 14 statin trials. Over five years, there were 8186 deaths, 14,348 individuals had CVD events, and 5103 developed cancer. The LDL-C differences ranged from 0.35 to 1.77 (mean 1.09) mmol/L. Mortality was reduced by 12 (9–16)% per 1 mmol/L reduction in LDL-C (p <0.0001) driven by a 19 (15–34)% reduction in CHD mortality (p <0.0001),

and non-significant 7 (-3–17)% reductions in non-coronary vascular mortality (p = 0.2) and 5%(-1–10)% in non-vascular mortality (p = 0.1). The CHD events were reduced by 33 (20–36)% (p <0.0001), revascularization by 34 (20–37)% (p <0.0001), stroke by 17 (12–22)% (p <0.0001), and all CVD by 21 (19–23)% (p <0.0001). The reduction in CVD events differed according to the absolute reduction in LDL-C achieved (p <0.0001), occurred within one year, and the event lines continued to diverge.

The second meta-analysis (2010) included trials of more versus less intensive statin therapy. The additional reduction in LDL-C was 0.51 mmol/L. More intensive regimens produced a 15(11–18)% (p <0.0001) reduction in CVD events (p <0.0001), 13 (7–19)% in CHD events (p <0.0001), 16 (5–26)% in stroke (p = 0.005) per 1.0 mmol/L reduction in LDL-C. Over all trials CVD events were reduced by 22 (20–34)%, and mortality by 10 (7–14)% per 1 mmol/L LDL-C reduction with the mortality reduction attributable to CHD deaths.

Strengths and limitations

The CTTC remains the largest and most comprehensive meta-analysis performed of lipid-lowering trials. It clearly shows the benefits of lipid-lowering therapy with statins on CVD events in all groups (male vs. female, elderly vs. young; patients with diabetes vs. normoglycaemia) in proportion to the absolute reduction in LDL-C and no other factor. Statins reduce mortality through an effect on CHD deaths and have no effect on fatal stroke, but do reduce non-fatal strokes. Statins have no effect on non-CVD mortality or on rates of incident or established cancer. The CTTC could not clearly address the effects of other parts of the lipid profile on CVD risk as its constituent trials usually had restrictions on entry triglycerides (<4–6 mmol/L) and also statins have only small and similar effects on HDL-C. It does demonstrate that lower HDL-C is associated with an increased risk both in the placebo and statin-treated groups.

Conclusion

This landmark meta-analysis demonstrated that statin therapy reduces mortality by 12% per 1 mmol/L of LDL-C reduction in secondary prevention and high-risk (diabetes) patients and all types of CVD events by 22% per 1 mmol/L of LDL-C reduction in all groups.

Learning points

- Statins reduce mortality by 12% per 1 mmol/L LDL-C in secondary prevention and by 9% in patients with diabetes.
- Statins reduce CVD morbidity by 22% per 1 mmol/L LDL-C reduction and by similar amounts for CHD and stroke in all populations, including secondary and primary prevention.
- Though CVD risk in the trial population is dependent on HDL-C the effect of statins are independent of this risk factor and do not significantly affect HDL-C levels.

Further reading

- Briel M, Ferreira-Gonzalez I, You JJ, *et al.* Association between change in high density lipoprotein cholesterol and cardiovascular disease morbidity and mortality: systematic review and meta-regression analysis. *BMJ* 2009; 338: b92.
- Bucher HC, Griffith LE, Guyatt GH. Systematic review on the risk and benefit of different cholesterol-lowering interventions. *Arterioscler Thromb Vasc Biol* 1999; 19(2): 187–95.
- Kearney PM, Blackwell L, Collins R, *et al.* Efficacy of cholesterol-lowering therapy in 18,686 people with diabetes in 14 randomised trials of statins: a meta-analysis. *Lancet* 2008; 371(9607): 117–25.

Veterans Administration HDL Intervention Trial (VA-HIT)

Rubins HB, Robins SJ, Collins D, Fye CL, Anderson JW, Elam MB. Gemfibrozil for the secondary prevention of coronary heart disease in men with low levels of high-density lipoprotein cholesterol. Veterans Affairs High-Density Lipoprotein Cholesterol Intervention Trial Study Group. *N Engl J Med* 1999; 341(6): 410–8.

Background

The LDL hypothesis has a long history in cardiovascular medicine and was finally proven by the statin trials starting with 4S. However, the original lipid lowering studies were performed with niacin and fibrates and many of these studies suggested that the drugs that raised HDL-C could potentially reduce CHD events as well. The Helsinki Heart Study had shown a benefit in reducing CHD events in a high-risk primary prevention group. Many patients with CHD have low HDL-C levels. The VA-HIT study was the first trial to specifically attempt to define the effects of lipid-lowering therapy in patients with low HDL-C.

Methods and results

The trial randomized 2531 men with CHD, HDL-C <40mg/dL (1.0 mmol/L) and LDL-C <140 mg/dL (3.6 mmol/L) to gemfibrozil 1200 mg or placebo. The primary end point was CHD events. Gemfibrozil increased HDL-C levels by 6%, reduced triglycerides by 31%, but had no effect on LDL-C. Gemfibrozil therapy reduced CHD events by 22% after 5.1 years (219 [17.3%] vs. 275 [21.7%]; p = 0.006) and CVD events by 24% (p <0.001). Event rates were related to baseline HDL-C, apolipoprotein A-1 and B-100 levels and LDL particle numbers, but failed to show any relationship to triglycerides. Only a change in HDL-C with fibrate therapy was associated with outcomes.

Strengths and limitations

The VA-HIT trial remains one of the only two trials (both using gemfibrozil) to show a benefit with fibrate therapy on CHD. It showed the effects of raising HDL-C as no effect was seen on LDL-C. There is debate about whether the actions of fibrates can be generalized given the differences between the actions of individual drugs on HDL-C, fibrinogen, and other peroxisomal proliferator activating receptor (PPAR)-alpha target genes. Later trials of bezafibrate in cardiovascular prevention and peripheral arterial disease failed to show any benefits. Fenofibrate has taken over from gemfibrozil given its better safety profile and dosing convenience but despite benefits on the progression of coronary atherosclerosis in the Diabetes Atherosclerosis Intervention Study (DAIS) study, it failed to reduce CHD events in patients with type 2 diabetes (p = 0.16) in the statin-confounded Fenofibrate Intervention on Endpoint Lowering in Diabetes (FIELD) study, but did reduce CVD events by 11% (p = 0.035). The FIELD sub-studies have shown that fenofibrate reduces microvascular disease including retinopathy and nephropathy. The addition of fenofibrate to statin therapy in type 2 diabetes in the Action to Control Risk in Diabetes (ACCORD) study failed to show any CVD benefit except possibly for a marginal effect in patients with high triglycerides and low HDL-C.

Conclusion

This was the first trial to show that treatment of patients with a HDL-C <0.90 mmol/L with a fibrate, had no effects in reducing LDL-C, but did reduce CHD events by 22%.

Learning points

◆ Patients with low HDL-C are at high risk of CHD events.
◆ Fibrate therapy in a population with low HDL-C reduced CHD and CVD events.
◆ The benefits of fibrate therapy were dependent on baseline and changes in HDL-C levels.

Further reading

- Bezafibrate Infarction Prevention Study Group. Secondary prevention by raising HDL cholesterol and reducing triglycerides in patients with coronary artery disease: the Bezafibrate Infarction Prevention (BIP) study. *Circulation* 2000; 102(1): 21–7.
- Frick MH, Elo O, Haapa K, *et al.* Helsinki Heart Study: primary-prevention trial with gemfibrozil in middle-aged men with dyslipidemia. Safety of treatment, changes in risk factors, and incidence of coronary heart disease. *N Engl J Med* 1987; 317(20): 1237–45.
- Ginsberg HN, Elam MB, Lovato LC, *et al.* Effects of combination lipid therapy in type 2 diabetes mellitus. *N Engl J Med* 2010; 362(17): 1563–74.
- Jun M, Foote C, Lv J, *et al.* Effects of fibrates on cardiovascular outcomes: a systematic review and meta-analysis. *Lancet* 2010; 375(9729): 1875–84.
- Keech A, Simes RJ, Barter P, *et al.* Effects of long-term fenofibrate therapy on cardiovascular events in 9795 people with type 2 diabetes mellitus (the FIELD study): randomised controlled trial. *Lancet* 2005; 366(9500): 1849–61.
- Wierzbicki AS. FIELDS of dreams, fields of tears: a perspective on the fibrate trials. *Int J Clin Pract* 2006; 60(4): 442–9.

Gruppo Italiano per lo Studio della Sopravvivenza nell'Infarto miocardico-Prevenzione (GISSI-P) trial

Gruppo Italiano per lo Studio della Sopravvivenza nell'Infarto miocardico. Dietary supplementation with n-3 polyunsaturated fatty acids and vitamin E after myocardial infarction: results of the GISSI-Prevenzione trial. *Lancet* 1999; 354(9177): 447–55.

Background

The Mediterranean diet was identified as being associated with lower rates of CVD events in the Seven Countries Study. The Lyon Heart Health study helped confirm that a Mediterranean diet was associated with lower event rates in an underpowered flax oil-controlled study.

Fish intake and the polyunsaturated fatty acid (PUFA; omega-3) content of the diet were associated with lower rates of CVD and also eating oily fish as opposed to a normal diet was associated with lower CHD event rates in the Diet and Re-infarction Trial (DART), which was not reproduced in a subsequent larger study. There was controvesry over whether these benefits were due to anti-oxidants or omega-3 fatty acids. The GISSI-P study investigated which was the beneficial component in patients with recent MI.

Methods and results

The trial randomized 11,324 patients <3 months post-myocardial infarction to n-3 PUFA (docosahexaenoic acid (DHA)/eicosapentaenoic acid (EPA) 1 g daily, n = 2836), vitamin E (300 mg daily, n = 2830), both (n = 2830), or placebo (control, n = 2828) for 3.5 years. The primary end point was CVD events. Vitamin E therapy had no effect. Omega-3 fatty acid therapy had no effect on lipid profiles. Treatment with PUFA reduced CVD events by 10 (1–18)% in a two-way analysis, and 15 (2–26)% by four-way analysis. This benefit was driven by a decrease in all deaths (14 [3–24]% two-way, 20 [6–33]% four-way) and CVD deaths (17 [3–29]% two way, 30 [13–44]% four-way). The effect of the PUFA was similar for the primary end point (14 [1–26]%) and for fatal events (20 [5–33]%). Survival curves for PUFA treatment diverged early, and total mortality was reduced by 41 (3–72)% after three months (p = 0.037). The 53 (0–78)% reduction in sudden death was significant at four months (p = 0.048). A similar pattern was observed after 6–8 months for cardiovascular deaths.

Strengths and limitations

The GISSI-P trial clearly demonstrated a significant reduction in CHD events with omega-3 fatty acid therapy, despite a lack of any clear effect on lipids. This study has proved controversial. It was first thought that it would only apply in patients with inadequate intake of omega-3 fatty acids and thus these were only recommended in those patients not consuming fish. Statin therapy increased rapidly in both arms of the trial from 8 to 44% by trial end and thus the effects of omega-3 fatty acid therapy might have been attenuated by these drugs. The Japan EPA Lipid Intervention Study (JELIS) study in 18,645 patients showed that even in patients with a high initial fish intake and receiving (low dose) statin therapy 1g EPA was associated with a 19% reduction in CVD events in patients with chronic CHD or in primary prevention. Again controversy has surrounded the relatively high final LDL-C level (3.3 mmol/L) attained in this trial. However, the GISSI-P trial in heart failure, again using a DHA-EPA regime, demonstrated that the DHA-EPA arm was associated with a 9% reduction in CVD events and hospitalizations. This was in contrast to the statin arm where no benefit was seen despite a 32% reduction in LDL-C. Thus there does seem to be clear though moderate benefits from omega-3 fatty acid therapy.

Conclusion

This trial showed that in an acute post-CHD event population a synthetic combination of omega-3 fatty acids reduces CVD events independently of any effects on hyperlipidaemia.

> ### Learning points
>
> ◆ Omega-3 fatty acids reduce CVD events by 15% safely at moderate doses (1g DHA+EPA).
> ◆ Omega-3 fatty acids have no effect on commonly measured lipid profiles.
> ◆ Omega-3 fatty acids reduce ACS CHD events and may reduce sudden cardiac deaths.

Further reading

- Tavazzi L, Maggioni AP, Marchioli R, *et al.* Effect of n-3 polyunsaturated fatty acids in patients with chronic heart failure (the GISSI-HF trial): a randomised, double-blind, placebo-controlled trial. *Lancet* 2008; 372(9645): 1223–30.
- Wierzbicki AS. A fishy business: omega-3 fatty acids and cardiovascular disease. *Int J Clin Pract* 2008; 62(8): 1142–6.
- Yokoyama M, Origasa H, Matsuzaki M, *et al.* Effects of eicosapentaenoic acid on major coronary events in hypercholesterolaemic patients (JELIS): a randomised open-label, blinded endpoint analysis. *Lancet* 2007; 369(9567): 1090–8.

The Framingham risk equation

Anderson KM, Odell PM, Wilson PW, Kannel WB. Cardiovascular disease risk profiles. *Am Heart J* 1991; 121(1 Pt 2): 293–8.

Background

Cardiovascular disease is multifactorial so the use of any single parameter does not predict future risk accurately unless the levels of a particular risk factor are dramatically elevated. Numerous epidemiological studies had defined cardiovascular risk factors and there was an increasing recognition that a method was required to identify patients at future risk of a CVD event prior to that event occurring as it might be possible to prevent them. This method was derived from the long-established Framingham cohort studies.

Methods and results

This paper derived prediction equations for several cardiovascular disease end points, based on measurements of known cardiovascular risk factors. The data was derived from 5573 subjects of the original and offspring groups from the Framingham Heart Study, aged 30–74 years, initially free of cardiovascular disease. Equations to predict risk for the following end points were developed: myocardial infarction, coronary heart disease (CHD), death from CHD, stroke, cardiovascular disease, and death from cardiovascular disease. The parametric model used was seen to have several advantages over existing standard regression models. Unlike logistic regression, it can provide predictions for different lengths of time, and probabilities can be expressed in a more straightforward way compared to the Cox proportional hazards model.

Strengths and limitations

This is the landmark paper that describes the first and still commonly used version of the Framingham risk equation. The only major modification in many countries has been the removal of the diabetes factor as all patients with diabetes are considered high risk now and

the reduced emphasis placed on the detection of left ventricular hypertrophy. The equations demonstrated the potential importance of controlling multiple risk factors (blood pressure, total cholesterol, high-density lipoprotein cholesterol, smoking, glucose intolerance, and left ventricular hypertrophy) as opposed to focusing on one single risk factor in the management of CVD risk. Subsequent versions of the equation were modified to include risk associated with glycaemia, LDL-C, and to provide specific tools for the identification of patients at risk of stroke and peripheral arterial disease. Other groups have defined measures of CVD risk to include markers of inflammation (Reynolds risk score) or used other epidemiological studies—Prospective Cardiovascular Münster study (PROCAM) to derive alternative risk calculators (see Table 2.1). Lately the availability of large primary care databases has allowed risk calculators to be derived for individual countries, for example QRISK for the UK. The latest versions of the equation are now being used to determine lifetime risk of CVD as the ten-year time horizon in the original equation tends to underestimate risk in young populations.

NB: diabetes is now considered a high-risk CVD parameter and is therefore no longer included in risk calculation. Both ethnicity and family history are added as post-hoc modifiers to the Framingham risk equation in some countries.

The limitations of the Framingham equation have been identified in clinical practice and in modeling and validation studies. The equation varies in its accuracy

Table 2.1 Characteristics of risk factors included in different CVD/CHD risk calculators

Risk factor	Framingham	Q-RISK	PROCAM	Reynolds
Age	Y	Y	Y	Y
Gender	Y	Y	Y	Y
Smoking	Y	Y	Y	Y
Blood pressure (systolic)	Y	Y	Y	Y
Total cholesterol: HDL-C ratio	Y	Y	Y	Y
Diabetes	Y	Y	Y	NA
Family history early CHD	(Y)	Y	Y	Y
Ethnicity	(Y)	N	Y	N
Deprivation score	N	Y	N	N
C-reactive protein	N	N	N	Y
eGFR	N	Y	N	N
ECG: left ventricular hypertrophy	Y	N	N	N

between populations—for instance overstating the risk in southern Europeans, and has wide confidence intervals. Many patients with intermediate risk predictions actually turn out to have high event rates, leading to the addition of secondary stratification tools to the Framingham equation, for example CRP, family history, ethnicity, and indirect or direct measures of atherosclerosis, such as carotid intima-media thickness or coronary calcium score.

Conclusion

This landmark paper established that epidemiological studies can be used to define methods of determining future CVD risk in individuals.

Learning points

- ◆ Epidemiological studies can be used to define risk equations to calculate the future risk of CVD in individuals.
- ◆ The CVD risk equations need to be validated in other populations to which they are applied.

- ◆ The CVD risk equations are subject to wide confidence intervals.
- ◆ Secondary risk stratification methods can be useful to identify more precisely individuals at increased CVD risk.

Further reading

- Hippisley-Cox J, Coupland C, Vinogradova Y, *et al*. Predicting cardiovascular risk in England and Wales: prospective derivation and validation of QRISK2. *BMJ* 2008; 336(7659): 1475–82.
- Lloyd-Jones DM, Leip EP, Larson MG, *et al*. Prediction of lifetime risk for cardiovascular disease by risk factor burden at 50 years of age. *Circulation* 2006; 113(6): 791–8.
- Ridker PM, Paynter NP, Rifai N, Gaziano JM, Cook NR. C-reactive protein and parental history improve global cardiovascular risk prediction: the Reynolds Risk Score for men. *Circulation* 2008; 118(22): 2243–51, 4p.
- Sheridan S, Pignone M, Mulrow C. Framingham-based tools to calculate the global risk of coronary heart disease: a systematic review of tools for clinicians. *J Gen Intern Med* 2003; 18(12): 1039–52.
- Wierzbicki AS, Reynolds TM. Vascular risk screening: possible or too much, too soon? *Int J Clin Pract* 2009; 63(7): 989–96.

European Action on Secondary Prevention through Intervention to Reduce Events (EuroASPIRE)

EUROASPIRE Study Group. European Action on Secondary Prevention through Intervention to Reduce Events. EuroASPIRE. A European Society of Cardiology survey of secondary prevention of coronary heart disease: principal results. *Eur Heart J* 1997; 18(10): 1569–82.

Background

Numerous trials have described the benefits of antiatherosclerotic interventions in clinical research settings. However, the effectiveness of translating these guidelines to the clinical forum was unclear. The Cardiovascular Hospitalization Atherosclerosis Management Program (CHAMP) suggested in 1993 that a simple audit of prescribed therapies at discharge increased the rates of appropriate prescribing. The Action on Secondary Prevention through Intervention to Reduce Events (ASPIRE) study investigated the effectiveness of CVD progression strategies in the UK. It surveyed the prevalence of smoking, obesity, family history of CHD, diabetes, dyslipidaemia (raised LDL-C), and hypertension in 2583 secondary

prevention patients recruited from multiple centres (12 sites with 25 male and 25 female records audited per site) in one country (UK). It also investigated the success of smoking cessation, blood pressure control (<90 mmHg diastolic); total cholesterol (<5.2 mmol/L), and glycaemic control (glucose <10 mmol/L) in this population at one year after the original presenting event. This study indicated a wide variance in the success of implementation of effetive strategies even within one country. The next task was to extend this to the international stage. The EuroASPIRE study audited CVD risk factors and the effects of implementation of anti-CVD progression strategies in nine European countries (not including the UK) with diverse health systems and wide variations in wealth.

Methods and results

The EuroASPIRE survey audited 4863 medical records: 75% male and 25% female. The 3569 patients were interviewed (response rate 85%) with an average age of 61 years. The prevalence of CVD risk factors in this secondary prevention population was smoking, at 19%; 25% were overweight (BMI >30kg/m²); 53% had raised blood pressure (systolic BP >140 and/or diastolic BP >90 mmHg); 44% had raised total plasma cholesterol (total cholesterol >5.5 mmol/L); and 18% had diabetes. The reported medications at the time of interview were: anti-thrombotic drugs 81%, beta blockers 54% (58% in post-infarction patients), ACE inhibitors 30% (38% in post-infarction patients), and lipid lowering drugs (the vast majority being statins in most countries), 32%. Of the patients receiving blood pressure lowering drugs (not always prescribed for the treatment of hypertension) 50% had a systolic BP >140 mmHg and 21% >160 mmHg, and of those receiving lipid lowering drugs, 49% had plasma total cholesterol >5.55 mmol/L and 13% >6.5 mmol/L. A family history of premature coronary heart disease in a first-degree blood relative was present in 37%, but only 21% of patients reported being advised to have their relatives screened for CVD risk factors.

Strengths and limitations

The EuroASPIRE audit was a landmark study as it demonstrated the extent of variation in risk prevalences and their control in high-risk secondary prevention populations that had been managed in specialist cardiology units. It highlighted the poor translation of guidelines into clinical practice. The strength of these types of studies is that they gather data from a wide variety of sources, but the episodic and selective nature of audit means that more comprehensive programmes are essential to ensure that all patients with CHD receive the appropriate care. A variety of national strategies have been implemented on a systematic basis to audit guidelines on a larger scale. In the UK these comprise the Myocardial Infarction National Audit Project (MINAP) mandated in the UK National Service Framework for Coronary Heart Disease and the Quality Outcomes Framework (QoF). Other countries have similar programmes, for example in the US 'Get with the Guidelines'. Subsequent audits (EuroASPIRE II and III) by the EuroASPIRE group show great improvements in reducing the prevalence of some CVD risk factors but failure in reducing obesity. Drug treatment has improved where successful therapies exist, but rates of smoking cessation still remain disappointing.

These audits are now being extended to primary prevention. It is notable that specific incentive systems such as the UK QoF have resulted in dramatic improvements in CVD risk factor control, compared to general statements of intent, for instance achieving rates of lipid control >90%.

Conclusion

This landmark audit of CVD risk factors and their treatment in secondary prevention demonstrated large variances within and between countries and later audits showed that these can be reduced by effective implementation of guidelines.

Learning points

- Audits of CVD risk factors and their treatment show large variances within and between countries.
- Cycles of audit show improvements in the control of most CVD risk factors with successive cycles.
- Simple implementation tools and appropriate incentive schemes seem to deliver quicker benefits in terms of ensuring effective implementation of guidelines.

Further reading

- Bowker TJ, Clayton TC, Ingham J, *et al.* A British Cardiac Society survey of the potential for the secondary prevention of coronary disease: ASPIRE (Action on Secondary Prevention through Intervention to Reduce Events). *Heart* 1996; 75(4): 334–42.
- Fonarow GC, Gawlinski A, Moughrabi S, Tillisch JH. Improved treatment of coronary heart disease by implementation of a Cardiac Hospitalization Atherosclerosis Management Program (CHAMP). *Am J Cardiol* 2001; 87(7): 819–22.
- Kotseva K, Stagmo M, de Baquer D, de Backer G, Wood D. Treatment potential for cholesterol management in patients with coronary heart disease in 15 European countries: findings from the EUROASPIRE II survey. *Atherosclerosis* 2008; 197(2): 710–7.
- Kotseva K, Wood D, de Backer G, de Baquer D, Pyorala K, Keil U. EUROASPIRE III: a survey on the lifestyle, risk factors and use of cardioprotective drug therapies in coronary patients from 22 European countries. *Eur J Cardiovasc Prev Rehabil* 2009; 16(2): 121–37.
- Kotseva K, Wood D, de Backer G, de Baquer D, Pyorala K, Keil U. Cardiovascular prevention guidelines in daily

practice: a comparison of EUROASPIRE I, II, and III surveys in eight European countries. *Lancet* 2009; 373(9667): 929–40.

- Kotseva K, Wood D, de Backer G, *et al*. EUROASPIRE III. Management of cardiovascular risk factors in asymptomatic high-risk patients in general practice: cross-sectional survey in 12 European countries. *Eur J Cardiovasc Prev Rehabil* 2010; 17(5): 530–40.

Conclusion

In the last 30 years a series of trials have established the widespread efficacy of statin therapy. However, statins are not successful in reducing CVD events in all groups. For instance, despite large reductions in LDL-C no benefit was seen in studies of established chronic renal failure (e.g. a Study to Evaluate the Use of Rosuvastatin in Subjects on Regular Hemodialysis: An Assessment of Survival and Cardiovascular Events (AURORA) and Die Deutsche Diabetes Dialyse Studie-4D), in chronic cardiac failure (e.g. Controlled Rosuvastatin in the Multinational Trial in Heart Failure (CORONA), and GISSI-Heart Failure Trial), or calcific aortic stenosis (e.g. Simvastatin and Ezetimibe in Aortic Stenosis: SEAS). However, the Study of Heart And Renal Protection (SHARP) showed the efficacy of a statin-ezetimibe combination in chronic renal failure, including a dialysis subgroup, by demonstrating a 17% reduction in CVD events.

Current trials underway include The IMProved Reduction of Outcomes: Vytorin Efficacy International Trial (IMPROVE-IT) investigating the role of ezetimibe added to baseline statin in ACS (due 2015). Already the Action to Control Cardiovascular Risk in Diabetes (ACCORD) tiral has shown no benefit of universal addition of fibrates to statins in type 2 diabetes, except possibly in the high triglyceride, low HDL-C subgroup and similar results were seen in the underpowered Active Intervention in Metabolism of Low HDL/High Triglycerides and Impact on Global Health Outcomes (AIM-HIGH) trial in patients with CVD and low HDL-C with niacin. The Heart Protection Study-2/Treatment of HDL to Reduce the Incidence of Vascular Events (HPS-2/THRIVE) are investigating the role of adding niacin to underlying statin therapy in a dyslipidaemic (low HDL-C) population and in a far larger general population with a high proportion of diabetes rspectively. These will report in 2013–14.

New drugs to raise HDL-C by inhibiting cholesterol ester transfer protein (CETP) or to lower LDL-C by interference with apolipoprotein B synthesis (mipomersen) or microsomal transfer protein (lomitapide) are in development. However, torcetrapib (the prototype CETP inhibitor) showed no benefits on surrogate outcomes and increased CVD events in the Investigation of Lipid Level Management to Understand Its Impact in Atherosclerotic Events (ILLUMINATE) study likely as a result of its hypertensive action. Other CETP inhibitors such as dalcetrapib—being trialled in the efficacy and safety of dalcetrapib in patients with recent acute coronary syndrome dal-OUTCOMES study in chronic CHD (results due 2015), and anacetrapib and evacetrapib show no hypertensive effects and raise HDL-C by 35–80%.

The trials of the future will answer how much of the residual risk of CVD events that occur even on high dose statin therapy can be attributed to LDL-C and more likely HDL-C or whether this risk arises from other sources, for example thrombosis-associated risk factors.

Further reading

- AIM-HIGH Investigators. Niacin in patients with low HDL cholesterol levels receiving intensive statin therapy. *N Engl J Med* 2011; 365(24): 2255–67.
- Baigent C, Landray MJ, Reith C, et al. The effects of lowering LDL cholesterol with simvastatin plus ezetimibe in patients with chronic kidney disease (Study of Heart and Renal Protection): a randomised placebo-controlled trial. *Lancet* 2011; 377(9784): 2181–92.
- Barter PJ, Caulfield M, Eriksson M, *et al*. Effects of torcetrapib in patients at high risk for coronary events. *N Engl J Med* 2007; 357(21): 2109–22.
- Wierzbicki AS, Hardman TC, Viljoen A. New lipid-lowering drugs: an update. *Int J Clin Pract* 2012; 66(3): 270–80.

Chapter 3

Myocardial ischaemia

Dr Kalpa De Silva and Dr Divaka Perera

Introduction

The fields of coronary physiology and interventional practice have evolved remarkably over the last forty years. Specifically in relation to the improved understanding of basic pathophysiological principles underpinning myocardial ischaemia and infarction, and also in the expansion of *in vivo* human research, allowing novel insights and increased understanding into the functioning of the coronary circulation. This period has, arguably, witnessed the most successful era of cardiovascular research; with effective translation seen in improvements in clinical practice disease, with particular relevance to the treatment of coronary artery disease.

The widespread implementation of cardiac catheterization has been a key development in the assessment and treatment of coronary artery disease. Whilst this has been the gold-standard diagnostic test for coronary disease in both the chronic and acute settings during this period, it

has also provided a platform for a new generation of research to be undertaken, which has broadened myocardial ischaemia research from the initial building blocks of cellular and molecular biology investigation to dynamic invasive coronary physiology, paralleled by the advent of unique clinical applications, such as pressure wire assessment of coronary stenoses.

Advancement in technology and methodological techniques has allowed more detailed investigation of the pathophysiological mechanisms at the root of myocardial ischaemia, which in turn has led to improved understanding of the phenomenon of ischaemia and subsequent development of various treatment and management strategies. A small proportion of the key breakthroughs of the last four decades are described in the chosen papers that follow.

Selecting ten 'landmark' papers in the field of myocardial ischaemia has been an extremely challenging task, as the topic encompasses many aspects of cardiovascular medicine, cross-cutting between themes, including basic science, interventional cardiology, and imaging sciences. The choice of papers considered to be suitable for review in this chapter were vast, and inevitably there are studies that have provided cutting edge research and moved the specialty forward, that have not been included. The papers finally chosen for inclusion encompass a range of topics, including the molecular basis of ischaemia and infarction, the discovery and potential clinical utility of myocardial pre- and post-conditioning[1], assessment, and prognostic value of myocardial viability[2], to recent large contemporary randomized controlled trials such as Fractional flow reserve versus Angiography for Multivessel Evaluation (FAME)[3]. Additionally, prominent literature review articles that were seminal in focusing, developing, and challenging the understanding of myocardial ischaemia and infarction are also included[4, 5]. The studies and articles outlined in the chapter, aim to provide a thread through the progressive advancement seen in the field, from the molecular understanding of ischaemia to the application of clinical tools in current practice. Whilst this entails a wide breadth of coverage, relevance and applicability to the practising cardiologist is maintained throughout.

Myocardial contractile function during ischaemia and hypoxia

Allen DG, Orchard, CH. *Circulation Research* 1987; 60: 153–68.

Background

This was a review article of a variety of experimental techniques, which aimed to improve the understanding of myocardial contractile function during ischaemia, and encompassed changes observed in the mechanical performance of the left ventricle, with the description of the metabolic and ionic changes seen as a result of an ischaemic insult.

Methods and results

The review detailed the various deleterious effects of ischaemia and hypoxia on the myocardium. From a cellular level, it is evident that depletion of adeonsine tri-phosphate (ATP), most notably at the beginning of an ischaemic cascade affects the underlying cellular function, with the reduction in ATP concentrations being a crucial factor in myocellular dysfunction and, ultimately, necrosis. Furthermore it highlighted the differences or 'compartmentation' in workload, blood supply, and metabolic demand between the endocardial and epicardial layers of the left ventricle and subsequently at a cellular level in these regions[6].

At an ionic level the article discusses the main constituents found within the myocardium; calcium, hydrogen, sodium, and potassium ions, and the effect ischaemia has on the relative concentrations and the subsequent effects on myocardial function. An example of this is with potassium, where an efflux, secondary to anaerobic respiration, is seen corresponding to the onset of an ischaemic insult. The consequent relative reduction in intracellular, and increase in extracellular, potassium concentrations, causing alterations in the depolorization potential, manifest by slowing in conduction and the proliferation of arrhythmias.[7].

The postulated mechanisms underlying acute ischaemic failure were also described, as underpinned by three pathophysiological principles of myocardial function. Though available data at this time was conflicting, the link between changes in the action potential and contractile function was recognized in this review. Ischaemia reduces the amplitude of the action potential and reduces its duration, causing a reduction in contractile pressure, ultimately causing complete failure of contraction after 10–15 minutes of ischaemia[8]. The tensile ventricular pressure developed in each contraction of the heart is also dependent on the amount of calcium delivered to the myoplasm. A reduction in intracellular calcium concentration leads to reduced myofibrillar contraction and reduced ventricular contraction. Despite the absence of direct experimental data at the time, extrapolation from data on hypoxia related to calcium concentration alterations and reduction in left ventricular function, suggested the importance of this phenomenon in the ischaemic cascade. The final pathophysiological component considered was the properties of myofibrils. Data obtained by Katz and Hecht[9] showed the effect of ischaemia in producing an increasingly acidotic intracellular environment leading to increased myocyte dyfunction, which was affirmed with nuclear magnetic resonance studies, showing that the pH decreased when the myocardium was in an ischaemic or hypoxic state[10].

Conclusions and clinical implications

This insightful review of the literature at the time, outlined the potential causal factors of acute ischaemic left ventricular dysfunction. It saliently described the basic pathophysiological principles of ischaemia, increasing the awareness of these principles and allowing treatment strategies and investigative modalities to target the various stages involved in the deleterious ischaemic cascade. These early findings underpinned the principle that increasing ischaemic time leads to increased myocardial necrosis and therefore heralded a new approach to the management of acute myocardial infarction with the subsequent advent of management strategies such as thrombolysis and latterly primary percutaneous intervention, in an attempt to mitigate the effects of acute, and subsequent chronic, left ventricular impairment.

Learning points

- The effects of ischaemia are apparent after even a brief ischaemic insult, at both a cellular and functional level.
- This study highlights the importance of rapid restoration of adequate oxygenation to myocytes, to prevent metabolic derangement and eventual (potentially permanent) functional ventricular impairment.

- Murphy JG, Marsh JD, Smith TW. The role of calcium in ischaemic myocardial injury. *Circulation* 1987; 75(2): V15–24.

Further reading

- Downar E, Janse MJ, Durrer D. The effect of acute coronary artery occlusion on subepicardial transmembrane potentials in the intact porcine heart. *Circulation* 1977; 56(2): 217–24.

Preconditioning with ischaemia: a delay of lethal cell injury in ischemic myocardium

Murry CE, Jennings RB, Reimer KA. *Circulation* 1986; 74: 1124–36.

Background

The effect of numerous brief periods of ischaemia on the myocardium, caused by occlusion of major epicardial arteries, was believed to cause incremental myocardial necrosis in a 'wavefront' fashion, beginning in the endocardium and extending outward to the epicardium[11]. However, Reimer *et al.* had previously demonstrated that, contrary to established consensus, brief ischaemic insults did not necessarily cause ATP depletion, a precursor for cell death and subsequent myocardial necrosis, concluding that that there may be an intrinsic protective mechanism preventing myocardial necrosis following ischaemia, remote in time to a severe, prolonged episode of ischaemia[12]. They postulated that intermittent ischaemia followed by reperfusion might, therefore, have a protective effect on the myocardium during a subsequent sustained ischaemic insult. This study attempted to experimentally determine the notion that brief periods of ischaemia and reperfusion, 'preconditioning', prior to a prolonged ischaemic insult would result in reduced infarct size compared to a control group of those undergoing infarction without preconditioning.

Methods and results

This was a descriptive study using a dog model, with 44 mongrel dogs selected for surgical ligation of their circumflex arteries in order to induce myocardial infarction, and was comprised of two independent studies. The primary study end point was to assess the histological infarct size determined on post-mortem assessment.

The first study selected a cohort of dogs to have four five-minute periods of ischaemia, followed by the same period of reflow and reperfusion, followed by a 40-minute period of persistent ischaemia, whilst the control group had a persistent 40-minute ischaemic insult. The second study used the same preconditioning protocol, but was followed by a more prolonged occlusion of three hours, with the control arm having a single three-hour occlusion (Figure 3.1). Furthermore, regional myocardial blood flow and collateral flow was measured before and after occlusion by using a microsphere injection technique, with myocardial blood flow being calculated according to a pre-defined relationship between tissue counts and reference flow, which would allow the effect of preconditioning on the collateral flow to be determined.

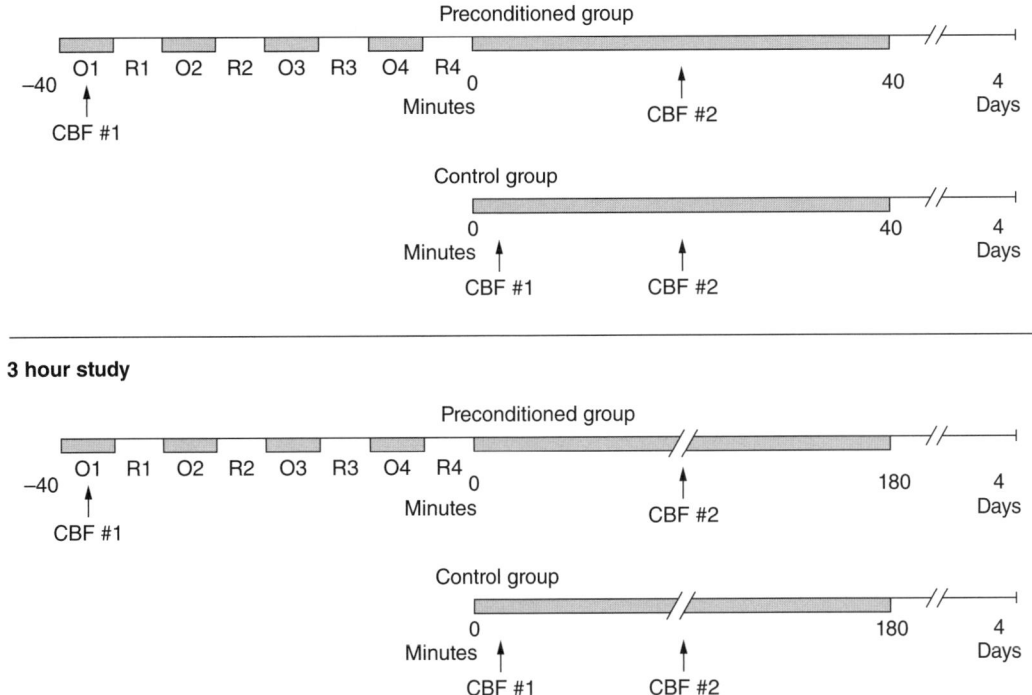

Figure 3.1 Preconditioning protocol used in the 40 minute and three-hour experiments.

Reproduced from Murry CE, Jennings RB, Reimer KA. Preconditioning with ischemia: a delay of lethal cell injury in ischemic myocardium. *Circulation* 1986, with permission of Wolters Kluwer Health.

An important initial observation was that with successive circumflex artery occlusions, the time taken for ST segment elevation to occur increased steadily, and the magnitude of ST deviation from baseline on the electrocardiogram was sequentially decreased following each occlusion. This was postulated to be as a result of the cellular adaptation that takes place in myocytes to allow preconditioning to occur. Reimer and Jennings had previously demonstrated that collateral blood flow (CBF) reduced the extent of myocardial infarction following prolonged ischaemia. However, the effect of preconditioning in this latter study was not thought to be driven by CBF, as sub-endocardial CBF was unchanged in both groups, and sub-epicardial flow increased in the preconditioned and control groups, in both (40-minute and three-hour occlusion) arms of the study. In the control animals in the 40-minute arm, sub-epicardial CBF tended to increase from 0.24 to 0.29 ml min^{-1}g (p = 0.06) but significantly increased in the three-hour arm of the study, from 0.28 to 0.42 ml min^{-1} g (p = 0.005).

The preconditioned animals had increases in sub-epicardial flow from the first occlusion to midway through the sustained occlusion that were similar to those in control animals: 0.30–0.41 ml min^{-1} g in the 40-minute group (p = 0.05) and 0.22 to 0.35 ml min^{-1} g in the three-hour group (p = 0.005). Since the increases in flow that occurred over time in the control animals were similar to those that occurred between the first and fifth occlusion in the preconditioned animals, it was supposed that preconditioning did not increase collateral flow.

Though there was a significant 75% reduction in infarct size in the pre-conditioned group in the 40-minute study, with average infarct size being 7.3 ± 2.1% of the anatomical area at risk, compared to 29.4 ± 4.4% in the control group, importantly no difference was seen in the infarct size (as a proportion of anatomic area at risk) in the prolonged three-hour ischaemia model (47.9 ± 6.6% in control group vs. 47.1 ± 4.8% in the pre-conditioned group) (Figure 3.2a and b). However, histological investigation revealed interesting differences in infarct morphology

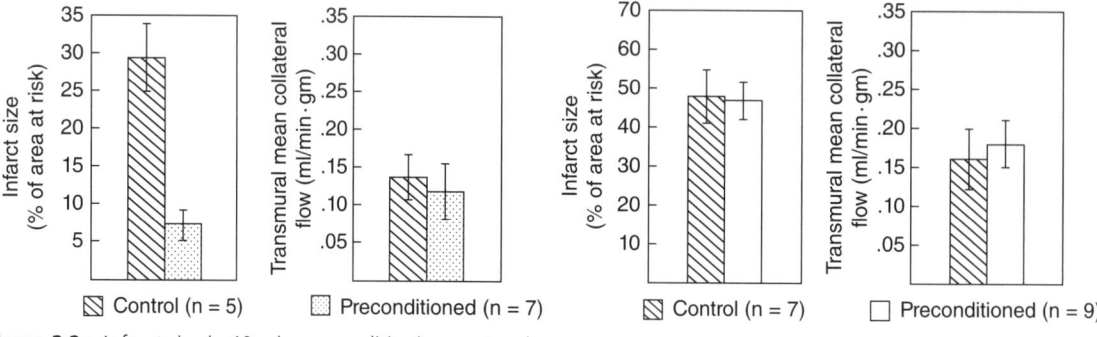

Figure 3.2a Infarct size in 40 min preconditioning protocol.
Reproduced from Murry CE, Jennings RB, Reimer KA. Preconditioning with ischemia: a delay of lethal cell injury in ischemic myocardium. *Circulation* 1986, with permission of Wolters Kluwer Health. **b** Infarct size in three-hour preconditioning protocol. Reproduced from Murry CE, Jennings RB, Reimer KA. Preconditioning with ischemia: a delay of lethal cell injury in ischemic myocardium. *Circulation* 1986, with permission of Wolters Kluwer Health.

between the two groups in the three-hour study. Infarcted areas in the control group showed dense confluent areas with clear boundaries, whilst the myocardium of those that underwent preconditioning had less dense patchy areas of infarction, with areas of normal myocardium interspersed, suggesting that preconditioning my be beneficial even after prolonged periods of ischaemia.

Study limitations

Whilst this study was seminal in demonstrating the concept of preconditioning, there were important limitations. This was a small animal study, which utilized a ligation model of infarction, which is pathophysiologically distinct from the process of athethero-thrombosis. Furthermore, dog hearts are not morphologically the same as human hearts, and tend to have a much greater degree of collaterization, which may exaggerate the differences in the CBF in the preconditioning arm of the study and is therefore not necessarily directly transferrable to humans.

Conclusions and clinical implications

This was the first study to demonstrate the protective effect of ischaemic preconditioning on the myocardium. It attempted to shed light on the pathophysiological alterations that may occur within the myocardium to allow reduced infarction size following brief episodes of ischaemia.

The study enabled, for the first time, extrapolation regarding the potential beneficial effect of episodic angina pectoris preceding myocardial infarction in humans, with corroborating animal evidence. The postulation was that preconditioning slowed the time taken to cell death, therefore increasing the time available and the opportunity for a successful reperfusion strategy to be initiated.

Learning points

- Preconditioning is the myocardium's intrinsic ability to protect itself from ischaemia.
- Utilizing an ischaemia/reperfusion model has the therapeutic potential of reducing infarct size.

Further reading

- Marber MS, Latchman DS, Walker JM, Yellon DM. Cardiac stress protein elevation 24 hours after brief ischaemia or heat stress is associated with resistance to myocardial infarction. *Circulation* 1993; 88(3): 1264–72.
- Reimer KA, Jennings RB. The 'wavefront phenomenon' of myocardial ischemic cell death. Transmural progression of necrosis within the framework of ischemic bed size (myocardium at risk) and collateral flow. *Lab Invest* 1979; 40: 633.

Postconditioning in the Human Heart

Staat P, Rioufol G, Piot C, Cottin Y, Cung T, L'Huillier I, Aupetit J, Bonnefoy E, Finet G, André-Fouët X, Ovize, M. *Circulation* 2005; 112: 2143–8.

Background

Over the last two decades the treatment of myocardial infarction has improved dramatically, with improving prognosis; however, it remains a major cause of death and morbidity from residual heart failure[13]. While improvements in the rapidity and quality of reperfusion therapies (thrombolysis or primary percutaneous coronary intervention) have reduced mortality from MI[14], there is evidence that the process of reperfusion itself may cause myocardial injury and contribute to final infarct size. Given that ischaemic preconditioning cannot be applied in the clinical setting of an acute MI, strategies for reducing infarct size after vessel occlusion have been termed post-conditioning[15]. This study was the first human study assessing the potential value of post-conditioning in MI, aimed at reducing reperfusion injury.

Methods and results

This was a prospective, multi-centre, randomized-controlled study, that recruited 33 patients who were included if they presented with an ST-elevation myocardial infarction within six hours of symptom onset, and if the culprit vessel, defined during coronary angiography, was either the left anterior descending artery or the right coronary artery, to ensure a large area at risk and had to be occluded (thrombolysis in myocardial infarction (TIMI) 0 flow) at the start of the PCI, with adequate restoration of flow (TIMI 2–3) after direct stenting PCI. Patients were randomized to either a post-conditioning protocol (by graded reperfusion) or a control group, which had no additional intervention performed. The post-conditioning protocol consisted of serial balloon inflations distal to the deployed stent, avoiding significant branching vessels, with each inflation at 4–6 atm, lasting one minute in duration, followed by reperfusion for one minute. This was carried out four times, with the ischaemia-reperfusion protocol lasting a total of eight minutes.

Patients were excluded if they had suffered a cardiac arrest, were in cardiogenic shock at presentation, or had a known previous MI or had pre-infarct angina within 48 hours, representing potential preconditioning. In addition, patients with significant angiographically visualized collaterization of the infarct territory defined Rentrop

grade ≥1 (Rentrop grade 0 = no angiographic visualization of collateral arteries, 1 = filling of the distal collateral branches of the recipient artery, but not the epicardial artery itself, 2 = partial filling of recipient epicardial artery via collaterals, 3 = complete filling of the epicardial artery via the collaterals) were also excluded.

The study end points were size of infarction and myocardial reperfusion. First, enzymatic size of infarction, using creatine kinase taken four hourly on day 1 after reperfusion, and then six hourly on days 2 and 3, up to 72 hours post infarction was considered. Myocardial blush grade (MBG) assessment of myocardial perfusion was used to compare the respective response to PCI reperfusion in both cohorts, along with left ventriculogram assessment of circumferential size of infarction. Further to this, maximal ST segment change was analysed, comparing admission 12-lead ECG with one obtained 48 hours after reperfusion.

The data analysis was from 30 patients, after three exclusions, and showed no significant differences in the patient population or the haemodynamic conditions of the two patient cohorts at the time of their infarct-related artery PCI. There was a 36% reduction in peak creatine kinase (CK) with those that underwent post-conditioning compared with the control arm, 2831 ± 404 IU/L vs. 4234 ± 722 IU/L, p = 0.05, respectively (Figure 3.3a). Furthermore, there was a strong negative correlation with the presence and severity of myocardial segment contraction seen on ventriculography in the post-conditioning arm (R^2 = 0.52, p <0.05). Further evidence of the potential benefit to the myocardium from post-conditioning was observed when myocardial blush grades were assessed; where significantly higher MBGs were seen in the post-conditioned group rather than in the control hearts, averaging 2.44 + 0.18 and 1.79 + 0.28, respectively (p = 0.02) (Figure 3.3b). However, there was no significant difference in ST segment elevation observed on 12-lead ECGs 48 hours after PCI.

Study limitations

This was a small study, with no clinical follow-up, therefore data relating to the apparent reduction in infarct size and likely positive remodelling in the post-conditioned arm could not be correlated with cardiovascular morbidity

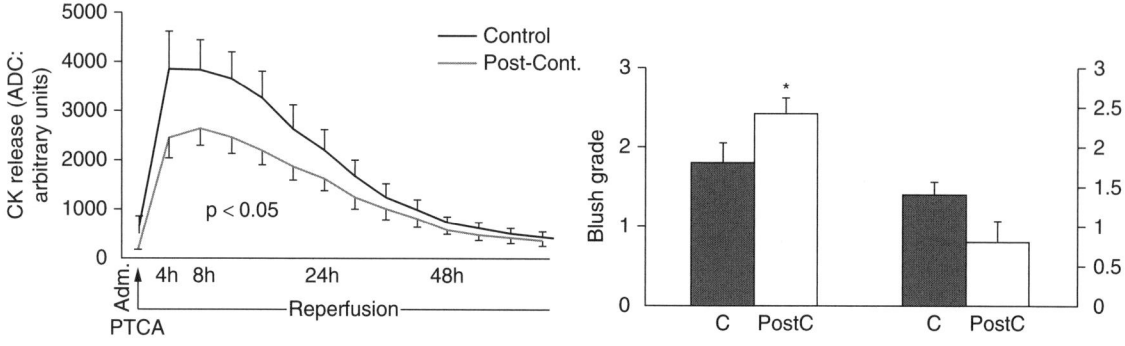

Figure 3.3a Peak creatine kinase in post-conditioned and routinely treated patients.
Reproduced from Staat, P. *et al.* Postconditioning the Human Heart. *Circulation* 2005, with permission of Wolters Kluwer Health. **b** Myocardial blush grade in post-conditioned and routinely treated patients. Reproduced from Staat, P. *et al.* Postconditioning the Human Heart. *Circulation* 2005, with permission of Wolters Kluwer Health.

or mortality end points. Furthermore, the surrogate of infarct size, and coronary and myocardial flow were not the most accurate methods of assessment, and may have been better served by non-invasive assessment with late-gadolinium enhancement cardiac magnetic resonance imaging and Doppler-pressure flow derived indices of flow and microvascular resistance, respectively.

Conclusions and clinical implications

The likely basis of the positive effect in the post-conditioned arm, is centred around the minimization of 'reperfusion injury', clinically seen as the angiographic observation of the 'no-reflow' phenomenon or reper-fusion arrhythmias[16, 17]. Whilst the most important factor in preventing myocyte death is restoration of flow, a variety of metabolic pathways are activated and are causal in myocardial injury during reperfusion, including the activation of oxidants[18], neutrophil adherence to endothe-lium, and subsequent endothelial dysfunction[19]. It had been previously demonstrated that slow onset, or 'ramped' reperfusion, reduces infarct size, which is the process likely to be the mediated and underpinning finding of this study[16].

Staat *et al.* provided an excellent example of bench-to-bedside translational research, bringing together basic science and clinical interventional cardiology, and pro-viding proof of concept in humans of the potential thera-peutic target of post-conditioning in the management of acute coronary syndromes. The study demonstrated the potential value of post-conditioning in reducing infarct size, and confirmed that the post-conditioning process, brief cycles of ischaemia/reperfusion, were safe and

feasible in patients undergoing primary PCI in the setting of an acute myocardial infarction, whilst highlighting the importance of further investigation into this mode of cardioprotection.

> **Learning points**
>
> ◆ The promising clinical utility of ischaemic post-conditioning as a potential adjunctive therapy during primary PCI in those having acute myocardial infarctions.
> ◆ Drawing attention to the importance of continued advancement of reperfusion strategies over and above current routine practice of primary PCI in the STEMI population to minimize left ventricular impairment.

Further reading

- Okamoto F, Allen BS, Buckberg GD, Bugyi H, Leaf J. Reper-fusion conditions: importance of ensuring gentle versus sudden reperfusion during relief of coronary occlusion. *J Thorac Cardiovasc Surg* 1986; 92(3 Pt 2): 613–20.
- Sato H, Jordan JE, Zhao ZQ, Sarvotham SS, Vinten-Johansen J. Gradual reperfusion reduces infarct size and endothelial injury but augments neutrophil accumulation. *Ann Thorac Surg* 1997; 64(4): 1099–107.
- Yellon D, Hausenloy D. Myocardial Reperfusion Injury. *NEJM* 2007; 357: 1121–35.

The hibernating myocardium

Rahimtoola SH. *Am Heart J.* 1989; 117(1): 211–21.

Background

This editorial article attempted to increase the awareness and understanding of the principles that underpin 'hibernating myocardium' and the value of viability assessment to identify patients who were most likely to have restoration or improvement of left ventricular function with revascularization. It reviewed research data, available at that time, demonstrating the pathophysiological basis of persistently impaired left ventricular function at rest due to a reduced coronary blood flow, and how this relationship can be altered if blood flow to the affected area of myocardium was restored. Investigative data was analysed from both animal and human coronary revascularization studies.

Methods and results

This paper details the various *in vivo* human and *ex vivo* animal evidence, present at the time, of improvement in regional myocardial dysfunction seen following restoration of adequate coronary blood flow to the 'hibernating myocardium'[20]. Hibernating myocardium refers to resting left ventricle (LV) dysfunction due to reduced coronary blood flow (or flow reserve) that can be partially or completely reversed by myocardial revascularization and/or by reducing myocardial oxygen demand 'hibernation' and its predilection to certain subgroups of patients. The review highlighted the clinical importance of this phenomenon, the potential to reverse it, and the methods available to detect hibernating myocardium.

Whilst left ventriculography was undertaken commonly to assess regional and global LV function, the technique could not discriminate scar from hibernating myocardium. However, ventriculography during nitroglycerin infusions was able to reduce oxygen demand, by reducing pre-load, therefore increasing contractility in previously dysfunctional areas. Those showing regional improvement had an 85% chance of long-term improvement following subsequent revascularization with CABG[21]. Indirect assessment of hibernation was considered, with the use of thallium and exercise echocardiography, for example, where, in the absence of prior myocardial infarction, worsening of a resting regional wall motion abnormality, under dynamic stimulation, would suggest myocardial dysfunction secondary to repetitive inducible ischaemic insults. Positron emission tomography (PET)

scanning to determine myocardial perfusion and metabolism was in its infancy, but was regarded as a promising technique in the assessment of myocardial viability, whereby detection of active metabolism in dysfunctional and under-perfused regions is used to determine hibernation, as distinct from areas of completed infarction which are characterized by a matched reduction in metabolism and perfusion.

Conclusions and clinical implications

In 1982, Rahimtoola *et al.* described the discovery of improvement or even normalization in pre-operative left ventricular dysfunction after myocardial revascularization with coronary artery bypass graft surgery (Figure 3.4)[21]; subsequently describing 'myocardial viability' and 'hibernating' myocardium. Despite this early clinical demonstration, there was a considerable time-lag before acceptance of these pathophysiological concepts. However, over the last three decades, an increasing body of research has fortified the utility and importance of viability assessment in mainstream clinical cardiology practice. Revascularization of hibernating, viable myocardium has been demonstrated to have numerous benefits, such as the improvement of regional and global LV systolic function[22], the reversal of negative remodelling[23,24], a reduction in mortality[25], and a decrease in the composite of myocardial infarction, heart failure, and unstable

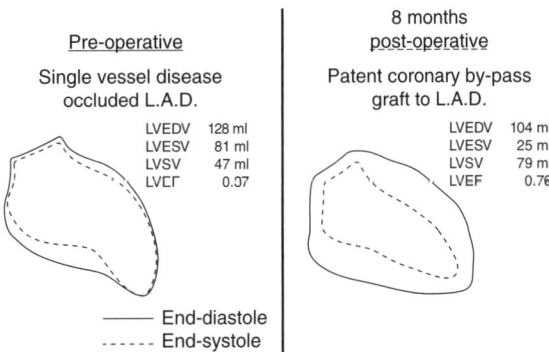

Figure 3.4 Preoperative and postoperative left ventricular function in a patient with hibernating myocardium.

Reproduced from Rahimtoola SH. The hibernating myocardium. *Am Heart J.* 1989; 117(1): 211–21, with permission of Elsevier.

angina[26]. However, most importantly, revascularization of patients with left ventricular dysfunction following stratification confirming the absence of significant amounts of viable myocardium, has no demonstrable clinical benefit[25].

Rahimtoola's work in the field of understanding the pathophysiological concepts involved in ischaemic ventricular dysfunction are illustrated by this literature review and were instrumental in defining the entity of hibernating myocardium, the concept of myocardial viability, and its prognostic importance afforded by its identification, in the context of coronary revascularization.

Learning points

- This raised the possibility of reversible left ventricular dysfunction due to a metabolic down-regulation of myocardial function (hibernation) in the presence of a flow-limiting coronary stenosis.
- Assessment of reversible myocardial dysfunction is an important clinical marker of success after all forms of coronary revascularization strategies.

Further reading

- Allman KC, Shaw LJ, Hachamovitch R, Udelson JE. Myocardial viability testing and impact of revascularization on prognosis in patients with coronary artery disease and left ventricular dysfunction: a meta-analysis. *J Am Coll Cardiol* 2002; 39(7): 1151–8.
- Tillisch J, Brunken R, Marshall R, *et al.* Reversibility of cardiac wall-motion abnormalities predicted by positron tomography. *N Engl J Med* 1986; 314(14): 884–8.

The use of contrast enhanced magnetic resonance imaging to identify reversible myocardial dysfunction

Kim RJ, Wu E, Rafael A, Chen E-L, Parker MA, Simonetti O, Klocke FJ, Bonow RO, Judd RM. *N Engl J Med* 2000; 343: 1445–53.

Background

In patients with CAD and LV dysfunction, the ability to distinguish patients who have suffered irreversible myocardial necrosis and scarring from those with potentially reversible contractile dysfunction is extremely valuable in predicting the potential success of revascularization procedures. Since the phenomenon of hibernating myocardium[5] and myocardial viability was introduced, a variety of non-invasive imaging modalities sought to differentiate patients with or without viability post-infarction. Techniques such as single positron emission tomography (SPECT), PET, and dobutamine echocardiography are useful but have limitations, including the dichotomous assignment of viability as an 'all-or-none' phenomenon, rather than being able to demonstrate the varying degrees of myocardial infarction and the variance in residual viability and subsequent recovery of function. This study aimed to identify viable myocardium in those patients with resting left ventricular dysfunction, in those who had suffered prior myocardial infarction, on the basis of the transmural extent of scar, by using and validating cardiac magnetic resonance (CMR) imaging in conjunction with an extravascular gadolinium contrast agent. The hypothesis was that transmural hyperenhancement in regions on the late gadolinium-enhanced CMR (LGE-CMR) corresponded to transmural myocardial infarction and thus non-viable territories, with the study looking at the utility of LGE-CMR in demonstrating viable myocardium in addition to visual and semi-quantitative analysis of regional wall motion abnormalities (RWMA) in patients undergoing planned PCI or CABG.

Methods and results

This was a prospective, single-blinded, non-randomized trial, where fifty patients (63 ± 11 years), scheduled to undergo PCI or CABG, with prior demonstration of LV dysfunction through either ventriculography or echocardiography were included into the study. In this study 42% (n = 21) had prior documented myocardial infarctions. Important and valid exclusions included those with unstable angina and New York Heart Association class IV heart failure.

They had semi-quantitivative CMR RWMA assessment, pre- and post-revascularization, with a grading of 0–4, which corresponded to a continuum of regional myocardial dysfunction, where 0 = normal, 1 = mild/moderate hypokinesia, 2 = severe hypokinesia, 3 = akinesia, and 4 = dyskinesia. Further to this, the degree of gadolinium hyperenhancement was also semi-quantitatively assessed, with a five-point transmurality scoring (TMS) system describing the varying percentage thickness of myocardial wall the contrast agent was localized to (where TMS 0 = 0%, 1 = 1–25%, 2 = 26–50%, 3 = 51–75%, 4 = 76–100%). The observers were blinded to the original CMR scan findings, and to whether the patient had undergone revascularization at all. In the analysis 13 patients were included who did not have revascularization, in an attempt to reduce the potential effect of study bias. Treatment was not altered as a consequence to initial CMR findings, with clinicians blinded to the results

and revascularization occurring as per the physician's original plan.

Follow-up CMR scans were performed at a mean of 76 ± 36 days after revascularization, demonstrating the variable relationship between the transmural extent of viability and the likelihood of functional improvement. In the study, 90% of those with greater than 51% LGE showed no functional recovery after revascularization, highlighting the importance of viability assessment post-MI, validating the use of LGE imaging techniques for this purpose (see Figure 3.5). The study also demonstrated the inherent inaccuracy of using a widely held convention that the presence of pathological Q waves on 12-lead electrocardiograms (ECG) as a surrogate, bedside measure of complete transmural infarction and inferring non-viability. The study showed that 89% of those with Q waves on their resting ECG post-MI, actually had CMR demonstrable evidence of non-transmural infarction,

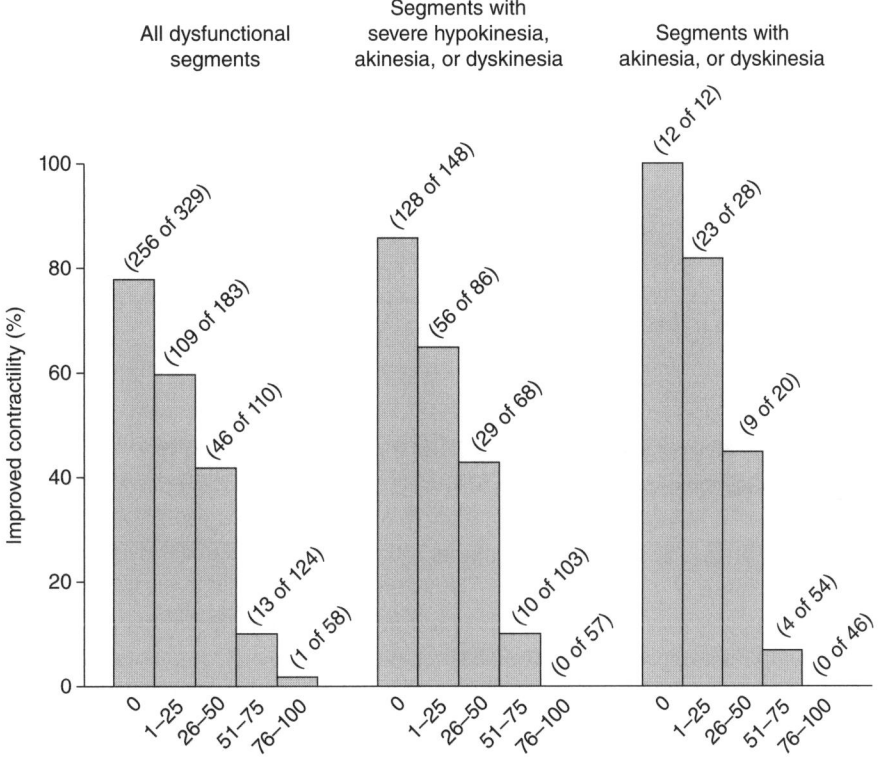

Figure 3.5 Relation between the transmural extent of hyperenhancement before revascularization and the likelihood of increased contractility after revascularization.

and showed subsequent improvement in function after revascularization.

Study limitations

Though the study highlighted the variability in LV recovery across a range of 'real-world' patients the study population had a mean LVEF of 43% before revascularization, higher than other contemporary viability assessment studies, introducing the possibility of LGE-CMR not necessarily having the same degree of accuracy in patients who have more severe left ventricular dysfunction. Additionally, assessment of regional wall motion abnormalities and transmurality of hyper-enhancement secondary to late-gadolinium imaging were through visual analyses rather than robustly quantitative methods.

Conclusions and clinical implications

This was the seminal CMR study to examine the value of late-gadolinium enhancement imaging, demonstrating that patients who have coronary artery disease and left ventricular dysfunction with residual viable myocardium before revascularization have a greater improvement in regional and global left ventricular function after revascularization than patients with predominantly nonviable myocardium, whilst demonstrating the predictive value of the high spatial and temporal resolution of functional and LGE-CMR techniques, which has subsequently become the gold-standard method of viability assessment.

The study highlighted the value of optimal non-invasive imaging to identify patients that are best served by coronary revascularization, aiding a paradigm shift in the assessment and treatment of patients with coronary artery disease, moving from strategies revolving around routine revascularization of all CAD patients, to a more careful assessment and individualization of management strategy, treating patients based on their residual viability and/or ischaemia rather than the presence of a stenosis alone per se.

Learning points

- The study shows the importance of non-invasive assessment in patients with known CAD, to allow accurate assessment of myocardial viability, with LGE-CMR being a particularly powerful method.
- It reaffirms that revascularization of coronary arteries subtending non-viable myocardium has no benefit in the recovery of left ventricular function.

Further reading

- Kwong RY, Schueeheim A, Rekhraj S, *et al*. Detecting Acute Coronary Syndrome in the Emergency Department with Cardiac Magnetic Resonance Imaging. *Circulation* 2003; 107: 531–7.
- Wellnhofer E, Olariu A, Klein C, *et al*. Magnetic resonance low-dose dobutamine test is superior to SCAR quantification for the prediction of functional recovery. *Circulation* 2004; 109(18): 2172–4.

Relation between Myocardial Blood Flow and the Severity of Coronary-Artery Stenosis

Uren NG, Melin JA, De Bruyne B, Wijns W, Baudhuin T, Camici PG. *N Eng J Med* 1994; 330: 1782–8.

Background

The correlation between the severity of a coronary artery stenosis and the consequent reduction in myocardial blood flow had been demonstrated in animal experimentation[27]. However, the relationship between angiographic stenosis severity and myocardial flow reduction had been investigated in humans with varying degrees of success[28, 29]. This study assessed the relationship between quantitatively assessed coronary artery stenoses compared to positron emission tomography (PET) assessment of myocardial blood flow.

Methods and results

This was a descriptive observational study. Thirty-five patients with varying degrees of angiographic single vessel CAD were recruited and underwent angiography with quantitative analysis of stenoses followed by PET imaging. Angiographic stenoses were categorized according to the percentage cross-sectional area reduction in luminal diameter, and grouped <40%, 40–59%, 60–79%, and >80%. In addition, a computerized endocardial contour detection system, was utilized to determine the ejection fraction using a modified Simpson's rule during left ventriculography.

The main trial end points were based upon the quantification of PET derived myocardial blood flow (ml/min/g) and coronary flow reserve (ratio of basal flow to hyperaemic flow) during intravenous dipyridamole and adenosine induced vasodilation, with variable independent stenosis features such as diameter and cross-sectional area of stenoses, in an attempt to define the angiographic stenosis threshold for causing a reduction in myocardial blood flow.

Patients with potentially increased microvascular resistance such as those with long-standing diabetes mellitus, systemic hypertension, or valvular disease were excluded, to avoid erroneous false positive results when examined by PET. A control group was recruited, who had normal ECGs and a normal exercise stress response at a high workload.

The majority of the cohort (n = 30) had left anterior descending artery disease; four had dominant right coronary artery disease and one had a dominant circumflex vessel stenosis. Mean stenosis was 56 ± 20% in the cohort, with a luminal diameter of 1.21 ± 0.61 mm. Haemodynamic measurements obtained from PET assessment showed that the heart rate at baseline in both study and control groups was similar, with significant increases in heart rate observed in both groups (from 63 ± 10 to 88 ± 16 in the patients and 65 ± 7 to 84 ± 10 in the controls, p = 0.001) during maximal vasodilatation. Despite actively excluding hypertensives, resting systolic blood pressure was significantly higher in the patients compared to the controls (148 ± 22 mmHg vs. 132 ± 19 mmHg, p = 0.01), though diastolic and mean arterial pressures were similar in the patient and control groups (74 ± 11 vs. 76 ± 8 mmHg and 98 ± 13 vs. 100 ± 13 mmHg), respectively.

The main end point of the study, regional myocardial blood flow, was observed to be similar at rest in patients and controls, (1.14 ± 0.42 and 1.13 ± 0.26 ml/min/g), but significantly lower in patients during hyperaemia (2.10 ± 1.16 vs. 3.37 ± 1.25 ml/min/g, p = 0.001). When myocardial blood flow was subcategorized according to the stenosis severity, no difference was seen in basal flow between the patient and control groups, irrespective of stenosis severity. Furthermore, flow during hyperaemia in those with <40% stenosis was not significantly different from flow in the controls (3.44 ± 1.47 vs. 3.37 ± 1.25 ml/min/g, respectively). In those with a stenosis diameter of 40% or more, the myocardial flow during hyperaemia progressively reduced with the increase in stenosis severity, with baseline flow being 3.37 ± 1.25 ml/min/g compared to 1.23 ± 0.50 ml/min/g in those with >80% stenoses. See Figure 3.6.

Study limitations

A minor criticism of this study was the surrogates used to assess coronary flow, with coronary flow reserve being a poor marker of flow, as individual patient haemodynamic alterations can cause aberration in CFR. Furthermore, the PET scans were performed at a remote time point to the coronary angiographic assessment, further confounding the variability in underlying baseline haemodynamic conditions.

Conclusions and clinical implications

Gould et al.[30] had provided early experimental evidence for the likely relation of stenosis severity to perfusion; however, this study was the earliest clinical demonstration

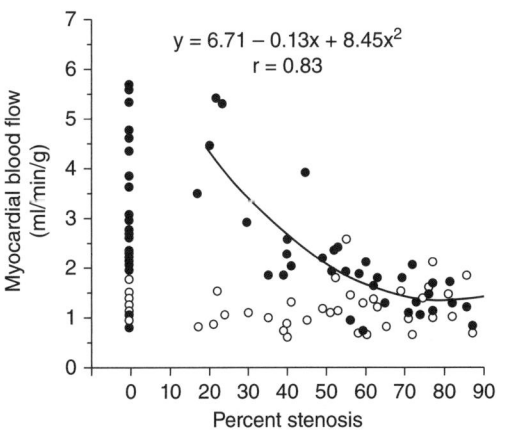 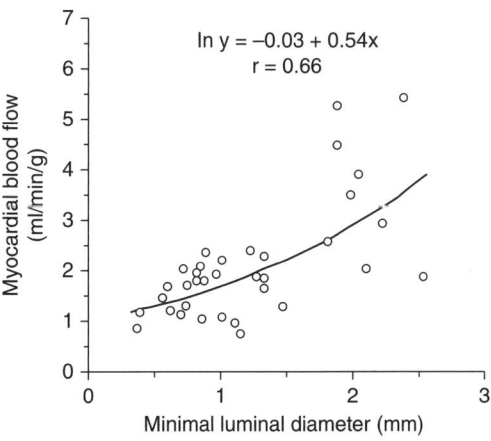

Figure 3.6 Effect of percent stenosis and angiographic luminal diamter on PET derived myocardial blood flow.

of the interplay between stenosis severity identified on coronary angiography and consequent myocardial perfusion.

This study demonstrated the inverse correlation between angiographic severity of coronary artery stenoses and underlying myocardial blood flow during hyperaemia. Their findings suggest that maximal flow decreases progressively if the stenosis is greater than 40%, with exhaustion of the coronary vasodilator reserve for stenosis greater than 80%. These data form the basis of the visual angiographic classification that is in use to date, whereby diameter stenoses below 40% are considered 'subcritical'. However, the study also demonstrated considerable variation in flow reserve between individuals who appeared to have similar angiographic lesion characteristics, highlighting the limitations of two-dimensional luminographic assessment of coronary disease and the importance of functional assessment of coronary artery stenoses, in this instance using PET imaging.

Learning points

- ◆ Ischaemia inducing stenoses can be accurately determined by non-invasive perfusion imaging, such as PET, and complement coronary angiographic assessment of CAD.
- ◆ Maximal coronary flow begins to diminish progressively if stenoses are >40%, with resting flow impaired in stenoses >80% diameter.

Further reading

- Gould KL, Kirkeeide RL, Buchi M. Coronary flow reserve as a physiologic measure of stenosis severity. *J Am Coll Cardiol* 1990; 15(2): 459–74.
- Gould KL, Lipscomb K, Hamilton GW. Physiologic basis for assessing critical coronary stenosis. Instantaneous flow response and regional distribution during coronary hyperemia as measures of coronary flow reserve. *Am J Cardiol* 1974; 33(1): 87–94.

Experimental basis of determining maximum coronary, myocardial, and collateral blood flow by pressure measurements for assessing functional stenosis severity before and after percutaneous transluminal coronary angioplasty

Pijls NH, van Son JA, Kirkeeide RL, De Bruyne B, Gould KL. *Circulation* 1993; 87: 1354–67.

Background

Coronary stenosis severity had previously been defined in terms of geometric dimensions, pressure gradient, resistance to flow, and CFR. However, angiographic lumen measures correlate poorly with the functional characteristics of a stenosis and CFR varies with prevailing haemodynamic conditions. This seminal paper describes a model of the coronary circulation that individually describes the relative contributions of epicardial artery, collateral, and myocardial blood flow, which, moreover, could be predicted from pressure measurements alone. This manuscript describes the experimental basis of fractional flow reserve (FFR), the most widely assessed physiological parameter in clinical interventional cardiology practice today.

Methods and results

The initial phase of the study revolved around the development of a theoretical model identifying the relationship between pressure and flow within different components of the coronary circulation. Three important conceptual obstacles that had undermined previous investigations were overcome during this study. The first was that previously invasive instruments available to measure intracoronary pressure were inadequate and were affected by the very pressure they were meant to measure, a problem negated by the development of a pressure sensor mounted on a 0.015 inch guide-wire. Second, previous investigation into the utility of pressure to determine flow had been done during basal coronary flow, which would therefore have been affected by the powerful and continually varying influences of epicardial and microvascular resistances. If resistance could be made minimal and constant, with the introduction of a vasodilating agent, such as a paparavine or adenosine, this would theoretically allow pressure to relate directly to flow. The third conceptual step forward was in the appreciation of the importance of collateral flow to the overall myocardial blood flow.

Subsequently, an equation was derived to describe the relationship between pressure and the regional distribution of maximal myocardial perfusion, incorporating the unique concept of maximum flow through a stenotic artery (Q_s), compared to hypothetical flow in the same artery, in the absence of a stenosis (Q_N). This ratio was termed FFR, where FFR $= Q_s/Q_N = (P_d-P_v)/(P_a-P_v)$, during maximal hyperaemia, when myocardial (microvascular) resistance is considered minimal and constant (see Figure 3.7).

The experimental phase of the study evaluated the mathematical model and the rigidity of the theoretical assumptions made regarding coronary resistance in an animal experimental model. Five anaesthetized dogs had surgical ligation of their left circumflex artery, with an extrinsic balloon occlusion device being attached to enable varying degrees of stenosis to be created. An external Doppler-flow velocity device was attached to the vessel and an intracoronary (IC) pressure sensing wire allowed measurements of the artery to be taken during twelve different degrees of stenosis, after 8 mg IC papavarine was administered to create a state of maximal hyperaemia. Additionally, continuous aortic and venous pressure recordings were obtained, via Millar catheters placed in the aortic root and right atrium respectively, enabling direct coronary flow reserve calculation (Q_s/Q_N). To assess for the independence of the FFR values from coexisting haemodynamic states, normotensive, hypertensive, and hypotensive conditions were mimicked using either vasopressor (phenylephrine) or vasodilatory (sodium nitroprusside) agents, respectively.

The study confirmed that pressure derived fractional coronary flow reserve correlated well with the directly measured (Qs/Q_N) equivalent, with a correlation coefficient of 0.98 ± 0.01. Furthermore, by direct experimentation it was determined that pharmacologically induced vasodilation, in this case with papavarine, could reliably induce hyperaemia, as evidenced by the ratio between maximum blood flow velocity and post-occlusion maximum blood flow velocity at the start of each series of measurements being 0.99 ± 0.0, confirming that maximum arterial vasodilatation had been obtained. The most notable finding was the indirect validation of FFR_{MYO} (P_d-P_v/P_a-P_v) as a surrogate of flow when correlated against the directly observed Doppler derived flow (Q_s/Q_N), confirming the validity of the principle that pressure derived markers of flow alone, under conditions of maximum vasodilatation are related to maximum flow. The study also provided the experimental basis for the first quantitative measure of coronary collateral flow (the Collateral Flow Index, CFI).

Study limitations

Whilst the study assessed the validity of the mathematical relationship between pressure and flow in coronary arteries, the major limitation of the technique is the

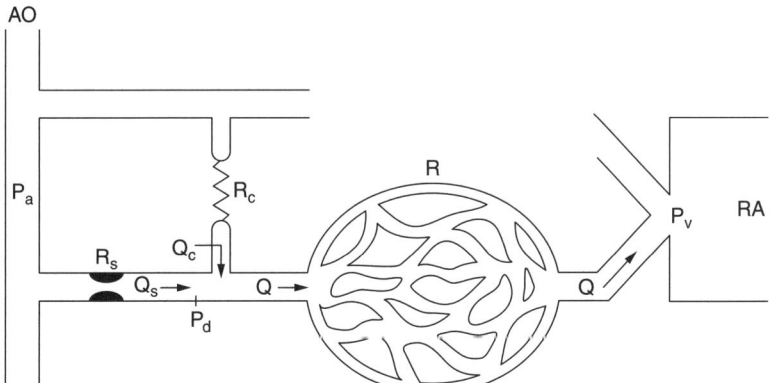

Figure 3.7 Schematic diagram representing the coronary circulation. AO, aorta; P_a, arterial pressure; P_d, distal coronary pressure, P_v, venous pressure; Q, blood flow through the myocardial vascular bed; Q_c, collateral blood flow; Q_s, epicardial blood flow; R, resistance of the myocardial vascular bed; R_s, resistance of the stenosis in the epicardial artery; RA, right atrium.

Reproduced from Pijls NH, *et al.*, Experimental basis of determining maximum coronary, myocardial, and collateral blood flow by pressure measurements for assessing functional stenosis severity before and after percutaneous transluminal coronary angioplasty. *Circulation* 1993; 87: 1354–67, with permission from Wolters Kluwer Health.

assumption that this relationship is entirely linear in all circumstances[31]. There is in fact a curvilinear relationship between pressure and flow, which becomes apparent at high pressures and may be confounded by inadequate hyperaemia.

Conclusions and clinical implications

This was the first description of the physiological basis of FFR, defined, in its simplest form, as P_d/P_a, and its utility in using it to assess the functional significance of a coronary stenosis in inducing myocardial ischaemia. It also underlined important differences between CFR and FFR, namely the dependence of CFR on salient haemodynamics, such as blood pressure and heart rate, whilst FFR determines maximum flow in a stenotic coronary artery as a fraction of normal maximum flow without a stenosis, independently of intrinsic haemodynamic conditions, negating the issue of indifferent reproducibility inherent to the previously used CFR measurement.

This study is yet another excellent example of 'bench-to-bedside' research in clinical cardiology. From the initial animal model described here, a safe, reliable clinical tool was developed, and was subsequently utilized in daily practice. The results of this study were critical to the understanding of invasive pressure-derived assessment of coronary stenosis, and allowed further clinical trial investigation, development, and validation of FFR as a technique to assess ischaemia.

Learning points

- ◆ Pressure measurements are equivalent to flow in the coronary circulation, during maximal hyperaemia, where resistance is minimal and constant.
- ◆ Fractional flow reserve was highlighted as a potential 'on-table' assessment of functional stenosis significance.

Further reading

- Bech GJ, De Bruyne B, Pijls NH, *et al*. Fractional flow reserve to determine the appropriateness of angioplasty in moderate coronary stenosis: a randomized trial. *Circulation*. 2001; 103(24): 2928–34.
- Pijls NH, De Bruyne B, Peels K, *et al*. Measurement of fractional flow reserve to assess the functional severity of coronary-artery stenoses. *N Engl J Med*. 1996; 334(26): 1703–8.

Comparison of the Short-Term Survival Benefit Associated With Revascularization Compared With Medical Therapy in Patients With No Prior Coronary Artery Disease Undergoing Stress Myocardial Perfusion Single Photon Emission Computed Tomography

Hachamovitch R, Hayes SW, Friedman JD, Cohen I, Berman DS. *Circulation* 2003; 107: 2900–07.

Background

The optimal mode of management, either revascularization or medical therapy, in patients with stable coronary artery disease has been subject to many trials, with conflicting conclusions and recommendations[33, 34]. This study aimed to define the ischaemia threshold required for patients to benefit from revascularization compared with medical management, as assessed by single photon emission computer tomography (SPECT) myocardial perfusion imaging.

Methods and results

This was a large retrospective observational analysis of patients with suspected CAD in a relatively contemporary setting, undergoing either exercise or adenosine SPECT scans and then either continued medical management or revascularization. Perfusion imaging was quantified according to the percentage severity of the reversible defect observed.

Patients were included if they had undergone clinically indicated SPECT perfusion imaging, and were subsequently divided into two groups—medical management (n = 9956) and revascularization with PCI or CABG (n = 671), occurring within 60 days of their scan. Patients were excluded if they had known prior myocardial infarctions and/or undergone previous revascularization procedures; those that were lost to follow-up were also excluded.

Follow-up was through telephone questionnaires used to determine death, or cardiovascular morbidity. To adjust for non-randomization of treatment, a propensity score was developed using logistic regression to model the decision to refer to revascularization. This model identified inducible ischaemia and anginal symptoms as the most powerful predictors and was incorporated into survival models.

The main end point of the study was cardiac death, defined as death attributable to any cardiovascular cause, with data ascertained through death certification or hospital records, to mode of therapy. All-cause mortality over the duration of the follow-up period was also analysed. There were a total of 492 (4.6%) all-cause deaths, with 146 (1.4%) of these being attributable to a cardiac cause in the entire cohort (Figure 3.8a).

Analysis of the cohort according to the presence and severity of ischaemic burden confirmed two important principles. The first was that mortality increased with increasing ischaemic burden, regardless of the treatment modality. The second was that survival was better with medical therapy in the setting of mild or no ischaemia, whereas it improved when a revascularization strategy was adopted, in the context of moderate or severe ischaemia. Furthermore, the study identified a critical ischaemic threshold or 'tipping point', observed at 12.5%, where revasculazation began to confer a mortality advantage over conservative management (Figure 3.8b). Increasing ischaemia, above this level, led to an additive benefit from adopting an invasive management strategy. Those with a 20% ischaemic burden showed a definitive survival advantage in favour of revascularization, with cardiac death rate being 2.0% vs. 6.7%, p = 0.02, respectively.

Study limitations

The results are limited by the non-randomized, retrospective observational nature of the study, which required complex statistical models to counteract the lack of randomization of therapeutic strategy, with potential intrinsic statistical errors.

Conclusions and clinical implications

This observational study first introduced the concept of a critical ischaemic threshold and the role of ischaemia assessment in patients with stable coronary artery disease, along with the demonstrable benefit obtained by revascularization in those with moderate to severe ischaemia. Hachamovatich et al. provide evidence that revascularization, in the correct setting, is likely to represent the optimal strategy in patients with stable CAD. The study also laid the foundation for subsequent prospective trials, such as COURAGE, to further assess this topic. The COURAGE study, itself a randomized control trial, which assigned patients with stable CAD, to a medical or invasive management strategy, subsequently reaffirmed the findings of the low ischaemia group in this earlier observational study[35].

Finally, the study alluded to a means of risk stratification of patients according to the severity of ischaemia observed, using complimentary non-invasive imaging, which are frequently discordant from the extent of CAD visualized on coronary angiography.

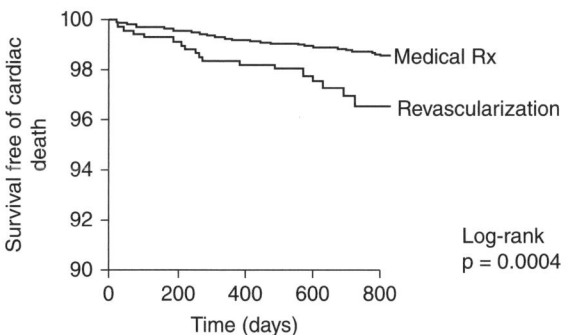
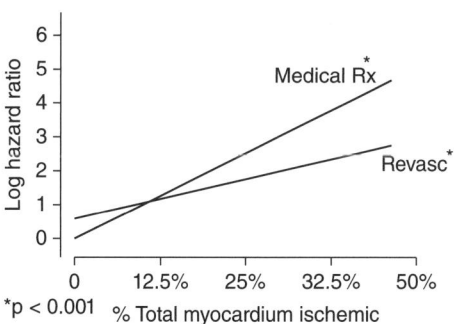

Figure 3.8a Unadjusted Kaplan-Meier survival in patients undergoing revascularization vs. medical. **b** Log hazard ratio of revascularization vs. medical management.

Reproduced from Hachamovitch R. Comparison of the Short-Term Survival Benefit Associated With Revascularization Compared With Medical Therapy in Patients With No Prior Coronary Artery Disease Undergoing Stress Myocardial Perfusion Single Photon Emission Computed Tomography. *Circulation* 2003, with permission from Wolters Kluwer Health.

Further reading

- Boden WE, O'Rourke RA, Teo KK, *et al.* Optimal medical therapy with or without PCI for stable coronary disease. *N Engl J Med* 2007; 356(15): 1503–16.
- Davies RF, Goldberg AD, Forman S, *et al.* Asymptomatic Cardiac Ischaemia Pilot (ACIP) study two-year follow-up: outcomes of patients randomized to initial strategies of medical therapy versus revascularization. *Circulation* 1997; 95: 2037–43.

Optimal Medical Therapy With or Without Percutaneous Coronary Intervention to Reduce Ischemic Burden: Results From the Clinical Outcomes Utilizing Revascularization and Aggressive Drug Evaluation (COURAGE) Trial Nuclear Substudy

Shaw LJ, Berman DS, Maron DJ, Mancini GBJ, Hayes SW, Hartigan PM, Weintraub WS, O'Rourke RA, Dad M, Spertus JA, Chaitman BR, Friedman J, Slomka P, Heller GV, Germano G, Gosselin G, Berger P, Kostuk WJ, Schwartz RG, Knudtson M, Veledar E, Bates ER, McCallister B, Teo KK, Boden WE; for the COURAGE Investigators. *Circulation* 2008; 117: 1283–91.

Background

The COURAGE trial[35] had previously randomized patients to medical management or percutaneous revascularization to assess and determine the optimal treatment strategy for stable coronary artery disease, concluding that medical management was non-inferior to an invasive strategy. However, this study had important limiting factors, principally, the exclusion of patients with highly positive stress tests or severe anginal symptoms, the cohort that might be expected to have benefited most from an invasive strategy[36, 37, 38]. In addition, there was a high therapy cross-over rate from those randomized initially to medical management subsequently requiring PCI. The COURAGE nuclear substudy was devised to determine the value and importance of ischaemia assessment in guiding what the optimal management strategy should be in stable coronary disease.

Methods and results

The study was a prespecified subgroup analysis of the COURAGE randomized control trial. Patients were eligible for the main RCT if they had an angiographically confirmed stenosis in one major epicardial artery of more 70% and had anginal symptoms, less than CCS class III in severity. From this 2287 patient cohort 314 patients formed the substudy, and included patients from 25 of the 50 COURAGE centres. Each patient underwent pre-treatment and follow-up nuclear myocardial perfusion scans (at 6–18 months) after randomization to either optimal medical management (OMT) or OMT + percutaneous coronary intervention (PCI). Optimal medical management was strictly defined as patients having ongoing therapy with a combination of multiple pharmacological agents: anti-platelet medication with low-dose aspirin; anti-ischaemic therapy with long-acting metoprolol; amlodipine and isosorbide mononitrate, alone or in combination; lisinopril or losartan for hypertension, left ventricular dysfunction, or secondary prevention. Further to this, target-based LDL cholesterol lowering (<85 mg/dL or 2.2 mmol/L) along with increasing HDL (>40 mg/dL or 1.0 mmol/L) and reducing triglycerides (<150 mg/dL or 1.70 mmol/L) was mandated using simvastatin in addition to ezetimibe, extended release niacin or fibrates. Successful PCI was defined as a normal arterial flow (TIMI 3) with <20% residual stenosis post-stent deployment, with procedural details and stent type used at the discretion of the operator.

Exclusions to the study included patients with refractory heart failure symptoms, cardiogenic shock, ejection fraction <30%, or coronary anatomy not amenable to PCI. As a substudy of the main COURAGE trial the inclusion criteria mirrored those used in that study, with the exclusion of patients with significant angina burden and more importantly those that had positive ischaemia stress tests.

The primary study end point was ≥5% reduction in ischaemic burden on the follow-up MPS, compared to the baseline study to determine which treatment modality (OMT or OMT + PCI) would confer the greatest percentage reduction in ischaemia. Other end points measured were anginal status at follow-up and also the number of anti-ischaemic therapies patients remained on and determining the clinical outcomes between the two groups.

Compared with the main trial, patients enrolled in this substudy had less severe angina (p = 0.013) and less multi-vessel CAD (p = 0.05). Of the 314 patients recruited (OMT = 155, OMT + PCI = 159) exercise stress testing pre- and post-treatment showed no difference in the frequency of exercise induced ST segment depression, and exercise capacity increased in both arms of treatment (approx. 1.1 minute in both groups, p <0.01). The median follow-up period was 4.6 years. The primary end point of ischaemia reduction was observed in 33% of OMT + PCI and only 19% in the OMT therapeutic arm (p = 0.0004) of the whole cohort. Whilst pre-treatment myocardial percentage ischemic burden was similar in both groups (8.2% vs. 8.6%, p = 0.63), post-treatment (mean = 374 ± 50 days) ischaemia reduction was noted to be greater in the OMT + PCI group compared to the OMT group (-2.7% vs. -0.5%, p <0.0001). Furthermore, more of the OMT + PCI group were rendered non-ischaemic (15.2% vs. 8.8%, p = 0.06), and fewer had >10% (severe) residual ischaemic myocardium (15.8% vs. 27.0%, p = 0.02). This reduction in ischaemic end points translated into a symptomatic improvement also, with a larger proportion of those treated with OMT + PCI having an improvement of ≥1 Canadian Cardiovascular Society class (82% vs. 70%, p = 0.007). This corresponded with a reduction in long-acting nitrate use in the OMT + PCI group (64% vs. 75%, p = 0.03).

With regards to the prognostic importance of ischaemia-guided therapy, the overall death and non-fatal MI rate was 21.7%, with an unadjusted death or non-fatal MI rate being 13.4% in those patients with significant ischaemia reduction compared to 24.7% for those without significant ischaemia reduction in either therapeutic arm, unadjusted it was statistically significant, p = 0.04. However, when risk-adjusted this trend was no longer significant (p = 0.26) which is likely to represent a function of the small numbers in the trial (Figure 3.9). Moreover, further analysis of the relationship between residual ischaemia and outcome suggested that there was a gradual

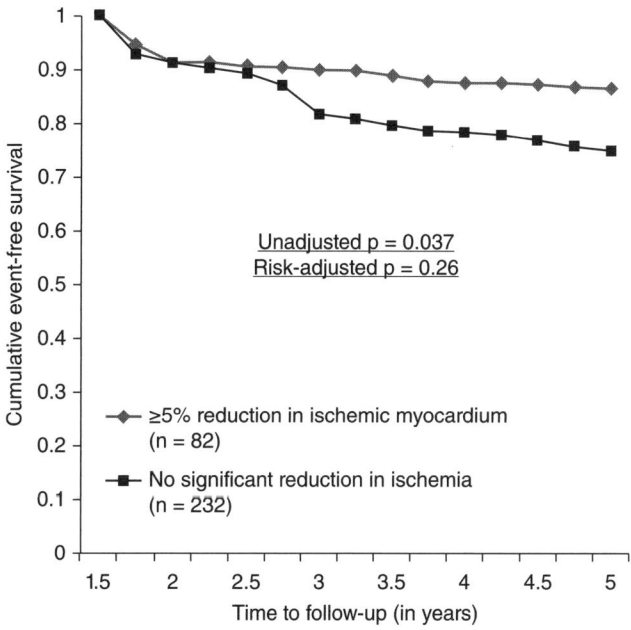

Figure 3.9 Kaplan-Meier survival for patients with >5% ischaemia reduction after 6–18 months on OMT or OMT + PCI.

Reproduced from Shaw L, *et al.* Optimal Medical Therapy With or Without Percutaneous Coronary Intervention to Reduce Ischemic Burden: Results From the Clinical Outcomes Utilizing Revascularization and Aggressive Drug Evaluation (COURAGE) Trial Nuclear Substudy. *Circulation* 2008, with permission from Wolters Kluwer Health.

incremental relationship between risk of events and the extent and severity of residual ischaemia, with rate of death increasing from 0% in those with no demonstrable ischaemia on MPS, to 39.3% in those where >10% of the myocardium is ischaemic (>10% ischaemia HR 7.5).

Study limitations

As this was a substudy of a large, randomized-controlled study, statistical conclusions cannot be made as it was not adequately powered to determine the prognostic value of ischaemia reduction in stable CAD. However, clear trends are evident from this data in favour of ischaemia-guided therapy. Furthermore, the vast majority of patients in this substudy had a baseline ischaemic burden below the prognostic threshold previously identified by Hachamovitch et al.[38]; therefore it is possible that inclusion of a higher risk cohort, with more ischaemia at baseline, would have shown even more dramatic effects.

Conclusions and clinical implications

The role of an invasive management strategy with PCI in patients with stable coronary artery disease has been disputed over the last twenty years[39, 40, 41, 42, 43]. The majority of the trial data available to date consisted of sub-optimal interventional strategies, prior to routine use of intracoronary stents, latterly with immunosuppressive drug eluting stents, aligned with little or no formal risk stratification with ischaemia assessment to inform clinical decision making regarding which patient population would benefit from PCI rather than medical management alone. This was the first randomized trial addressing the

value of risk assessment of patients with stable CAD with ischaemia testing. Though not statistically powered to address the prognostic implications of ischaemia-driven treatment of CAD, it provided a clear trend toward assessing patients more rigorously, with incremental benefits seen in those treated with an invasive strategy with high ischaemic burdens compared to optimal medical management alone.

Learning points

- Ischaemia guided therapy of stable CAD with PCI in those with moderate to severe ischaemia (>5%) is likely to represent the best therapeutic option prognostically and in improving symptoms.
- This trial helped to increase awareness of the importance of routine ischaemia assessment, allowing improved risk assessment and optimal treatment of patients with CAD.

Further reading

- Hachamovitch R, Berman DS, Kiat H, *et al*. Exercise myocardial perfusion SPECT in patients without known coronary artery disease: incremental prognostic value and use in risk stratification. *Circulation* 1996; 93: 905–14.
- Shaw LJ, Hachamovitch R, Berman DS, *et al*. The economic consequences of available diagnostic and prognostic strategies for the evaluation of stable angina patients: an observational assessment of the value of pre-catheterization ischaemia. *J Am Coll Cardiol* 1999; 33: 661–9.

Fractional Flow Reserve versus Angiography for Guiding Percutaneous Coronary Intervention (FAME)

Tonino PAL, De Bruyne B, Pijls NHJ, Siebert U, Ikeno F, van 't Veer M, Klauss V, Manoharan G, Engstrøm T, Oldroyd KG, Ver Lee PN, MacCarthy PA, Fearon WF; for the FAME Study Investigators. *N Eng J Med* 2009; 360: 213–24.

Background

The presence and extent of myocardial ischaemia on non-invasive testing determines prognosis in CAD[38]. The multi-centre randomized study to compare deferral vs. performance of PCI of non-ischaemic-producing stenoses (DEFER) trial had previously investigated the utility of invasive physiological assessment to guide management of single vessel coronary disease. Patients with

angiographically intermediate stenoses had pressure wire based assessment of FFR. Lesions with a FFR ≤0.75 were treated by PCI and those with a FFR >0.75 were randomly assigned to have PCI or to have medical therapy. Event-free survival was better in the group treated with medical therapy compared to those randomized to have PCI, demonstrating that deferring PCI based on FFR was a safe strategy and that a dichotomous FFR threshold of 0.75 could be used to determine the need for revascularization[32]. However, in clinical practice, a significant proportion of patients have multi-vessel coronary artery disease and the utility of FFR in this setting was unclear. Additionally, revascularization decisions are frequently based upon angiographic morphology of stenoses alone, without prior non-invasive ischaemia testing. The FAME study[3], aimed to compare a strategy of revascularization based on angiographic appearances alone versus one based on physiological lesion assessment by FFR, in patients with multi-vessel disease.

Methods and results

The FAME study was a multi-centre, prospective RCT, which recruited a total of 1005 patients with multi-vessel CAD. The primary end point was a composite of rate of death, non-fatal myocardial infarction, and repeat revascularization at one year. Secondary end points included procedure time, the amount of contrast agent used and questionnaire based functional classification at one-month and one-year. Patients were included, if they had a visual angiographic stenosis of >50% in two or more vessels, and were scheduled to have PCI.

Patients were then randomly assigned to either angiography-guided PCI or FFR-guided PCI. Fractional flow reserve was measured in all vessels thought to have a significant lesion, and treatment (with a drug-eluting stent) recommended only if FFR ≤0.80. Fractional flow reserve was determined with an intracoronary pressure wire during maximal hyperaemia induced by an intravenous infusion of adenosine (140 mcg/kg/min) through a central vein. For instances where multiple focal coronary lesions or diffuse atheroma, was present, pressure pullback recordings were performed. Those randomized to the angiography-guided arm underwent PCI to all lesions identified before randomization.

An important cohort included into this trial were patients who had suffered prior myocardial infarction, both ST-elevation (STEMI) and non-ST elevation infarction (NSTEMI), if the infarct was greater than five days remote to the planned PCI; and if the CK was less 1000 units per litre in the case of NSTEMI, therefore addressing a more 'real-world' population. However, those with left main stem disease, previous coronary artery bypass grafts, severely calcific coronary disease, or those in cardiogenic shock were excluded. A total of 496 patients were assigned to the angiography-guided treatment arm, and 509 to the FFR-guided arm. A history of previous MI was seen in 36.3% and 36.7% in the angiography-guided arm and FFR-guided arm, respectively.

The primary composite end point of death, MI, CVA, and revascularization in the FFR group was significantly lower than in the angiographically-guided PCI group (13.2% vs. 18.3%, p = 0.02). In addition to this, the FFR-guided approach was shown to be equivalent or better than the traditional approach, when the numerous secondary end points were considered; with all-cause mortality at one year and rate of myocardial infarction rate being similar in both the FFR and angiographic arm, 1.8% vs. 3.0%, p = 0.19, and 5.7% vs. 8.7%, p = 0.07 respectively (see Figure 3.10). Furthermore, when two important procedural end points, procedure duration and number of stents used per patient, are considered, strategic PCI via FFR guidance results in similar procedure times (70 ± 44 minutes angiography group vs. 71 ± 43 minutes in the FFR group, p = 0.71) and significantly reduced stent use per patient (2.7 ± 1.2 vs. 1.9 ± 1.3, p = 0.001), with importantly, no difference in anginal burden seen between the patient cohorts at one year (73% vs. 67.6 p = 0.07).

Study limitations

The revascularization strategies adopted in the study may not have been representative of routine practice, with 40.7% of lesions in the angiography group and 44.1% in the FFR group having intermediate severity stenoses of 50–70%. Furthermore, approximately 55% of patients only had class I or II angina, with no prior non-invasive evidence of inducible ischaemia being mandated before coronary angiography was undertaken. In the absence of demonstrable ischaemia or a large area of at-risk myocardium, PCI is not recommended for these lesions[44]. Routine use of PCI for these lesions in the angiography group could have contributed to the worse outcomes in that group. Furthermore, the cohort in the study excluded important subsets of patients, including patients with previous bypass grafts and acute phase myocardial infarctions. Therefore extrapolation to 'real-world' practice and the validity of ischaemia assessment with FFR in PCI in these two large populations remains unclear.

Conclusions and clinical implications

Coronary angiography has been deemed the gold-standard method of investigation of coronary disease, after its initial demonstration of safety by Werner Forssmann in 1929[45]; followed by Andreas Gruentzig highlighting the clinical utility of coronary angioplasty in 1977[46]. However, the two-dimensional nature of angiographic assessment of coronary disease has been subject to rigorous investigation, demonstrating that visual assessment of a

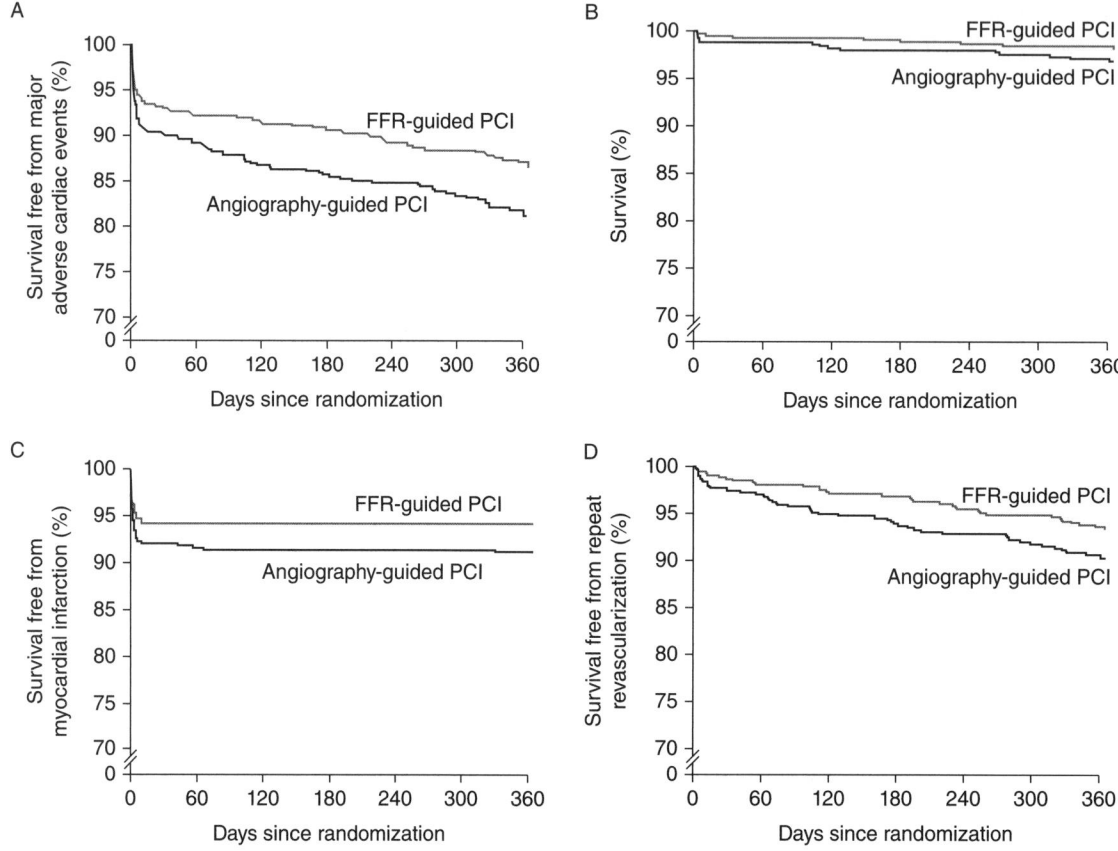

Figure 3.10 Kaplan-Meier survival curves according to study group in the FAME trial.

stenosis alone, inaccurately estimates the functional ischaemia-inducing significance of a stenosis[47, 48]. The relationship between the fluid dynamics exerted by a stenosis in an epicardial coronary vessel on coronary flow and the resultant myocardial perfusion deficiency are multifactorial, and therefore require a more physiological basis of evaluation[32, 49]. The FAME study demonstrates the strengths of 'on-line' physiological stenosis assessment with FFR in addition to routine anatomical considerations, in determining functionally significant coronary stenoses, along with reasserting the safety of selective stenting according to physiological significance. It has built on the body of evidence of the limitations of coronary angiography in identifying ischaemia-inducing stenoses and highlighted the importance of ischaemia assessment prior to revascularization, via FFR or non-invasive modalities to guide stenosis selection.

Learning points

◆ Fractional flow reserve is a robust clinical tool to assess the physiological significance of a coronary stenosis in a wide variety of multi-vessel PCI patients.

◆ It provides further evidence that ischaemia assessment of stenosis is of paramount importance prior to, or when, undertaking revascularization procedures.

Further reading

● Bech GJ, De Bruyne B, Pijls NH, *et al*. Fractional flow reserve to determine the appropriateness of angioplasty in moderate coronary stenosis: a randomized trial. *Circulation*. 2001; 103(24): 2928–34.

- Berger A, Botman KJ, MacCarthy P, *et al.* Long term clinical outcome after fractional flow reserve-guided percutenaous coronary intervention in patients with multivessel disease. *J Am Coll Cardiol* 2005; 46: 438–42.

- Pijls NH, van Schaardenburgh P, Manoharan G, *et al.* Percutenous coronary intervention of functionally nonsignificant stenosis: 5 year follow-up of the DEFER study. *J Am Coll Cardiol* 2007; 49: 2105–11.

Final thoughts

Vast progress has been made in numerous facets of investigation relating to coronary artery disease and myocardial ischaemia, which have been encapsulated in the seminal papers described in this chapter. Further discoveries in basic science, adjunctive pharmacology, and the physiological behaviour of the coronary circulation will continue to grow at a rapid rate in the coming years.

The sophistication of interventional practice will also continue to increase; the utilization of technologies such as optical coherence tomography, high definition intravascular ultrasound, and the potential of MRI-guided interventional procedures are likely to find important niches in invasive management strategies of both CAD and in the growing field of structural heart intervention. The role of improved adjuvant pharmacotherapy and stent technology will continue to evolve, allowing further reductions in the continually improving morbidity and

mortality secondary to CAD. Furthermore, the development of computational modelling, providing a multiplicity of haemodynamic and functional parameters, in a single amalgamated modality, may allow a novel approach, and true individualization of management decisions with regard to coronary revascularization in the future.

It is evident that during the last four decades many pathophysiological quandaries relating to coronary artery disease and ischaemia have been, to varying degrees, unravelled. However, many unanswered questions and challenges remain, from understanding the molecular basis of plaque formation and subsequent rupture, to the ability to accurately investigate and treat the coronary microcirculation as a therapeutic target in acute coronary syndromes, rather than focused treatment of epicardial artery disease. With this in mind, the next four decades may prove to be the most innovative yet.

References

1. Murry CE, Jennings RB, Reimer KA. Preconditioning with ischaemia: a delay of lethal cell injury in ischemic myocardium. *Circulation* 1986; 74(5): 1124–36.
2. Kim RJ, Wu E, Rafael A, *et al.* The use of contrast-enhanced magnetic resonance imaging to identify reversible myocardial dysfunction. *N Engl J Med* 2000; 343(20): 1445–53.
3. Tonino PA, De Bruyne B, Pijls NH, *et al.* Fractional flow reserve versus angiography for guiding percutaneous coronary intervention. *N Engl J Med* 2009; 360(3): 213–24.
4. Allen DG, Orchard CH. Myocardial contractile function during ischaemia and hypoxia. *Circ Res* 1987; 60(2): 153–68.
5. Rahimtoola SH. The hibernating myocardium. *Am Heart J* 1989; 117(1):211–21.
6. Boerth RC, Covell JW, Seagren SC, Pool PE. High-energy phosphate concentrations in dog myocardium during stress. *Am J Physiol* 1969; 216(5): 1103–6.
7. Harris AS, Bisteni A, Russell RA, Brigham JC, Firestone JE. Excitatory factors in ventricular tachycardia resulting from myocardial ischaemia; potassium a major excitant. *Science* 1954; 119(3085): 200–3.
8. Downar E, Janse MJ, Durrer D. The effect of acute coronary artery occlusion on subepicardial transmembrane potentials in the intact porcine heart. *Circulation* 1977; 56(2): 217–24.
9. Katz AM, Hecht HH. Editorial: the early 'pump' failure of the ischemic heart. *Am J Med* 1969; 47(4): 497–502.
10. Bailey IA, Williams SR, Radda GK, Gadian DG. Activity of phosphorylase in total global ischaemia in the rat heart. A phosphorus-31 nuclear-magnetic-resonance study. *Biochem J* 1981; 196(1): 171–8.
11. Reimer KA, Jennings RB. The 'wavefront phenomenon' of myocardial ischemic cell death. II. Transmural progression of necrosis within the framework of ischemic bed size (myocardium at risk) and collateral flow. *Lab Invest* 1979; 40(6): 633–44.
12. Reimer KA, Murry CE, Yamasawa I, Hill ML, Jennings RB. Four brief periods of myocardial ischaemia cause no cumulative ATP loss or necrosis. *Am J Physiol* 1986; 251(6 Pt 2): H1306–15.
13. McGovern PG, Pankow JS, Shahar E, *et al.* Recent trends in acute coronary heart disease—mortality, morbidity,

medical care, and risk factors. The Minnesota Heart Survey Investigators. *N Engl J Med* 1996; 334(14): 884–90.

14. Grines CL, Browne KF, Marco J, *et al.* A comparison of immediate angioplasty with thrombolytic therapy for acute myocardial infarction. The Primary Angioplasty in Myocardial Infarction Study Group. *N Engl J Med* 1993; 328(10): 673–9.

15. Zhao ZQ, Corvera JS, Halkos ME, *et al.* Inhibition of myocardial injury by ischemic postconditioning during reperfusion: comparison with ischemic preconditioning. *Am J Physiol Heart Circ Physiol* 2003; 285(2): H579–88.

16. Okamoto F, Allen BS, Buckberg GD, Bugyi H, Leaf J. Reperfusion conditions: importance of ensuring gentle versus sudden reperfusion during relief of coronary occlusion. *J Thorac Cardiovasc Surg* 1986; 92(3 Pt 2): 613–20.

17. Sato H, Jordan JE, Zhao ZQ, Sarvotham SS, Vinten-Johansen J. Gradual reperfusion reduces infarct size and endothelial injury but augments neutrophil accumulation. *Ann Thorac Surg* 1997; 64(4): 1099–107.

18. Zweier JL, Flaherty JT, Weisfeldt ML. Direct measurement of free radical generation following reperfusion of ischemic myocardium. *Proc Natl Acad Sci USA* 1987; 84(5): 1404–7.

19. Tsao PS, Aoki N, Lefer DJ, Johnson G, 3rd, Lefer AM. Time course of endothelial dysfunction and myocardial injury during myocardial ischaemia and reperfusion in the cat. *Circulation* 1990; 82(4): 1402–12.

20. Tillisch J, Brunken R, Marshall R, *et al.* Reversibility of cardiac wall-motion abnormalities predicted by positron tomography. *N Engl J Med* 1986; 314(14): 884–8.

21. Rahimtoola SH. Coronary bypass surgery for chronic angina—1981. A perspective. *Circulation* 1982; 65(2): 225–41.

22. Rahimtoola SH, Dilsizian V, Kramer CM, Marwick TH, Vanoverschelde JL. Chronic ischemic left ventricular dysfunction: from pathophysiology to imaging and its integration into clinical practice. *JACC Cardiovasc Imaging* 2008; 1(4): 536–55.

23. Carluccio E, Biagioli P, Alunni G, *et al.* Patients with hibernating myocardium show altered left ventricular volumes and shape, which revert after revascularization: evidence that dyssynergy might directly induce cardiac remodeling. *J Am Coll Cardiol* 2006; 47(5): 969–77.

24. Rahimtoola SH, La Canna G, Ferrari R. Hibernating myocardium: another piece of the puzzle falls into place. *J Am Coll Cardiol* 2006; 47(5): 978–80.

25. Allman KC, Shaw LJ, Hachamovitch R, Udelson JE. Myocardial viability testing and impact of revascularization on prognosis in patients with coronary artery disease and left ventricular dysfunction: a meta-analysis. *J Am Coll Cardiol* 2002; 39(7): 1151–8.

26. Allman KSL, Hachamovitch R, Udelson JE. Prognostic valve of myocardial viability testing: a meta-analysis. *Circulation* 2000; 102(Suppl II): 576.

27. Gould KL, Kelley KO, Bolson EL. Experimental validation of quantitative coronary arteriography for determining pressure-flow characteristics of coronary stenosis. *Circulation* 1982; 66(5): 930–37.

28. Gould KL. Identifying and measuring severity of coronary artery stenosis. Quantitative coronary arteriography and positron emission tomography. *Circulation* 1988; 78(2): 237–45.

29. Gould KL, Kirkeeide RL, Buchi M. Coronary flow reserve as a physiologic measure of stenosis severity. *J Am Coll Cardiol* 1990; 15(2): 459–74.

30. Gould KL, Lipscomb K, Hamilton GW. Physiologic basis for assessing critical coronary stenosis. Instantaneous flow response and regional distribution during coronary hyperemia as measures of coronary flow reserve. *Am J Cardiol* 1974; 33(1): 87–94.

31. Kern MJ, Lerman A, Bech JW, *et al.* Physiological assessment of coronary artery disease in the cardiac catheterization laboratory: a scientific statement from the American Heart Association Committee on Diagnostic and Interventional Cardiac Catheterization, Council on Clinical Cardiology. *Circulation* 2006; 114(12): 1321–41.

32. Bech GJ, De Bruyne B, Pijls NH, *et al.* Fractional flow reserve to determine the appropriateness of angioplasty in moderate coronary stenosis: a randomized trial. *Circulation* 2001; 103(24): 2928–34.

33. Varnauskas E. Twelve-year follow-up of survival in the randomized European Coronary Surgery Study. *N Engl J Med* 1988; 319(6): 332–7.

34. Alderman EL, Bourassa MG, Cohen LS, *et al.* Ten-year follow-up of survival and myocardial infarction in the randomized Coronary Artery Surgery Study. *Circulation* 1990; 82(5): 1629–46.

35. Boden WE, O'Rourke RA, Teo KK, *et al.* Optimal medical therapy with or without PCI for stable coronary disease. *N Engl J Med* 2007; 356(15): 1503–16.

36. Beller GA, Zaret BL. Contributions of nuclear cardiology to diagnosis and prognosis of patients with coronary artery disease. *Circulation* 2000; 101(12): 1465–78.

37. Shaw LJ, Iskandrian AE. Prognostic value of gated myocardial perfusion SPECT. *J Nucl Cardiol* 2004; 11(2): 171–85.

38. Hachamovitch R, Hayes SW, Friedman JD, Cohen I, Berman DS. Comparison of the short-term survival benefit associated with revascularization compared with medical therapy in patients with no prior coronary artery disease undergoing stress myocardial perfusion single photon emission computed tomography. *Circulation* 2003; 107(23): 2900–7.

39. Parisi AF, Folland ED, Hartigan P. A comparison of angioplasty with medical therapy in the treatment of single-vessel coronary artery disease. Veterans Affairs ACME Investigators. *N Engl J Med* 1992; 326(1): 10–6.

40. Coronary angioplasty versus medical therapy for angina: the second Randomised Intervention Treatment of Angina (RITA-2) trial. RITA-2 trial participants. *Lancet* 1997; 350(9076): 461–8.

41. Pitt B, Waters D, Brown WV, *et al*. Aggressive lipid-lowering therapy compared with angioplasty in stable coronary artery disease. Atorvastatin versus Revascularization Treatment Investigators. *N Engl J Med* 1999; 341(2): 70–6.

42. Hueb W, Soares PR, Gersh BJ, *et al*. The medicine, angioplasty, or surgery study (MASS-II): a randomized, controlled clinical trial of three therapeutic strategies for multivessel coronary artery disease: one-year results. *J Am Coll Cardiol* 2004; 43(10): 1743–51.

43. Henderson RA, Pocock SJ, Clayton TC, *et al*. Seven-year outcome in the RITA-2 trial: coronary angioplasty versus medical therapy. *J Am Coll Cardiol* 2003; 42(7): 1161–1170.

44. Patel MR, Dehmer GJ, Hirshfeld JW, Smith PK, Spertus JA. ACCF/SCAI/STS/AATS/AHA/ASNC 2009 Appropriateness Criteria for Coronary Revascularization: A Report of the American College of Cardiology Foundation Appropriateness Criteria Task Force, Society for Cardiovascular Angiography and Interventions, Society of Thoracic Surgeons, American Association for Thoracic Surgery, American Heart Association, and the American Society of Nuclear Cardiology: Endorsed by the American Society of Echocardiography, the Heart Failure Society of America, and the Society of Cardiovascular Computed Tomography. *Circulation* 2009; 119(9): 1330–52.

45. Forssmann-Falck R. Werner Forssmann: a pioneer of cardiology. *Am J Cardiol* 1997; 79(5): 651–60.

46. Hurst JW. The first coronary angioplasty as described by Andreas Gruentzig. *Am J Cardiol* 1986; 57(1): 185–6.

47. Fischer JJ, Samady H, McPherson JA, *et al*. Comparison between visual assessment and quantitative angiography versus fractional flow reserve for native coronary narrowings of moderate severity. *Am J Cardiol* 2002; 90(3): 210–5.

48. Topol EJ, Nissen SE. Our preoccupation with coronary luminology. The dissociation between clinical and angiographic findings in ischemic heart disease. *Circulation* 1995; 92(8): 2333–42.

49. Pijls NH, van Schaardenburgh P, Manoharan G, *et al*. Percutaneous coronary intervention of functionally nonsignificant stenosis: 5-year follow-up of the DEFER Study. *J Am Coll Cardiol* 2007; 49(21): 2105–11.

Chapter 4

Thrombosis, haemostasis, and platelet biology

Dr Paul Gurbel, Dr Dean Kereiakes, and Dr Udaya Tantry

Introduction

Coronary heart disease (CHD) is the leading cause of morbidity and mortality worldwide[1]. An enhanced understanding of platelet receptor physiology and the development of new platelet inhibitors has led to a resurgence in the pharmacologic treatment of CHD in the past four decades. Overwhelming evidence suggests that platelet activation and aggregation at the sites of endothelial cell erosion and plaque rupture are the primary processes responsible for the development of ischaemic events in patients with CHD[2,3]. Two major agonists—thromboxane A_2 (TXA_2) and adenosine diphosphate (ADP), released from activated platelets are responsible for amplifying platelet activation and aggregation and generation of a stable thrombus at the site of vascular injury.[2,3] Therefore, pharmacologic management of patients with CHD mainly consists of aspirin and clopidogrel to inhibit TXA_2 generation and the ADP-$P2Y_{12}$ interaction, respectively[4-6]. In addition, inhibition of the GPIIb/IIIa receptor, the final common pathway of platelet aggregation, is also an important treatment strategy in high risk CHD patients during acute conditions[4-6].

Aspirin (acetylsalicylic acid—ASA) is the bedrock of all antithrombotic therapies for both primary and secondary prevention of CHD[7,8]. All new antiplatelet agents are combined with aspirin in the treatment of high-risk CHD patients. However, the demonstration of various limitations of clopidogrel and aspirin therapy (i.e. dual antiplatelet therapy—DAPT) such as continued ischaemic event occurrence, clopidogrel response variability and resistance, as well as the relationship of high on-treatment platelet reactivity in response to ADP have stimulated two recent important developments: (1) the development of more potent $P2Y_{12}$ receptor blockers such as prasugrel and ticagrelor and (2) the advent of a personalized antiplatelet therapy concept based on objective measurement of platelet function in the individual patient[4]. However, current treatment guidelines of the American Heart Association and the American College of Cardiology still recommend a 'one size fits all' strategy for oral antiplatelet therapy[5]. Based on the results from numerous observational studies, recent treatment guidelines have given a Class IIb recommendation to perform genotyping or phenotyping in high risk PCI patients if a change in antiplatelet therapy will ensue based on the test results.[5,9].

The latter may be due to a lack of consensus on the optimal method(s) to quantify high platelet reactivity in addition to cutoff values associated with clinical risk, as well as the availability of limited data to show that alterations of therapy based on platelet function measurements actually improve clinical outcomes[9].

Aggregation of blood platelets by adenosine diphosphate and its reversal

Born GVR. *Nature* 1962; 194: 927–9.

Background

Laboratory evaluation of platelet function by *in vitro* methods is very challenging since platelets can be activated easily during blood drawing and laboratory processing and samples need to be processed within a short period of time to avoid spontaneous activation of platelets. Earlier, it was suggested that ADP may play a crucial role in the initial stages of thrombosis[10]. *In vitro* assessment of platelet function by a simple laboratory method is crucial to understand the role platelets play during normal haemostasis and ischaemic heart disease.

Methods

In this landmark study, human blood samples were collected and sodium citrate (3.8 mg/ml) or heparin (0.01 mg/ml) was used to prevent clotting. Platelet rich plasma at a concentration of 10^8–10^9/ml was separated by centrifuging the blood at 500G and further centrifugation then yielded platelet poor plasma. After measuring the optical density of platelet poor plasma at 600 μm using a unicam *SP* 400 absorptiometer, platelet rich plasma was stirred at a rate of 1000 rotations per minute using a small polythene covered iron rod. Different concentrations of ADP (1×10^{-7} to 1×10^{-6} M) were added and the optical density (OD) was measured continuously for up to 20 minutes.

Results

The OD decreased immediately after the addition of ADP and platelet aggregation was observed. It was also demonstrated that the rate and extent of decrease in OD was proportional to the ADP concentration with maximal and least decreases observed at $>1 \times 10^{-6}$ M and 1×10^{-7} M ADP, respectively. At lower than 1×10^{-6} M ADP, the decrease in OD (platelet aggregation) was transient, that is, after 1–2 minutes the OD started increasing and at 10 minutes it was almost at baseline. It was suggested that platelet aggregation was reversible due to disappearance

of ADP by conversion to adenosine monophosphate (AMP). It was further demonstrated that the addition of AMP at similar concentrations reversed the platelet aggregation induced by ADP.

Limitations

The Born method may not completely reflect *in vivo* platelet activation. Artificial platelet activation during blood drawing and sample processing and the effects of lipaemia, haemolysis, or contamination with other blood cells that are known to modulate platelet function are major limitations of this method.

Conclusions

The specificity of ADP in platelet aggregation indicated that ADP may play a crucial role during *in vivo* platelet aggregation that is essential for normal haemostasis and thrombosis. This investigation stimulated further research in understanding the role of ADP and other agonists during platelet activation and aggregation and also facilitated the discovery of new antiplatelet agents.

Learning points

- Adenosine diphosphate-induced platelet aggregation can be quantified by an *in vitro* method. This is still considered the 'gold-standard' to measure ADP-induced platelet aggregation despite numerous limitations. It has been the most widely used technique to assess the pharmacodynamic response to ADP-receptor blockers and was the primary method used to correlate platelet function to adverse ischaemic clinical outcomes.
- This method is the standard used for the quantification of antiplatelet response to P2Y$_{12}$ receptor blockers.

Further reading

- Gurbel PA, Becker RC, Mann KG, Steinhubl SR, Michelson AD. Platelet function monitoring in patients with coronary artery disease. *J Am Coll Cardiol* 2007; 50: 1822–34.

- Michelson AD. Platelet function testing in cardiovascular diseases. *Circulation* 2004; 110: e489–93.

Inhibition of prostaglandin synthesis as a mechanism of action for aspirin-like drugs

Vane JR. *Nat New Biol* 1971; 231: 232–5.

Background

Aspirin, also known as acetylsalicylic acid, is an anti-inflammatory drug used extensively to relieve minor aches and pains and to reduce fever[11]. The antithrombotic effect of aspirin, and associated prevention of myocardial infarction (MI), was first reported in 1950 by Craven *et al*[12]. In addition to aspirin, the mechanism of action of other anti-inflammatory drugs was unclear. Potential antiplatelet effects of aspirin were described by Weiss and Aldort in 1967[13]. Earlier, Piper and Vane demonstrated that aspirin-like drugs antagonized the release of prostaglandins from isolated perfused lungs of guinea pigs and stimulated bronchoconstriction. It was hypothesized that aspirin-like drugs inhibit the enzymes that generate prostaglandins from arachidonic acid[14].

Methods

Initially guinea pig lung homogenates were incubated with arachidonic acid to synthesize prostaglandins PGE_2 and $F_{2\alpha}$. The extracts were quantified for prostaglandin E_2 and $F_{2\alpha}$ using thin-layer chromatography. 'Prostaglandin-like activity' assays based on the contraction of isolated rat stomach with pure prostaglandin E_2 and colon with prostaglandin $F_{2\alpha}$ were standardized. The PGE_2 and $PGF_{2\alpha}$ strips from the thin-layer chromatography were incubated with rat colon and stomach strips to measure 'prostaglandin-like activity' after incubation with lung homogenates with varying amounts of aspirin-like drugs: indomethacin, sodium acetyl salicylate, and sodium salicylate.

Results

Indomethacin, sodium acetyl salicylate, and sodium salicylate all inhibited the generation of PGE_2- and $PGF_{2\alpha}$-like activity, exhibiting a linear relationship between percentage inhibition and log concentration of the drugs, with aspirin being the most potent inhibitor.

Hydrocortisone was a weak inhibitor, whereas morphine and mepyramine had no effect.

Conclusions

Aspirin and aspirin-like drugs inhibit prostaglandin synthesis from arachidonic acid, whereas hydrocortisone, morphine, and mepyramine may have a different mechanism of action to attenuate inflammation. The major actions of aspirin-like drugs (antipyretic, anti-inflammatory, and analgesic) can be explained by inhibition of prostaglandins. Further experiments from the same institute demonstrated the inhibition of prostaglandin biosynthesis by aspirin and indomethacin in human platelets and perfused dog spleens.

Learning points

- This and related groundbreaking experiments explained the mechanism of action of aspirin as an antiplatelet agent.
- These experiments also explained why aspirin-like drugs shared similar pharmacologic actions and side effects.
- Sir John R. Vane won a Nobel Prize in Physiology or Medicine in 1982 for this work on aspirin.

Further reading

- Ferreira SH, Moncada S, Vane JR. Indomethacin and aspirin abolish prostaglandin release from the spleen. *Nat New Biol* 1971; 231: 237–9.
- Roth GJ, Stanford N, Majerus PW. Acetylation of prostaglandin synthase by aspirin. *Proc Natl Acad Sci USA* 1975; 72: 3073–6.
- Smith JB, Willis AL. Aspirin selectively inhibits prostaglandin production in human platelets. *Nat New Biol* 1971; 231: 235–7.

Identification of the platelet ADP receptor targeted by antithrombotic drugs

Hollopeter G, Jantzen HM, Vincent D, Li G, England L, Ramakrishnan V, Yang RB, Nurden P, Nurden A, Julius D, Conley PB. *Nature* 2001; 409: 202–7.

Background

Pharmacological evidence at the time indicated that ADP acted on three receptors on human platelets, namely $P2Y_1$, $P2X_1$, and a hitherto unidentified third receptor[15]. Although the two important drugs ticlopidine and clopidogrel were used to prevent heart attack and stroke in patients with CHD, the ADP receptor that these two drugs inhibited was incompletely defined[16, 17].

Method and results

Initially rat $P2Y_{12}$ receptor cDNA was identified and used to construct human full length $hP2Y_{12}$ cDNA. The latter was injected into Xenopus oocytes to allow the detection of G_i-linked responses (known to be associated with ADP-receptor) through an electrophysiological assay. Receptor specificity was evaluated by using other agents in addition to ADP, such as 2–2-methylthioadenosine 5'-monophosphate (2MeSAMP), a non-nucleotide inhibitor C1330–7, and a $P2Y_1$-selective antagonist A3P5P. G_i-mediated effects of ADP on cAMP levels were demonstrated using Chinese hamster ovary (CHO) cells expressing the $hP2Y_{12}$ receptor. Northern blot analysis was used to demonstrate that the $P2Y_{12}$ receptor was expressed extensively in human platelets and to a smaller extent in the brain. Chromosomal localization of the $P2Y_{12}$ receptor gene using a Stanford G3 panel found that the $P2Y_{12}$ receptor gene was located along with the UDP-glucose and $P2Y_1$ receptors; all of these receptors are G-protein coupled receptors (GPCRs). A critical role of the cysteine residues containing a thiol-group in the ADP-$P2Y_{12}$ receptor interaction was also demonstrated using thiol reagent p-chloromercuriphenylsulphonic acid (pCMBS) that eliminated ADP-evoked current responses in oocytes. Finally, the investigators provided the evidence that a patient with a bleeding disorder had a defect in the $P2Y_{12}$ receptor gene.

Limitations

The mechanism of action of the $P2Y_{12}$ receptor was not directly demonstrated in human platelets.

Conclusion

With their ground breaking study, Hallopeter *et al.* identified the elusive ADP-receptor that they termed the '$P2Y_{12}$' receptor. They provided the conclusive evidence for the specificity of this receptor for ADP, the mechanism of action—a cysteine residue mediated ADP-$P2Y_{12}$ receptor interaction and involvement of the G_i coupled adenylate cyclase enzyme. They also provided evidence that the $P2Y_{12}$ receptor is exclusively expressed in platelets and to a smaller extent in the human brain.

Learning points

- The study identified the $P2Y_{12}$ receptor that explained the mechanism of action of ticlopidine and clopidogrel.
- This study facilitated the development of more potent $P2Y_{12}$ receptor blockers—prasugrel and ticagrelor.

Further reading

- van Giezen JJ, Humphries RG. Preclinical and clinical studies with selective reversible direct $P2Y_{12}$ antagonists. *Semin Thromb Hemost* 2005; 31: 195–204.
- Hasegawa M, Sugidachi A, Ogawa T, Isobe T, Jakubowski JA, Asai F. Stereoselective inhibition of human platelet aggregation by R-138727, the active metabolite of CS-747 (prasugrel, LY640315), a novel $P2Y_{12}$ receptor inhibitor. *Thromb Haemost* 2005; 94: 593–8.
- Murugappa S, Kunapuli SP. The role of ADP receptors in platelet function. *Front Biosci* 2006; 11: 1977–86.
- Savi P, Zachayus JL, Delesque-Touchard N, *et al.* The active metabolite of Clopidogrel disrupts $P2Y_{12}$ receptor oligomers and partitions them out of lipid rafts. *Proc Natl Acad Sci USA* 2006; 103: 11069–74.

Platelet activation in unstable coronary disease

Fitzgerald DJ, Roy L, Catella F, FitzGerald GA. *N Engl J Med* 1986; 315: 983–9.

Background

Detailed histological and angioscopic studies highlighted the pivotal role of platelets during thrombus generation in conditions associated with unstable angina[18, 19, 20, 21]. Specific factors that control platelet activation and aggregation during *in vivo* thrombus generation are unknown. However, demonstration of attenuation of myocardial infarction with aspirin treatment suggested an essential role for TXA_2—an important platelet agonist, during occlusive thrombus generation[22].

Methods and results

Thirty six patients with chest pain (16 and 14 patients diagnosed as having unstable angina and MI, respectively) who had not taken aspirin or other cyclooxygenase inhibitor for the past ten days were enrolled. Serial determination (every 6 hours for the first 48 hours after admission and on day 5) of urine 2,3-dinor thromboxane B_2 and 2,3 dinor-keto-prostaglandin $F_{1\alpha}$, and also plasma 11-dehydro thromboxane B_2 immediately after admission were determined. In addition, urine thromboxane and prostaglandin metabolites and plasma 11-dehydro thromboxane B_2 were determined in male patients with stable coronary artery disease before and after exercise induced myocardial ischaemia. Plasma and urine thromboxane and prostaglandin metabolites were significantly elevated in admitted patients with MI and also correlated with plasma creatinine kinase levels (r = 0.795; p <0.001). The maximum rise in thromboxane synthesis was observed in patients with UA, where most of the episodes of chest pain were associated with a phasic increase in the excretion of thromboxane and prostaglandin metabolites.

Limitations

A small number of patients were studied; the source of the plasma and urine prostanoid metabolites was not determined. It was assumed that thromboxane metabolites were generated solely by activated platelets. However, upstream intermediates derived from inflammatory cells can be converted to TXA_2 in unactivated platelets by transcellular mechanisms.

Conclusions

This was the initial study that demonstrated that platelet activation, marked by elevated *in vivo* excretion of thromboxane metabolites, occurs during spontaneous ischaemia in the setting of unstable angina as compared to stable angina. These data supported the role of TXA_2 inhibition in the treatment of acute coronary syndromes (ACS) and remain the bedrock therapy to this date.

Learning points

- Platelet activation is critically important for the development of ischaemia in the setting of unstable angina.
- Targeted inhibition of platelet activation pathways is critical for the prevention of acute ischaemic complications.

Further reading

- Antithrombotic Trialists' (ATT) Collaboration, Baigent C, Blackwell L, Collins R, *et al.* Aspirin in the primary and secondary prevention of vascular disease: collaborative meta-analysis of individual participant data from randomised trials. *Lancet* 2009; 373: 1849–60.
- Second International Study of Infarct Survival Collaborative Group. Randomised trial of intravenous streptokinase, oral aspirin, both, or neither among 17,187 cases of suspected acute myocardial infarction: ISIS-2. ISIS-2 (Second International Study of Infarct Survival) Collaborative Group. *Lancet* 1988; 2: 349–60.
- Tantry US, Mahla E, Gurbel PA. Aspirin resistance. *Prog Cardiovasc Dis* 2009; 52: 141–52.
- Undas A, Brummel-Ziedins KE, Mann KG. Antithrombotic properties of aspirin and resistance to aspirin: beyond strictly antiplatelet actions. *Blood* 2007; 109: 2285–92.

Early potent antithrombotic effect with combined aspirin and a loading dose of clopidogrel on experimental arterial thrombogenesis in humans

Cadroy Y, Bossavy JP, Thalamas C, Sagnard L, Sakariassen K, Boneu B. *Circulation* 2000; 101: 2823–8.

Background

The Dual Antiplatelet Therapy Study (DAPT) composed of aspirin and ticlopidine was associated with a significant decrease in thrombotic events in patients treated with coronary stenting and after ACS[23]. However, ticlopidine was associated with neutropenia and gastrointestinal and other side effects[24]. The addition of the new more potent thienopyridine, clopidogrel, a compound now known to have fewer side effects, enhanced the antithrombotic effect of aspirin in experimental animals[24, 25]. Cadroy's study was the first in-human evaluation of the antithrombotic effect of a loading dose of clopidogrel added to aspirin.

Methods and results

In this single centre, randomized, double-blind, non-placebo controlled study, 18 male volunteers were treated with three regimens for ten days followed by a 3–6 week washing period: 325 mg/d ASA, 325 mg/d ASA + 75 mg/day clopidogrel, and 325 mg/day ASA + clopidogrel 300 mg loading dose followed by 75 mg/d maintenance dose. Blood samples were collected at baseline, 1.5, 6, and 24 hours after drug intake on day 1 and 6 hours after drug intake on day 10. Adenosine diphosphate, collagen, and arachidonic acid-induced platelet aggregation were determined by light transmittance agregometry (LTA). *Ex vivo* perfusion chamber analysis studies using collagen-coated cover slips under arterial shear rate to induce thrombus formation and immunological determinations of fibrin and platelet depositions were performed to assess the antithrombotic effects of the various regimens. In the *ex vivo* perfusion chamber experiments, the antithrombotic effect of ASA plus clopidogrel was superior to ASA administration alone. The antithrombotic effect without loading was observed within six hours and was maximum at day 10. However, after loading, the antithrombotic effect was observed within 90 minutes, and a superior antithrombotic effect was observed within six hours and was comparable to the maximum inhibitory effect observed at day 10 (p ≤0.01) without loading. Similar time and dose-dependent antithrombotic effects of ASA plus clopidogrel therapy were replicated in platelet aggregation and immunological experiments.

Limitations

The study involved only healthy volunteers. Long-term antiplatelet effects of clopidogrel therapy were not measured.

Conclusions

Aspirin has a moderate inhibitory effect on collagen and ADP-induced aggregation, and superior effects on arachidonic acid-induced platelet aggregation in all subjects. The addition of clopidogrel provides a moderately superior antithrombotic effect compared to aspirin alone early after treatment. A faster antithrombotic effect can be achieved with loading. These results provided a rationale for loading with clopidogrel and demonstrate the central role of the P2Y$_{12}$ receptor in the attenuation of platelet-mediated thrombosis. To this date clopidogrel therapy is instituted with a loading dose and added to aspirin in order to achieve rapid antithrombotic effects that are superior to those achieved with aspirin therapy alone.

Learning points

- Addition of clopidogrel with a loading dose produces superior and faster antithrombotic effects compared to aspirin therapy alone.
- This strategy is widely recommended in all of the guidelines and remains the current standard of care to treat the high-risk CHD patient.

Further reading

- Mehta SR, Yusuf S, Peters RJ, et al.; for the Clopidogrel in Unstable Angina to Prevent Recurrent Events Trial (CURE) Investigators. Effects of pretreatment with clopidogrel and aspirin followed by long-term therapy in patients undergoing percutaneous coronary intervention: the PCI-CURE study. *Lancet* 2001; 358: 527–33.
- Sabatine MS, Cannon CP, Gibson CM, et al.; for the Clopidogrel as Adjunctive Reperfusion Therapy (CLARITY)–Thrombolysis in Myocardial Infarction (TIMI) 28 Investigators. Effect of clopidogrel pretreatment before percutaneous coronary intervention in patients with ST-elevation myocardial infarction treated with fibrinolytics: the PCI-CLARITY study. *JAMA* 2005; 294: 1224 –32.

- Steinhubl SR, Berger PB, Mann JT, Fry ET, DeLago A, Wilmer C; for the CREDO Investigators. Clopidogrel for the Reduction of Events During Observation. Early and sustained dual oral antiplatelet therapy following percutaneous coronary intervention: a randomized controlled trial. *JAMA* 2002; 288: 2411–20.

- Yusuf S, Zhao F, Mehta SR, Chrolavicius S, Tognoni G, Fox KK; for the Clopidogrel in Unstable Angina to Prevent Recurrent Events Trial Investigators. Effects of clopidogrel in addition to aspirin in patients with acute coronary syndromes without ST-segment elevation. *N Engl J Med* 2001; 345: 494–502.

Clopidogrel for coronary stenting: response variability, drug resistance, and the effect of pretreatment platelet reactivity

Gurbel PA, Bliden KP, Hiatt BL, O'Connor CM. *Circulation* 2003; 107: 2908–13.

Background

Large-scale clinical trials have established the clinical efficacy of DAPT with clopidogrel and aspirin in the settings of percutaneous coronary intervention (PCI) and ACS[26, 27]. The results of these trials based on clinical outcomes overwhelmingly supported the 'one size fits all' strategy of DAPT and this strategy has been adopted widely in clinical practice. However, treatment failure persisted and the mechanism to explain it was unclear. Despite the absence of clinical utility, a loading dose of clopidogrel was extensively administered to patients undergoing PCI to achieve faster and superior inhibition of platelet function[5, 6]. However, the pharmacodynamic response in the individual patient and the stability of the response over time was unknown.

Methods and results

Patients undergoing stenting were treated with 325 mg aspirin and a 300 mg clopidogrel loading dose in the catheterization laboratory followed by 75 mg maintenance dose for 30 days. Platelet aggregation (5 and 20 µmol/L ADP), the activation of glycoprotein IIb/IIIa (PAC-1 antibody), and the expression of P-selectin were measured at baseline and at 2 hours, 24 hours, 5 days, and 30 days after stenting to evaluate the antiplatelet response. Marked inter-individual variability in clopidogrel antiplatelet response was demonstrated by a bell-shaped, normal distribution curve measured by all markers. Most interestingly, some patients were found to have no measurable antiplatelet effect; the absolute difference between pre-and post-treatment platelet aggregation was ≤10% and this phenomenon was described as 'clopidogrel non-responsiveness or resistance'. In this study, measurable platelet inhibition was observed at two hours post-300 mg clopidogrel loading, and a steady state of ~30–40% inhibition was reached at 24 hours that remained stable for ~30 days when followed by a 75 mg/day dose. Moreover, the prevalence of non-responsiveness was 53–63% at 2 hours, 31–35% at 24 hours and 5 days, and 13–21% at 30 days post-treatment.

Limitations

The study included only patients undergoing stenting, which is known to increase platelet reactivity. The definition of resistance mentioned in the study involves the amplitude of maximal platelet aggregation and can be influenced by various factors, including intra-patient variability. The current rates of stent thrombosis observed in elective stenting are much lower than the incidence of clopidogrel resistance in the present study, which suggests that our definition may be an overestimate or that resistance to clopidogrel is not a primary factor influencing stent thrombosis in these patients.

Conclusions

Clopidogrel response following loading and maintenance doses is not uniform and there is a wide response variability, with nearly 30% of patients exhibiting 'non-responsiveness or resistance'. This study also suggested that clopidogrel responsiveness is dependent on time of measurement in relation to clopidogrel administration and post-treatment platelet reactivity is critically dependent on pre-treatment reactivity. Based on the study results, it was hypothesized that the occurrence of clopidogrel resistance was related to the inadequacy of a 300 mg loading dose to provide sufficient active metabolite generation to arrest platelet reactivity in selected patients and that patients with high pre-treatment platelet reactivity are least protected from ischaemic event occurrence.

Learning points

♦ Clopidogrel responsiveness is variable and a substantial percentage of patients exhibit 'non-responsiveness or resistance' and may be least protected from post-PCI ischaemic event occurrence.

♦ This first demonstration of clopidogrel response variability and resistance challenged the concept of a 'one size fits all' strategy. It stimulated further research to study the pharmacodynamic utility of higher dosing, the mechanisms behind the variable response, the relation of high on-treatment platelet reactivity to adverse clinical event occurrence, and

the development of new $P2Y_{12}$ receptor blockers to overcome non-responsiveness and provide a more uniform antiplatelet effect.

Further reading

- Gurbel PA, Tantry US. Drug insight: Clopidogrel nonresponsiveness. *Nat Clin Pract Cardiovasc Med* 2006; 3: 387–95.
- Järemo P, Lindahl TL, Fransson SG, Richter A. Individual variations of platelet inhibition after loading doses of clopidogrel. *J Intern Med* 2002; 252: 233–8.
- Müller I, Seyfarth M, Rüdiger S, *et al.* Effect of a high loading dose of clopidogrel on platelet function in patients undergoing coronary stent placement. *Heart* 2001; 85: 92–3.

Platelet reactivity in patients and recurrent events post-stenting: results of the PREPARE POST-STENTING Study

Gurbel PA, Bliden KP, Guyer K, Cho PW, Zaman KA, Kreutz RP, Bassi AK, Tantry US. *J Am Coll Cardiol* 2005; 46: 1820–6.

Background

Although various clinical trials have demonstrated the efficacy of DAPT with aspirin and clopidogrel, recurrent ischaemic event occurrence is a major concern. Pharmacodynamic studies have demonstrated clopidogrel resistance and hypothesized its relation to increased ischaemic risk in PCI patients[28, 29, 30]. Given the inherent variability in platelet aggregation levels, it was hypothesized that measurement of platelet reactivity during clopidogrel therapy may better predict ischaemic risk than the measurement of clopidogrel resistance[31, 32]. Moreover, physical properties of the thrombin mediated platelet-fibrin clot may also affect the occurrence of ischaemic events[33, 34].

Methods and results

The following were measured by thrombelastography (TEG) in patients undergoing PCI (n = 192): 20µM ADP-induced platelet aggregation measured by LTA, and thrombin-induced platelet fibrin clot strength (MA) and the time to initial fibrin generation (R), a marker of thrombin activity. The relation of these measurements to six-month ischaemic event occurrence (death secondary to cardiovascular causes, MI, UA, and stroke) were evaluated. The odds ratio with respect to each measurement

was calculated based on a logistic regression model; the sensitivity and specificity of each measurement in predicting events was calculated using receiver operating characteristic (ROC) curve analysis.

At six months' follow up, 44 events occurred in 38 patients. Patients with ischaemic events had higher on-treatment ADP-induced aggregation (63 ± 12% vs. 56 ± 15%, p = 0.02) and clot strength (maximal amplitude—MA) (74 ± 5 mm vs. 65 ± 4 mm, p < 0.001) and shorter time to initial fibrin generation (R) (4.3 ± 1.3 min vs. 5.9 ± 1.5 min, p <0.001). The event rates in the highest quartiles of LTA (>67% 20 µM ADP) and MA (>72 mm) were 32% and 58%, respectively. The most prevalent risk factor in patients with ischaemia was high MA (71%) with odds ratio estimate of 22.6, followed by a low R (42%) with odds ratio estimate of 4.4, and high LTA with odds ratio estimate of 2.7. The presence of all three risk factors was 100% predictive of an ischaemic event. The ROC curve analysis showed that high TEG MA has 74% sensitivity and 89% specificity; low TEG R has 42% sensitivity and 79% specificity; high LTA has 37% sensitivity and 79% specificity. Interestingly, ischaemic events were associated with a threshold of on-treatment platelet aggregation (~50% induced by 20 µM ADP) suggesting a therapeutic target for $P2Y_{12}$ blockers.

Limitations

Patients were not stratified before clinical events to different degrees of platelet reactivity or MA. It is uncertain whether improvements in the degree of platelet reactivity or MA before and after the procedure would help an individual patient in reducing their risk of a future ischaemic event.

Conclusions

High platelet reactivity and clot strength, and rapid fibrin formation are novel risk factors for ischaemic events within six months of PCI.

Learning points

◆ This is the first prospective study to demonstrate the relation of ADP-induced platelet aggregation to post-PCI ischaemic event occurrence during therapy with clopidogrel and aspirin.

◆ This study gave birth to the 'threshold' concept and the field of personalized antiplatelet therapy in the PCI patient.

Further reading

- Barragan P, Bouvier JL, Roquebert PO, *et al.* Resistance to thienopyridines: clinical detection of coronary stent thrombosis by monitoring of vasodilator-stimulated phosphoprotein phosphorylation. *Catheter Cardiovasc Interv* 2003; 59: 295–302.
- Geisler T, Langer H, Wydymus M, *et al.* Low response to clopidogrel is associated with cardiovascular outcome after coronary stent implantation. *Eur Heart J* 2006; 27: 2420–5.
- Gurbel PA, Bliden KP, Samara W, *et al.* Clopidogrel effect on platelet reactivity in patients with stent thrombosis: results of the CREST Study. *J Am Coll Cardiol* 2005; 46: 1827–32.
- Gurbel PA, Bliden KP, Zaman KA, Yoho JA, Hayes KM, Tantry US. Clopidogrel loading with eptifibatide to arrest the reactivity of platelets: results of the Clopidogrel Loading With Eptifibatide to Arrest the Reactivity of Platelets (CLEAR PLATELETS) study. *Circulation* 2005; 111: 1153–9.

Association of cytochrome P450 2C19 genotype with the antiplatelet effect and clinical efficacy of clopidogrel therapy

Shuldiner AR, O'Connell JR, Bliden KP, Gandhi A, Ryan K, Horenstein RB, Damcott CM, Pakyz R, Tantry US, Gibson Q, Pollin TI, Post W, Parsa A, Mitchell BD, Faraday N, Herzog W, Gurbel PA. *JAMA* 2009; 302: 849–57.

Background

Clopidogrel response variability and the relation of high on-treatment platelet reactivity to ischaemic events are well established[35]. Insufficient active metabolite generation leading to diminished platelet inhibition has been suggested as a main reason for clopidogrel non-responsiveness[36]. A diminished pharmacodynamic response to clopidogrel has been observed with co-administration of proton pump inhibitors, lipophilic statins, and calcium channel blockers that are metabolized by the CYP2C19 and CYP3A4 isoenzymes[37]. However, the contribution of these factors may be minimal. Candidate gene analysis demonstrated the influence of single nucleotide polymorphisms of genes encoding CYP2C19 isoenzymes on clopidogrel metabolism and antiplatelet response[38, 39, 40].

Methods and results

In the Pharmacogenomics of Antiplatelet Intervention (PAPI) study, clopidogrel antiplatelet response was measured by *ex vivo* ADP-induced platelet aggregation following administration of clopidogrel (300 mg loading dose followed by 75 mg/day for seven days) in old order healthy Amish persons (n = 429) a relatively homogeneous founder population in which confounding factors, including medication usage and lifestyle variability, are minimized. A genome-wide association study (GWAS) was performed followed by genotyping the loss of function cytochrome P450 (CYP) *2C19*2* variant (rs4244285). Findings in the PAPI study were extended by examining the relation of *CYP2C19*2* genotype to platelet function and cardiovascular outcomes in an independent sample of 227 patients undergoing PCI.

In this study, 13 nucleotide polymorphisms on chromosome 10q24 within the *CYP2C18–CYP2C19–CYP2C9–CYP2C8* cluster were associated with diminished clopidogrel response, with a high degree of statistical significance (p = 1.5 x 10^{-13} for rs12777823, additive model). The rs12777823 polymorphism was in strong linkage disequilibrium with the *CYP2C19*2* variant, and was associated with diminished clopidogrel response, accounting for 12% of the variation in platelet aggregation to ADP (p = 4.3 x10^{-11}). In clopidogrel-treated patients undergoing PCI, *CYP2C19*2* was associated with greater on-treatment platelet aggregation compared to platelet aggregation in patients without *CYP2C19*2* allele (p = 0.02). Moreover, risk of one-year cardiovascular ischaemic event or death was higher in *CYP2C19*2* allele carriers compared to non-carriers (event rate 20.9% vs. 10.0%; hazard ratio = 2.42; 95% confidence interval = 1.18–4.99; p = 0.02).

Conclusions

This was the first GWAS conducted in clopidogrel treated subjects. It demonstrated that the heritability of clopidogrel response is approximately 70%, the *CYP2C19*2* genotype accounts for only about 12% of clopidogrel response variability and *CYP2C19*2 allele* exhibits a gene-dose response (ADP-stimulated platelet aggregation was reduced to 40.7%, 47.1%, and 65.4% of baseline in response to clopidogrel in participants with 0, 1, and 2 *CYP2C19*2* alleles, respectively). The majority of factors, both genetic and non-genetic, influencing clopidogrel response variability remain unexplained. The *CYP2C19*2* allele is associated with increased risk for post-PCI ischaemic event occurrence.

Learning points

◆ Clopidogrel response variability was linked to a single nucleotide polymorphism in this first GWAS.

◆ The *CYP2C19*2* allele was linked strongly to the pharmacodynamic effect of clopidogrel and clinical outcomes in a PCI population.

Further reading

- Brandt JT, Close SL, Iturria SJ, *et al*. Common polymorphisms of CYP2C19 and CYP2C9 affect the pharmacokinetic and pharmacodynamic response to clopidogrel but not prasugrel. *J Thromb Haemost* 2007; 5: 2429–36.
- Bouman HJ, Schömig E, van Werkum JW, *et al*. Paraoxonase-1 is a major determinant of clopidogrel efficacy. *Nat Med* 2011; 17: 110–6.
- Hulot JS, Collet JP, Silvain J, *et al*. Cardiovascular risk in clopidogrel-treated patients according to cytochrome P450 CYP2C19*2 loss-of-function allele or proton pump inhibitor co-administration: a systematic meta-analysis. *J Am Coll Cardiol* 2010; 56: 134–43.
- Mega JL, Close SL, Wiviott SD, *et al*. Cytochrome p-450 polymorphisms and response to clopidogrel. *N Engl J Med* 2009; 360: 354–62.

Comparison of platelet function tests in predicting clinical outcome in patients undergoing coronary stent implantation

Breet NJ, van Werkum JW, Bouman HJ, Kelder JC, Ruven HJ, Bal ET, Deneer VH, Harmsze AM, van der Heyden JA, Rensing BJ, Suttorp MJ, Hackeng CM, ten Berg JM. *JAMA* 2010; 303: 754–62.

Background

The P2Y$_{12}$ receptor plays a critical role in amplifying platelet activation in response to numerous agonists and the ADP-P2Y$_{12}$ interaction is central to the genesis of thrombosis[41]. These pivotal properties of the P2Y$_{12}$ receptor provide the rationale for *ex vivo* quantification of the intensity of the ADP-P2Y$_{12}$ interaction as a means to identify patients at increased thrombotic risk who require adjustment in antiplatelet therapy. To support the latter hypothesis, numerous small-scale translational research studies have established a threshold level of ADP-induced platelet reactivity in clopidogrel treated patients above which higher risk of ischaemic event occurrence is observed[35,36].

Methods and results

In this prospective, observational, single-centre cohort study, 1069 consecutive patients with established coronary artery disease who were scheduled to undergo elective PCI were treated with clopidogrel (75 mg/d for >5 days or a loading dose of 300 mg ≥24 hours or 600 mg ≥4 hours before PCI) and aspirin (8–100 mg/day for ≥10days). Following PCI, all patients were treated with 75 mg/d clopidogrel dose and 75–100 mg aspirin/day for at least one year. Before PCI, blood samples were collected and on-treatment platelet function was measured by LTA (5 and 20 μM ADP-induced aggregation), VerifyNow P2Y$_{12}$ assay, the Plateletworks assay using ADP tubes, the IMPACT-R assay (with and without ADP prestimulation), and PFA-100 assay with Dade PFA collagen/ADP cartridges and the Innovance PFA P2Y. Patients were followed up for the following ischaemic end points—composite of all-cause death, MI, stent thrombosis, and ischaemic stroke. The primary safety end point was major or minor bleeding according to Thrombolysis in Myocardial Infarction study group criteria. Cutoff values for high on-treatment platelet reactivity were established by ROC curve analysis.

At one-year follow-up, patients with high on-treatment platelet reactivity (HPR) when assessed by LTA, VerifyNow, and Plateletworks were significantly associated with a higher ischaemic event rate compared to patients without HPR. The platelet reactivity measured by the IMPACT-R assay (with and without ADP prestimulation) and PFA-100 assay with Dade PFA collagen/ADP cartridge and the Innovance PFA P2Y assay did not show any relation to ischaemic events. With the ROC curve analysis, only the LTA, the VerifyNow and the Plateletworks assays were able to distinguish between patients with and without ischaemic events. High on-treatment platelet reactivity cutoff points of 42.9% maximal aggregation induced by 5µM ADP and 64.5% by 20 µM ADP; 236 $P2Y_{12}$ reaction units measured by VerifyNow $P2Y_{12}$ assay; and 80.5% aggregation by Plateletworks all correlated with the occurrence of the composite primary end point, with an area under the curve of ~0.62 for each assay. The addition of HPR as measured by the noted platelet assays to more classical clinical and procedural risk factors improved the area under the curve to ~0.73. None of these assays were able to identify patients at high risk for bleeding.

Limitations

Platelet function was measured only once following clopidogrel administration and the stability of platelet reactivity over time is not known. Vasodilator stimulated phosphoprotein phosphorylation assay, a more specific laboratory assay to evaluate $P2Y_{12}$ receptor response to ADP was not implemented in this study. Patients received three different clopidogrel regimens which may have affected HPR differently.

Conclusions

The on-treatment platelet function measured by LTA, the VerifyNow assay, and Plateletworks was significantly associated with one year clinical outcome with a modest predictability in the largest prospective PD-clinical event relation study thus far. The relation of platelet reactivity and bleeding is still unclear.

Learning points

- This is the largest prospective clinical trial that established the link between HPR and one-year clinical outcomes in a PCI population.
- This study also provided specific cutoff points for high platelet reactivity to be used in the future clinical trials of personalized antiplatelet therapy.

Further reading

- Bonello L, Tantry US, Marcucci R, *et al.*; Working Group on High On-Treatment Platelet Reactivity. Consensus and future directions on the definition of high on-treatment platelet reactivity to adenosine diphosphate. *J Am Coll Cardiol.* 2010; 56: 919–33.
- Kereiakes DJ, Gurbel PA. Peri-procedural platelet function and platelet inhibition in percutaneous coronary intervention. *JACC Cardiovasc Interv* 2008; 1: 111–21.
- Patrono C, Rocca B. The future of antiplatelet therapy in cardiovascular disease. *Annu Rev Med* 2010; 61: 49–61.
- Verstuyft C, Simon T, Kim RB. Personalized medicine and antiplatelet therapy: ready for prime time? *Eur Heart J* 2009; 30(16): 1943–63.

A murine monoclonal antibody that completely blocks the binding of fibrinogen to platelets produces a thrombasthenic-like state in normal platelets and binds to glycoproteins IIb and/or IIIa

Coller BS, Peerschke EI, Scudder LE, Sullivan CA. *J Clin Invest* 1983; 72: 325–38.

Background

Fibrinogen binding to the platelet receptor is essential for platelet aggregation in response to ADP, epinephrine, thrombin, or arachidonic acid metabolites, adhesion of platelets to glass surfaces and normalization of skin bleeding time[42]. Moreover, in patients with Glanzmann's thrombasthenia, platelets are unable to bind to fibrinogen since they have deficient membrane glycoproteins IIb and IIIa[43]. These latter glycoproteins, (IIb and IIIa) exist together in a complex that has been tentatively referred to as the 'fibrinogen receptor'[44].

Methods and results

A monoclonal antibody to the GPIIb/IIIa receptor was developed by hybrodoma technology. Initially, washed platelets were injected into BALB/C mice and spleen cells were isolated and fused with myeloma cells. Supernatant from the cultured hybridized cells was screened for anti-fibrinogen receptor activity based on the inhibition of the interaction of platelet with fibrinogen-coated beads in the presence of the antibody. The hybridized cells producing monoclonal antibodies with >99% specificity were isolated and propagated; 10E5 antibodies and F(ab')2 fragments specific for GPIIb/IIIa receptor were purified from culture supernatants. Antibodies were covalently iodinated with ^{125}I using immobilized lactoperoxidase and glucose oxidase. Binding of purified and labelled antibodies to the GPIIb/IIIa receptor on platelets in platelet rich plasma was studied. Effects of 10E5 antibody on platelet aggregation in response to ADP, epinephrine, thrombin, and collagen and on the secretion of ATP from platelets were also studied. Further characterization of the fibrinogen receptor was evaluated by studying the binding of the ^{125}I-fibrinogen antibody binding to platelets. Finally, the inhibition of ^{125}I-fibrinogen binding to platelets by 10E5 antibody was correlated with the inhibition of ADP-induced platelet aggregation.

Both purified F(ab')2 fragments and/or intact antibody were effective in inhibiting ADP- thrombin or epinephrine-induced platelet aggregation as well as the binding of ^{125}I-fibrinogen to ADP-induced platelets. The antibody did not have any effect on ristocetin-induced agglutination of formaldehyde fixed platelets or agonist-induced platelet shape change. Moreover, platelet secretion induced by ADP or epinephrine was completely blocked by antibody, whereas its influence on collagen and thrombin induced platelet secretion was partial and dose dependent. Finally, the platelet adhesion to glass and clot retraction were significantly inhibited by the 10E5 antibody, indicating a thrombasthenic-like state induced by the antibody. The specificity of antibody to platelets and megakaryocytes expressing GPIIb/IIIa receptor was confirmed by immunofluorescent studies. In patients with thrombasthenia, it was demonstrated that radiolabelled antibody bound to <2000 receptor sites compared to ~40,000 in platelets isolated from normal individuals. Finally, it was suggested that the both GPIIb and GPIIIa proteins coexist, since both the glycoproteins were co-precipitated with 10E5 antibody.

Conclusions

The 10E5 antibody completely blocked the binding of fibrinogen to platelets and produced rapid dissociation of fibrinogen from platelets that had been pre-treated with ADP. These data suggest that the glycoproteins IIb and IIIa exist as a complex and are the platelet receptor for fibrinogen. Furthermore, thrombasthenic platelets cannot bind fibrinogen because they lack these glycoproteins.

> ### Learning points
>
> - These experiments identified the platelet glycoprotein IIb and IIIa receptors for fibrinogen.
> - This research stimulated the development of antibodies and receptor antagonists for GPIIb/IIIa receptor which are currently used in high-risk CHD patients.

Further reading

- Bennett JS, Hoxie JA, Leitman GV, Vilaire G, Cines DB. Inhibition of fibrinogen binding to stimulated human platelets by a monoclonal antibody. *Proc Natl Acad Sci USA* 1983; 80: 2417–21.
- Goto S, Tamura N, Ishida H. Ability of anti-glycoprotein IIb/IIIa agents to dissolve platelet thrombi formed on a collagen surface under blood flow conditions. *J Am Coll Cardiol* 2004; 44: 316–23.
- Reverter JC, Béguin S, Kessels H, Kumar R, Hemker HC, Coller BS. Inhibition of platelet-mediated, tissue factor-induced thrombin generation by the mouse/human chimeric 7E3 antibody. Potential implications for the effect of c7E3 Fab treatment on acute thrombosis and 'clinical restenosis'. *J Clin Invest* 1996; 98: 863–74.

Conclusions

In the past four decades, there has been a resurgence in the pharmacologic treatment of CHD with the development of new antiplatelet and antithrombotic agents. The pharmacologic management of patients with CHD mainly consists of inhibition of thromboxane synthesis by aspirin and inhibition of the ADP-$P2Y_{12}$ interaction by $P2Y_{12}$ receptor blockers. Aspirin (acetylsalicylic acid—ASA) is the bedrock of all antithrombotic therapies for both primary and secondary prevention of CHD. The efficacy of new oral antiplatelet agents has been studied on top of aspirin in clinical trials and the new agents are always prescribed in addition to aspirin in common clinical practice. Clopidogrel, a second-generation thienopyridine, is the widely prescribed $P2Y_{12}$ receptor, and is associated with better clinical outcomes in a wide range of patients with CHD, compared to therapy with aspirin alone. However, clopidogrel therapy is associated with numerous limitations, including high on-treatment platelet reactivity that has been linked to increased ischaemic event occurrence. Both of the new $P2Y_{12}$ inhibitors: prasugrel—an irreversible, third-generation thienopyridine and ticagrelor—a reversibly binding, direct acting agent, are associated with a faster onset of action, greater platelet inhibition, lower on-treatment platelet reactivity than clopidogrel, and are associated with improved clinical outcomes, including less stent thrombosis compared to clopidogrel. However, increased major bleeding associated with prasugrel and ticagrelor therapies is a major concern. In selected CHD patients with high on-treatment platelet reactivity during clopidogrel therapy, treatment with new more potent antiplatelet agents may be an effective strategy. Selecting the patient for treatment with the new more potent therapies may be assisted by genotyping and platelet function testing. Understanding the mechanisms of treatment failure and bleeding during dual antiplatelet is a major area of ongoing investigations. The use of prasugel or ticagrelor, $P2Y_{12}$ inhibitors with a rapid onset of potent pharmacodynamic effects, may also influence the future role of GPIIb/IIIa inhibitors. Finally, clopidogrel is pharmacodynamically effective in about two thirds of patients undergoing PCI; these patients do not have HPR. Ischemic risk is much greater in patients with HPR. Therefore, selectively treating two thirds of patients with generic clopidogrel at this time may provide significant cost savings. Unselected therapy with the new $P2Y_{12}$ receptor blockers is associated with increased bleeding. Therefore, clinicians should strive to find the antiplatelet therapy that achieves the optimal level of platelet inhibition for the patient, regardless of cost.

References

1. World Health Organization. *World Health Statistics* 2008. Geneva: WHO; 2008.
2. Davi G, Patrono C. Platelet activation and atherothrombosis. *N Engl J Med* 2007; 357: 2482–94.
3. Gurbel PA, Bliden KP, Hayes KM, Tantry U. Platelet activation in myocardial ischemic syndromes. *Expert Rev Cardiovasc Ther* 2004; 2: 535–45.
4. Gurbel PA, Tantry US. Do platelet function testing and genotyping improve outcome in patients treated with antithrombotic agents?: Platelet function testing and genotyping improve outcome in patients treated with antithrombotic agents. *Circulation*. 2012; 125: 1276–87.
5. Levine GN, Bates ER, Blankenship JC, et al. 2011 ACCF/AHA/SCAI Guideline for Percutaneous Coronary Intervention: a report of the American College of Cardiology Foundation/American Heart Association Task Force on Practice Guidelines and the Society for Cardiovascular Angiography and Interventions. *Circulation* 2011; 124: e574–651.
6. Patrono C, Baigent C, Hirsh J, Roth G; American College of Chest Physicians. Antiplatelet drugs: American College of Chest Physicians Evidence-Based Clinical Practice Guidelines. 8th edn. *Chest* 2008; 133: 199S-233S.
7. Randomised trial of intravenous streptokinase, oral aspirin, both, or neither among 17,187 cases of suspected acute myocardial infarction: ISIS-2. ISIS-2 (Second International Study of Infarct Survival) Collaborative Group. *Lancet* 1988; 2: 349–60.
8. Antithrombotic Trialists' (ATT) Collaboration, Baigent C, Blackwell L, Collins R, *et al.* Aspirin in the primary and secondary prevention of vascular disease: collaborative meta-analysis of individual participant data from randomised trials. *Lancet* 2009; 373: 1849–60.
9. Bonello L, Tantry US, Marcucci R, *et al.*; Working Group on High On-Treatment Platelet Reactivity. Consensus and future directions on the definition of high on-treatment platelet reactivity to adenosine diphosphate. *J Am Coll Cardiol* 2010; 56: 919–33.

10. Gaarder A, Jonsen J, Laland S, Owren PA. Adenosine diphosphate in red cells as a factor in the adhesiveness of human blood platelets. *Nature* 1961; 192: 531–2.

11. Cheng TO. 'The History of Aspirin'. *Texas Heart Institute Journal* 2007; 34: 392–3.

12. Craven LL. Acetylsalicylic acid, possible preventive of coronary thrombosis. *Ann West Med Surg* 1950; 4: 95.

13. Weiss HJ, Aledort LM. Impaired platelet-connective-tissue reaction in man after aspirin ingestion. *Lancet* 1967; 2: 495–7.

14. Piper PJ, Vane JR. Release of additional factors in anaphylaxis and its antagonism by anti-inflammatory drugs. *Nature* 1969; 223: 29–35.

15. Gachet C, Savi P, Ohlmann P, Maffrand JP, Jakobs KH, Cazenave JP. ADP receptor induced activation of guanine nucleotide binding proteins in rat platelet membranes—an effect selectively blocked by the thienopyridine clopidogrel. *Thromb Haemost* 1992; 68: 79–83.

16. Gachet C, Cazenave JP, Ohlmann P, *et al.* The thienopyridine ticlopidine selectively prevents the inhibitory effects of ADP but not of adrenaline on cAMP levels raised by stimulation of the adenylate cyclase of human platelets by PGE$_1$. *Biochem Pharmacol* 1990; 40: 2683–7.

17. Mills DC, Puri R, Hu CJ, *et al.* Clopidogrel inhibits the binding of ADP analogues to the receptor mediating inhibition of platelet adenylate cyclase. *Arterioscler Thromb* 1992; 12: 430–6.

18. Vetrovec GW, Leinbach RC, Gold HK, Cowley MJ. Intracoronary thrombolysis in syndromes of unstable ischemia: angiographic and clinical results. *Am Heart J* 1982; 104: 946–52.

19. Mandelkorn JB, Wolf NM, Singh S, *et al.* Intracoronary thrombus in nontransmural myocardial infarction and in unstable angina pectoris. *Am J Cardiol* 1983; 52: 1–6.

20. Gotoh K, Katoh O, Fukui S, Hamano Y, Minamino T. Angiographic visualization of coronary thrombus during anginal attack in unstable angina. *Circulation* 1985; 72: Suppl III: 111–2. Abstract.

21. Sherman CT, Litvack F, Grundfest W, *et al.* Coronary angioscopy in patients with unstable angina pectoris. *N Engl J Med* 1986; 315: 913–9.

22. Lewis HD Jr, Davis JW, Archibald DG, *et al.* Protective effects of aspirin against acute myocardial infarction and death in men with unstable angina: results of a Veterans Administration cooperative study. *N Engl J Med* 1983; 309: 396–403.

23. Patrono C, Coller B, Dalen JE, *et al.* Platelet-active drugs: the relationships among dose, effectiveness, and side effects. *Chest* 1998; 114: 470S–88S.

24. Bertrand ME, Rupprecht HJ, Urban P, Gershlick AH. CLASSICS Investigators. Double-blind study of the safety of clopidogrel with and without a loading dose in combination with aspirin compared with ticlopidine in combination with aspirin after coronary stenting: the clopidogrel aspirin stent international cooperative study (CLASSICS). *Circulation* 2000; 102: 624–9.

25. Herbert JM, Dol F, Bernat A, *et al.* The antiaggregating and antithrombotic activity of clopidogrel is potentiated by aspirin in several experimental models in the rabbit. *Thromb Haemost* 1998; 80: 512–8.

26. Yusuf S, Zhao F, Mehta SR, *et al.* Clopidogrel in Unstable Angina to Prevent Recurrent Events Trial Investigators. Effects of clopidogrel in addition to aspirin in patients with acute coronary syndromes without ST-segment elevation. *N Engl J Med* 2001; 345: 494–502.

27. Sabatine MS, Cannon CP, Gibson CM, *et al.* CLARITY-TIMI 28 Investigators. Addition of clopidogrel to aspirin and fibrinolytic therapy form myocardial infarction with ST segment elevation. *N Engl J Med* 2005; 352: 1179–89.

28. Müller I, Seyfarth M, Rüdiger S, *et al.* Effect of a high loading dose of clopidogrel on platelet function in patients undergoing coronary stent placement. *Heart* 2001; 85: 92–3.

29. Gurbel PA, Bliden KP, Samara W, *et al.* Clopidogrel effect on platelet reactivity in patients with stent thrombosis: results of the CREST Study. *J Am Coll Cardiol* 2005; 46: 1827–32.

30. Barragan P, Bouvier JL, Roquebert PO, *et al.* Resistance to thienopyridines: clinical detection of coronary stent thrombosis by monitoring of vasodilator-stimulated phosphoprotein phosphorylation. *Catheter Cardiovasc Interv* 2003; 59: 295–302.

31. Samara WM, Bliden KP, Tantry US, Gurbel PA. The difference between clopidogrel responsiveness and posttreatment platelet reactivity. *Thromb Res* 2005; 115: 89–94.

32. Tantry US, Bliden KP, Gurbel PA. What is the best measure of thrombotic risks—pre-treatment platelet aggregation, clopidogrel responsiveness, or post-treatment platelet aggregation? *Catheter Cardiovasc Interv* 2005; 66: 597–8.

33. Rivard GE, Brummel-Ziedins KE, Mann KG, Fan L, Hofer A, Cohen E. Evaluation of the profile of thrombin generation during the process of whole blood clotting as assessed by thromboelastography. *J Thromb Haemost* 2005; 3: 2039–43.

34. Khurana S, Mattson JC, Westley S, O'Neill WW, Timmis GC, Safian RD. Monitoring platelet glycoprotein IIb/IIIa-fibrin interaction with tissue factor-activated thromboelastography. *J Lab Clin Med* 1997; 130: 401–11.

35. Gurbel PA, Becker RC, Mann KG, Steinhubl SR, Michelson AD. Platelet function monitoring in patients with coronary artery disease. *J Am Coll Cardiol* 2007; 50: 1822–34.

36. Gurbel PA, Tantry US. Drug insight: Clopidogrel nonresponsiveness. *Nat Clin Pract Cardiovasc Med* 2006; 3: 387–95.

37. Gurbel PA, Antonino MJ, Tantry US. Recent developments in clopidogrel pharmacology and their relation to

clinical outcomes. *Expert Opin Drug Metab Toxicol* 2009; 5: 989–1004.

38. Brandt JT, Close SL, Iturria SJ, *et al.* Common polymorphisms of CYP2C19 and CYP2C9 affect the pharmacokinetic and pharmacodynamic response to clopidogrel but not prasugrel. *J Thromb Haemost* 2007; 5: 2429–36.

39. Mega JL, Close SL, Wiviott SD, *et al.* Cytochrome p-450 polymorphisms and response to clopidogrel. *N Engl J Med* 2009; 360: 354–62.

40. Trenk D, Hochholzer W, Fromm MF, *et al.* Cytochrome P450 2C19 681G>A polymorphism and high on-clopidogrel platelet reactivity associated with adverse 1-year clinical outcome of elective percutaneous coronary intervention with drug-eluting or bare-metal stents. *J Am Coll Cardiol* 2008; 51: 1925–34.

41. Murugappa S, Kunapuli SP. The role of ADP receptors in platelet function. *Front Biosci* 2006; 11: 1977–86.

42. Coller BS, Peerschke EI, Scudder LE, Sullivan CA. A murine monoclonal antibody that completely blocks the binding of fibrinogen to platelets produces a thrombasthenic-like state in normal platelets and binds to glycoproteins IIb and/or IIIa. *J Clin Invest* 1983; 72: 325–38.

43. Coller BS. Interaction of normal, thrombasthenic, and Bernard-Soulier platelets with immobilized fibrinogen: defective platelet fibrinogen interaction in thrombasthenia. *Blood* 1980; 55: 169–78.

44. Nachman, RL, Leung LKK. Complex formation of platelet membrane glycoproteins IIb and IIIa with fibrinogen. *J Clin Invest* 1982; 69: 263–9.

Chapter 5

Medical versus invasive management of coronary heart disease

Dr William Moody and Professor Bernard Gersh

Introduction

The era of coronary revascularization has entered its fifth decade and despite its undeniable impact on the outcomes of acute and chronic coronary artery disease (CAD), the indications for revascularization versus medical therapy remain an area somewhat shrouded by controversy. In this chapter, the pivotal trials of revascularization versus medical therapy in patients with stable disease are presented and discussed, and it is the data from these trials that have shaped current approaches on the *indications* for revascularization as opposed to other chapters which deal with the *preferred method* of revascularization, whether coronary artery bypass graft (CABG) surgery, or percutaneous coronary intervention (PCI).

Trials of revascularization are difficult to perform and are often perhaps unfairly criticized in that many patients are screened and relatively few are enrolled—the issue of 'entry' bias in trials as opposed to 'selection' bias in registries[1]. One has to remember, however, that in order for patients to be ethically enrolled in a trial of revascularization

versus medical therapy or trials of PCI versus CABG, there has to be clinical equipoise which automatically excludes those patients who are particularly suited for any one form of therapy as opposed to the alternative. A second limitation of these trials is that they take time to complete the follow-up, which in a way dooms them to relative obsolescence at the time of publication. This is basically an inescapable fact of clinical trial life since these trials take place upon a changing canvas of rapid technological advances, changing attitudes towards secondary prevention and the development of a host of new antithrombotic and platelet inhibitor drugs. After all, during the 1970s and early 1980s, during the era of the earliest and perhaps the most influential trials of bypass surgery and medical therapy, the left internal mammary artery was not used by the majority, and medical therapy was limited to beta blockers, aspirin, and long-acting nitrates; the last treatment often taken around the clock, resulting in probable tolerance in many. Perhaps the defining difference between the two approaches during that time period (namely surgery versus medical therapy) is that one group had an operation and the other did not, until the time of cross-over. A third aspect of the design of these trials is that randomization took place *after* the performance of coronary angiography; with one exception, namely the TIME trial.

Despite these caveats, however, the trials when taken in conjunction with registry studies such as the CASS registry, have provided us with a rational framework for establishing the indications for revascularization over medical therapy in regard to survival and symptom relief. What we have learned is the concept of 'gradient of risk' and that the major benefit of CABG over medical therapy and survival is in 'sicker' patients as defined by the severity of symptoms and ischaemia, the location and severity of stenoses (i.e. left main disease, proximal left anterior descending (LAD)), the number of vessels diseased, and the presence of left ventricular dysfunction. We have also learned that symptom relief is greater after CABG versus medical therapy, but that many patients do improve symptomatically under medical programmes, with the option of revascularization for those who fail medical therapy, providing they do not fall into the anatomic subgroup in which there is a survival benefit for surgery. In addition, the early advantage in terms of symptom relief following CABG is blunted over time.

Despite the major impact on prognosis of PCI in patients with acute coronary syndromes including ST-elevation myocardial infarction (STEMI) and non-STEMI (NSTEMI), no trial has shown in *angiographically-selected* patients with stable coronary disease that PCI improves survival as opposed to symptoms in comparison with medical therapy. The TIME trial, in which 52% of the invasive arm did receive PCI, demonstrated in severely symptomatic patients aged 75 years and older a probable survival benefit at four years and a reduction in subsequent MI. The COURAGE and BARI-2D trials have been polarizing, and the debate among interventionalists, non-interventional cardiologists, policy makers, professional associations, and the media has been spirited to say the least. Nonetheless, the conclusions from these large studies remain in place and that is that in angiographically-selected patients with stable coronary-artery disease and preserved left ventricular function, there is no benefit from PCI over medical therapy upon death and MI.

There are several explanations for the lack of benefit from PCI which is directed towards a 'culprit lesion' or 'culprit lesions', whereas disease progression and non-obstructive future culprits are factors perhaps more amenable to aggressive secondary prevention. It is also important to emphasize that 'cross-overs' might dilute the end point, but these are not so much trials of a specific therapy as of an initial therapeutic strategy.

From the early days of angiography, left ventricular dysfunction has been recognized as a major prognostic factor in patients with coronary disease. Moreover, as revascularization techniques improved, left ventricular dysfunction has emerged as a prime therapeutic target as opposed to its prior status as a relative contraindication to revascularization. The recently published Surgical Treatment for Ischaemic Heart Failure (STICH) trial of patients with stable coronary disease (Class III angina excluded) and more severe left ventricular dysfunction (ejection fraction — EF <35%) whose anatomy was suitable for surgery, did not demonstrate any difference in all-cause mortality (the primary end point) at five years between CABG and optimal medical therapy. Nonetheless, cardiovascular mortality was reduced, as was cardiovascular hospitalization. Additional analyses based on protocol or treatment received, which was performed because of the large numbers of cross-overs in both groups, did reach statistical significance in regard to all cause mortality. In this respect, I would consider the trial as demonstrating a modestly positive result. From a clinical perspective, there should be a heightened awareness of the potential for CABG to improve survival in suitable patients: patients with congestive heart failure and/or severe left ventricular dysfunction due to CAD, and among whom distal vessels are suitable targets for coronary bypass. The role of viability testing requires further clarification and investigation.

See Table 5.1 for a summary of trials comparing medical therapy with revascularization for stable CAD.

Table 5.1 Summary of trials comparing medical therapy versus revascularization for stable coronary artery disease

	VACS	CASS	DANAMI	RITA-2	AVERT	TIME	MASS II	SWISSI II	COURAGE	BARI-2D
Year of original publication	1977	1983	1997	1997	1999	2001	2004	2007	2007	2009
Years of enrolment	1970–74	1975–79	1990–94	1992–96	1995–96	1996–2000	1995–2000	1991–97	1999–2004	2001–05
Total no. of patients	596	780	1008	1018	341	301	611	201	2287	2368
Medical therapy	310	390	505	514	164	148	203	105	1149	1192
Revascularisation	286	390	503	504	177	153	408	96	1138	1176
Primary end point	Death	Death	Death/MI/ Admission for UA	Death/MI	Ischaemic event	Symptoms, QoL	Death, MI, Refractory angina	Death, MI, Revascularisation	Death, MI	Death
Secondary end point(s)	Perioperative MI Graft patency	Perioperative MI Graft patency	Angina	Angina	Angina, QoL, LDL, TC	Survival	Angina, Stroke	Ischaemia	Symptoms	Death, MI, Stroke
Patient selection	CAD by angio Suitable anatomy	CAD by angio Suitable anatomy	Post infarct ischaemia	CAD by angio Suitable anatomy	CAD by angio Suitable anatomy and LDL >3 mmol/L	Clinical presentation	Proximal 2–3VD with angina or stress ischaemia	Silent ischaemia CAD by angio Suitable anatomy	CAD by angio Suitable anatomy	T2DM CAD by angio
Angina CCS	I–II	0–II	I–III	0–III	0–III	II–IV	II–III	0	0–III	0–II (82% I–II)
Exclusions	Unstable angina Recent MI Low EF, Female	NYHA III–IV UA	UA Previous MI, PCI or CABG	CCS IV, ACS <7d, LM, Previous PCI or CABG	LM, 3VD, UA, MI in last 2/52 EF < 40%	Age <75 yrs ACS <10d	Unstabilized ACS, <2VD, EF<40%	CCS ≥1, ACS <10d, LM or 3VD	CCS IV, severe ischaemia	LM, NYHA ≥III Immediate need for PCI
Type of revascularisation	CABG	CABG	PCI/CABG	PCI	PCI	PCI/CABG	PCI/CABG	PCI	PCI	PCI/CABG
Stents (%)	NA	NA	0	8	30	44	68	0	90	91
Initial follow-up (years)	3	5	2.4	7	1.5	4.1	5	10	4.6	5

VACS, Veterans Association Cooperative Study; CASS, Coronary Artery Surgery Study; DANAMI, DANish trial in Acute Myocardial Infarction; RITA-2, second Randomized Intervention Treatment of Angina; AVERT, Atorvastatin Versus Revascularization Treatments; TIME, Trial of Invasive versus Medical therapy in Elderly patients with chronic symptomatic coronary artery disease; MASS II, Medicine, Angioplasty, or Surgery Study; SWISSI II, Swiss Interventional Study on Silent Ischaemia type II; COURAGE, Clinical Outcomes Utilizing Revascularization and Aggressive Drug Evaluation; BARI-2D, Bypass Angioplasty Revascularization Investigation 2 Diabetes; T2Di, type 2 diabetes mellitus; CCS, Canadian Cardiovascular Society classification; ACS, acute coronary syndrome; d, day; LM, left main coronary disease; NYHA, New York Heart Association classification; EF, ejection fraction; PCI, percutaneous coronary intervention; CABG, coronary artery bypass grafting.

The Veterans Affairs (VA) cooperative study of coronary artery bypass surgery for stable angina

Murphy M, Hultgren H, Detre K, Thomsen J, Takaro T, and participants of the Veterans Administration Cooperative Study. Treatment of chronic stable angina; a preliminary report of survival data of the randomized Veterans Administration cooperative study. *N Engl J Med* 1977; 297: 621–7.

Background

Following its introduction in 1960, CABG surgery had improved considerably, but results from studies addressing its long-term outcomes had been difficult to interpret for several reasons. First, a 'steady state' had not been reached for long enough to begin accumulating meaningful data. Second, the rates of cross-over between treatment arms from medical to surgical therapy had been high because of a perceived improvement in symptoms when anti-anginal medications failed. Third, there was significant heterogeneity among patients with stable coronary artery disease (CAD) which had not until now been appreciated. Thus, in most previous studies the variables that could affect survival were not initially defined and then not rigorously controlled for, so that small differences in baseline characteristics were just as likely to account for differences in survival as were the interventions patients were assigned to. Finally, since the differences in survival between surgically or medically treated patients were small, if present at all, greater numbers were required to adequately power the studies to demonstrate statistically significant differences in outcomes. The VA Cooperative Study was the first randomized clinical trial (RCT) large enough to address these issues and determine whether CABG offered any additional benefit over medical therapy alone in patients with stable angina.

Methods

Only patients with stable angina without a recent MI were included. After subgrouping the patients with left main coronary artery stenosis, a total of 596 patients were entered into this study; 310 patients were randomly assigned to medical therapy and 286 patients to saphenous-vein-CABG. All patients were men aged less than 65 years who had mild-to-moderate angina pectoris, at least two-vessel disease, and good left ventricular function. Following randomization, clinical and angiographic baseline variables were comparable between the two treatment arms.

Results

Operative mortality at 30 days was as high as 5.6%. At an average of one year after operation, 69% of all grafts were patent, and 88% of the surgical patients had at least one patent graft. At 36 months, 87% of the medical group and 88% of the surgical group were alive. While there was no statistically significant difference in survival between patients treated medically and those treated with saphenous vein CABG at a minimum follow-up interval of 21 months, after four years, the surgical treatment group showed significantly better survival than the medical treatment group in the total patient population (p <0.001), particularly among patients with three-vessel disease (p <0.001).

In a study by Takaro et al., subset analysis of 91 patients with left main disease demonstrated a four-year survival of 90% when treated surgically, but only 60% when treated medically (p <0.001). This was later supported by the six years' follow up data. In patients with left main lesions, surgery significantly improved survival in the two-thirds of those characterized as middle or high risk by four simple non-invasive predictors of prognosis (New York Heart Association (NYHA) functional class III or IV, history of MI, history of hypertension, and ST-segment depression on the resting baseline electrocardiogram (ECG)). Patients with three-vessel disease and no significant disease of the left main coronary artery also had better survival rates when treated surgically. At six years, however, this was only statistically significant in the ten hospitals in which the aggregate operative mortality was 3.3%.

Limitations

While enrolment took place between 1970 and 1974, only data from the last two years were published because the operative mortality was excessively high in the earlier operations, which may have led to considerable selection bias. Even in the last two years of the study, 3 of the 13 collaborating VA hospitals reported a 23% operative mortality, while the remaining 10 reported a 3.4% operative mortality. This study has also been criticized for using stringent inclusion and exclusion criteria that resulted in a very specific, albeit well-defined population. The criteria excluded patients with unstable angina or recent MI, a population that frequently undergoes CABG today. Of the surgical group, 6% refused operation but

17% of the medical group eventually had bypass procedures. It could be argued that the patients who refused operation were probably minimally symptomatic and therefore low-risk patients, while the medical to surgical cross-overs were more symptomatic and, therefore, higher risk patients, thus biasing the results away from surgical therapy. Nonetheless, the three-year survival results of the VA Cooperative Study were the same whether the cross-over patients were left in their original groups, placed in the group to which they crossed over or eliminated from the analysis altogether. The short-term surgical results reflecting operative technique and perioperative care, perioperative mortality, perioperative infarction rate, and graft patency rate have justifiably been the most criticized aspects of the study. Specifically, the 30-day mortality in the VA Cooperative Study was 5.6%, while a perioperative mortality of approximately 1% is closer to the norm in today's practice. At worst, given that the short-term results reflecting operative technique and perioperative care in the VA Cooperative Study do not compare with those being achieved today in major medical centres, these results could well be deemed obsolete.

Conclusions

There is increased survival of patients with symptomatic left main CAD treated surgically as compared with medical therapy alone. After long-term follow-up of trial participants (see Further reading list below), however, it began to emerge that CABG surgery did not confer a survival benefit over medical therapy.

Learning points

◆ Surgery remains the 'gold standard' intervention for haemodynamically significant left main coronary artery lesions and extensive three-vessel disease.

Further reading

- Peduzzi P, Kamina A, Detre K. Twenty-two-year follow-up in the VA Cooperative Study of Coronary Artery Bypass Surgery for Stable Angina. *Am J Cardiol* 1998; 81: 1393–9. This study offers the longest follow-up data from the original VA Cooperative Study. It confirmed that initial CABG surgery with saphenous vein grafts does not improve survival for low-risk patients, and that it does not reduce the overall risk of MI. Despite an early survival benefit with surgery in high-risk patients (up to a decade), long-term survival rates began to converge in both treatment groups.
- Takaro T, Hultgren HN, Detre KM, Peduzzi P. The Veterans Administration Cooperative Study of stable angina: current status. *Circulation* 1982; 65: 60–6. These six-year follow-up data confirmed not only patients with left main coronary-artery disease, but also those with three three-vessel disease have better survival rates when treated surgically as compared with medical therapy alone.
- Takaro T, *et al.* and participants in the VA Cooperative Study. Results of a randomized study of medical and surgical management of angina pectoris. *World J Surg* 1978; 2: 797–807. This was the first study to demonstrate a survival benefit of CABG over medical therapy alone in high risk patients with left main coronary-artery disease.
- The VA Coronary Artery Bypass Surgery Cooperative Study Group. Eighteen-year follow-up in the Veterans Affairs Cooperative Study of Coronary Artery Bypass Surgery for stable angina. *Circulation* 1992; 86: 121–130. This provided evidence that the benefits of CABG on survival, symptoms, and post-infarction mortality were transient, lasting fewer than 11 years. The benefits began to diminish after five years, when graft closure accelerated. Surgery was only effective in reducing mortality for high-risk patients with a poor natural history.
- The Veterans Administrations Coronary Artery Bypass Surgery Study Group. Eleven-year survival in the Veterans Administration randomized trial of coronary bypass surgery for stable angina. *N Engl J Med* 1984; 311: 1333–9. Patients had been followed-up for an average of 11.2 years. In a primary analysis of all 686 patients and including the 595 without left main coronary-artery disease, cumulative survival did not differ significantly at 11 years compared with medical therapy.

The Coronary Artery Surgery Study (CASS)

CASS Prinicipal Investigators and their Associates. Coronary artery surgery study (CASS): a randomized trial of coronary artery bypass surgery. Survival data. *Circulation* 1983; 68: 939–50.

Background

The marked relief of angina after CABG, the improving perioperative mortality, and the increasingly widespread availability of experienced surgical teams led to an upsurge in the number of operations performed in the United States, from an estimated 24,000 in 1971 to an estimated 159,000 a decade later. The controversy sparked by the initially negative three-year results of the VA Cooperative Study Group, meant physicians were still unsure whether CABG conferred a survival advantage over medical therapy alone in the absence of severe left main CAD. Thus in 1973, the National Heart, Lung and Blood Institute organized a patient registry and a randomized trial designed to compare results of medical and surgical therapy in patients with CAD. The primary aim of this trial was to evaluate the effect of assigned treatment on total mortality in well-characterized subsets of patients with CAD.

Methods

The CASS registry included 16,626 patients who were screened to determine their eligibility for entry into the randomized trial. Inclusion criteria included an age of 65 years or less, angina that was Canadian Cardiovascular Society (CCS) class I or II with or without a history of MI or, a well-documented MI more than three weeks old. Clinical criteria for exclusion included prior CABG, unstable or progressive angina and congestive heart failure (NYHA class III or IV). During the recruitment period, 2099 (12.7%) CASS registry patients met the criteria for participation in this study; 780 patients, 37% of those eligible, were randomly assigned to receive medical or surgical therapy. Randomisation was stratified by clinical site, number of diseased vessels, and ejection fraction.

Results

In patients randomly assigned to undergo surgery, operative mortality, defined as death occurring in hospital or within 30 days of surgery, was 1.4% (5 out of 357 patients). At five years, there were no significant differences in survival for the two treatment groups. There were no statistically significant differences among survival curves for pharmacological and surgical groups when patients were grouped according to presence of single, double, or triple-vessel disease, by ejection fraction, or by a combination of number of diseased vessels and ejection fraction. In patients with unimpaired ventricular performance on entry into the study (ejection fraction of at least 50%), the survival curves were indistinguishable. In those with impaired left ventricular function, a statistically non-significant trend in favour of surgery was evident.

Limitations

The annual mortality in patients assigned to medical therapy was 1.6%, a figure considerably lower than that estimated during trial design and the 4.3% reported in

the Veterans Administration Study. The excellent long-term results in CASS patients assigned to medical therapy reduced the power of the study to detect a reduction in mortality afforded by prompt elective CABG. Beta-blockers were used with equal frequency in both groups at entry, but were subsequently given more frequently to patients assigned to medical therapy, which may have biased results in favour of pharmacotherapy alone. The survival curves revealed a statistically non-significant advantage for the patients assigned to surgical therapy, especially in those with three-vessel disease. In view of the small sample size, a significant improvement in survival due to immediate surgical intervention cannot be excluded as a possibility.

Conclusions

The CASS trial is most applicable to mild to moderate angina and asymptomatic patients following MI. The authors concluded that in these patients a treatment strategy of prompt elective CABG does not result in improved survival when compared with an aggressive medical strategy and thus, revascularisation should be reserved for those with worsening symptoms.

Learning points

- In patients with mild to moderate angina and in asymptomatic patients post-MI, elective CABG does not confer a survival benefit when compared with medical therapy alone.
- After extended follow-up, the CASS trial did reveal a significant advantage favouring surgical therapy in patients with three-vessel disease and impaired ventricular function.

Further reading

- Alderman EL, Bourassa MG, Cohen LS, *et al*. Ten-year follow-up of survival and MI in the randomized Coronary Artery Surgery Study. *Circulation*. 1990; 82: 1629–46. The ten-year follow-up results confirmed earlier reports from CASS that patients with left ventricular dysfunction exhibit long-term benefit from an initial strategy of surgical intervention. Patients with mild stable angina and normal left ventricular function randomized to initial medical treatment (with an option for later surgery if symptoms progressed) had survival comparable to those patients randomized to initial CABG.
- Killip T, Passamani E, Davis K. Coronary artery surgery study (CASS): a randomized trial of coronary bypass surgery.

Eight years follow-up and survival in patients with reduced ejection fraction. *Circulation*. 1985; 72: V102–9. After eight years, survival curves are not significantly different between medical and surgical groups. However, a significant advantage favouring surgical assignment was observed in patients with three-vessel disease and reduced ejection fractions (35–50%).

The DANish trial in Acute Myocardial Infarction (DANAMI)

Madsen JK, Grande P, Saunamäki K, Thayssen P, Kassis E, Eriksen U, Rasmussen K, Haunsø S, Nielsen TT, Haghfelt T, Fritz-Hansen P, Hjelms E, Paulsen PK, Alstrup P, Arendrup H, Niebuhr-Jørgensen U, Andersen LI. Danish multicenter randomized study of invasive versus conservative treatment in patients with inducible ischaemia after thrombolysis in acute myocardial infarction (DANAMI). DANish trial in Acute Myocardial Infarction. *Circulation* 1997; 96: 748–55.

Background

Thrombolytic therapy was the conventional strategy for patients with STEMI before primary PCI became the treatment of choice. Patients had been shown to gain improved survival after thrombolytic therapy at long-term follow-up. It was already known that PCI immediately after thrombolysis did not result in a lower morbidity or mortality compared with conservative treatment or deferred PCI. It had been hypothesized that in patients with documented post-infarction ischaemia, revascularization might reduce the incidence of future coronary events. To date, other studies comparing an early invasive versus a non-invasive strategy had not shown a difference in outcome, although these studies had received considerable criticism, with only 56–61% of patients originally allocated to the invasive group undergoing such intervention. Furthermore, 5–20% of those in the conservative treatment group were noted to have crossed over to the intervention arm.

The DANAMI study was designed to compare a deferred invasive strategy comprising either PCI or CABG with a conservative strategy in patients with documented myocardial ischaemia within weeks of an acute MI.

Methods

Forty-three hospitals in Denmark participated in this multi-centre study. Patients ≤69 years old were included in the study if they presented with an acute MI (significant elevation of creatine kinase—MB, defined as an increase to at least twice the upper limit of normal), ST deviation or T wave changes, and/or Q waves developed, and thrombolytic treatment was commenced within 12 hours of symptom onset. To be included in the study patients had to demonstrate inducible post-infarction ischaemia, which was usually defined during a compulsory pre-discharge, symptom-limited bicycle exercise test. Patients with unstable angina who would have ordinarily required intervention were excluded, as were patients with a history of MI, PCI, or CABG. The primary end points consisted of death, acute MI, and admission with unstable angina pectoris. Revascularization was scheduled within 2–5 weeks of discharge and follow-up was for at least 12 months.

Percutaneous coronary intervention was performed within two weeks of randomization in patients with either one or two-vessel disease and a maximum of three significant stenoses or occlusion of the infarct-related artery. Conventional PCI *without* stent implantation was performed. Coronary artery bypass grafting was performed within five weeks of randomization in all patients with left main coronary-artery stem stenosis, two-vessel disease with a total of more than three stenoses, three-vessel disease, and occlusion of a non-infarct-related artery. Medical therapy, including the choice of anti-ischaemic medication, was prescribed according to local practice.

Results

The study included 1008 patients, of which 505 were randomized to conservative treatment and 503 to invasive treatment. The invasive-strategy patients underwent 266 angioplasty procedures and 147 bypass operations. There was no significant difference in mortality between the two groups at a median of 2.4 years. However, the rates of re-infarction and of readmission for unstable angina were 5.6% and 17.9%, respectively, for the invasive strategy and 10.5% and 29.5%, respectively, for the conservative strategy (p = 0.0038 and p = 0.00001, respectively). The number of patients in the conservative treatment group with CCS class II or III angina declined from 23% at three months' follow-up to 15% after one year (p = 0.001), although the proportion in class I remained almost constant.

Limitations

Revascularization was only performed in 413 (82.1%) of the 503 patients randomized to invasive treatment, whereas 17.9% in the invasive treatment group received no revascularization. The median time to PCI and CABG was 18 days and 38 days after randomization, respectively. Eight patients (1.6%) randomized to conservative therapy had PCI (n = 5) or CABG (n = 3) performed during the first two months of follow-up, and 76 patients (n = 33) had PCI or CABG (n = 43) during the first year due to worsening angina. The study failed to address how patients with different thresholds of inducible ischaemia should be managed. In addition, less than half of the conservatively treated patients were taking beta-blockers post-infarction with inducible ischaemia. Data on the use of lipid-lowering drugs, despite their well-established benefits in secondary prevention, was also lacking.

Conclusions

The DANAMI study was the first to show a small but significant benefit of revascularization in selected patients after acute MI. Specifically, the invasive strategy (PCI or CABG) in patients with inducible ischaemia after MI was associated with a reduction in recurrent infarction and admissions for unstable angina as well as a reduction in

prevalence and severity of angina. There was, however, no difference in mortality between the two groups.

Learning points

♦ The DANAMI study supports the current practice of angiography for all post-infarction patients with ischaemia, who subsequently undergo revascularization.

Further reading

Other trials comparing early invasive with non invasive strategies include:
- Barbash GL, Roth A, Hod H, *et al.* Randomized controlled trial of late in-hospital angiography and angioplasty versus conservative management after treatment with recombinant tissue-type plasminogen activator in acute myocardial infarction. *Am J Cardiol* 1990; 66: 538–45.
- SWIFT (Should We Intervene Following Thrombolysis?) Trial Study Group. SWIFT trial of delayed elective intervention versus conservative treatment after thrombolysis with anistreplase in acute myocardial infarction. *Br Med J* 1991; 302: 555–60.
- The TIMI Study Group. Comparison of invasive and conservative strategies after treatment with intravenous tissue plasminogen activator in acute myocardial infarction: results of the Thrombolysis In Myocardial Infarction (TIMI) phase II trial. *N Engl J Med* 1989; 320: 618–27.

The second Randomized Intervention Treatment of Angina (RITA-2) trial

RITA-2 trial participants. Coronary angioplasty versus medical therapy for angina: the second Randomized Intervention Treatment of Angina (RITA-2) trial. *Lancet* 1997; 350: 461–8.

Background

The role of PCI in the management of patients with angina remained subject to question, particularly in patients whose symptoms were adequately controlled by medical treatment. Until this point, no large-scale study had addressed the management of patients with stable CAD admitted to hospital for chronic or unstable angina.

Methods

This multi-centre trial included 1018 patients with angiographically-proven CAD, irrespective of symptoms, and coronary anatomy considered suitable for PCI without ongoing instability, and without previous revascularization

or left main coronary-artery disease. Subjects were randomized to either PCI (504) or continued medical therapy (514).

Results

After a median follow up of 2.7 years, the combined primary end point of all cause mortality or MI occurred in 6.3% of patients treated with PCI compared with 3.3% on drug therapy (a beta-blocker, calcium antagonist or long-acting nitrate in maximum tolerated doses; p = 0.02). This difference was largely driven by an early intervention hazard, with seven intervention-related MIs in patients treated with PCI.

Angina improved in both groups, but more so in the PCI group. There was a 16.5% absolute excess of CCS class II or worse angina in the medical group three months after randomization (p <0·001), which attenuated to 7.6% after two years. Total exercise time (Bruce protocol) also improved in both groups, again with a treatment difference in favour of PCI: mean advantage of 35 seconds at three months (p <0·001). On subgroup analysis, for patients with baseline angina grade 2 or more there was a marked benefit of PCI at six months, with a 20% lower frequency of angina and a one-minute longer mean exercise time than in patients on medical therapy. By contrast, for patients with no angina or grade 1 angina at baseline, there was negligible difference between the PCI and medical arms (interaction tests for angina and exercise outcomes respectively, p = 0.03 and p = 0.01).

After an extended follow up of seven years (Henderson *et al.*, 2003), the rate of cardiac death was similar in patients randomly assigned to PCI (20/504; 4.0%) and drug therapy (24/514; 4.7%). At late follow-up, 43% of patients in the medical group needed revascularization for medically uncontrollable symptoms, which was significantly more than in the PCI group (32.5%; p <0.01).

Limitations

Patients ranged from those with no angina and single vessel disease to those with severe symptoms and multi-vessel disease. The majority had mild symptoms, one-vessel or two-vessel disease, and preserved left-ventricular function, and were therefore at low cardiovascular risk. It is important to emphasize that these patients were therefore not representative of all patients undergoing percutaneous coronary intervention, but represented a substantial group for whom either medical therapy or angioplasty appeared appropriate.

Conclusions

The investigators concluded that medical therapy versus PCI in patients with stable CAD have equivalent long-term survival outcomes, although there is a greater symptomatic improvement after early intervention, especially if symptoms are severe. This symptomatic benefit which persisted for up to two years after randomization has to be weighed against a small, early intervention hazard associated with PCI. It must be remembered, however, that this trial was conducted during a time when the pharmaco-therapeutic armamentarium available to clinicians was significantly restricted compared to the drugs we have available today and PCI was also not performed as it is practiced now.

Learning points

- There was no additional long-term mortality benefit from PCI versus medical therapy alone in patients with stable CAD.
- Early intervention with PCI was associated with greater symptomatic improvement in patients with more severe angina or limited exercise tolerance.
- Patients without severe angina do not initially gain substantial symptomatic benefit from PCI, suggesting that in these patients revascularization may reasonably be deferred unless more severe symptoms supervene.
- Exercise tolerance does not improve appreciably in patients with already good exercise capacity at baseline, and since these patients are at low cardiovascular risk they are unlikely to gain major prognostic advantage from PCI.

Further reading

- Henderson RA, Pocock SJ, Clayton TC, *et al.*; Second Randomized Intervention Treatment of Angina (RITA-2) Trial Participants. Seven-year outcome in the RITA-2 trial: coronary angioplasty versus medical therapy. *J Am Coll Cardiol* 2003; 42: 1161–70.

The Atorvastatin Versus Revascularization Treatments (AVERT) trial

Pitt B, Waters D, Brown WV, van Boven AJ, Schwartz L, Title LM, Eisenberg D, Shurzinske L, McCormick LS. Aggressive lipid lowering therapy compared with angioplasty in stable coronary-artery disease. *N Engl J Med* 1999; 341: 70–6.

Background

Data from studies which compared medical therapy with PCI, such as RITA-2, suggested that patients with stable CAD who underwent revascularization benefited from improvements in quality of life and exercise performance. However, the effect of medical treatment, as compared with PCI, on the incidence of ischaemic events and the frequency of subsequent revascularization procedures was still debatable. Lipid-lowering treatment had been proven to significantly reduce the incidence of cardiovascular events, overall mortality, and the need for revascularization. Pitt *et al.* hypothesized that in patients with stable CAD (those with one or two-vessel CAD, relatively normal left ventricular function, and no severe symptoms of angina pectoris), treatment with atorvastatin would delay or prevent the need for revascularization without increasing the risk of ischaemic events.

Study design

The study was an open-label, randomized, multi-centre study of 341 patients with stable CAD, a serum level of low-density lipoprotein cholesterol (LDL-C) of at least 3.0 mmol/l (115 mg/dl), and a serum level of triglycerides of no more than 5.6 mmol per litre (500 mg/dl). Patients had been recommended for treatment with PCI following angiography demonstrating a stenosis of 50% or more in at least one coronary artery. Patients included were able to complete at least four minutes of the Bruce protocol on treadmill without marked electrocardiographic changes indicative of ischaemia and virtually all were either asymptomatic or had CCS class I or II angina. Participants were randomized to receive either medical treatment with atorvastatin 80 mg per day (164 patients), or to undergo the recommended PCI followed by usual care, which could include lipid-lowering treatment (177 patients). There was no washout period for patients already receiving lipid-lowering medication. Patients assigned to receive atorvastatin discontinued any other lipid-lowering medication they might have been taking, whereas patients assigned to angioplasty and usual care were allowed to continue their current drug regimen. The primary efficacy parameter was the incidence of an ischaemic event, defined as any of the following: cardiovascular death, cardiac arrest, non-fatal MI, the need for CABG or angioplasty, cerebrovascular accident, and worsening angina verified by objective evidence requiring hospitalization (including unstable angina). The follow-up period was 18 months.

Results

Twenty two (13%) of the patients who received aggressive lipid-lowering treatment with atorvastatin (resulting in a 46% reduction in the mean serum LDL cholesterol level to 2.0 mmol/l (77 mg/dl)) had ischaemic events, as compared with 37 (21%) of the patients who underwent angioplasty (who had an 18% reduction in the mean serum LDL-C level, to 3.0 mmol/l (119 mg/dl)). The incidence of ischaemic events was thus 36% lower in the atorvastatin group over an 18-month period (p = 0.048). This reduction in events was due to a smaller number of angioplasty procedures, CABG operations, and hospitalizations for worsening angina. Due to concerns over the safety of patients not undergoing PCI as the initial treatment, two interim analyses were performed using the O'Brien–Fleming stopping rule. Consequently, the significance level for the final analysis of the incidence of ischaemic events was adjusted from 5% to 4.5%. Thus, the result for the study's primary end point was not deemed to be statistically significant. Nevertheless, this represents an important study since, as compared with the patients who were treated with angioplasty and usual care, the patients who received atorvastatin had a significantly longer time to the first ischaemic event (p = 0.03).

Limitations

The second Randomized Intervention Treatment of Angina trial showed that the three-year cumulative incidence of death or non-fatal MI was greater in those undergoing PCI as compared with those on medical therapy (6.3% vs. 3.3%). Thus, the selection of a PCI-based strategy as the control therapy in patients with minimal (if any) myocardial ischaemia could be criticized for inherently biasing the study toward a positive result for medical therapy, with or without aggressive lipid lowering. The benefits of statin therapy may also have been exaggerated by the use of less-than-standard medical therapy. For example, less than 70% of the patients in the study received beta-adrenergic antagonists, an important therapy for angina and CAD. More importantly, less than 50% received antiplatelet therapy, an effective preventive therapy against cardiac events for patients with angina. By today's standards, the study also tended to use outdated PCI techniques and only a small proportion of patients received intracoronary stenting and platelet glycoprotein IIb/IIIa receptor blockade. Long-term outcome studies always tend to be criticized for not using the most up-to-date therapies, but the irony is that by the time the 'modern' therapies undergo the proof of long-term outcomes, they themselves are no longer contemporary.

As was the case for RITA-2, these results do not provide evidence with regard to the importance of angioplasty in those with severe symptoms and/or those at high cardiovascular risk. However, as has now been proven, aggressive lowering of lipid levels complements angioplasty in such patients particularly by stabilizing untreated lesions (Patti *et al.*, 2007). The follow-up period was relatively short at 18 months. It is improbable that a longer follow-up would have uncovered a benefit of angioplasty in comparison with medical therapy. The authors highlight the serial angiographic studies which have shown that MI occurs most often in lesions that originally appear to be haemodynamically unimportant and that would therefore not be subject to angioplasty.

Conclusion

The authors concluded that aggressive lipid-lowering therapy with atorvastatin is as effective as PCI followed by usual care in reducing the frequency of ischaemic events in low-risk patients who have been referred for revascularization.

Learning points

◆ Low-risk patients compliant with optimal medical therapy (OMT) may choose to defer revascularization until symptoms worsen or exercise performance deteriorates to the extent that it interferes with the quality of life, without any apparent adverse effect on morbidity or mortality.

Further reading

- LaRosa JC, Grundy SM, Waters DD, *et al.* Treating to New Targets (TNT) Investigators. Intensive lipid lowering with atorvastatin in patients with stable coronary disease. *N Engl J Med* 2005; 352: 1425–35.
- Patti G, Pasceri V, Colonna G, *et al.* Atorvastatin pre-treatment improves outcomes in patients with acute coronary syndromes undergoing early percutaneous coronary intervention: results of the ARMYDA-ACS randomized trial. *J Am Coll Cardiol* 2007; 49: 1272–8.

The Trial of Invasive versus Medical therapy in Elderly patients with chronic symptomatic coronary-artery disease (TIME)

The TIME investigators. Trial of invasive versus medical therapy in elderly patients with chronic symptomatic coronary-artery disease (TIME): a randomised trial. *Lancet* 2001; 358: 951–7.

Background

For patients with symptomatic chronic coronary-artery disease, revascularization therapy had already been shown to improve symptoms as well as survival among high-risk subsets. However, since these data had been based almost exclusively on middle-aged populations, it may not have been applicable to elderly patients. Indeed, only 6.7% of 719,922 patients enrolled in 593 published trials of ACS from 1966 to 2000 were 75 years or older, despite an increased risk of mortality and disability from revascularization procedures in this population. Elderly patients were known to have an increased risk of several of the complications of acute MI, such as congestive heart failure, cardiogenic shock, myocardial rupture, hypotension, and arrhythmias. More than a third of the total healthcare expenditure was, and continues to be, spent on individuals over the age of 75 years. In view of such public health costs and an increasingly ageing population, the TIME investigators were commended for addressing the debate on relevant management strategies in elderly patients with symptomatic CAD.

Methods

Pfisterer and colleagues performed a prospective, randomized, multi-centre study in 301 patients aged 75 years or older with angina pectoris of CCS class II or more despite treatment with at least two anti-anginal drugs. On the basis of their clinical presentation, patients were randomized to either optimum pharmacological therapy consisting of an increase in anti-ischaemic drugs and drug doses, or an invasive strategy of left-heart catheterization followed by either PCI or CABG surgery, which was undertaken for 74% of patients (54% percutaneous intervention, 20% bypass grafting). Of note, angiography was performed before randomization.

Results

After six months, severity of angina decreased and measures of quality of life increased in both treatment groups (p <0.01). However, these improvements in the combined primary end point were significantly greater for those in the revascularization group. Death, non-fatal MI, or hospital admission for acute coronary syndrome with or without the need for revascularization occurred in 49% of the medical group and in 19% of the invasive group (p <0·0001). The rate of major adverse cardiac events, a secondary end point, was elevated in patients given pharmacological therapy, mainly because of a need for revascularization; 46% of patients in this group underwent revascularization during the first 12 months for symptoms refractory to pharmacotherapy. While there was a trend towards an increased early mortality at six months in the invasive group as compared with the medical group (8.4% vs. 4.1%) this result did not reach statistical significance and the study was not powered to detect such a difference. After four years of follow-up, patients who had been revascularized within the first year of the study had a significantly improved long-term survival compared with those on drug therapy (76% vs. 46%, p < 0.01).

Limitations

The investigators use the term 'optimized medical therapy' but no evidence is included to show that this was achieved. As with almost all of these studies, since masking of therapy was not possible, any superiority of PCI compared to medical therapy as an anti-anginal strategy may at least in part be due to the placebo effect.

Conclusions

Revascularization was associated with improvements in quality of life and a lower frequency of events in the composite end point than medical therapy. Thus, despite their high-risk profile, patients over 75 years should be offered invasive evaluation and coronary revascularization procedures as clinically indicated. One reason to withhold revascularization to elderly patients is the increased risk of such procedures in this population. The TIME data confirmed there is an appreciable risk in the elderly population undergoing PCI, but it was lower than had been expected. Intervention-related mortality was far lower (2.5%) than noted in previous registries. A six-month mortality of 8.4% in the invasive group was low given that about half the cardiac deaths occurred in patients unsuitable for revascularization.

Learning points

- Patients aged 75 years or older suffering with angina refractory to standard medical therapy benefit from both optimized medical and revascularization strategies in terms of symptom relief and quality of life.
- Symptomatic elderly patients at high cardiovascular risk should be offered an invasive assessment, although they need to be counselled on the small peri-interventional mortality hazard.

The Medicine, Angioplasty, or Surgery Study (MASS II) trial

Hueb W, Soares PR, Gersh BJ, César LA, Luz PL, Puig LB, Martinez EM, Oliveira SA, Ramires JA. The medicine, angioplasty, or surgery study (MASS II): a randomized, controlled clinical trial of three therapeutic strategies for multivessel coronary-artery disease: one-year results. *J Am Coll Cardiol* 2004; 43: 1743–51.

Background

Trials from the 1970s had clearly demonstrated that CABG reduced mortality in patients with extensive coronary-artery disease which included significant obstruction of the left main coronary-artery, triple-vessel CAD and left ventricular systolic dysfunction, and two-vessel CAD plus proximal left anterior descending coronary artery stenosis (the VA Cooperative Study of patients with chronic stable angina, the European Coronary Surgery Study, and CASS). By the turn of the century, however, the use of PCI was increasing more rapidly than CABG despite a lack of conclusive evidence regarding its superiority to modern pharmacological therapy alone or surgical approaches. This study sought to address the question of whether PCI or CABG offers any advantage over medical therapy in patients with stable angina and multi-vessel disease.

Methods

In the MASS II trial, 611 patients with multi-vessel CAD and stable angina of CCS class II–III or stress ischaemia, or both, were randomly assigned to CABG surgery, PCI, or medical therapy. The primary end point was cardiac mortality, Q-wave MI, or refractory angina necessitating revascularization.

Results

In this single-site study, the authors demonstrated a statistically significant lower rate of one-year mortality in the medical therapy group (1.5%), whereas the death rates for the PCI (4.5%) and CABG surgery (4.0%) groups were comparable. At 12 months, the frequency of the primary end point was significantly different (p <0.0001) across the three groups: 7% for CABG, 12% for medical therapy, and 14% for PCI. After five years, the primary end point occurred in 21% of patients assigned to CABG, 33% to PCI, and 36% to pharmacological therapy (p = 0.0026), with no significant difference in mortality rates among the three groups. However, only 55% of patients on medical therapy were free from angina after five years, compared with 74% after CABG and 71% after PCI (p <0.001). At ten years, there was no significant difference in the survival rates between groups (74.9% with CABG, 75.1% with PCI, and 69% with medical therapy (p = 0.089)) although the ten-year rates of freedom from angina did reach significance and were 64% with CABG, 59% with PCI, and 43% with medical therapy (p <0.001).

Limitations

First, the number of patients in each study group was small, about 200 each, which limited the observed event rates. Second, as in any trial of this type, blinding is difficult such that biases could influence end points such as angina or the indication for a subsequent revascularization procedure. Third, patients were enrolled at a single centre and the quality of treatments offered elsewhere may differ. Finally, medical therapy may not have been as aggressive as currently advised. A major strength of the study, however, was the completeness of follow-up, which was 100% for vital status, a critically important feature of a trial when differences in survival were observed.

Conclusions

At ten years, compared with CABG, medical therapy was associated with a significantly higher incidence of subsequent MI, a higher rate of additional revascularization, a higher incidence of cardiac death, and consequently a 2.3-fold increased risk of combined events. In addition, CABG was better than medical therapy at reducing angina. Findings from the ten-year follow-up report were similar to those reported at five years. At both intervals the composite end point favoured CABG, primarily due to differences in rates of subsequent revascularization. The rate of subsequent revascularization was lowest among patients with CABG (<10%) and similar (about 40%) in patients with PCI and medical therapy. Stroke was relatively infrequent, but appeared highest among patients with CABG (8.4%). Importantly, no difference across the three treatment arms for total mortality was noted at either time point.

Learning points

♦ In patients with extensive multi-vessel disease, CABG compared with medical therapy alone, appears to be associated with a significantly lower incidence of subsequent MI, a lower rate of additional revascularization, and a lower incidence of cardiac death.

Further reading

● Hueb W, Lopes NH, Gersh BJ, Soares PR, Machado LA, Jatene FB, Oliveira SA, Ramires JA. Five-year follow-up of the Medicine, Angioplasty, or Surgery Study (MASS II): a randomized controlled clinical trial of 3 therapeutic strategies for multivessel coronary-artery disease. *Circulation* 2007; 115: 1082–1089.
● Hueb W, Lopes NH, Gersh BJ, Soares PR, Ribeiro EE, Pereira AC, Favarato D, Rocha AS, Hueb AC, Ramires JA. Ten-year follow-up of survival of the Medicine, Angioplasty, or Surgery Study (MASS II): a randomized controlled clinical trial of three therapeutic strategies for multi-vessel coronary-artery disease. *Circulation* 2010; 122: 949–957.

The Swiss Interventional Study on Silent Ischemia type II (SWISSI II) trial

Erne P, Schoenenberger AW, Burckhardt D, Zuber M, Kiowski W, Buser PT, Dubach P, Resink TJ, Pfisterer M. Effects of percutaneous coronary interventions in silent ischaemia after myocardial infarction: the (SWISSI II) randomized controlled trial. *JAMA* 2007; 297: 1985–91.

Background

The presence of silent ischaemia had already been shown to predict an adverse prognosis after MI, CABG, and PCI with or without stenting. However, the effect of PCI on the long-term prognosis of patients with silent ischaemia post-MI was unknown and it was not known whether PCI in addition to secondary preventive measures was superior to anti-ischaemic drug therapy in such patients.

Methods

Patients with a documented, first STEMI or non-ST-segment elevation MI (NSTEMI) within the preceding three months were eligible for enrolment. They had to undergo a maximal symptom-limited exercise test without chest pain and have significant ST depression as a sign of silent ischaemia. Silent ischaemia was subsequently confirmed by stress myocardial perfusion scintigraphy in 98 patients, stress echocardiography in 91 patients, and stress radionuclide angiography in 12 patients. Patients with any angina or three-vessel disease were excluded. Patients with verified silent ischaemia underwent diagnostic coronary angiography. If they had one or two-vessel CAD suitable for PCI, they were randomized to balloon angioplasty (PCI group; n = 96) or medical management (intensive anti-ischaemic drug therapy group; n = 105). Percutaneous coronary intervention (according to standard techniques but without stents during that period) was performed with the aim of attaining full revascularization without residual coronary stenoses of more than 75%. Anti-ischaemic drug therapy consisted of either 5–10 mg/d of bisoprolol, 5–10 mg/d of amlodipine, 4–12 mg of molsidomine twice daily, or combinations thereof, aiming to eliminate or maximally reduce silent ischaemia during bicycle ergometry. Angiotensin converting enzyme inhibitors were recommended as an antihypertensive drug therapy. In addition, *both* patient groups received secondary preventive advice regarding weight control, eating habits, smoking cessation, daily exercise, and were treated with 100 mg/d of aspirin and a statin.

Results

The primary end point, survival free of major adverse cardiac events (defined as cardiac death, non-fatal (recurrent) MI, and/or symptom-driven revascularization (PCI or CABG)) was significantly better in the PCI group compared with the drug therapy group over a ten-year, follow-up (p <0.001). In addition, in patients treated with PCI, the frequency of objective ischaemia during repeated stress testing, was significantly lower throughout the entire study period than it was for patients on drug therapy.

Limitations

This study enrolled patients who were in the recovery phase of an MI and it is, therefore, inappropriate to generalize the results to all patients with chronic stable angina. Further, ACE inhibitors were recommended to treat hypertension and heart failure but were not administered routinely to all patients despite this history of MI. The HOPE trial was published in 2000 long after the protocol had been originally developed. Neither was any stenting performed as part of PCI therapy. Thus, as is often the case in studies with long-term follow-up, by the end of the study the protocol had effectively become outdated following the publication of new available evidence. Nevertheless, at the end of the SWISSI II study period, 42 patients in the medical treatment group and 41 patients in the angioplasty group were receiving an ACE inhibitor or angiotensin II receptor blocker.

Conclusions

This was the first long-term outcome study of an invasive therapy compared with an intensive anti-ischaemic drug therapy in asymptomatic patients with silent ischaemia after a recent MI. In patients with one or two-vessel CAD, with silent ischaemia verified by stress imaging following a recent MI, PCI reduced the long-term rate of major adverse cardiac events and mortality compared with pharmacological therapy. It also reduced signs of exercise ischaemia, the need for anti-ischaemic therapy, and follow-up revascularizations.

<table>
<tr><td>

Learning points

◆ In those patients with residual reversible ischaemia in the immediate aftermath of an MI, PCI is warranted for one or two-vessel disease above and beyond intensive medical therapy alone.

</td></tr>
</table>

Further reading

- Schoenenberger AW, Kobza R, Jamshidi P, *et al.* Sudden cardiac death in patients with silent myocardial ischemia after myocardial infarction (from the Swiss Interventional Study on Silent Ischemia Type II [SWISSI II]). *Am J Cardiol* 2009; 104: 158–163. This study showed that the prevention of residual myocardial ischaemia and recurrent MI using PCI resulted in better long-term left ventricular function and a reduced incidence of sudden cardiac death.

The Clinical Outcomes Utilizing Revascularization and Aggressive drug Evaluation (COURAGE) trial

Boden WE, O'Rourke RA, Teo KK, Hartigan PM, Maron DJ, Kostuk WJ, Knudtson M, Dada M, Casperson P, Harris CL, Chaitman BR, Shaw L, Gosselin G, Nawaz S, Title LM, Gau G, Blaustein AS, Booth DC, Bates ER, Spertus JA, Berman DS, Mancini GB, Weintraub WS; COURAGE Trial Research Group. Optimal medical therapy with or without PCI for stable coronary disease. *N Engl J Med* 2007; 356: 1503–16.

Background

Percutaneous coronary intervention had been clearly shown to reduce the incidence of death and MI in patients presenting with acute coronary syndromes, although a similar benefit had not been shown in patients with stable CAD. Nevertheless, the issue of a possible benefit of revascularization in stable CAD remained hotly debated as there had been a number of limitations in earlier randomized trials. First, this issue had been studied in fewer than 3000 patients in total, many of whom had been treated in the pre-stenting era and with less aggressive standards of medical management than were now accepted as routine. Earlier studies had been designed to compare revascularization versus optimized medical therapy, which does not accurately describe an appropriate standard therapy. In clinical practice, any intervention would be carried out in a background of aggressive medical therapy. Thus, to truly determine the incremental benefit of revascularization over medical therapy alone, revascularization had to proceed on top of optimized medical therapy rather than as an independent entity. Finally, 'conventional medical therapy' had often been relegated to the routine discretion of the supervising physician rather than being implemented via a protocol driven, robust strategy that actively involved healthcare professionals to achieve nationally recognized targets for secondary prevention. The Clinical Outcomes Utilizing Revascularization and Aggressive Drug Evaluation trial was designed as a much larger-scale RCT to determine whether PCI coupled with optimal medical therapy reduced the risk of death and non-fatal MI in patients with stable CAD, as compared with optimal medical therapy alone.

Methods

The Clinical Outcomes Utilizing Revascularization and Aggressive Drug Evaluation trial included 2287 patients with stable angina or ischaemia and coronary anatomy appropriate for PCI. Patients with persistent severe angina (CCS grade IV), a positive stress test, severe left ventricular failure, extensive CAD not suitable for PCI and those in need of urgent PCI were excluded. However, those in whom initial CCS class IV angina subsequently stabilized medically were included. The study population had a mean age of 62 years and overall baseline characteristics were consistent with at least an intermediate-risk profile for cardiac events. All patients underwent angiography before being randomized to undergo PCI and optimal medical therapy (PCI group), or OMT alone (medical-therapy group). Optimal medical therapy in both groups included a beta blocker, amlodipine, and isosorbide mononitrate, alone or in combination, along with either lisinopril or losartan as standard secondary prevention. All patients received aggressive therapy to lower LDL-C and triglyceride levels and increase HDL levels to pre-specified target levels using simvastatin, ezetimibe, extended-release niacin, or fibrates, alone or in combination. In patients undergoing PCI, target-lesion revascularization was always attempted, and complete revascularization was performed as clinically appropriate.

Results

The primary composite end point of all cause death or non-fatal MI did not differ between the two treatment arms over a mean follow-up of 4.6 years (p = 0.62). When analysed independently, all-cause mortality for PCI plus medical therapy was 5.9% as compared with 6.5% for medical therapy alone (p = 0.38). The prespecified secondary end point of the cumulative cardiovascular event rate of death, MI, or stroke also failed to show statistical significance (20% in the PCI plus medical therapy group versus 19.5% in the medical therapy alone; p = 0.62) and neither was there a significant difference in the rate of hospitalization for ACS or MI. In patients who received PCI, however, the secondary end point of freedom from angina was significantly higher at up to three years (p <0.005). In addition, follow-up revascularizations were needed less frequently during the first 12 months (p <0.001), and anti-ischaemic therapy could be reduced significantly throughout the study.

A later subgroup analysis of 264 high risk patients (Shaw et al., 2008) showed OMT alone did not increase long-term mortality or rates of MI, but it was associated with a high rate of cross-over to revascularization (30% within 12 months). Importantly, patients with greater than 10% residual ischaemia on stress perfusion imaging had a higher rate of death or MI than did those without ischaemia (p <0.001) suggesting a key role of imaging in the risk stratification of patients with a higher ischaemic burden.

Conclusions

Overall these data support the concept that in patients with stable CAD, there is no clear benefit of early PCI strategy over OMT alone in terms of hard clinical end points, including mortality, non-fatal MI, or cumulative major cardiovascular events.

Learning points

♦ As an initial management strategy in patients with stable CAD, PCI did not reduce the risk of death, MI, or other major cardiovascular events when added to OMT.

♦ In symptomatic angina patients with chronic stable angina, however, PCI appears to reduce the need for escalating anti-anginal drug therapy and the need for subsequent revascularizations.

♦ Those patients with a high ischaemic burden on stress perfusion scintigraphy (>10%) warrant timely intervention to prevent early mortality.

Further reading

● Maron DJ, Boden WE, O'Rourke RA, et al.; COURAGE Trial Research Group. Intensive multifactorial intervention for stable coronary-artery disease: optimal medical therapy in the COURAGE (Clinical Outcomes Utilizing Revascularization and Aggressive Drug Evaluation) trial. *J Am Coll Cardiol.* 2010; 55: 1348–58.

● Shaw LJ, Berman DS, Maron DJ, et al. Optimal medical therapy with or without percutaneous coronary intervention to reduce ischemic burden: results from the Clinical Outcomes Utilizing Revascularization and Aggressive Drug Evaluation (COURAGE) trial nuclear substudy. *Circulation.* 2008; 117: 1283–91.

● Teo KK, Sedlis SP, Boden WE, et al.; COURAGE Trial Investigators. Optimal medical therapy with or without percutaneous coronary intervention in older patients with stable coronary disease: a pre-specified subset analysis of the COURAGE (Clinical Outcomes Utilizing Revascularization and Aggressive druG Evaluation) trial. *J Am Coll Cardiol.* 2009; 54: 1303–8.

The Bypass Angioplasty Revascularization Investigation 2 Diabetes (BARI 2D) trial

BARI 2D Study Group, Frye RL, August P, Brooks MM, Hardison RM, Kelsey SF, MacGregor JM, Orchard TJ, Chaitman BR, Genuth SM, Goldberg SH, Hlatky MA, Jones TL, Molitch ME, Nesto RW, Sako EY, Sobel B. A randomized trial of therapies for type 2 diabetes and coronary-artery disease. *N Engl J Med* 2009; 360: 2503–15.

Background

The prevalence of diabetes in the western world is ever increasing and expected to double by 2030. Insulin resistance is established as a major determinant of accelerated CAD and its complications. Meanwhile, the advent of insulin sensitizers has enabled clinicians to begin targeting insulin resistance as treatment, as well as hyperglycaemia and dyslipidaemia. Patients with type 2 diabetes mellitus (T2DM) are known to have worse outcomes following PCI and CABG as compared with non-diabetic patients. All of these issues led to the initiation of the Bypass Angioplasty Revascularization Investigation 2 Diabetes (BARI 2D) trial, designed to specifically investigate patients with T2DM and assess whether early revascularization, either in the form of PCI or CABG, reduced mortality and morbidity in patients whose cardiac symptoms were mild and stable. It also sought to determine whether treatment targeted to attenuate insulin resistance could arrest or retard progression of CAD compared with treatment targeted to the same level of glycaemic control with an insulin-providing approach.

Methods

The trial included patients with type 2 diabetes mellitus and documented stable CAD who were eligible for elective PCI or CABG (≥50% stenosis of a major epicardial coronary artery associated with a positive stress test or ≥70% stenosis of a major epicardial coronary artery and classic angina). Over 80% of patients had mild to moderate angina of CCS class I–II. Patients with left main coronary-artery disease, those in need of immediate revascularization, dyspnoea of NYHA classification III or IV were excluded. Patients were randomized to either prompt revascularization (either PCI or CABG depending on the referring physician's preference) combined with medical therapy, or to medical therapy alone.

Results

Of the 2368 patients enrolled, 1176 patients were randomly assigned to the revascularization arm (approximately two-thirds of which underwent PCI and one-third CABG) and 1192 to the medical therapy arm. The primary end point of all-cause mortality after five years did not significantly differ between the two treatment arms (p = 0.97), nor did survival free from MI or stroke (p = 0.70). Consistent with the findings from COURAGE, when analysed separately according to the type of revascularization, patients who underwent PCI plus medical therapy had the same rates of all-cause mortality and major adverse cardiovascular events as the medical therapy alone group. In the CABG group, there was no significant difference in overall mortality compared with the medical therapy group, but there were fewer major cardiovascular events (22.4% vs. 30.5%; p = 0.01), driven mainly by the reduced number of non-fatal MIs. In addition, there was no significant difference between the insulin sensitization and insulin provision groups with respect to rates of death and cardiovascular events at five years (p = 0.89 and 0.13, respectively).

Limitations

Despite large numbers of patients, in view of the low mortality rate in patients with stable CAD, much of the opposition to this trial has accused it of being underpowered. It is also worth noting that 42% of patients originally in the medical therapy arm crossed over and underwent subsequent revascularization. Only one-third of patients in the PCI stratum who were assigned to undergo revascularization received a drug eluting stent, which may have masked some of the potential benefit of 'contemporary' PCI. Patients selected to undergo CABG rather than PCI were a higher-risk group with much higher event rates leading to considerable entry bias. Indeed, it is worth remembering that this study was designed to compare coronary revascularization with intensive medical therapy, not CABG with PCI.

Conclusions

These findings suggest that in diabetic patients with stable CAD, upfront PCI in addition to aggressive medical therapy does not confer an incremental benefit in terms of all-cause mortality or the composite of major cardiovascular events. It is also suggested from subset analysis that early CABG, although it did not reduce mortality, significantly reduced the rate of non-fatal MI compared with an initial medical therapy approach.

Learning points

- In diabetic patients with stable CAD, there is no significant difference in the rates of death and major cardiovascular events between those undergoing prompt revascularization and those undergoing medical therapy.
- Revascularization of diabetic patients with stable CAD should be considered for patients with severe or refractory symptoms despite a trial of medical therapy.
- In higher-risk diabetic patients with extensive CAD early CABG appears to offer additional benefits to intensive medical therapy alone.

Further reading

- Chaitman BR, Hardison RM, Adler D, *et al.*; Bypass Angioplasty Revascularization Investigation 2 Diabetes (BARI 2D) Study Group. The Bypass Angioplasty Revascularization Investigation 2 Diabetes randomized trial of different treatment strategies in type 2 diabetes mellitus with stable ischaemic heart disease: impact of treatment strategy on cardiac mortality and myocardial infarction. *Circulation* 2009; 120: 2529–40.

- Maron DJ, Boden WE, Spertus JA, *et al.*; COURAGE Trial Research Group. Impact of metabolic syndrome and diabetes on prognosis and outcomes with early percutaneous coronary intervention in the COURAGE (Clinical Outcomes Utilizing Revascularization and Aggressive Drug Evaluation) trial. *J Am Coll Cardiol* 2011; 58: 131–7. The addition of early PCI to optimal medical therapy did not significantly reduce the risk of death or MI regardless of the presence of metabolic syndrome or diabetic status.

Conclusion

It is to the credit of the cardiovascular community that the development of new therapies such as CABG, fibrinolytic therapy, coronary angioplasty and the implantable cardiovertor defibrillator have all been closely followed by well-designed trials. We have, therefore, had the luxury of an abundant amount of data upon which to build evidence-based approaches to treatment, and there is no reason to believe that this trend will not continue into the future.

In regard to revascularization versus medical therapy the National Heart, Lung, and Blood Institute (NHLBI) sponsored ISCHEMIA trial, which is just beginning, is pivotal. Patients will be enrolled after a stress test demonstrating significant ischaemia to a strategy of optimal medical therapy alone or optimal medical therapy and angiography with a view to coronary revascularization. This trial could answer the crucial question as to whether patients with mild to moderate stable angina but moderate to severe ischaemia, will fare better with revascularization in regard to survival, but the answer is several years away.

The SYNTAX trial is nearing its final year of follow-up, and this has been helpful by stratifying patients using the SYNTAX score, which is a measure of anatomic complexity, into subsets of risks. Approximately two-thirds of patients with left main coronary and three-vessel disease fall into higher risk subsets which clearly benefit from CABG surgery, and in the tercile of lowest risk, PCI, however, seems a reasonable option. It is unlikely that this score will be useful, however, in decisions regarding PCI and medical therapy.

Another area which is rapidly evolving is that of plaque characterization based upon fractional flow reserve, intravascular ultrasound, optical coherence tomography, and cardiac magnetic resonance among other technologies. We are moving away from the angiographic definition of stenosis severity, and it is clearly conceivable that we will see trials of PCI versus medical therapy targeted towards 'future culprits' based upon the characterization of plaques and not their stenotic severity as defined angiographically. Small studies are ongoing, which should shape the design of future large trials. Whether some of these techniques will be integrated into the SYNTAX anatomic score so as to develop an anatomic/functional, plaque characteristic score is uncertain.

In diabetics, the largest ongoing trial is Future Revascularization Evaluation in Patients with Diabetes Mellitus: Optimal Management of Multi-vessel Disease (FREEDOM), which is comparing drug-eluting stents versus bypass surgery on the hard end points of death and MI. It should be emphasized that in this trial, patients were enrolled after angiography and as such there was both clinical and anatomic equipoise, and the extent to which these data will be generalizable to the population at large is uncertain, pending publication.

It is unlikely that another trial of revascularization versus medical therapy in patients with left main coronary-artery disease will ever be performed, even though the original subset from the Veterans Administration cooperative study was only 91 patients. The key question here is what will be the future role of PCI versus CABG in left main coronary-artery disease. The ongoing EXCEL trial of 3600 patients (G. Stone personal communication) will be the key to answering this question.

An area that is less amenable to clinical trials but of great importance is the appropriateness of performing revascularization as determined by stress testing and other imaging modalities. Appropriateness criteria suggests that in acute coronary syndromes, PCI in the United States has been performed appropriately in the vast majority, but there is certainly room for improvement in patients with chronic coronary-artery disease.

Nonetheless, appropriateness criteria only look at one side of the spectrum and do not address the issue of *underutilization* of therapy. What is of concern are data from the United States and Europe that demonstrate a marked variability among regions in regard to the performance of coronary angiography, PCI, CABG, stress testing, and functional imaging. Many of the factors which determine utilization appear to be unrelated to disease severity, that is, race, socioeconomic status, age, number of catheterization facilities per size of the population, etc. It is also difficult to determine 'optimal' utilization rates. Nonetheless, we are in an era in which the cost of healthcare is of major concern around the world, and resource allocation has to balance the demands and attractions of new technology with the potential rewards and costs of primary and secondary prevention.

In summary, the last few decades have been a triumph for proponents of evidence-based practice in cardiovascular diseases. The onus of responsibility to practice in this fashion and to follow the guidelines is on our shoulders as cardiovascular healthcare providers, and it is intrinsic to our credibility as a profession. It would be a tragedy if it is felt that we are relinquishing the responsibility and if the decisions were driven by payers and not by ourselves.

Reference

1. Brown ML, Gersh BJ, Holmes DR, Bailey KR, Sundt TM III. From randomized trials to registry studies: translating data into clinical information. *Nature Clinical Practice Cardiovascular Medicine* 2008; 5: 613–20.

Chapter 6

Percutaneous coronary intervention

Dr Nalyaka Sambu and Professor Nicholas Curzen

Introduction

Over the past three decades, there have been major advances in the field of interventional cardiology that have revolutionized the treatment of coronary heart disease (CHD). Grüentzig and Myler performed the first coronary angioplasty in 1977 and, since then, the practice of percutaneous coronary intervention (PCI) has undergone a dramatic transformation brought about by:

◆ the transition from balloon angioplasty to drug eluting stents.
◆ the use of adjunctive techniques during PCI such as the pressure wire, intravascular ultrasound, rotablator, laser, and the manual aspiration catheter.
◆ the redundancy of thrombolytic therapy and its replacement with primary PCI as the gold-standard treatment for ST-elevation myocardial infarction (STEMI).
◆ a shift in focus away from PCI driven by angiographic lesion severity towards ischaemia-driven intervention instead.

◆ the development and widespread use of more potent and effective antiplatelet and antithrombotic agents, including more rigorous therapeutic regimes.
◆ the role of PCI as first line revascularization strategy in patients with more complex coronary disease who would have traditionally undergone coronary artery bypass surgery.

The vast body of clinical research in interventional cardiology over the years has led to a significant expansion in the envelope of patients referred and accepted for PCI due to significant improvements in techniques, devices, and adjunctive pharmacotherapy. This chapter describes some of the truly landmark papers in the field of interventional cardiology that have had a clinical impact on our everyday practice. Of note, we have not specifically discussed landmark studies comparing PCI versus coronary artery bypass surgery as this is discussed in detail in Chapter 7.

Primary angioplasty versus intravenous thrombolytic therapy for acute myocardial infarction: a quantitative review of 23 randomized trials

Keeley EC, Boura JA, Grines CL. *Lancet* 2003; 36: 13–20.

Background

Large, randomized, placebo-controlled trials conducted in the 1980s to investigate the beneficial effects of thrombolytic therapy in acute STEMI unequivocally showed that prompt restoration of coronary blood flow salvages myocardium, reduces infarct size, and improves survival. Immediate thrombolysis thus became the standard of care in suitable patients with STEMI. However, there were shortcomings of thrombolysis, which included failure to achieve infarct-related artery (IRA) patency in up to 20% of cases, serious bleeding complications such as fatal intracerebral haemorrhage, and recurrent ischaemia. These limitations led to a growing interest in the role of immediate angioplasty as an alternative reperfusion strategy in STEMI patients.

A large number of randomized trials comparing short and long-term benefits of thrombolysis versus primary angioplasty in acute STEMI rapidly emerged. Whilst almost universally positive in favour of PCI, particularly in terms of reduced re-infarction rates, demonstration of mortality benefit remained elusive. Keeley and colleagues provided a quantitative analysis of 23 such studies. This paper galvanized the primary PCI movement.

Methods

Data from 23 trials comparing primary angioplasty versus thrombolytic therapy in patients with acute STEMI were analysed. Eligibility criteria differed between studies but typically included ischaemic symptoms associated with either ST-segment elevation of at least 1 mm in two contiguous leads or left bundle branch block on ECG, and no contraindications to thrombolytic treatment. The following outcomes were compared based on an intention-to-treat analysis: death, non-fatal reinfarction, stroke, recurrent ischaemia and major bleeding. *Short-term* follow-up was defined as 4–6 weeks and *long-term* follow-up was defined as 6–18 months. Subgroup analyses were undertaken to assess the effect on clinical outcome of (1) the specific thrombolytic regimen used, and (2) the strategy of emergent hospital transfer for primary angioplasty compared with on-site thrombolysis.

Results

In total, 7739 patients were randomly assigned to either primary angioplasty (n = 3872) or thrombolytic therapy (n = 3867). Most patients assigned to thrombolysis received a fibrin-specific agent (76%), stents were used in 12 trials, and glycoprotein IIb/IIIa inhibitors were used in 8. The criterion for time to treatment was ≤ 6 hours in 9 trials, 12 hours in 13 trials and up to 36 hours in 1 trial (Should We Emergently Revascularize Occluded Coronaries for Cardiogenic Shock (SHOCK) study). Overall, primary angioplasty was more effective than thrombolysis at reducing mortality (7% vs. 9%, p = 0.0002), non-fatal re-infarction (3% vs. 7%, p <0.0001), stroke (1% vs. 2%, p = 0.0004) and the combined end point of death, non-fatal re-infarction, and stroke (8% vs. 14%, p <0.0001). These results were consistent at both short and long-term follow-up and were irrespective of thrombolytic agent used and whether or not reperfusion was delayed because of transfer to another hospital for primary angioplasty.

Limitations

There were inevitable differences among the individual trials with regards to study design, patient population, and time to treatment, which should be taken into consideration when interpreting the data. For example, the SHOCK study specifically enrolled high risk patients in cardiogenic shock and was therefore not representative of the wider patient population. Furthermore, 11 out of the 23 studies used balloon angioplasty alone without stents, 15 did not use glycoprotein IIb/IIIa inhibitors, and none used thrombectomy. This is not representative of current day practice.

Conclusions and clinical implications

Primary angioplasty is the most effective reperfusion strategy in acute STEMI. The Keeley *et al.* paper revealed a mortality benefit, as well as significant reduction in re-infarction and stroke compared with thrombolysis. The results are tempered by the fact that studies of fibrinolysis were not always contemporary (i.e. absent angiographic follow-up) and the differences between strategies were less robust when fibrin-specific studies alone were compared. With recent improvements in PCI technique and the expansion of dedicated and experienced heart attack centres, thrombolytic treatment is already redundant in many areas of the UK and Europe as a whole.

Learning points

◆ Primary angioplasty is the gold-standard treatment in acute STEMI.
◆ Timely angioplasty results in more effective restoration of vessel patency, less re-occlusion and better clinical outcome compared with thrombolytic treatment.

Further reading

● de Boer SP, Barnes EH, Westerhout CM, *et al.* High-risk patients with ST-elevation myocardial infarction derive greatest absolute benefit from primary percutaneous coronary intervention: Results from the Primary Coronary Angioplasty Trialist versus Thrombolysis (PCAT)-2 Collaboration. *Am Heart J* 2011; 161: 500–7.
● Grines CL, Browne KF, Marco J, *et al.* for the Primary Angioplasty in Myocardial Infarction Study Group. A comparison of immediate angioplasty with thrombolytic therapy for acute myocardial infarction. *N Engl J Med* 1993; 328: 673–9.
● Weaver WD, Simes RJ, Betriu A, *et al.* Comparison of primary coronary angioplasty and intravenous thrombolytic therapy for acute myocardial infarction: a quantitative review. *JAMA* 1997; 278: 2093–8.

A comparison of coronary angioplasty with fibrinolytic therapy in acute myocardial infarction

Andersen HR, Nielsen TT, Rasmussen K, Thuesen L, Kelbaek H, Thayssen P, Abildgaard U, Pedersen F, Madsen JK, Grande P, Villadsen AB, Krusell LR, Haghfelt T, Lomholt P, Husted SE, Vigholt E, Kjaergard HK, Mortensen LS; for the DANAMI-2 Investigators. *N Engl J Med* 2003; 349: 733–42.

Background

Primary PCI is the gold standard treatment in acute STEMI. It reduces the risk of death, re-infarction, and stroke and has been shown to be superior to thrombolysis in patients admitted directly to hospitals with PCI facilities. However, clinical outcome in patients with STEMI is directly related to the time taken to receive definitive treatment. Concerns regarding the safety and feasibility of transportation of patients with STEMI from their local community or admitting hospital to the nearest PCI centre, and the inevitable associated treatment delays, was perceived to be a major limitation to the widespread implementation of primary PCI. The Danish Multicentre Randomized Study on Fibrinolytic Therapy versus Acute Coronary Angioplasty in Acute Myocardial Infarction (DANAMI-2) study investigated whether transfer of patients with acute STEMI to their nearest PCI centre, with all its logistic challenges, resulted in better clinical outcomes compared with receiving immediate on-site thrombolysis. This landmark study broke down geographical barriers and firmly established primary PCI as a safe and feasible option for STEMI patients presenting to a non-PCI centre.

Methods

A group of 1572 patients with STEMI presenting within 12 hours of symptom onset were randomly assigned to either thrombolysis with altepase (n = 782) or transfer to the nearest PCI centre (n = 790) with a target transportation time of no greater than three hours. The transfer time was defined as the time from randomization at the referral hospital to arrival in the cardiac catheterization laboratory. Patients deemed to be too high risk for transportation due to cardiogenic shock, severe heart failure, persistent life-threatening arrhythmias, or requiring mechanical ventilation were excluded. All patients received a loading dose of aspirin and the PCI group received ticlopidine or clopidogrel daily for one month. The primary end point was a composite of death from any cause, re-infarction (not including procedural related infarction), or disabling stroke at 30 days.

Results

The median transfer time was 67 minutes (interquartile range 50–85). Among those patients presenting to a non-PCI centre, the median time difference between thrombolysis and primary PCI was 55 minutes. Only 4% of patients were considered unsuitable for transfer. The primary composite end point occurred in 8% of patients in the PCI group, versus 13.7% in the thrombolysis group (p <0.001) (see Figure 6.1). This was driven by a significant reduction in re-infarction rates (1.6% vs. 6.3%; p <0.001) and 30-day mortality was significantly higher

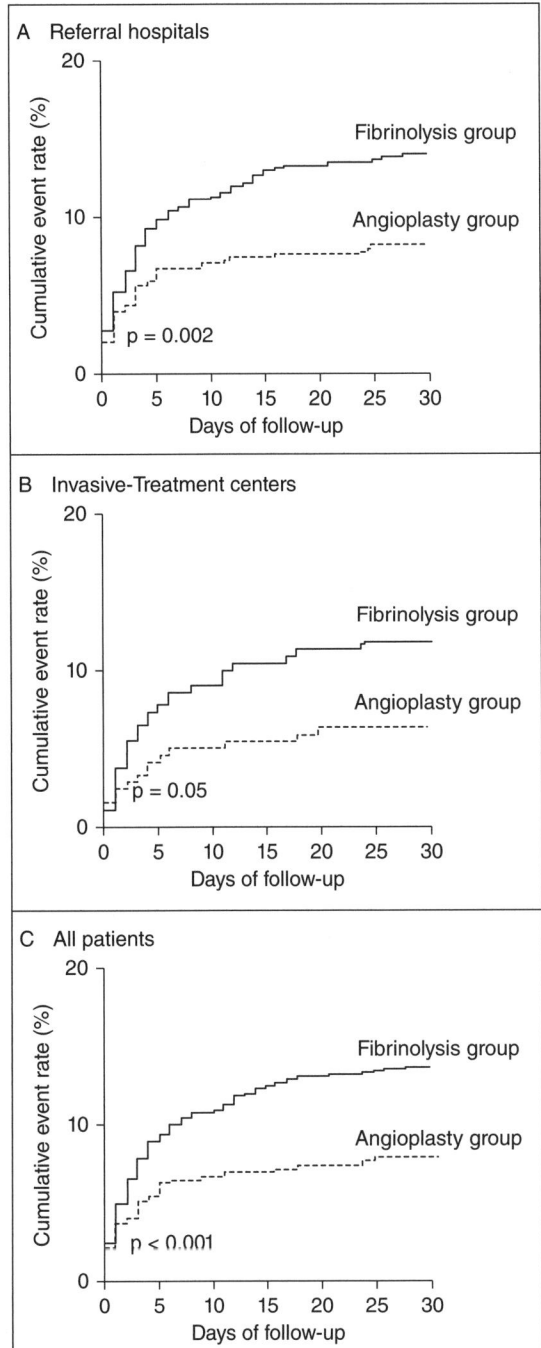

Figure 6.1 Kaplan-Meir curves showing cumulative event rates for the primary composite end point of death, clinical re-infarction, or disabling stroke during 20 days follow-up.

among patients with re-infarction. However, there was no difference in overall mortality or disabling stroke between the two treatment groups.

Limitations

In the thrombolysis group, failed reperfusion or recurrent ischaemia with ST-segment elevation was treated with repeat thrombolysis in the first instance rather than rescue PCI, which has subsequently been shown to be superior. Furthermore, in the PCI group none of the patients were pre-loaded with clopidogrel. This protocol is not consistent with current recommended evidence-based clinical guidelines.

Conclusions and clinical implications

Inter-hospital transfer of patients with acute STEMI is safe and feasible. The clinical benefit of primary PCI versus thrombolysis is maintained even if they require transportation to the nearest unit, provided the transfer takes no more than two hours. These results are consistent with findings from the PRAGUE-2 study which also showed that long distance transport (up to 120 km) for primary PCI significantly reduces major adverse cardiovascular events compared to immediate thrombolysis. These findings paved the way towards the widespread implementation of a 24-hour primary PCI service and have led to national guidance which recommends that primary PCI is the gold-standard treatment strategy in patients with acute STEMI provided it can be undertaken within two hours of first contact with the medical team.

Learning points

- Primary PCI is the gold-standard treatment for acute STEMI if offered in a timely manner.
- Inter-hospital transfer of patients with STEMI to their nearest PCI centre within two hours of call-for-help results in improved clinical outcome compared to immediate thrombolysis.

Further reading

- Department of Health. Treatment of heart attack national guidance: Final report of the National Infarct Angioplasty Project (NIAP). October 2008. http://www.dh.gov.uk/ prod_consum_dh/groups/dh_digitalassets/@dh/@en/ documents/digitalasset/dh_089454.pdf
- Van de Werf F, Bax J, Betriu A, *et al.*; ESC Committee for Practice Guidelines (CPG). Management of acute myocardial infarction in patients presenting with persistent

ST-segment elevation: the Task Force on the management of ST-segment elevation acute myocardial infarction of the European Society of Cardiology. *Eur Heart J* 2008; 29: 2909–45.

• Widimský P, Budesínský T, Vorác D, *et al.* for the 'PRAGUE' Study Group Investigators. Long distance transport for primary angioplasty vs. immediate thrombolysis in acute myocardial infarction. Final results of the randomized national multicentre trial—PRAGUE-2. *Eur Heart J* 2003; 24: 94–104.

A comparison of balloon-expandable-stent implantation with balloon angioplasty in patients with coronary artery disease

Serruys PW, de Jaegere P, Kiemeneij F, Macaya C, Rutsch W, Heyndrickx G, Emanuelsson H, Marco J, Legrand V, Materne P, Belardi J, Sigwart U, Colombo A, Goy JJ, van den Heuvel P, Delcan J, Morel MA. for the BENESTENT study group. Benestent Study Group. *N Engl J Med* 1994; 331: 489–95.

Background

Grüentzig performed the first coronary artery balloon angioplasty in 1977. The main shortcomings associated with plain old balloon angioplasty (POBA) include acute vessel closure and early re-stenosis and this is largely due to the injury introduced to the diseased arterial segment during balloon inflation. Early registry data demonstrated an incidence of acute vessel closure following balloon dilatation in the range of 4–8%, with more than 20% of patients requiring emergency coronary artery bypass surgery. Furthermore, beyond the acute complications, the observed re-stenosis rates in POBA were 30–50%. In an attempt to alleviate the high observed rates of acute vessel closure and re-stenosis, coronary artery stents were developed to provide a scaffolding that maintained arterial lumen integrity following balloon dilatation. The first human coronary stent was deployed in 1986 and seven years later, bare metal stents were subsequently approved in the United States for the treatment of acute or threatened vessel closure following failed balloon angioplasty. The Belgium Netherlands Stent Arterial Revascularization Therapies Study (BENESTENT) was a multicentre, randomized study that investigated whether coronary stent implantation improved long-term angiographic and clinical outcomes compared with POBA alone. This study changed PCI practice forever.

Methods

A total of 520 patients with stable angina and a single *de novo* lesion <15 mm in length and >3 mm in diameter in a native coronary artery were randomly assigned to either Palmaz-Schatz stent implantation (n = 262) or POBA (n = 258). Exclusion criteria included ostial lesions, bifurcation disease, a lesion within a previously grafted vessel, or suspected intracoronary thrombus. All patients received aspirin and dipyridamole for six months and the stent group were anticoagulated with warfarin in addition to dual antiplatelet therapy. The primary clinical end points included all cause death, major adverse cardiovascular events and target lesion revascularization (TLR) at seven-month follow-up. The primary angiographic end point was minimal lumen diameter at up to six months follow-up, determined by quantitative coronary angiography.

Results

Acute angiographic and procedural success rates were similar between the two groups. At seven-month follow-up, the primary clinical end point was achieved in 30% of patients in the balloon angioplasty group versus 20% of patients in the stent group (p = 0.02). The difference in primary end point was largely driven by the significant reduction in TLR in the stent group (10% vs. 21%; p = 0.001). Furthermore, the incidence of re-stenosis was 22% in the stent group versus 32% in the POBA group (p = 0.002). Bleeding and vascular complications were significantly higher in the stent group who received warfarin in addition to dual antiplatelet therapy (13.5% vs. 3.1%; p <0.001). In addition, the mean hospital stay was significantly longer in the stent group compared with the POBA group (8.5 vs. 3.1 days; p <0.001).

Limitations

Patients included in the study had stable angina symptoms and single-vessel coronary disease with simple target lesions only. In addition, adjunctive pharmacotherapy differed between the two groups. Specifically, the stent group received warfarin in addition to dual antiplatelet therapy and this is likely to have accounted for the increased rate of bleeding, vascular complications, and prolonged hospital stay observed in this group.

Conclusions and clinical implications

Stenting versus POBA in patients with *de novo* coronary lesions reduces the incidence of major adverse cardiac events and TLR at seven-month follow-up. Longer-term follow-up of the BENESTENT trial showed that the improvement in TLR remained unchanged at five years, but there was no significant difference in event-free survival rates between the stent and POBA groups. This, and similar studies, revolutionized the outcome of PCI and was the first major step forward in making PCI a viable 'mainstream' revascularization strategy.

Further reading

● Fischman DL, Leon MB, Baim DS, *et al.* for the Stent Restenosis Study Investigators. A randomized comparison of coronary-stent placement and balloon angioplasty in the treatment of coronary artery disease. Stent Restenosis Study Investigators. *N Engl J Med* 1994; 331: 496–501.
● Kiemeneij F, Serruys PW, Macaya C, *et al.* Continued benefit of coronary stenting versus balloon angioplasty: five-year clinical follow-up of Benestent-I trial. *J Am Coll Cardiol* 2001; 37: 1598–600.

Learning points

◆ Stenting of *de novo* coronary lesions compared with POBA alone reduces the incidence of target lesion revascularization and this benefit is maintained at up to five-year follow-up.

Safety and efficacy of drug-eluting and bare metal stents: comprehensive meta-analysis of randomized trials and observational studies

Kirtane AJ, Gupta A, Iyengar S, Moses JW, Leon MB, Applegate R, Brodie B, Hannan E, Harjai K, Jensen LO, Park SJ, Perry R, Racz M, Saia F, Tu JV, Waksman R, Lansky AJ, Mehran R, Stone GW.
Circulation 2009; 119: 3198–206.

Background

The main clinical limitation of bare metal stenting (BMS) was a real world target vessel revascularization (TVR) rate of 10–15%. The RAndomized study with the sirolimus-eluting VElocity balloon-expandable stent in the treatment of patients with de novo native coronary artery Lesions (RAVEL) study was the first randomized double-blind trial comparing BMS with drug eluting stenting (DES) in 238 patients with single vessel coronary disease. Morice *et al.* demonstrated a significant difference in the rate of

Table 6.1 Summary of the meta-analyses of DES versus BMS

End point	RCTs	Observational studies
All cause mortality	n = 8867 No significant difference HR 0.97, 95% CI 0.81–1.15, p = 0.72	n = 169,595 22% reduction with DES HR 0.78, 95% CI 0.71–0.86, p <0.001
Myocardial infarction	n = 8850 No significant difference HR 0.95, 95% CI 0.79–1.13, p = 0.54	n = 130,191 13% reduction with DES HR 0.87, 95% CI 0.78–0.97, p = 0.014
Target vessel revascularization	n = 7291 55% reduction with DES HR 0.55, 95% CI 0.37–0.54, p <0.001	n = 74,154 46% reduction with DES HR 0.54, 95% CI 0.48–0.61, p <0.001

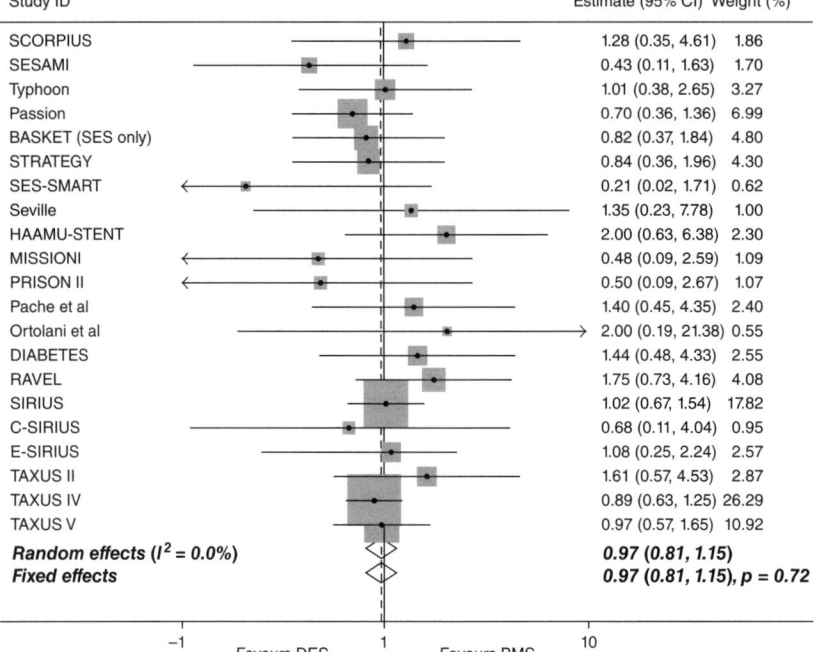

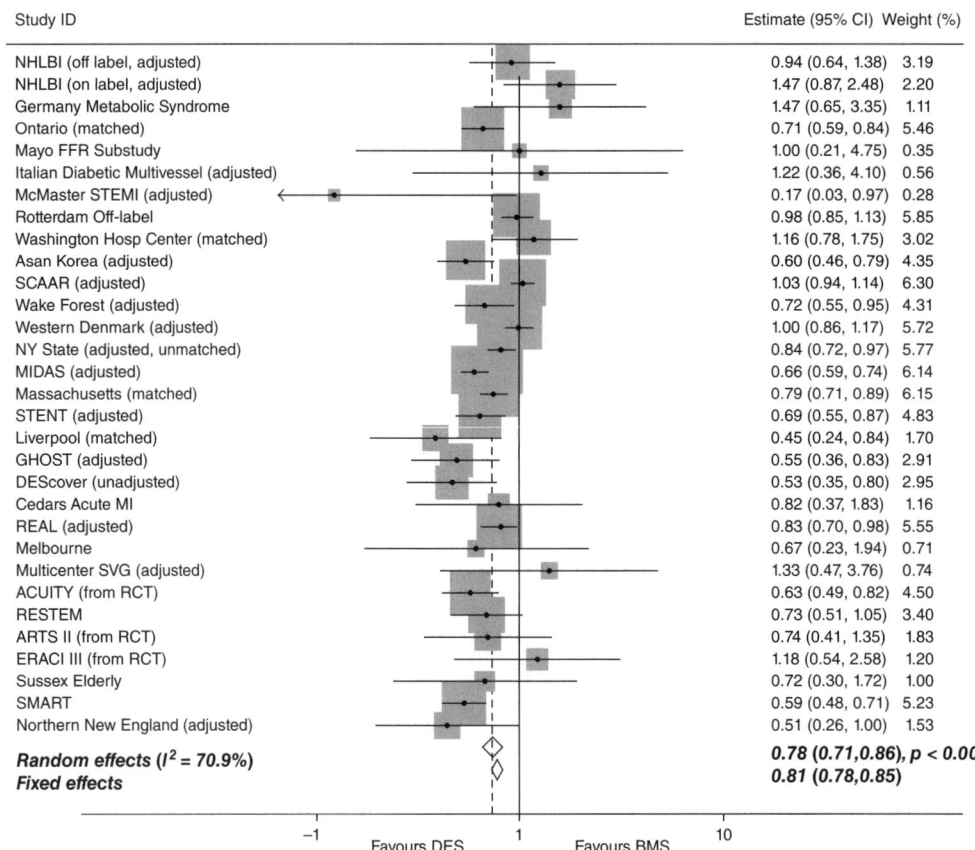

Figure 6.2 Meta-analysis of TVR with DES vs. BMS. (A) RCTs; (B) observational studies. Dots represent the individual study estimates, boxes, study weights, and lines, 95% CIs.

Reproduced from Kirtane AJ, *et al*. Safety and efficacy of drug-eluting and bare metal stents: comprehensive meta-analysis of randomized trials and observational studies. *Circulation* 2009; 119: 3198–206, with permission from Wolters Kluwer Health.

in-stent restenosis between BMS versus DES (27% vs. 0%; p <0.001) at six months and at one year overall major adverse cardiac events (MACE) rate of 29% versus 6%, respectively, which was entirely driven by higher rates of TVR in the BMS group. The study investigators concluded that the use of DES resulted in the 'virtual elimination of in-stent neointimal hyperplasia' and one of the study group members was famously quoted to have said at a scientific meeting 'if I am dreaming, please don't wake me up …'. The significant and dramatic improvement in TVR with DES, was accompanied by the requirement for prolonged dual antiplatelet therapy. Despite the latter, there have been lingering doubts about the safety of DES with regard to stent thrombosis (ST) in particular. Definitive data to address the issue of safety between BMS and DES was required. This need was satisfied by this landmark study conducted by Kirtane *et al.* The inclusion of both observational and randomized trial data was extremely valuable. It allowed an understanding of the comparative safety and efficacy of DES versus BMS, both from the perspective of scientific credibility *and* real world impact.

Methods

Studies eligible for inclusion were all comparative DES versus BMS RCT and observational studies published or presented at major cardiovascular meetings through to February 2008 in which more than 100 patients were enrolled and in which mortality data at greater than one-year follow-up were available. The primary end points were all-cause mortality, myocardial infarction, and TVR. Off-label indications were classified as treatment of patients with myocardial infarction or complex disease, including chronic total occlusions and bifurcation lesions.

Results

Data from 9470 patients in 22 RCTs and from 182,901 patients in 34 observational studies were included. Analyses of RCTs and observational studies were undertaken separately and the results are summarized in Table 6.1. In the RCTs, treatment with DES compared with BMS was associated with a significant reduction in TVR (see Figure 6.2), but no detectable difference in all-cause mortality or myocardial infarction. By contrast, the observational data analyses showed that treatment with DES resulted in a significant reduction in all three study end points (see Table 6.1).

Limitations

Although the large observational studies are more representative of real world clinical practice and subject to less enrolment bias, they are of course subject to treatment selection bias. By contrast, RCTs represent the most scientifically robust comparison, but in the process of recruitment exclude over 90% of potentially eligible patients.

Conclusions and clinical implications

In this analysis, PCI with DES consistently resulted in a significant reduction in TVR compared with BMS across a broad spectrum of patients and coronary lesion subsets. In the RCTs, there was no significant difference between DES and BMS in the rates of death or myocardial infarction for either off-label or on-label indications. By contrast, the larger observational studies demonstrated a significant reduction in both all cause mortality and myocardial infarction in patients treated with DES compared with BMS. The observational data included nearly 20 times more patients than the RCTs.

Learning points

- Percutaneous coronary intervention with DES is safe and efficacious for both on-label and off-label use, including complex coronary interventions and in acute MI.
- Use of DES compared with BMS significantly reduces the rate of recurrent ischaemia, necessitating target vessel revascularization.
- The enormous observational analysis indicates a mortality advantage for DES in the 'real world'.

Further reading

- Marroquin OC, Selzer F, Mulukutla SR, *et al.* A comparison of bare metal and drug eluting stents for off-label indications. *N Engl J Med* 2008; 358: 342–52.
- Morice MC, Serruys PW, Sousa JE, *et al.*; RAVEL Study Group. Randomized Study with the Sirolimus-Coated Bx Velocity Balloon-Expandable Stent in the Treatment of Patients with de Novo Native Coronary Artery Lesions. A randomised comparison of a sirolimus-eluting stent with a standard stent for coronary revascularization. *N Engl J Med* 2002; 346: 1773–80.
- Shishehbor MH, Goel SS, Kapadia SR, *et al.* Long-Term Impact of Drug-Eluting Stents Versus Bare-Metal Stents on All-Cause Mortality. *J Am Coll Cardiol* 2008; 52: 1041–48.

Optimal Medical Therapy with or without PCI for Stable Coronary Disease

Boden WE, O'Rourke RA, Teo KK, Hartigan PM, Maron DJ, Kostuk WJ, Knudtson M, Dada M, Casperson P, Harris CL, Chaitman BR, Shaw L, Gosselin G, Nawaz S, Title LM, Gau G, Blaustein AS, Booth DC, Bates ER, Spertus JA, Berman DS, John Mancini J, Weintraub WS; for the COURAGE Trial Research Group. *N Engl J Med* 2007; 356: 1503–16.

Background

Clinical studies have established that PCI reduces the incidence of death and myocardial infarction in patients with acute coronary syndromes and decreases the frequency of angina in stable coronary artery disease (CAD). However, the potential prognostic benefit of PCI in stable CAD is unproven, particularly in the absence of documented evidence of ischaemia. Furthermore, the prognostic benefit of optimal medical therapy (OMT) consisting of antiplatelets, statins, ACE inhibitors, and/or beta blockers is unequivocal. Nonetheless, PCI is frequently undertaken in stable patients, potentially exposing them to procedure-related complications even when their symptoms on medical treatment are absent or mild. The Clinical Outcomes Utilizing Revascularization and Aggressive Drug Evaluation (COURAGE) trial was a large multicentre study that investigated whether PCI with OMT reduces the risk of adverse cardiac events in patients with stable CAD compared with OMT alone. This paper has (appropriately) sparked debate regarding the role of PCI in stable CAD and led to marked scrutiny of current PCI practice, especially in the United States.

Methods

Patients with stable angina symptoms or documented myocardial ischaemia and at least one angiographically significant coronary lesion were included in the study. Main exclusion criteria were persistent Canadian Cardiovascular Society (CCS) class IV angina, a markedly positive stress test, refractory heart failure, an ejection fraction of less than 30%, and revascularization within the previous six months. A total of 2287 patients were randomized to PCI with OMT (n = 1149) versus OMT alone (n = 1138). In those patients undergoing PCI, target lesion revascularization was always attempted and complete revascularization only undertaken if clinically appropriate. The primary outcome was a composite of death from any cause and non-fatal MI during a median follow-up period of 4.6 years.

Results

Mean age was 61 years, 85% were male, 35% were diabetic, and 70% had multi-vessel coronary disease.

Drug eluting stenting was used in only 3% of patients, and BMS in the remaining 97%. At median follow up of 4.6 years, there were no significant differences between the PCI and OMT groups in the incidence of the primary composite end point of death and MI (211 versus 202 events; p = 0.62), mortality alone (7.6% vs. 8.3%; p = 0.38) or hospitalization for acute coronary syndromes (12.4% vs. 11.8%; p = 0.56) (see Figure 6.3). However, additional revascularization for angina unresponsive to medical therapy or for objective evidence of worsening ischaemia was significantly higher in the OMT alone versus PCI group (33% vs. 21%; p <0.001).

Limitations

Over 35,000 patients were screened and assessed for study suitability, but only 3071 (9%) met the eligibility criteria. This study cannot therefore be entirely representative of real world clinical practice, in common with all the other randomized trial data in this field. In addition, 97% of patients randomized to PCI were treated with BMS and this inevitably will have contributed to the relatively high rate of repeat revascularization in the PCI group.

Conclusions and clinical implications

In patients with stable coronary artery disease, PCI in addition to OMT reduces the prevalence of angina symptoms, but does not reduce the risk of major adverse cardiovascular events. The lack of prognostic benefit with PCI in addition to OMT is consistent across all patient groups regardless of the extent, severity of coronary artery disease or the presence of comorbid conditions such as diabetes. Following on from COURAGE, the COURAGE nuclear substudy showed that PCI in addition to OMT resulted in a greater reduction in ischaemic burden compared with OMT alone, particularly in patients with moderate to severe baseline pre-treatment ischaemia. In this small subset of patients, the reduction in ischaemic burden was directly proportional to improvement in angina class and to the reduction in risk of death and myocardial infarction. This paper appropriately encourages careful patient selection for PCI in stable disease and has stimulated the need for more data about the prognostic value of PCI directed at

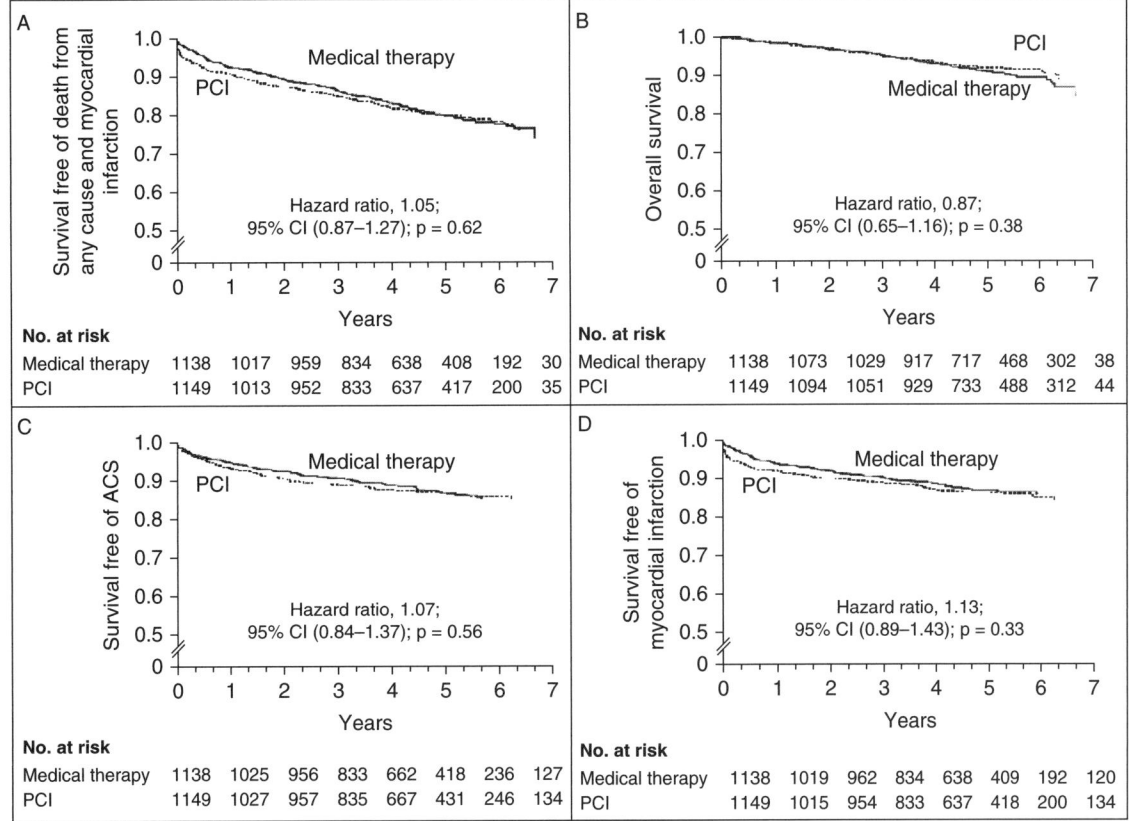

Figure 6.3 Kaplan–Meier Survival Curves. In Panel A, the estimated 4.6-year rate of the composite primary outcome of death from any cause and non-fatal myocardial infarction was 19.0% in the PCI group and 18.5% in the medical-therapy group. In Panel B, the estimated 4.6-year rate of death from any cause was 7.6% in the PCI group and 8.3% in the medical-therapy group. In Panel C, the estimated 4.6-year rate of hospitalization for acute coronary syndrome (ACS) was 12.4% in the PCI group and 11.8% in the medical-therapy group. In Panel D, the estimated 4.6-year rate of acute myocardial infarction was 13.2% in the PCI group and 12.3% in the medical-therapy group.

lesion-level ischaemia. Ongoing studies such as the 'Fractional Flow Reserve versus Angiography for Multivessel Evaluation' (FAME) 2 study and the 'does RoutIne Pressure wire assessment influence management strategy at COROnary angiography for DIagnosIs of chest pain' (RIPCORD) study may well help to improve our understanding.

Learning points

◆ Percutaneous coronary intervention in addition to OMT in patients with stable coronary artery disease is associated with an improvement in angina symptoms, but does not confer any prognostic benefit.

◆ Percutaneous coronary intervention in addition to medical therapy is of particular benefit in patients with objective evidence of inducible ischaemia.

Further reading

● Katritsis DG, Ioannidis JP. Percutaneous coronary intervention versus conservative therapy in non-acute coronary artery disease: a meta-analysis. *Circulation* 2005; 111: 2906–12.

● Shaw LJ, Berman DS, Maron DJ, *et al*.; COURAGE Investigators. Optimal medical therapy with or without percutaneous coronary intervention to reduce ischemic burden: results from the Clinical Outcomes Utilizing Revascularization and Aggressive Drug Evaluation (COURAGE) trial nuclear substudy. *Circulation* 2008; 117: 1283–91.

Fractional flow reserve versus angiography for guiding percutaneous coronary intervention

Tonino PA, De Bruyne B, Pijls NH, Siebert U, Ikeno F, van' t Veer M, Klauss V, Manoharan G, Engstrøm T, Oldroyd KG, Ver Lee PN, MacCarthy PA, Fearon WF; for the FAME Study Investigators. *N Engl J Med* 2009; 360: 213–24.

Background

It is widely accepted that revascularization of coronary lesions causing ischaemia not only relieves angina symptoms but also improves clinical outcome. However, in patients with stable CAD, although revascularization may improve symptoms it has not been clearly shown to confer any prognostic benefit, but does expose the patient to potentially unnecessary procedural risk. However, 'circumstantial' evidence from observational data suggests that it is ischaemia that determines clinical outcome.

Specifically, in patients with multi-vessel coronary disease referred for PCI, determining which lesion is ischaemic and thus warrants revascularization cannot be established from angiographic images alone. Furthermore, simple non-invasive tests of ischaemia are often limited in their ability to accurately localize lesion-level ischaemia, and more sophisticated non-invasive tests are not widely available and are used predominantly for research purposes at present.

Fractional flow reserve (FFR) is a robustly validated invasive index that can be used to accurately determine the functional significance of a coronary lesion at the time of angiography. Fractional flow reserve is defined as the ratio of maximal myocardial blood flow supplied by a stenotic artery to normal maximal blood flow and is measured using a coronary pressure guidewire. It is calculated by dividing mean distal coronary pressure by mean aortic pressure during maximal hyperaemia. The FFR value in a normal coronary artery is 1.0 and an FFR value of 0.8 or less has been shown to be representative of ischaemia with a high degree of diagnostic accuracy.

The multi-centre Fractional Flow Reserve versus Angiography for Multi-vessel Evaluation (FAME) study investigated whether FFR-guided PCI in patients with multi-vessel coronary disease could lead to improved clinical outcome. Together with the earlier DEFER study, this trial has almost universally changed clinical practice and strongly reinforced the concept of 'lesion-level' ischaemia.

Methods

The study recruited patients being considered for PCI with coronary stenoses of at least 50% of the vessel diameter in at least two of the three major epicardial arteries. Main exclusion criteria were angiographically significant left main coronary artery disease and STEMI within the previous five days. A group of 1005 patients were randomly assigned to undergo either (1) angiography-guided PCI, where all indicated lesions were stented, or (2) FFR-guided PCI in which lesions were only stented if the FFR value was 0.8 or less. The primary end point was a composite of death, MI, and repeat revascularization at one year.

Results

Ninety-seven per cent of lesions were treated with drug eluting stents and all patients received aspirin and clopidogrel for at least one year after PCI. Sixty- three per cent of all lesions had an FFR value of 0.8 or less. The primary end point occurred in 18.3% of patients in the angiography group and 13.2% of patients in the FFR group (p = 0.02). Furthermore, 78% of patients in the angiography group and 81% of patients in the FFR group were free from angina at one year (p = 0.20). Compared with angiography-guided PCI, the FFR-guided strategy utilized fewer number of stents per patient (2.7 ± 1.2 versus 1.9 ± 1.3; p <0.001) and significantly less contrast agent (302 ± 127 ml versus 272 ± 133 ml; p <0.001).

Limitations

Longer-term follow up data is required to determine whether the benefit of FFR-guided PCI is maintained.

Conclusions and clinical implications

In patients with multi-vessel coronary disease, routine measurement of FFR at the time of coronary angiography and subsequent revascularization of ischaemic lesions not only reduces the number of lesions being stented but also significantly reduces the rate of death, MI, and repeat revascularization at one year. The absolute risk reduction of major adverse cardiac events was 5%. Furthermore, FFR-guided PCI allows for the more appropriate and judicious use of stents, thus avoiding unneccesary patient exposure to procedural and stent-related complications. The FAME investigators recently published two-year follow-up data which showed that the benefit of FFR-guided PCI in reducing adverse cardiac events is maintained.

Further reading

- Pijls NH, De Bruyne B, Peels K, *et al.* Measurement of fractional flow reserve to assess the functional severity of coronary-artery stenoses. *N Engl J Med* 1996; 334: 1703–8.
- Pijls NH, van Schaardenburgh P, Manoharan G, *et al.* Percutaneous coronary intervention of functionally non-significant stenosis: 5-year follow-up of the DEFER Study. *J Am Coll Cardiol.* 2007; 49: 2105–11.
- Pijls NH, Fearon WF, Tonino PA, *et al.*; FAME Study Investigators. Fractional flow reserve versus angiography for guiding percutaneous coronary intervention in patients with multi-vessel coronary artery disease: 2-year follow-up of the FAME (Fractional Flow Reserve Versus Angiography for Multivessel Evaluation) study. *J Am Coll Cardiol* 2010; 56: 177–84.

Routine versus selective invasive strategies in patients with acute coronary syndromes

Mehta SR, Cannon CP, Fox KA, Wallentin L, Boden WE, Spacek R, Widimsky P, McCullough PA, Hunt D, Braunwald E, Yusuf S. A collaborative meta-analysis of randomized trials. *JAMA* 2005; 293: 2908–17.

Background

The most appropriate management strategy in patients with non-ST-elevation myocardial infarction (NSTEMI) has been a contentious issue, particularly with regards to the role and timing of coronary angiography in those patients who are considered to be at low to moderate risk. Previous clinical guidelines recommended either a routine invasive strategy, whereby all patients with NSTEMI undergo early coronary angiography with a view to revascularization, or a conservative approach which involves selective angiography restricted only to those NSTEMI patients with refractory or inducible ischaemia. These recommendations were based on conflicting data from various randomized trials and large-scale registries and led to significant discrepancies in the way in which NSTEMI patients were managed during their initial hospitalization. This landmark paper was an early meta-analysis of randomized trials designed to evaluate the benefits and risks of early routine versus selective coronary angiography in patients with unstable angina and NSTEMI. The data confirmed that, in most patients, an early invasive strategy was superior and thereby contributed to a change in routine clinical practice.

Methods

All RCTs identified through a literature search of Medline and Cochrane databases from 1970 through to 2004 were

included if they enrolled patients with unstable angina or NSTEMI and randomly allocated them to undergo either a routine invasive or a selective invasive strategy. The meta-analysis included The Framingham and Fast Revascularization During Instability in Coronary Artery Disease (FRISC II) II Trial, Treat angina with Aggrastat and determine Cost of Therapy with an Invasive or Conservative Strategy-Thrombolysis in Myocardial Infarction 18 (TACTICS-TIMI 18), RITA 3, Veterans Affairs Non-Q-Wave Infarction Strategies In-Hospital (VANQWISH), Medicine versus Angiography in Thrombolytic Exclusion (MATE), Thrombolysis in Myocardial Infarction IIIB (TIMI IIIB), and Value of first day angiography/angioplasty In evolving Non-ST segment elevation myocardial infarction, an Open multicenter randomized trial (VINO) trials. Routine strategy was defined as coronary angiography with a view to revascularization, and a selective strategy was defined as medical therapy in the first instance, followed by coronary angiography only in those patients with recurrent symptoms or objective evidence of inducible ischaemia. Data on mortality (in-hospital and long term), MI, CCS class angina, and rehospitalization were analysed.

Results

A total of seven randomized trials involving 9208 patients were included. Mean age was 62.4 years, 18.9% were diabetic, 59% had an NSTEMI, and 41% had unstable angina. Mean duration of follow-up was 17.3 months. Overall, there was a significant reduction in major adverse cardiovascular events in the routine invasive compared with the selective invasive group: specifically, there was a significant reduction in the composite of death or MI (12.2% vs. 14.4%; p = 0.001), refractory angina (11.2% vs. 14%; p <0.001) and rehospitalization (32.5% vs. 41.3%; p <0.001) in the routine invasive versus selective invasive groups, respectively. However, the routine invasive strategy was associated with a significantly higher early mortality (1.8% vs. 1.1%; p = 0.007), but subsequent fewer deaths following discharge. Of note, the long-term benefits associated with a routine invasive strategy were observed in patients with elevated baseline cardiac enzyme levels.

Limitations

Between the seven trials, there were inevitable differences in study design, inclusion criteria, adjunctive therapy, and cardiac marker thresholds for defining MI.

Conclusions and clinical implications

In patients with unstable angina and NSTEMI, routine early coronary angiography with a view to revascularization is associated with a significant reduction in long-term major adverse cardiovascular events, refractory angina, and rehospitalization, compared with the more conservative, selective approach. The clinical benefit of early revascularization is most evident in higher-risk patients with elevated baseline cardiac enzymes. The precise optimal timing of angiography is less clear from the data, particularly given the observed increased early hazard associated with routine intervention. As such, current clinical guidelines recommend risk stratification

in all patients with NSTEMI. Those deemed to be high risk, that is, ongoing or recurrent ischaemia, dynamic ECG changes, and/or haemodynamic instability, should be referred for urgent coronary angiography, whereas the lower-risk group should undergo angiography within 72 hours of hospital admission. Meta-analyses of data at five-year follow-up (including two of the seven studies analysed by Mehta *et al.*) has shown a 14.7% versus 17.9% incidence in cardiovascular death or MI in the routine invasive versus selective invasive groups respectively (p = 0.002).

Learning points

- Patients with unstable angina or NSTEMI should undergo risk stratification at presentation in order to determine the optimal timing of coronary angiography and revascularization.
- Early revascularization in patients with NSTEMI is associated with a reduction in the incidence of re-infarction, refractory angina, and rehospitalization.

Further reading

- Fox KAA, Clayton TC, Damman P, *et al.*; for the FIR Collaboration. Long term outcome of a routine versus selective invasive strategy in patients with non ST-segment elevation acute coronary syndrome: a meta-analysis of individual patient data. *J Am Coll Cardiol* 2010; 55: 2435–45.
- Wijns W, Kolh P, Danchin N, *et al.* Guidelines on myocardial revascularization: The Task force on myocardial revascularization of the European Society of Cardiology (ESC) and the European Association for Cardiothoracic Surgery (EACTS). *Eur Heart J* 2010; 31: 2501–55.

Randomized trial of simple versus complex drug-eluting stenting for bifurcation lesions: the British bifurcation coronary study: old, new, and evolving strategies

Hildick-Smith D, de Belder A, Cooter N, Curzen N, Clayton TC, Oldroyd KG, Bennett L, Holmberg S, Cotton JM, Glennon PE, Thomas MR, MacCarthy PA, Baumbach A, Mulvihill NT, Henderson RA, Redwood SR, Starkey IR, Stables RH. *Circulation* 2010; 121: 1235–43.

Background

The optimal treatment of complex coronary artery bifurcation lesions remains a contentious and challenging

issue. In the early angioplasty and bare metal stent era, bifurcation compared with straightforward non-bifurcation interventions were associated with (1) lower procedural success due to high rates of dissection and acute vessel closure, and (2) poorer long-term outcome due to high rates of re-stenosis at the ostium of the side branch. With the advent of DES and significantly lower observed rates of in-stent restenosis, more complex bifurcation stenting techniques have been developed in order to optimize treatment of this relatively complex lesion subset and thus improve outcome. The British Bifurcation Coronary Study (BBC ONE) is a randomized, multicentre study that investigated whether complex versus simple stenting strategies for the treatment of bifurcation disease offers any clear benefit with regards to clinical outcome.

Methods

A group of 500 patients with coronary bifurcation lesions were randomized to either a simple or complex stenting strategy with DES. Patients were eligible for study inclusion if they had bifurcation disease requiring PCI in which the main vessel reference diameter was ≥2.5 mm and the side branch reference diameter was ≥2.25 mm. Main exclusion criteria were unprotected left main stem narrowing ≥50%, primary angioplasty for acute STEMI, cardiogenic shock, chronic total occlusions, additional type C or bifurcation lesion that required PCI, and left ventricular ejection fraction ≤20%. The simple arm of the study involved the provisional T-stent strategy where the main vessel was stented followed by optional kissing balloon dilatation or T-stent. In the complex arm, both vessels were systematically stented with either the 'crush' or 'culotte' technique, followed by mandatory kissing balloon dilatations. The primary end point was a composite of all-cause death, target vessel failure (revascularization or inadequate Thrombolysis in Myocardial Infarction – TIMI– flow), or MI at nine months.

Results

Mean age was 64 years and 77% were male. True bifurcation lesions, defined as greater than 50% narrowing in the main vessel and side branch, were seen in over 80% of cases in both study arms. The primary end point occurred in 8% in the simple strategy group versus 15.2% in the complex strategy group (p = 0.009). As illustrated in Table 6.2, the difference in primary end point between the two groups was largely driven by peri-procedural and in-hospital MI. Cumulative risk of primary outcome, MI, and target vessel failure is shown in Figure 6.4.

As expected, procedural differences were marked between the two groups, with the more complex group having longer procedural times, greater stent length, more radiation exposure, higher contrast load, and longer duration of vessel instrumentation, with more frequent wire, balloon, and stent exchanges. In-hospital major adverse cardiovascular events occurred in 2.0% versus 8.0% in the simple and complex groups, respectively (p = 0.002).

Limitations

A limitation of the study design is that not all patients included in the study had true bifurcation lesions. Furthermore, the principal investigators in the study had access to their own patient's data, which may have introduced selection bias.

Conclusions and clinical implications

For treatment of coronary artery bifurcation lesions, the simple single stent strategy with provisional bailout T-stent is preferable to the more complex systematic two-stent strategy. The latter approach is associated with higher rates of MACE and increased procedural complications. The findings from this study suggest that the more simple approach to bifurcation lesions should be the default strategy in most instances and this is now becoming an accepted method of clinical practice.

The results of BBC ONE are similar to the NORDIC Bifurcation study findings which showed no significant advantage of complex versus simple stenting strategies in

Table 6.2 BBC ONE study end points

End point	Complex strategy (%)	Simple strategy (%)	p value
Death	0.8	0.4	NS
Target vessel failure	7.2	5.6	NS
Myocardial infarction	11.2	3.6	0.001
Primary end point	15.2	8.0	0.009

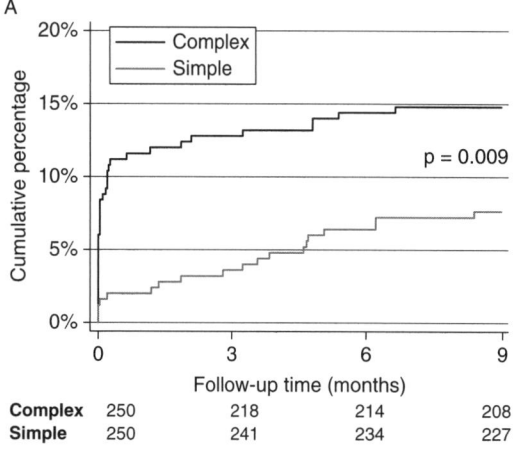

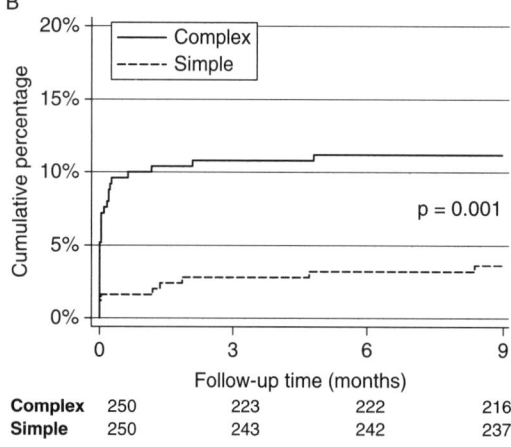

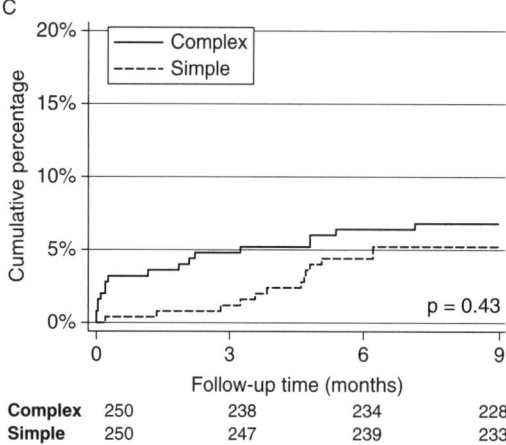

Figure 6.4 Outcome measures. (A) cumulative risk of primary outcome; (B) Cumulative risk of myocardial infarction; and, (C), cumulative risk of target vessel failure.

Reproduced from Hildick-Smith D, *et al*. Randomized trial of simple versus complex drug-eluting stenting for bifurcation lesions. The British Bifurcation Coronary Study: Old, New and Evolving Strategies. *Circulation* 2010; 121: 1235–43, with permission from Wolters Kluwer Health.

bifurcation disease. The NORDIC study did not include peri-procedural MI in their primary end point. Further studies are required to determine whether there are specific subsets of bifurcation lesions that may do better with the more complex systematic two-stent approach, although subsequent meta-analyses combining data from BBC ONE and NORDIC Bifurcation studies have not identified any subset differences.

Learning points

◆ For bifurcation lesions in which the main vessel diameter is ≥2.5 mm and the side branch diameter is ≥2.25 mm, a stepwise provisional T-stent strategy is superior to a systematic complex strategy.

◆ The complex systematic two-stent approach is associated with a higher rate of major adverse cardiac events, target vessel failure, and procedural complications.

Further reading

● Colombo A, Bramucci E, Sacca S, *et al*. Randomized study of the crush technique versus provisional side-branch stenting in true coronary bifurcations: the CACTUS (Coronary Bifurcations: Application of the Crushing Technique Using Sirolimus-Eluting Stents) Study. *Circulation* 2009; 119: 71–78.

● Steigen TK, Maeng M, Wiseth R, *et al*. Randomized study on simple versus complex stenting of coronary artery bifurcation lesions: the Nordic bifurcation study. *Circulation* 2006; 114: 1955–61.

● Iakovou I, Ge L, Colombo A. Contemporary stent treatment of coronary bifurcations. *J Am Coll Cardiol* 2005; 46: 1446–55.

Thrombus aspiration during primary percutaneous coronary intervention

Svilaas T, Vlaar PJ, van der Horst IC, Diercks GF, de Smet BJ, van den Heuvel AF, Anthonio RL, Jessurun GA, Tan ES, Suurmeijer AJ, Zijlstra F. *N Engl J Med* 2008; 358: 557–67.

Background

Primary PCI is the gold-standard treatment for acute STEMI. The latter is caused by rupture of an atherosclerotic plaque leading to platelet-rich thrombus overlying the culprit lesion, causing severe narrowing or complete occlusion of the vessel. However, despite successful restoration of blood flow down the infarct related artery following primary PCI, embolization of atherothrombotic material downstream leads to microvascular obstruction and can result in suboptimal reperfusion of viable myocardium. This is associated with increased infarct size, diminished recovery of left ventricular function and poorer prognosis. In order to overcome this problem, various devices, including the relatively flexible and non-traumatic manual-aspiration catheter have been developed to protect the microcirculation during PCI. The Thrombus Aspiration during Percutaneous Coronary Intervention in Acute Myocardial Infarction Study (TAPAS) was a single-centre, prospective, randomized trial that evaluated the use of a manual aspiration catheter to improve myocardial perfusion during primary PCI in patients with acute STEMI. The data presented in this paper precipitated widespread uptake in routine thrombus aspiration by primary angioplasty operators.

Methods

Patients presenting with STEMI within 12 hours of symptom onset were eligible for study inclusion. A total of 1071 patients were randomized to undergo either thrombus aspiration during PCI or conventional PCI. Randomization was undertaken prior to coronary angiography. The target lesion was crossed with a guidewire, and in the conventional PCI group, was followed by balloon dilatation. In the thrombus aspiration group, the first manipulation was the passage of a six-French Export® Aspiration Catheter (Medtronic, Minneapolis, USA) into the target coronary segment during continuous aspiration. Balloon dilatation was undertaken in the aspiration group only when necessary. All aspirated material underwent histological examination and was defined as effective on the basis of the presence of atherothrombotic material in the aspirate samples. All patients received bare metal stents, were pre-loaded with aspirin and clopidogrel and received a glycoprotein IIb/IIIa inhibitor unless contraindicated.

The primary end point was myocardial blush grade of 0 or 1, which is representative of absent or minimal myocardial perfusion, respectively. Secondary end points included post-procedural TIMI flow grade 3, complete resolution of ST-segment elevation, the absence of persistent ST-segment deviation, TVR, re-infarction, death, and the combination of major adverse cardiac events at 30 days.

Results

A myocardial blush grade of 0 or 1 occurred in 17% of patients in the thrombus-aspiration group, compared with 26% of patients in the conventional PCI group (p <0.001) and complete resolution of ST-segment elevation occurred in 57% and 44% of patients, respectively (p <0.001). At 30 days, the rates of death and major adverse cardiac events were both significantly related to myocardial blush grade (p = 0.003 and p <0.001 respectively). Histopathological examination confirmed successful aspiration in 73% of patients.

Limitations

This study was a single-centre experience that used surrogate end points (myocardial blush grade and ECG criteria) and was not powered for mortality. However, these end points were clearly linked to clinical outcome, thus indicating their validity. Furthermore, no systematic and objective measurement of infarct size or left ventricular function was undertaken, which could have provided useful information with regards to the mechanism behind the observed clinical benefit seen in the thrombus aspiration group.

Conclusions and clinical implications

Effective manual aspiration of thrombus material immediately prior to balloon angioplasty or direct stenting in patients with STEMI results in improved myocardial reperfusion indicated by the myocardial blush grade and ST-segment analysis. This is directly linked to clinical outcome. The beneficial effect of aspiration is consistently observed in all patients, regardless of their clinical and angiographic characteristics at baseline. By contrast to previous studies involving manual aspiration devices, this study randomized patients prior to coronary angiography and showed that angiographic variables such as TIMI flow and thrombotic burden are not predictors of patients in whom aspiration will be effective. Histopathological examination of the aspirate confirmed that thrombi were predominantly composed of platelets, underlining the important role of antiplatelet therapy in STEMI. One-year follow-up results of the TAPAS study have shown that the reduction in mortality and re-infarction in the manual aspiration versus conventional PCI group is maintained (5.6% vs. 9.9% respectively; p = 0.009). Uncertainty regarding the unplanned mortality benefit outcome has led to two much larger studies being initiated. Both the TOTAL (n=4000) and TASTE studies (n=5000) are well underway in terms of recruitment.

Learning points

◆ Myocardial blush grade is an important measure of myocardial perfusion following PCI and is a predictor of infarct size, recovery of left ventricular function, and mortality.

◆ Manual aspiration of atherothrombotic material prior to PCI in patients with acute STEMI results in improved myocardial blush grade and better clinical outcome at 30-day and one-year follow-up.

Further reading

- Brodie BR. Aspiration thrombectomy with primary PCI for STEMI: review of the data and current guidelines. *J Invasive Cardiol* 2010; 22(10 Suppl B): 2B–5B.
- Henriques JP, Zijlstra F, van 't Hof AW, *et al*. Angiographic assessment of reperfusion in acute myocardial infarction by myocardial blush grade. *Circulation* 2003; 107: 2115–19.
- Vlaar PJ, Svilaas T, van der Horst IC, *et al*. Cardiac death and reinfarction after 1 year in the Thrombus Aspiration during Percutaneous coronary intervention in Acute myocardial infarction Study (TAPAS): a 1-year follow-up study. *Lancet* 2008; 371: 1915–20.

Conclusion: the future

The landmark papers we have selected illustrate the significant progress that has been made in PCI and the treatment of CHD over the last three decades. These studies have paved the way towards better standards of patient care and improved clinical outcomes. They provide the essential evidence base that clinicians require to determine the optimal treatment strategy in CHD patients in both the acute and elective setting as well as when faced with more challenging complex cases.

Future challenges and landmark studies in interventional cardiology are likely to be focused on:

◆ Improvement in stent technology and adjunctive devices.

◆ Selection of the most appropriate antiplatelet agent based on individual patient response.
◆ The use of more sophisticated non-invasive tests of ischaemia in routine practice to identify those patients in whom revascularization is warranted.

For now, the challenge is to adopt and implement evidence-based cardiology in our day-to-day clinical practice.

Chapter 7

Percutaneous coronary intervention versus coronary artery bypass graft surgery

Dr Richard Varcoe and Dr Robert Henderson

Introduction

Obstructive coronary artery disease causing symptomatic myocardial ischaemia can be treated with anti-anginal medication or by myocardial revascularization, with either coronary artery bypass graft (CABG) surgery or percutaneous coronary intervention (PCI). Coronary artery bypass graft surgery began in the 1960s[1] and rapidly became a routine treatment for patients with symptomatic coronary artery disease. Long-term clinical outcomes have improved with advances in surgical technique, particularly the use of internal mammary artery grafts[2].

Percutaneous coronary intervention was first performed in 1977[3] and was initially considered appropriate only in patients with an isolated proximal coronary artery stenosis[4]. Technological advances, particularly the introduction of bare metal then drug eluting stents[5], together with developments in adjunctive pharmacology[6] have improved clinical outcomes and expanded the indications for PCI to the treatment of more complex lesions and patient subsets, including those with multi-vessel and left main stem disease.

For some patients with multi-vessel coronary artery disease (CAD) both methods of myocardial revascularization may be technically feasible, but the optimal treatment strategy is uncertain. A number of randomized controlled trials have compared initial treatment strategies of CABG and PCI in patients who were considered to be clinically and angiographically suitable for either procedure and in whom there is equipoise about the most appropriate method of myocardial revascularization. These trials fall into several distinct eras as PCI technology has developed from balloon angioplasty, to bare metal, and then drug eluting stents. This chapter reviews the landmark trials from each of these three eras.

Coronary artery bypass graft surgery versus percutaneous coronary intervention with balloon angioplasty

Bypass Angioplasty Revascularization Investigation (BARI)

The Bypass Angioplasty Revascularization Investigation (BARI) Investigators. Comparison of coronary bypass surgery with angioplasty in patients with multivessel disease. *N Eng J Med* 1996; 335: 217–25.

The BARI trial enrolled patients with multi-vessel CAD and severe angina or objective evidence of myocardial ischaemia who were suitable for either CABG or PCI. The trial was designed to test the hypothesis that an initial treatment strategy of coronary balloon angioplasty does not compromise clinical outcomes at five years compared to an initial treatment strategy of CABG[7]. Patients over 80 years, with single vessel or left main stem disease were ineligible. The primary end point was all-cause mortality at five years, but ten-year follow-up data are also available[8,9]. The initial recruitment target was 2400 patients, but recruitment was terminated prematurely after 1829 patients were enrolled at 18 North American centres from 1988 to 1991.

A group of 914 patients were randomized to CABG with a mean of 2.8 grafts per patient, including at least one internal mammary graft in 82%[10]. A group of 915 patients were randomized to PCI with a mean of 2.4 lesions attempted per patient, multi-vessel PCI in 70%, and staged procedures in 17%[11].

In-hospital mortality was 1.3% in the CABG group and 1.1% in the PCI group. Periprocedural Q wave myocardial infarction (MI) occurred in 4.6% of CABG patients and 2.1% of PCI patients. Emergency CABG was required in 6.3% of PCI patients.

The survival rate was 89.2% in the CABG group and 86.3% in the PCI group at five years (difference 2.9%, 95% confidence interval [CI] -0.2–6.0%, p = 0.19) and 73.5% and 71.0% respectively at ten years (relative risk [RR] 1.09 for PCI, p = 0.18). In a retrospective subgroup analysis of 353 patients with treated diabetes mellitus CABG was associated with a survival advantage over PCI at five years (80.6% vs. 65.5%, difference 15.1%, 99.5% CI 1.4–28.9%, p = 0.003) and at ten years (57.8% vs. 45.5%, RR 1.29 for PCI, p = 0.025), but at ten years the treatment subgroup interaction was not statistically significant (p = 0.12)[9].

There was a significantly greater rate of repeat revascularization in the PCI group, with 54% of patients undergoing an additional procedure within five years versus 8% of CABG patients. This increased to 66.8% versus 20.3% respectively at ten years. Both procedures improved symptoms, but mild stable angina (Canadian Cardiovascular Society (CCS) class I or II) was more prevalent in the PCI group within the first five years, but this difference attenuated over time and was no longer significant at seven years[12]. Patients returned to work an average of six weeks after PCI, compared to eleven weeks after CABG, but there was no difference in long-term employment status. The mean costs of initial revascularization were US$32347 for CABG patients and US$21113 for PCI patients (p <0.001). At five years costs increased to US$58889 for CABG and US$56225 for PCI (p = 0.047) mainly due to repeat revascularizations[13].

Coronary Artery Bypass Revascularization Investigation (CABRI)

CABRI trial participants. First-year results of CABRI (Coronary Angioplasty versus Bypass Revascularization Investigation). *Lancet* 1995; 346: 1179–84.

The CABRI study was a multi-national European randomized trial designed to compare initial strategies of CABG and coronary balloon angioplasty in the treatment of patients with symptomatic multi-vessel CAD[14]. Patients with angina or ischaemia on stress testing were randomized if coronary angiography showed a >50% stenosis in two or more major epicardial vessels (>2 mm diameter). Patients with left main stem disease, occlusion of two

major epicardial vessels, an ejection fraction <35% or previous revascularization were ineligible. The primary end points were mortality and angina status at one and five years.

The CABRI study recruited 1054 patients at 26 centres from July 1988 to December 1992. A group of 513 patients were assigned to CABG and 541 patients to PCI. In the CABG group 1318 out of 1601 diseased coronary segments were grafted, with a mean of 2.8 grafts per patient and at least one arterial graft in 81%. In the PCI group balloon dilatation was attempted in 1072 of 1815 diseased coronary segments, with procedural success of 91.7%, and an average of 2.1 successfully dilated stenoses per patient.

At one year there were 14 deaths in the CABG group (2.7%) and 21 deaths in the PCI group (3.9%) (RR 1.42, 95% CI 0.73–2.76, p = 0.297). Symptoms improved in both groups during follow-up but PCI patients were more likely to have significant angina (CCS class II or worse, 13.9% versus 10.1%, p = 0.012) and to be taking antianginal medication (70% versus 53%, p <0.001). Repeat revascularization was more frequent in the PCI group, with 66%

of such patients reaching one year with only one revascularization procedure compared to 93% of CABG patients. In a small subgroup analysis (147 Belgian patients), initial costs were 11870 European currency units (ECU) for CABG and 5624 ECU for PCI, increasing to 11966 ECU and 10326 ECU respectively at 20 months follow-up[15]. Four-year follow-up data confirmed no statistically significant difference in mortality between CABG and PCI in the entire patient cohort and in a subgroup of 125 diabetic patients[16].

Randomized Intervention Treatment of Angina Trial (RITA)

Coronary angioplasty versus coronary artery bypass surgery: the Randomized Intervention Treatment of Angina (RITA) trial. *Lancet* 1993; 341: 573–80.

The RITA study was a United Kingdom trial involving 16 centres that compared an initial treatment strategy of CABG with coronary balloon angioplasty[17]. Patients with angiographically proven CAD were eligible for randomization if a cardiologist and a cardiac surgeon agreed that equivalent revascularization could be achieved by either procedure. Patients with more than three vessels requiring treatment, left main stem disease, or previous revascularization were ineligible. The primary end point was the combined rate of death and non-fatal MI at five years. A cohort of 1011 patients were randomized from March 1988 to November 1991, including 45% with single-vessel disease.

A group of 501 patients were randomized to CABG with a mean of 2.1 grafts per patient and at least one internal mammary artery graft in 74%. Another group of 510 patients were randomized to PCI with balloon dilatation attempted in 779 vessels, an average of 1.6 vessels per patient and an angiographic success rate of 87% (90% excluding occluded vessels). Staged procedures were required in 7%.

At a median of 6.5 years follow-up there were 45 deaths in the CABG group versus 39 deaths in the PCI group

(p = 0.51)[18]. The primary end point occurred in 80 CABG patients and 87 PCI patients (p = 0.64), and there was no treatment difference among patients with single vessel or multi-vessel disease. A non-randomized CABG was required in 26% of the PCI group compared to 3% of the CABG group, whereas a non-randomized PCI was required in 27% of the PCI group compared to 9% of the CABG group. The prevalence of angina (CCS class II or worse) was greater among PCI patients than CABG patients with an excess prevalence of 9.8% at one year (95% CI 5.3–14.3, p <0.001) and 9.0% at five years (95% CI 3.8–14.2, p <0.001). At one month, return to work, physical activity, and exercise treadmill times were lower in CABG patients, but these differences decreased over time, with no long-term differences between the two treatment groups. Over two years of follow-up there were only small differences in perceived health status (assessed with the Nottingham Health Profile (NHP)) between the two groups, reflecting the increased prevalence of angina in PCI patients[19]. Initial treatment costs were £6520 for CABG compared to £3389 for PCI[20], but at five years there was no significant difference in total health-service costs between the two strategies (mean difference £426, 95% CI -£383 to £1235, p = 0.30)[18].

Coronary artery bypass graft surgery versus percutaneous coronary intervention with bare metal stents

Argentine Randomized Trial of Coronary Angioplasty with Stenting versus Coronary Bypass Surgery in patients with multivessel disease (ERACI II)

Rodriguez AE, Baldi J, Fernandez Pereira C, Navia J, Rodriguez Alemparte M, Delacasa A, Vigo F, Vogel D, O'Neill W, Palacios IF; ERACI II Investigators. Five-year follow-up of the Argentine randomized trial of coronary angioplasty with stenting versus coronary bypass surgery in patients with multiple vessel disease (ERACI II). *J Am Coll Cardiol* 2005; 46: 582–8.

This trial compared initial strategies of CABG and PCI using bare metal stents in patients with multi-vessel disease and a clinical indication for revascularization[21]. Eligible patients had limiting angina (CCS class III/IV), unstable angina, or mild symptoms with a large area of myocardium at risk judged by thallium scintigraphy. Patients were required to have >50% stenosis in two or more major epicardial vessels or >70% stenosis in at least one vessel. Target stenoses had to be suitable for stent deployment and unprotected left main stenoses could be included if they were amenable to a single-stent procedure. Patients with single-vessel disease, more than two chronic total occlusions, ejection fraction <35%, or previous revascularization were excluded from the trial. The primary end point was a composite of death, non-fatal Q wave MI, stroke, and repeat revascularization (event-free survival) at five years.

From October 1996 to September 1998, 450 patients were randomized to CABG or PCI at seven centres in Argentina, with unstable angina (Braunwald IIb, IIIa and C) in 91.1% of the entire cohort. A group of 225 patients were assigned to CABG and at least one arterial conduit was used in 88.5%. Another group of 225 patients were assigned to PCI with 91.5% of planned target vessels being successfully treated, with a mean of 1.4 stents per patient.

At five years the primary end point occurred significantly more frequently in the PCI group than the CABG group (34.7% vs. 23.6%, p = 0.019) but this difference was solely due to the increased incidence of repeat revascularization in the PCI arm. After five years, mortality was 11.5% in the CABG group versus 7.1% in the PCI group (p = 0.182). The rates of non-fatal Q wave MI were 6.2% and 2.8% in the CABG and PCI groups respectively (p = 0.128). There was a significantly greater need for repeat revascularization in the PCI group (28.4% vs. 7.2%, p = 0.0002) predominantly in the form of repeat PCI procedures, with only 19 patients (8.4%) in the PCI group requiring CABG during the follow-up period. At five years 86% of the PCI group and 82% of the CABG group were asymptomatic or had CCS class I angina (p = 0.916). At five years the economic cost per patient was significantly higher for PCI than CABG ($13,584 vs. $11,362, p = 0.04).

Stent or Surgery trial (SoS)

SoS Investigators. Coronary artery bypass surgery versus percutaneous coronary intervention with stent implantation in patients with multi-vessel coronary artery disease (the Stent or Surgery trial): a randomized controlled trial. *Lancet* 2002; 360: 965–70.

The SoS trial was a multi-centre trial involving 53 sites in Europe and Canada. Patients with multi-vessel CAD were considered for inclusion if revascularization was clinically indicated and could be achieved by either CABG or PCI. Patients were excluded if they had had previous coronary revascularization, or required intervention to valves, great vessels, or aorta. The primary end point was repeat revascularization, with secondary end points including death or non-fatal MI, all-cause mortality, angina status, and cost.

From November 1996 to December 1999, 988 patients were randomized to CABG or PCI. A group of 500 patients were assigned to CABG, with a mean of 2.8 bypass grafts per patient and an internal mammary artery conduit in 93%. Another group of 488 patients were assigned to PCI, with a mean of 2.7 treated lesions per patient, a success rate of 94%, and stent placement in 78% of lesions.

At a median follow-up of two years the primary end point occurred more frequently in the PCI arm (20.7%) than in the CABG arm (6.0%) (HR 3.85, 95% CI 2.56–5.79, p <0.001) but there was a similar incidence of death or non-fatal MI (p = 0.8). At a median follow-up of six years there was a statistically significant mortality benefit for CABG over PCI (6.8% vs. 10.9%, HR 1.66, 95% CI 1.08–2.55, p = 0.022)[22], but this treatment difference was not influenced by baseline angina grade (interaction test p = 0.52), severity of coronary disease (interaction test p = 0.92), or diabetic status (interaction test p = 0.15). Moreover, this apparent mortality benefit of CABG may be partly explained by an excess of non-cardiovascular deaths in the PCI group (25 vs. 11, of which 20 and 8, respectively, were cancer-related deaths).

At one year the cost of CABG was higher than PCI (£8905 versus £6296, cost difference £2609, 95% CI £1769–3314)[23]. A substudy in 145 patients showed no difference in neuropsychological outcome at six and twelve months[24].

Arterial Revascularization Therapies Study I (ARTS I)

Serruys PW, Unger F, Sousa JE, Jatene A, Bonnier HJ, Schönberger JP, Buller N, Bonser R, van den Brand MJ, van Herwerden LA, Morel MA, van Hout BA; Arterial Revascularization Therapies Study Group; for the Arterial Revascularization Therapies Study Group. Comparison of coronary-artery bypass surgery and stenting for the treatment of multi-vessel disease. *N Engl J Med* 2001; 344: 1117–24.

The ARTS study was a multi-centre trial involving 67 sites worldwide. Patients with multi-vessel disease and stable angina, unstable angina, or silent ischaemia were eligible if either CABG or PCI could achieve equivalent revascularization. Exclusion criteria included an ejection fraction <30% and left main stem disease. The primary end point was a composite of death, stroke, MI, and repeat revascularization at twelve months.

From April 1997 to June 1998, 1205 patients were randomized. A group of 605 patients were assigned to CABG, with a mean of 2.5 conduits per patient and at least one arterial conduit in 93%. Another group of 600 patients were assigned to PCI, with a mean of 2.6 treated lesions per patient, stent placement in 89% (mean stent length 47.5 mm), and balloon angioplasty in 11%.

At one and five years survival free of the primary end point was higher in the CABG group than in the PCI group (87.8% vs. 73.8% at one year [RR 2.14, 95% CI 1.66–2.75] and 78.2% vs. 58.3% at five years). This difference was driven by a significantly higher rate of repeat revascularization in the PCI group (21.0% vs. 3.8% at one year [RR 5.52, 95% CI 3.59–8.49] and 30.3% vs. 8.8% at five years). There was no difference in death, stroke, or non-fatal MI between the two groups.

Quality of life, assessed using the self-rated EuroQol questionnaire, was better after PCI than CABG at one month and equivalent at six and twelve months[25]. Angina symptoms were significantly more frequent in the PCI group than in the CABG group (21.2% vs. 15.5% at five years, p <0.05), as was the use of anti-anginal medications (nitrates, beta blockers, and calcium channel antagonists)[26]. Costs at one year were significantly higher in the CABG group by approximately $2973 (p <0.001).

Coronary artery bypass grafting versus percutaneous coronary intervention with drug eluting stents

Synergy between PCI with Taxus and Cardiac Surgery trial (SYNTAX)

Serruys PW, Morice M-C, Kappetein P, Colombo A, Holmes DR, Mack MJ, Ståhle E, Feldman TE, van den Brand M, Bass EJ, Van Dyck N, Leadley K, Dawkins KD, Mohr FW; for the Syntax Investigators. Percutaneous coronary intervention versus coronary-artery bypass grafting for severe coronary artery disease. *N Eng J Med* 2009; 360: 961–72.

Sianos G, Morel MA, Kappetein AP, Morice MC, Colombo A, Dawkins K, van den Brand M, Van Dyck N, Russell ME, Mohr FW, Serruys PW. The SYNTAX score: an angiographic tool grading the complexity of coronary artery disease. *Eurointervention* 2005; 1: 219–27.

The SYNTAX trial was a multi-centre trial involving 85 sites in Europe and the United States, designed to test the hypothesis that PCI using paclitaxel-eluting stents is non-inferior to CABG in patients with three vessel or left main stem disease[27]. Eligible patients had stable angina, unstable angina, atypical chest pain, or asymptomatic myocardial ischaemia, but patients having had previous revascularization, recent acute MI, or the need for concomitant cardiac surgery were excluded. A surgeon and an interventional cardiologist had to agree that CABG or PCI could achieve equivalent anatomical revascularization. The primary end point was a composite of major adverse cardiac and cerebrovascular events (MACCE) comprising death, MI, stroke, and repeat revascularization.

From March 2005 to April 2007 1800 patients were randomized. A group of 897 patients were assigned to CABG, with an average of 2.8 conduits and 3.2 distal anastomoses per patient. One or more arterial grafts were used in 97.3% of patients and 15.0% had surgery without cardiopulmonary bypass. Another group of 903 patients were assigned to PCI using paclitaxel-eluting stents, with an average of more than four stents per patient, a mean stent length of 86.1 mm, and a total stent length of >100mm in one third. Overall, more than four significant coronary lesions were treated per patient (4.4 for CABG and 4.3 for PCI) with a chronic occlusion in 23.1% and a bifurcation lesion in 72.8%. A greater proportion of patients had complete revascularization after CABG than PCI (63.2% vs. 56.7%, p = 0.005).

At 12 months there was a significantly higher incidence of MACCE in the PCI group than in the CABG group (17.8% vs. 12.4%, p = 0.002), largely driven by a significantly higher rate of repeat revascularization in the PCI group (13.5% vs. 5.9%, p <0.001). There was no difference in the incidence of death or MI between the two groups. Stroke was significantly more frequent after CABG than PCI (2.2% vs. 0.6%, p = 0.003), but the diagnosis was made on clinical grounds and not confirmed by cranial imaging. In addition, the rates of symptomatic graft occlusion and stent thrombosis were almost identical (3.3% vs. 3.4%, p = 0.89).

More CABG patients were angina free at 12 months and amongst symptomatic patients, angina frequency was significantly lower in CABG patients at 6 and 12 months. Nevertheless a similar proportion of patients in the CABG and PCI groups reported a significant improvement in angina frequency.

The SYNTAX trial employed a standardized angiographic scoring system (SYNTAX score) that was developed from an amalgamation of seven pre-existing anatomical classification systems[28, 29, 30, 31, 32, 33, 34, 35]. Each lesion with ≥50% luminal obstruction in a coronary vessel ≥1.5 mm in diameter is scored separately for side branch involvement or aorto-ostial location, presence of chronic occlusion, vessel tortuosity, lesion length, calcification, and presence of thrombus, with the eventual SYNTAX score calculated by summation of the scores. Patients enrolled in the SYNTAX trial were stratified into tertiles with low, intermediate, and high SYNTAX scores.

In the CABG group there was no difference in MACCE at 12 months between patients with low, intermediate, or high SYNTAX scores, whereas in the PCI group MACCE rates increased with increasing SYNTAX scores (23.4% with high vs. 16.7% with intermediate [p = 0.04] and 13.6% with low [p = 0.002] SYNTAX scores). There was a significant interaction between SYNTAX score and treatment group with similar MACCE rates for patients with low (13.6% vs. 14.7%, p = 0.71) and intermediate (16.7% vs. 12.0%, p = 0.10) SYNTAX scores, but significantly higher MACCE rates in the PCI group than the CABG group with high SYNTAX scores (23.4% vs. 10.9%, p <0.001). This difference was mainly due to the increased rate of repeat revascularization.

Coronary artery bypass grafting was significantly more expensive at 12 months ($39581 versus $35991 for PCI,

p <0.001) in the entire trial cohort, but when analysed according to SYNTAX scores the difference remained significant for low and intermediate risk patients, but not for those in the highest tertile of SYNTAX score[36].

Results of SYNTAX have also been presented separately for 705 patients with left main stem[37] and 1095 patients with three-vessel disease (see Table 7.1). At three years the MACCE rate in patients with left main stem disease was similar in both treatment groups[38]. The rate of CVA was significantly higher in the CABG group driven mainly by a difference in stroke rate in the first year. There was no difference between CABG and PCI in MACCE or any of its individual components for patients with left main disease and low or intermediate SYNTAX scores. For patients with left main disease and high SYNTAX scores, however, MACCE was significantly higher in the PCI group (21.2% for CABG vs. 37.3% for PCI, p = 0.003) driven predominantly by an increased revascularization rate (9.2% for CABG vs. 27.7% for PCI, p <0.001) (see Table 7.2).

For the subset of patients with triple vessel disease at three years there was a significantly greater incidence of MACCE, all-cause death, cardiac death, MI, all-cause

Table 7.1 Three-year results in the left main, triple-vessel disease, and diabetic subgroups of the SYNTAX trial

		CABG	PCI	p value
All cause death	LM	8.4%	7.3%	0.64
	3VD	5.7%	9.5%	0.02
CVA	LM	4.0%	1.2%	0.02
	3VD	2.9%	2.6%	0.64
MI	LM	4.1%	6.9%	0.14
	3VD	3.3%	7.1%	0.005
All cause death/CVA/MI	LM	14.3%	13.0%	0.60
	3VD	10.6%	14.8%	0.04
	DM	14.0%	16.3%	0.53
Repeat revascularization	LM	11.7%	20.0%	0.004
	3VD	10.0%	19.4%	<0.001
	DM	12.9%	28.0%	<0.0001
MACCE	LM	22.3%	26.8%	0.20
	3VD	18.8%	28.8%	<0.001
	DM	22.9%	37.0%	0.002

LM—left main, 3VD—triple vessel disease, DM—diabetes mellitus
CVA—cerebrovascular accident, MI—myocardial infarction
MACCE—major adverse cardiac and cerebrovascular events = composite of death, CVA, MI, and repeat revascularization

Table 7.2 Three-year MACCE rates in the left main, triple vessel disease, and diabetic subgroups of the SYNTAX trial by SYNTAX score

SYNTAX score		MACCE		p value
		CABG	PCI	
≤22	LM (n = 222)	23.0%	18.0%	0.33
	3VD (n = 352)	22.2%	25.8%	0.45
	DM (n = 136)	30.5%	29.8%	0.98
23–32	LM (n = 195)	23.4%	23.4%	0.90
	3VD (n = 415)	16.8%	29.4%	0.003
	DM (n = 156)	21.0%	36.2%	0.04
≥33	LM (n = 284)	21.2%	37.3%	0.003
	3VD (n = 321)	17.9%	31.4%	0.004
	DM (n = 157)	18.5%	45.9%	<0.001

LM—left main, 3VD—triple vessel disease, DM—diabetes mellitus
MACCE—major adverse cardiac and cerebrovascular events = composite of death, CVA, MI, and repeat revascularization, n—numbers

death/MI/CVA, and repeat revascularization in PCI patients compared to CABG patients[38] (see Table 7.1). In contrast to the left main results there was no difference in the incidence of CVA between CABG and PCI in patients with triple-vessel disease at three years. When analysed according to the SYNTAX score (see Table 7.2) MACCE was significantly higher in the PCI arm for patients with intermediate and high SYNTAX scores, whereas MACCE was equivalent for patients with low SYNTAX scores.

The SYNTAX trial enrolled 452 patients with medically treated *diabetes*[39, 40], of which 221 were assigned to CABG and 231 to PCI. At three years in this cohort the MACCE rate was significantly higher in the PCI arm (see Table 7.1), driven predominantly by an increased rate of repeat revascularization, but there was no difference between CABG and PCI for a composite of all-cause death/MI/CVA. There was no difference in MACCE for diabetic patients with low SYNTAX scores (see Table 7.2), whereas MACCE was significantly higher with PCI in diabetic patients with intermediate and high SYNTAX scores, although patient numbers in these subgroups were small.

Coronary Artery Revascularization in Diabetes Trial (CARDia)

Kapur A, Hall RJ, Malik IS, Qureshi AC, Butts J, de Belder M, Baumbach A, Angelini G, de Belder A, Oldroyd KG, Flather M, Roughton M, Nihoyannopoulos P, Bagger JP, Morgan K, Beatt KJ. Randomized comparison of percutaneous coronary intervention with coronary artery bypass grafting in diabetic patients: 1-year results of the CARDia (Coronary Artery Revascularization in Diabetes) trial. *J Am Coll Cardiol* 2010; 55: 432–40.

The CARDia trial was a multi-centre trial conducted at 24 sites in the United Kingdom. Patients were eligible if they had diabetes mellitus (type 1 or type 2) and symptomatic multi-vessel or complex single-vessel disease (ostial or proximal left anterior descending artery disease). A cardiac surgeon and an interventional cardiologist had to agree that the risks and benefits of CABG and PCI were equivalent before a patient could be randomized. Exclusion criteria included age >80 years, previous revascularization, left main stem disease, cardiogenic shock, recent STEMI, LVEF <20%, and contraindications to

antiplatelet therapy. The primary end point was a composite of death, MI, and CVA at one year with repeat revascularization as the major secondary end point[41].

510 patients were randomized from January 2002 to May 2007. Of these, a group of 254 patients were assigned to CABG with an average of 2.9 grafts per patient, a left internal mammary graft in 94%, at least two arterial grafts in 17%, and off-pump surgery in 31%. Another group of 256 patients were assigned to PCI, with an average of 3.6 stents (mean total stent length 71 mm) per patient, with a sirolimus-eluting stent in 69% and bare metal stents in 31%.

At one year there was no difference between CABG and PCI for the primary end point (10.5% for CABG vs. 13.0% for PCI, HR 1.25, 95% CI 0.75–2.09). This failed to meet the pre-specified criterion to demonstrate non-inferiority of PCI. Repeat revascularization was significantly higher in the PCI group (11.8% vs. 2.0% for CABG, HR 5.31, 95% CI 2.0–14.11) and patients in the CABG group had significantly less angina.

Meta-analyses

Coronary artery bypass surgery compared with percutaneous coronary interventions for multivessel disease: a collaborative analysis of individual patients' data from ten randomized trials

Hlatky MA, Boothroyd DB, Bravata DM, Boersma E, Booth J, Brooks MM, Carrié D, Clayton TC, Danchin N, Flather M, Hamm CW, Hueb WA, Kähler J, Kelsey SF, King SB, Kosinski AS, Lopes N, McDonald KM, Rodriguez A, Serruys P, Sigwart U, Stables RH, Owens DK, Pocock SJ. Coronary artery bypass surgery compared with percutaneous coronary interventions for multivessel disease: a collaborative analysis of individual patient data from ten randomized trials. *Lancet* 2009; 373: 1190–97.

By combining data from several trials, meta-analysis can increase the statistical power to detect differences in outcomes. Twelve trials comparing CABG and PCI in the treatment of multi-vessel CAD, with at least three years of follow-up were identified. Individual patient level data (7812 patients) were made available from ten of these trials (six balloon angioplasty vs. CABG, four bare metal stents versus CABG) and analysed for mortality[42]. These included BARI, CABRI, RITA, ERACI II, SoS and ARTS I. After a median follow-up of 5.9 years, 575 of 3889 patients (15%) assigned to CABG had died compared to 628 of 3923 patients (16%) assigned to PCI (HR 0.91, 95% CI 0.82–1.02, p = 0.12). In subgroup analyses there was an interaction between diabetes and treatment, such that in patients with diabetes, mortality was significantly lower in those assigned to CABG compared with those assigned to PCI (HR 0.70, 95% CI 0.56–0.87, p = 0.014 for interaction). This held true after adjustment for age, sex, smoking, hypertension, previous MI, heart failure, and three-vessel

Table 7.3 Key objectives, inclusion, and exclusion criteria of trials of CABG versus PCI in the treatment of multi-vessel disease

	Objectives	Inclusion	Exclusion	Left main stem	LV dysfunction
BARI	Relief of ischaemia/ symptoms	MVD, objective ischaemia, angina (unstable in 70%)	Age >80 yrs, recent MI, prior CABG/PCI	Excluded	Mean EF c. 57%
CABRI	Relief of ischaemia/ symptoms	MVD, objective ischaemia, angina (unstable in 15%)	Age>75 yrs, ≥2 CTOs, recent MI/CVA, prior CABG/PCI	Excluded	EF <35% excluded Mean EF c. 63%
RITA	Equivalent revascularization	CAD (45% SVD), CABG/PCI clinically indicated (unstable% not specified)	>3VD, recent MI, prior CABG/PCI	Excluded	Mean EF c. 56%
ERACI II	Complete functional revascularization	MVD, objective ischaemia, angina (unstable in 90%)	Prior CABG/PCI	5% of patients	EF <35% excluded
SoS	Equivalent revascularization	MVD, CABG/PCI clinically indicated (unstable in 24%)	Prior CABG/PCI	1% of patients	Mean EF c. 57%
ARTS I	Equivalent revascularization	MVD, objective ischaemia, angina (unstable in 35%)	Recent MI/CVA, prior CABG/PCI	Excluded	EF <30% excluded Mean EF c. 61%
SYNTAX	Equivalent revascularization	MVD, objective ischaemia, angina (unstable in 28%)	Recent MI, prior CABG/PCI	Specific subset of 705 patients	EF <30% c. 2% of patients
CARDia	Complete revascularization	DM, MVD (or prox LAD), CABG/PCI clinically indicated (unstable in 23%)	Age >80yrs, recent MI, prior CABG/PCI	Excluded	EF <20% excluded Mean EF c. 60%

MVD—multi-vessel disease, CABG—coronary artery bypass graft, PCI—percutaneous coronary intervention, EF—ejection fraction, CTO—chronic total occlusion, CVA—cerebrovascular accident, CAD—coronary artery disease, SVD—single vessel disease, 3VD—triple-vessel disease, DM—diabetes mellitus disease (p = 0.008), and after exclusion of data from the BARI trial (p = 0.048 for interaction). For patients without diabetes there was no difference in mortality between CABG and PCI. Age also had a significant interaction with treatment, with a mortality benefit of CABG emerging with age over 65 years (HR 0.82, 95% CI 0.70–0.97, p = 0.002 for interaction). No other variables, including proximal LAD disease, triple vessel disease, impaired LV function, or type of PCI (balloon angioplasty or bare metal stents) influenced the effect of treatment on mortality.

Discussion

The trials of CABG versus PCI included in this chapter all enrolled patients with multi-vessel CAD who were considered eligible for either procedure. The individual trials have provided very similar results and failed to show significant differences in the end points of death or MI, although a large individual patient data meta-analysis does suggest a mortality benefit for CABG over PCI in patients with diabetes or aged over 65 years[42]. Both treatments provide effective relief from angina, but to a greater degree following CABG. Repeat revascularization remains more frequent after PCI, although rates have decreased significantly with the introduction of first bare-metal and then drug-eluting stents. Initial costs are higher for CABG, but the cost difference attenuates over time, mainly because of repeat revascularization procedures in patients initially treated with PCI.

The consistency of these results is remarkable, particularly considering the differences between the trials in objectives, inclusion, and exclusion criteria, end point definitions (particularly for MI) and length of follow-up (see Table 7.3). In addition there has been a significant evolution of interventional and surgical techniques over the last 30 years with the introduction of bare metal and drug eluting stents, thienopyridines, glycoprotein IIbIIIa inhibitors, 'off-pump' surgery, and the greater use of arterial bypass conduits. These technological advances mean the earliest trials have less relevance to current practice.

The patients included in these trials were highly selected and many 'high-risk' patients were systematically excluded. The proportion of patients enrolled in the trials with an acute coronary syndrome as the initial presentation ranged from 15–35% in some of the trials to 70% in BARI and 90% in ERACI-II. Patients with left main stem disease were ineligible or poorly represented (5% of patients in ERACI II and 1% in SoS), with the exception of SYNTAX, where a left main stem group was pre-specified. Impaired left ventricular systolic function was similarly either excluded or poorly represented, with mean ejection fractions (EF) of between 56% and 63% in the different trial populations, and an EF of <30% in only 2% of patients in the SYNTAX trial. The patients enrolled in the trials are therefore not likely to be representative of patients undergoing revascularization in contemporary practice.

The individual trials comparing initial treatment strategies of CABG and PCI were small and had limited follow-up. The trials therefore all had limited statistical power to detect small but potentially important differences in outcomes, particularly mortality. Any mortality benefit of one treatment over the other will play out over the lifetime of an individual patient rather than the limited follow-up period of a clinical trial and it remains possible that small but potentially important differences do exist and might have emerged with longer-term follow-up.

With regards to overall MACCE, subgroup analyses from SYNTAX at three years suggest that for patients with left main disease, CABG and PCI may be equivalent in those with low or intermediate SYNTAX scores, whereas CABG appears to be superior in patients with high SYNTAX scores. For patients with triple vessel disease or medically treated diabetes, CABG and PCI may be equivalent in those with low SYNTAX scores, but CABG appears to be superior in patients with intermediate or high SYNTAX scores. These subgroup analyses, however, are based on small patient numbers (see Table 7.2) and are statistically underpowered, particularly for individual components of a composite end point. They should be interpreted with caution, and considered to be hypothesis generating, rather than definitive evidence of superiority of one strategy over another. In addition, whilst the SYNTAX score appears to provide useful information about risk, it was not prospectively derived from a cohort of unselected patients with CAD, nor has it been formally validated in populations outside the SYNTAX trial to assess discrimination and calibration. The SYNTAX score may simply be a marker for disease severity and a complex way of predicting total stent length required to revascularize the patient (which is likely to be a powerful predictor of PCI outcome)[43]. The SYNTAX trial also included patients at one end of a spectrum of disease severity suitable for either procedure and may not be applicable to the wider population of patients undergoing revascularization in routine clinical practice.

The role of PCI in diabetics has been controversial since the subgroup analysis of BARI was reported[8], but the meta-analysis described above[42] provides strong evidence of an interaction between diabetic status and revascularization strategy. The CARDia trial was underpowered for the primary composite outcome and achieved only 85% of the intended sample size, but is still the largest individual study of revascularization in diabetic patients. Further information is required and the results of the FREEDOM trial (Future REvascularization Evaluation in patients with Diabetes mellitus: Optimal Management of multi-vessel disease) will provide further data on the best interventional strategy for this important and complex patient subgroup[44]. This multi-centre trial of CABG versus PCI (with drug-eluting stents) in patients with diabetes mellitus and multi-vessel CAD is aiming to enroll 2400 patients and results are expected in 2012.

Longer-term results of contemporary trials of CABG versus PCI are required to further define the role of revascularization procedures in patients with angina. Ongoing follow-up of the SYNTAX trial suggests that those with the most complex CAD may have better outcomes with CABG than PCI. Coronary artery bypass grafting is,

however, a major operation, with a longer initial period of convalescence, followed by a relatively stable clinical course with relief of angina and a low requirement for additional procedures over several years. Percutaneous coronary intervention is a much less invasive procedure with a much shorter hospital stay and rapid return to normal activity, but with the increased likelihood for additional revascularization procedures in the short to medium term. Patients will differ in how they view the impact of the two procedures and some patients will happily accept the risk of several revascularizations to avoid bypass surgery, whereas for others this risk will be prohibitive. The SYNTAX score, despite its lack of formal derivation and validation, can be useful as a tool to aid decision making when choosing a revascularization strategy for individual patients, helping to identify those in whom CABG and PCI are likely to provide broadly similar outcomes at equivalent long-term cost. The SYNTAX score should not, however, be the sole determinant of whether a patient is referred for CABG or PCI. Age, diabetic status, and comorbidities are other important variables and where significant doubt exists as to the optimal revascularization strategy, patient preference and informed consent, together with the consensus opinion from a joint cardiology/cardiothoracic surgery multidisciplinary team meeting, should remain the final arbiters.

References

1. Favaloro RG. Saphenous vein autograft replacement of severe segmental coronary artery occlusion: operative technique. *Ann Thorac Surg* 1968; 5: 334–9.
2. Loop FD, Lytle BW, Cosgrove DM, *et al.* Influence of the internal-mammary-artery graft on 10 year survival and other cardiac events. *N Eng J Med* 1986; 314: 1–6.
3. Grüntzig A. Transluminal dilatation of coronary-artery stenosis. *Lancet* 1978; 1; 263.
4. Faxon DP, Kelsey SF, Ryan TJ, *et al.* Determinants of successful percutaneous transluminal coronary angioplasty: report from the National Heart, Lung and Blood Institute registry. *Am J Heart* 1984; 108: 1019–23.
5. Serruys PW, Kutryk MJ, Ong AT. Coronary-artery stents. *N Eng J Med* 2006; 354: 483–95.
6. Cohen M. Antiplatelet therapy in percutaneous coronary intervention: a critical review of the 2007 AHA/ACC/SCAI guidelines and beyond. *Catheter Cardiovasc Interv* 2009; 74: 579–97.
7. Anonymous. Protocol for the Bypass Angioplasty Revascularization Investigation. *Circulation* 1991; 84(Suppl V): 1–27.

8. The Bypass Angioplasty Revascularization Investigation (BARI) Investigators. Comparison of coronary bypass surgery with angioplasty in patients with multivessel disease. *N Eng J Med* 1996; 335: 217–25.
9. The BARI Investigators. The final 10-year follow-up results from the BARI randomized trial. *J Am Coll Cardiol* 2007; 49: 1600–6.
10. Schaff HV, Rosen AD, Shemin RJ, *et al.* Clinical and operative characteristics of patients randomized to coronary artery bypass surgery in the Bypass Angioplasty Revascularization Investigation (BARI). *Am J Cardiol* 1995; 75: 18C–26C.
11. Williams DO, Baim DS, Bates E, *et al.* Coronary anatomic and procedural characteristics of patients randomized to coronary angioplasty in the Bypass Angioplasty Revascularization Investigation (BARI). *Am J Cardiol* 1995; 75: 27C–33C.
12. The BARI Investigators. Seven-year outcome in the Bypass Angioplasty Revascularization Investigation (BARI) by treatment and diabetic status. *J Am Coll Cardiol* 2000; 35: 1122–9.

13. Hlatky MA, Rogers WJ, Johnstone I, *et al*. Medical care costs and quality of life after randomization to coronary angioplasty or coronary bypass surgery. *N Eng J Med* 1997; 336: 92–9.

14. CABRI trial participants. First-year results of CABRI (Coronary Angioplasty versus Bypass Revascularization Investigation). *Lancet* 1995; 346: 1179–84.

15. De Coster P, Malhomme B, Lejeune M, *et al*. Respective costs of percutaneous transluminal coronary angioplasty versus coronary artery bypass surgery: a substudy of the CABRI trial. *Eur Heart J* 1994; 15(Suppl): 32(abstract).

16. Kurbaan AS, Bowker TJ, Ilsley CD, *et al*. Difference in the mortality of the CABRI diabetic and nondiabetic populations and its relation to coronary artery disease and the revascularization mode. *Am J Cardiol* 2001; 87: 947–50.

17. Henderson RA. The Randomized Intervention Treatment of Angina (RITA) trial protocol: a long-term study of coronary angioplasty and coronary artery bypass surgery in patients with angina. *Br Heart J* 1989; 62: 411–4.

18. Henderson RA, Pocock SJ, Sharp SJ, *et al*. Long-term results of RITA-1 trial: clinical and cost comparisons of coronary angioplasty and coronary-artery bypass grafting. *Lancet* 1998; 352: 1419–25.

19. Pocock SJ, Henderson RA, Seed P, *et al*. Quality of life, employment status and anginal symptoms after coronary angioplasty or bypass surgery: 3-year follow-up in the Randomized Intervention Treatment of Angina (RITA) trial. *Circulation* 1996; 94: 135–42.

20. Sculpher MJ, Seed P, Henderson RA, *et al*. Health service costs of coronary angioplasty and coronary bypass surgery: the Randomized Intervention Treatment of Angina (RITA) trial. *Lancet* 1994; 344: 927–30.

21. Rodriguez AE, Baldi J, Fernandez Pereira C, *et al*. Five-year follow-up of the Argentine randomized trial of coronary angioplasty with stenting versus coronary bypass surgery in patients with multiple vessel disease (ERACI II). *J Am Coll Cardiol* 2005; 46: 582–8.

22. Booth J, Clayton T, Pepper J, *et al*. Randomized, controlled trial of coronary artery bypass surgery versus percutaneous coronary intervention in patients with multivessel coronary artery disease: six-year follow-up from the Stent or Surgery trial (SoS). *Circulation* 2008; 118: 381–8.

23. Weintraub WS, Mahoney EM, Zhang Z, *et al*. One year comparison of costs of coronary surgery versus percutaneous coronary intervention in the stent or surgery trial. *Heart* 2004; 90: 782–8.

24. Währborg P, Booth JE, Clayton T, *et al*. Neuropsychological outcome after percutaneous coronary intervention or coronary artery bypass grafting: results from the Stent or Surgery (SoS) Trial. *Circulation* 2004;110:3411–7.

25. Serruys PW, Unger F, Sousa JE, *et al* for the Arterial Revascularization Therapies Study Group. Comparison of coronary-artery bypass surgery and stenting for the treatment of multi-vessel disease. *N Engl J Med* 2001; 344: 1117–24.

26. Serruys PW, Ong AT, van Herwerden LA, *et al*. Five-year outcomes after coronary stenting versus bypass surgery for the treatment of multi-vessel disease: the final analysis of the Arterial Revascularization Therapies Study (ARTS) randomized trial. *J Am Coll Cardiol* 2005; 46: 575–81.

27. Serruys PW, Morice MC, Kappetein AP, *et al*. Percutaneous coronary intervention versus coronary-artery bypass grafting for severe coronary artery disease. *N Eng J Med* 2009; 360: 961–72.

28. Sianos G, Morel MA, Kappetein AP, *et al*. The SYNTAX score: an angiographic tool grading the complexity of coronary artery disease. *Eurointervention* 2005; 1: 219–27.

29. American Heart Association Grading Committee. Coronary Artery Disease Reporting System. *Circulation* 1975; 51: 31–3.

30. Serruys PW, Unger F, van Hout BA, *et al*. The ARTS study (Arterial Revascularization Therapies Study). *Semin Interv Cardiol* 1999; 4: 209–19.

31. Leaman DM, Brower RW, Meester GT, *et al*. Coronary artery atherosclerosis: severity of the disease, severity of angina pectoris and compromised left ventricular function. *Circulation* 1981; 63: 285–99.

32. Ryan TJ, Faxon DP, Gunnar RM, *et al*. Guidelines for percutaneous transluminal coronary angioplasty. A report of the American College of Cardiology/American Heart Association Task Force on assessment of diagnostic and therapeutic cardiovascular procedures (subcommittee on percutaneous transluminal coronary angioplasty). *Circulation* 1988; 78: 486–502.

33. Hamburger JN, Serruys PW, Scabra-Gomes R, *et al*. Recanalization of total coronary occlusions using a laser guidewire (the European TOTAL Surveillance Study). *Am J Cardiol* 1997; 80: 1419–23.

34. Topol EJ. *Textbook of Interventional Cardiology*. 3rd edn. Philadelphia: WB Saunders Co 1998. p. 728.

35. Lefevre T, Louvard Y, Morice MC, *et al*. Stenting of bifurcation lesions: classification, treatments, and results. *Catheter Cardiovasc Interv* 2000; 49: 274–83.

36. Cohen DJ, Lavelle TA, Serruys PW, *et al*. Health related quality of life and US economic outcomes of PCI with drug-eluting stents vs bypass surgery: 1-year results from the SYNTAX trial. American College of Cardiology scientific sessions late breaking clinical trials 2009.

37. Morice MC, Serruys PW, Kappetein AP, *et al*. Outcomes in patients with *de novo* left main disease treated with either percutaneous coronary intervention using paclitaxel-eluting stents or coronary artery bypass graft treatment in the Synergy Between Percutaneous Coronary Intervention with TAXUS and Cardiac Surgery (SYNTAX) trial. *Circulation* 2010; 121: 2645–53.

38. Kappetein AP, Feldman TE, Mack MJ, *et al*. Comparison of coronary bypass surgery with drug-eluting stenting for the treatment of left main and/or three-vessel disease: 3-year

follow-up of the SYNTAX trial. *Eur Heart J*. 2011; 32: 2125–34.

39. Banning AP, Westaby S, Morice MC, *et al*. Diabetic and non-diabetic patients with left main and/or 3-vessel coronary artery disease: comparison of outcomes with cardiac surgery and paclitaxel-eluting stents. *J Am Coll Cardiol* 2010; 55: 1067–75.

40. Kappetein AP. The 3-year outcomes of the SYNTAX trial focus on diabetes. Transcatheter Cardiovascular Therapeutics (TCT) 2010.

41. Kapur A, Hall RJ, Malik IS, *et al*. Randomized comparison of percutaneous coronary intervention with coronary artery bypass grafting in diabetic patients: 1-year results of the CARDia (Coronary Artery Revascularization in Diabetes) trial. *J Am Coll Cardiol* 2010; 55: 432–40.

42. Hlatky MA, Boothroyd DB, Bravata DM, *et al*. Coronary artery bypass surgery compared with percutaneous coronary interventions for multivessel disease: a collaborative analysis of individual patient data from ten randomized trials. *Lancet* 2009; 373: 1190–97.

43. Cutlip DE, Baim DS, Ho KK, *et al*. Stent thrombosis in the modern era: a pooled analysis of multicenter coronary stent clinical trials. *Circulation* 2001; 103: 1967–71.

44. Farkouh ME, Dangas G, Leon MB, *et al*. Design of the Future REvascularization Evaluation in patients with Diabetes mellitus: Optimal management of Multivessel disease (FREEDOM) Trial. *Am Heart J* 2008; 155: 215–23.

Part II

Cardiac electrophysiology and heart rhythm disturbances

Chapter 8

Epidemiology and molecular foundation

Dr Fu Siong Ng and Professor Nicholas Peters

Introduction

The past four decades have witnessed significant progress in the fields of basic science and epidemiology of cardiac electrophysiology. As demonstrated by the landmark papers in this chapter [1, 2, 3, 4, 5, 6, 7, 8, 9, 10, 11], advances and discoveries in basic science and epidemiology over this period have not only greatly enhanced our understanding of arrhythmia mechanisms, but importantly, these advances have been successfully translated into clinical practice in the form of new pharmacological therapies, diagnostic tools, and novel approaches to managing and treating arrhythmias.

These breakthroughs in basic science electrophysiology have been driven in no small part by methodological advances and the development of new research tools to study cardiac electrophysiology. For example, the voltage-clamp technique, first developed in the 1940s and then refined in the subsequent decades [12, 13, 14], was invaluable in helping researchers describe the ionic currents that contribute to the cardiac action potential, during the early second half of the twentieth century. One example of such voltage-clamp studies is the work paper

by Brown *et al.*[5], describing the pacemaker I_f current, discussed in the landmark papers section below.

By the 1980s, a great proportion of sarcolemmal ionic currents had been described and there was a move away from the more reductionist approach of focusing on electrophysiology at the cellular level, towards studying arrhythmia mechanisms at the tissue and organ level. The timely development of new *in vivo* disease models made possible experiments that have improved our understanding of disease-specific, arrhythmogenic processes [15, 16]. In the following section, we describe two landmark papers which utilized novel animal disease models to study arrhythmia mechanisms in atrial fibrillation [1] and post-myocardial infarction ventricular tachycardia [3].

Our ability to study arrhythmogenic processes at the intact tissue and whole organ level was further enhanced by methodological advances that have allowed for the imaging of cellular and electrophysiological processes of the heart. This included the development and refinement of optical techniques for imaging the heart [17, 18], which have provided a non-invasive method of detecting transmembrane voltage changes, as well as studying calcium homeostasis and metabolic processes in intact tissue and whole hearts.

Another factor in the advance of basic science cardiac electrophysiology has been the burgeoning of genetic research over the past two decades, which has greatly enhanced our understanding of pathophysiological processes in general as well as factors that predispose to disease[19]. Here we describe two landmark papers, which have utilized novel genetic research tools to identify arrhythmia determinants, one study in the 1990s using a candidate gene approach to identify causative genes in long QT syndrome[7], the other a genome-wide association study in the 2000s in atrial fibrillation[8].

All the above methodological advances, in parallel with the growth of molecular biological and epidemiological techniques, have provided researchers with a vast arsenal of tools and techniques to probe the mechanisms of arrhythmias and develop novel therapies. Some of the key breakthroughs of the last four decades using these tools are described in more detail below.

Selection of landmark papers

Selecting a short list of landmark basic science and epidemiology papers in the field of cardiac electrophysiology for this chapter has been no easy task. For every paper listed in the following section, we have had to leave out several other equally important, high-impact papers. To help narrow down the list, we have had to come up with a restrictive definition of what makes a landmark paper.

Here we describe basic science and epidemiology papers that are not only of high impact in terms of introducing novel concepts and opening up new fields of research, but these are papers that also have clear clinical implications that a reader can relate to. These clinical implications include the introduction of novel therapeutic agents or targets, the introduction of new diagnostic tools, or the changing of clinical practice in terms of the way we view, approach, and manage a particular disease.

As a result of these strict definitions, we have had to leave out many key papers that have introduced important electrophysiological concepts. These include the work of Antzelevitch and colleagues in investigating the transmural differences in electrophysiological properties between epicardial and endocardial cells[20] and the discovery of M cells[21], and the work of Kleber and colleagues on the novel concept of source-sink mismatch[22], to name but a few.

In order to ensure that we present a good spread of papers that cover a wide range of electrophysiological concepts and clinical arrhythmias, we have selected a single landmark paper for each of the subcategories listed below, so that these landmark papers cover a range of clinical entities such as atrial fibrillation, ventricular tachycardia, and inherited arrhythmia syndromes, different arrhythmia determinants, such as ionic currents, gap junctional coupling, and intracellular calcium, as well as important epidemiological studies.

Atrial fibrillation

Wijffels MC, Kirchhof CJ, Dorland R, Allessie MA. Atrial fibrillation begets atrial fibrillation. A study in awake chronically instrumented goats. *Circulation* 1995; 92: 1954–68.

Background

The past 30 years have seen significant advances in our understanding of the pathophysiology of atrial fibrillation (AF), culminating in successful, new treatments for this condition, including the ever-increasing use of catheter ablation. The seminal basic science paper relating to the pathophysiology of AF is the one from the lab of Maurits Allesie, which coined the now famous phrase 'AF begets AF'.

It had been previously observed that paroxysmal AF often progresses to chronic, persistent AF regardless of underlying aetiology[23, 24]. Anecdotal evidence also pointed to AF being a progressive disease, with reducing success rates of restoring sinus rhythm during cardioversion in patients with longer histories of AF[25]. As a result, the authors hypothesized that atrial fibrillation begets atrial fibrillation, and explored the potential electrophysiological remodeling processes that contributed to this phenomenon.

Methods and results

A goat model of AF was used, where 12 goats were chronically instrumented with multiple epicardial atrial electrodes, which were connected to a fibrillation pacemaker that artificially maintained AF in these animals. Electrophysiological parameters such as atrial effective refractory periods (AERP), conduction velocity, and inducibility of AF were studied at various time-points up to four weeks of continuous pacemaker-maintained AF.

Even during the first 24 hours of AF, significant electrophysiological changes were observed. At 24 hours, there was a significant shortening of AERP, a surrogate for action potential duration, from 146 ± 19 msec to 95 ± 20 msec. This corresponded with increased inducibility of AF by a single premature stimulus from 24% to 76%. In addition, the normal physiological adaptation of AERP to heart rate changes was lost. Conduction velocities were unchanged compared to baseline. Over the course of the following four weeks, the atrial fibrillation cycle lengths shortened and atrial electrograms became progressively more fractionated. Importantly, when the fibrillation pacemaker was switched off and sinus rhythm restored after four weeks of AF, the above electrophysiological changes were found to be reversible within one week.

Conclusions and clinical implications

These findings confirm that atrial fibrillation produces a series of electrophysiological changes that further increase the likelihood of sustaining AF. Specifically, the shortening of AERP allows for the formation of greater numbers of meandering wavelets in the atrium, thus reducing the likelihood of AF termination.

These insights into the electrical remodelling processes that occur in AF have significantly impacted on clinical practice and the way we manage this condition. They confirmed that AF is a progressive disease and, by extension, that paroxysmal AF and persistent AF are distinct entities, which require different management approaches. For example, electrical isolation of the pulmonary veins responsible for triggering AF is the conventional approach to catheter ablation of paroxysmal AF[26]. However, this approach is accepted to be insufficient for patients with persistent AF because of the super-added atrial electrical remodelling processes, and such patients often require a substrate-based approach to catheter ablation in addition to pulmonary vein isolation[27].

The other major insight provided by these experiments is that the electrical remodelling is fully reversible after four weeks of AF. This has influenced a recent shift in clinical practice towards treating and ablating AF earlier in its natural history to prevent progression to chronic, persistent AF, which is more difficult to treat.

Learning points

- ◆ Atrial fibrillation is a progressive disease.
- ◆ Atrial fibrillation induces electrical remodelling processes that increase the likelihood of AF maintenance and recurrence, and reduce the likelihood of termination—that is, 'AF begets AF'.
- ◆ The atrial electrophysiological substrate is different between paroxysmal and persistent AF, and they require different management approaches.

Further reading

- Potential causes of atrial remodelling in AF:
  Wijffels MC, Kirchhof CJ, Dorland R, Power J, Allessie MA. Electrical remodelling due to atrial fibrillation in chronically instrumented conscious goats: roles of neurohumoral changes, ischemia, atrial stretch, and high rate of electrical activation. *Circulation* 1997; 96(10): 3710–20.
- Evidence of electrical remodelling in human AF:
  Franz MR, Karasik PL, Li C, Moubarak J, Chavez M. Electrical remodelling of the human atrium: similar effects in patients with chronic atrial fibrillation and atrial flutter. *J Am Coll Cardiol* 1997; 30: 1785–92.

Post-myocardial infarction ventricular tachycardia

de Bakker JM, van Capelle FJ, Janse MJ, Wilde AA, Coronel R, Becker AE, Dingemans KP, van Hemel NM, Hauer RN. Re-entry as a cause of ventricular tachycardia in patients with chronic ischemic heart disease: electrophysiologic and anatomic correlation. *Circulation* 1988; 77: 589–606.

Background

Survivors of myocardial infarction are predisposed to developing ventricular tachyarrhythmias and sudden cardiac death[11]. It has been estimated that more than 50% of all deaths in individuals who have previously developed myocardial infarction are attributable to arrhythmic deaths[28]. However, the mechanisms of ventricular arrhythmias that occur in the chronic healed infarct remained unclear in the late 1980s.

Previous studies using programmed stimulation and endocardial catheter mapping in humans had suggested that the mechanism of arrhythmias post-infarction was predominantly re-entrant in nature[29], although it was difficult to reconcile this with the observation that these arrhythmias appeared to arise from focal circumscribed areas of myocardium[30].

To elucidate the mechanism of ventricular tachycardia post-infarction, de Bakker *et al.* carried out a series of electrophysiological experiments intra-operatively and on *in vitro* preparations, as well as histological analysis of the arrhythmic substrate.

Methods and results

The authors performed intra-operative mapping of endocardial activity using an endocardial balloon electrode in 72 patients undergoing surgery for refractory ventricular tachycardia (VT). In these patients, 139 different tachycardias were mapped. Of these only three tachycardias were of a macro-re-entrant nature around the infarct scar. The other 136 tachycardias were found to spread centrifugally on the endocardial surface from a small site of origin <1.4 cm^2.

Of interest, the authors were able to record small electrograms of low amplitude preceeding the main activation at the endocardial site of origin, which they termed 'presystolic activity'. Histological analysis of seven endocardial resected preparations revealed the presence of viable myocardial fibres in areas where presystolic activity was recorded. These surviving myocardial fibres were located subendocardially and intramurally. These bundles had slower macroscopic conduction velocities in the order of 25 cm/s and gave rise to fragmented electrograms as recorded during *in vitro* eletrophysiological experiments on resected myocardial preparations.

In addition to intra-operative activation mapping, *ex vivo* human Langendorff experiments and histology were also performed in two hearts from transplant patients. The findings from these experiments concur with the above findings that there are surviving bundles of myocardium within dense scar that form the circuit for re-entrant arrhythmias.

Conclusions and clinical implications

The authors provide experimental evidence that suggests that ventricular tachycardias in chronic post-infarction patients are predominantly re-entrant in nature. The apparent focal nature of these tachycardias as detected by endocardial mapping catheters reflects the fact that these tachycardia circuits involve surviving bundles of myocytes that traverse dense scar tissue and emerge on the endocardial surface at distinct exit points.

This landmark study is the first to provide a correlation between electrophysiological and histological data in humans showing the nature of post-infarction VT. It provided a crucial insight into the anatomical substrates that support post-infarction VT, specifically the involvement of surviving myocardial bundles in the VT circuit and the possibility of multiple circuits being present in the infarct scar. These data have informed the VT ablation procedures that have become far more widespread in the past decade, specifically the ablative strategy of targeting diastolic pathways[31], which consist of the surviving myocardial bundles demonstrated elegantly in this paper.

Learning points

◆ Post-infarction VT is predominantly re-entrant in nature.

◆ These arrhythmias are not re-entrant around the entire scar. Instead the re-entrant circuit tends to involve intramural and subendocardial surviving bundles of myocytes that exist within areas of dense scar.

◆ These surviving bundles of myocardium that support the re-entrant arrhythmias have slower conduction and give rise to small amplitude electrograms as detected by endocardial catheters.

Further reading

• Cause of slow conduction in infarcted hearts:
de Bakker JM, van Capelle FJ, Janse MJ, *et al.* Slow conduction in the infarcted human heart. 'Zigzag' course of activation. *Circulation* 1993; 88: 915–26.

• Review of post-infarction VT substrate:
Haqqani HM, Marchlinski FE. Electrophysiologic substrate underlying postinfarction ventricular tachycardia: characterization and role in catheter ablation. *Heart Rhythm* 2009; 6(8 Suppl): S70–6.

Gap junctions and arrhythmias

Peters NS, Coromilas J, Severs NJ, Wit AL. Disturbed connexin43 gap junction distribution correlates with the location of re-entrant circuits in the epicardial border zone of healing canine infarcts that cause ventricular tachycardia. *Circulation* 1997; 95: 988–96.

Background

The previous landmark paper by de Bakker *et al.*[2] described the importance of surviving bundles of myocytes within the infarct scar in forming the circuits of ventricular tachycardia (VT) and in sustaining VT. Although the nature of the macroscopic VT circuits was well-described by the 1990s, little was known about the microscopic and molecular changes within the re-entrant circuits, which can affect and alter conduction.

Gap junctions consist of clusters of transmembrane channels that connect the cytoplasmic compartments of adjacent cells, and consist of connexin43 (Cx43) protein subunits in ventricular myocardium[32]. They play an important role in the electrical coupling of cardiomyocytes and the conduction of the electrical impulse through the myocardium. It was previously noted that alterations in gap junctional distribution were found in the infarct border zone[33], although the electrophysiological consequences of this were unknown. The authors used a four-day canine infarct model to assess the link between Cx43 gap junctional maldistribution and VT circuits.

Methods and results

Six mongrel dogs underwent surgical left anterior descending artery ligation to generate myocardial infarction. At four days post-myocardial infarction, dogs were re-anaesthetized for open-chest electrophysiological studies. A flexible polymer sheet containing 292 bipolar electrodes was sutured to the left ventricular epicardial surface to record epicardial activation. Programmed electrical stimulation protocols were used to induce VT and the VT circuits were mapped using the electrode array.

Following the electrophysiological study, tissue corresponding to the 6 cm x 6 cm central electrode array was excised, divided into 25 equal squares and fixed. Tissue was sectioned and then stained with Masson's trichrome and immunolabelled to localize gap junctional Cx43 distribution on adjacent sections.

The results showed marked disturbance of Cx43 immunolabel localization in the epicardial infarct border zone. Significant 'lateralization' of Cx43, that is, presence of Cx43 immunolabel on the lateral membranes of cardiomyocytes as opposed to their usual location at the intercalated disks, was seen. Most regions of the epicardial border zone demonstrated partial-thickness gap junctional disarray, though in some areas there was full-thickness disarray. Importantly, location of areas of full-thickness gap junctional disarray correlated anatomically with the location of the central common pathway of the figure-of-eight re-entrant circuits.

Conclusions and clinical implications

This was the first study to correlate areas of gap junctional disturbance with the location of electrophysiological re-entrant circuits. The authors showed that altered gap junctional distribution is an early remodelling process post-infarction, and may be a determinant of VT susceptibility post-infarction, given its spatial correlation with re-entrant circuits.

This study revealed that the re-entrant VT circuits are not merely anatomically-defined and fixed substrates, but that there are also remodelling processes at the molecular level that can affect conduction in these re-entrant circuits. These early insights into the molecular changes occurring at the location of VT circuits were subsequently confirmed by studies showing abnormal slowing of conduction in these circuits[34], and there is currently significant interest in novel therapeutic strategies, both pharmacological[35] and biological[36], that seek to improve conduction within the border zone as a way to reduce susceptibility to post-infarction VT.

Learning points

- Gap junctional disarray occurs at the epicardial border zone.
- The location of the central common pathway in VT circuits correlates to regions with full thickness gap-junctional disarray.
- Remodelling occurs at the molecular level within the re-entrant VT circuits, which may affect conduction and increase susceptibility to VT.

Further reading

- Heterogeneous remodelling of gap junctions:
  Cabo C, Yao J, Boyden PA, *et al*. Heterogeneous gap junction remodeling in re-entrant circuits in the epicardial border zone of the healing canine infarct. *Cardiovasc Res* 2006; 72: 241–9.

- Review of gap junctional remodelling.
  Severs NJ, Bruce AF, Dupont E, Rothery S. Remodeling of gap junctions and connexin expression in diseased myocardium. *Cardiovasc Res* 2008; 80: 9–19.

Calcium and arrhythmias

Watanabe H, Chopra N, Laver D, Hwang HS, Davies SS, Roach DE, Duff HJ, Roden DM, Wilde AA, Knollmann BC. Flecainide prevents catecholaminergic polymorphic ventricular tachycardia in mice and humans. *Nat Med* 2009; 15: 380–3.

Background

Catecholaminergic polymorphic ventricular tachycardia (CPVT) is an inherited arrhythmia syndrome which predisposes to life-threatening ventricular arrhythmias. This disorder is characterized by the development of polymorphic ventricular tachycardia during adrenergic stress[37]. At present, the mainstay of treatment for CPVT is beta blockade to reduce adrenergic tone, in conjunction with implantation of implantable cardioverter defibrillators (ICDs) in selected patients to prevent sudden death, though these options have their limitations and are not completely effective.

The pathophysiology of CPVT relates to leaky ryanodine receptor (RyR2) Ca^{2+} channels, as a result of mutations that destabilize the RyR2 Ca^{2+} release complex[38]. This leads to spontaneous Ca^{2+} release from the sarcoplasmic reticulum (SR) and causes delayed after-depolarizations and polymorphic VT. In this study, the authors employed a bench-to-bedside approach to identify a therapy for CPVT based on knowledge of its pathophysiology.

Methods and results

First, the authors screened well-known clinically available anti-arrhythmic drugs to identify agents that possess inhibitory effects on RyR2. In this first set of experiments, they found that flecainide, a sodium channel blocking antiarrhythmic drug, also inhibited RyR2, as evidenced by a dose-dependent reduction in RyR2 open probability and mean open time when studying its effects on single sheep RyR2 channels incorporated in lipid bilayers.

Next, they tested if this inhibition of RyR2 translated into inhibition of spontaneous Ca^{2+} release. Using ventricular myocytes isolated from a CPVT mouse model, it was shown that 6 μM flecainide significantly reduced spontaneous SR Ca^{2+} leak (p <0.01), and reduced the number of triggered beats (p <0.001) through its dual action of inhibiting Ca^{2+} leak and blocking Na^+ channels.

Subsequently, the effects of flecainide were assessed *in vivo* in a mouse model of CPVT. In this model, a catecholamine challenge consistently Provoked bidirectional VT. Flecainide was successful in completely suppressing VT in 11/12 mice in response to catecholamine challenge.

Finally, given the efficacy in the mouse model, the authors then tested flecainide in two patients with drug-refractory CPVT, and showed marked clinical efficacy of flecainide in preventing exercise-induced ventricular arrhythmias in these two patients, each carrying a different CPVT mutation (CASQ2 and RyR2).

Conclusions and clinical implications

The authors show that flecainide, in addition to its well-known sodium channel blockade effect, also inhibits RyR2. This effect translated into a reduction in Ca^{2+} release at the myocyte level, a reduction in bidirectional VT in response to catecholamines in an *in vivo* mouse model, and finally a reduction in exercise-induced VT in two patients with drug-refractory CPVT.

This paper is a classic example in which understanding the pathophysiology and molecular mechanisms of a disease have led to the discovery of a potentially novel therapy. An elegant set of studies was performed along the bench-to-bedside experimental spectrum to prove a novel concept. Based on the result of these key studies, clinical trials are now ongoing to assess the effects of flecainide in a wider population of CPVT patients.

Of course, CPVT is not the only condition in which altered calcium handling leads to arrhythmias. Heart failure is another syndrome characterized by calcium leaks and in which calcium sparks can lead to triggered activity and arrhythmias. Ryanodine-receptor stabilzation has also been shown to reduce arrhythmias in animal models[39], and may be a novel therapeutic strategy for patients with heart failure[40].

Learning points

♦ Flecainide inhibits RyR2, in addition to its well-known effect of blocking sodium current.

♦ Flecainide was able to suppress isoprenaline-induced VT in a mouse model of VT.

♦ Flecainide can suppress exercise-induced VT in two patients with drug-refractory CPVT.

Further reading

● Ryanodine-receptor stabilization to prevent arrhythmias: Wehrens XH, Lehnart SE, Reiken SR, *et al*. Protection from cardiac arrhythmia through ryanodine receptor-stabilizing protein calstabin2. *Science* 2004; 304: 292–6.

● Mechanims of action of flecainide in reducing SR Ca^{2+} release: Hilliard FA, Steele DS, Laver D, *et al*. Flecainide inhibits arrhythmogenic Ca^{2+} waves by open state block of ryanodine receptor Ca2+ release channels and reduction of Ca^{2+} spark mass. *J Mol Cell Cardiol*. 2010; 48(2): 293–301.

Ionic currents (pacemaker I_f current)

Brown HF, DiFrancesco D, Noble SJ. How does adrenaline accelerate the heart? *Nature* 1979; 280: 235–6.

Background

Our understanding of the different ionic currents that determine and govern the cardiac action potential has been greatly enhanced by the wealth of data generated from voltage-clamp experiments in the past few decades[14]. One such landmark study by Brown *et al*. has had a particularly significant impact on recent clinical practice.

Although by the late 1970s, the majority of ionic currents responsible for the cardiac action potential had been elucidated[41], there remained some uncertainty regarding ion channels that determine sinoatrial node pacemaker function. Specifically, the mechanism by which a positive chronotropic agent such as adrenaline accelerates heart rate remained unclear.

Methods and results

The authors used a then novel method of voltage-clamping of sinoatrial nodal tissue to address this question. Very small (0.3 mm x 0.3 mm) preparations were dissected from rabbit sinoatrial node and voltage clamped using two microelectrodes. These preparations maintained spontaneous activity and voltage-clamp results were obtained over a range of potentials, including the pacemaker range.

In these experiments, the authors discovered that in addition to increasing the slow inward (Ca^{2+}/Na^+) current of the sinoatrial node, adrenaline also activated a previously unknown current, which they named the I_f current, or the pacemaker current. Activation of this newly-discovered current occurred in the range of voltage where the pacemaker depolarization occurs.

Conclusions and clinical implications

The authors postulated, based on these experimental data, that the I_f current may be important in normal sinoatrial node pacemaking. This has since been confirmed in other experimental studies[42]. This initial discovery of the I_f pacemaker current opened the way for the development of ivabradine, the first selective and specific I_f current inhibitor, which is now currently prescribed clinically to chronic stable angina patients[43, 44], and was also recently shown to improve outcomes in chronic heart failure in the SHIFT study[45]. This landmark paper is an excellent example of how the understanding of basic cardiac electrophysiology, specifically the function of sarcolemmal ionic currents, has led to the discovery of a novel drug target and the development of a novel pharmaceutical agent.

Learning points

♦ The I_f current (or the pacemaker current) is a slowly depolarizing current that activates within the voltage range where pacemaker depolarization occurs.

♦ The I_f current is responsible for sinoatrial node pacemaking.

Further reading

- Review of the I_f current in cardiac pacemaking: DiFrancesco D. The role of the funny current in pacemaker activity. *Circ Res* 2010; 106: 434–46.
- Ivabradine in chronic heart failure:

Swedberg K, Komajda M, Böhm M, *et al.*; SHIFT Investigators. Ivabradine and outcomes in chronic heart failure (SHIFT): a randomised placebo-controlled study. *Lancet* 2010; 376: 875–85.

Cardiac resynchronization therapy (CRT)

Chakir K, Daya SK, Tunin RS, Helm RH, Byrne MJ, Dimaano VL, Lardo AC, Abraham TP, Tomaselli GF, Kass DA. Reversal of global apoptosis and regional stress kinase activation by cardiac resynchronization. *Circulation* 2008; 117: 1369–77.

Background

Cardiac resynchronization therapy (CRT) has been the major advance in heart failure management in the past decade. Large clinical trials such as COMPANION[46] and CARE-HF[47] have showed significant mortality and morbidity benefits of resynchronizing ventricular contraction in patients with dyssnchronous heart failure (DHF).

Studies looking at possible mechanisms by which CRT confers mortality and morbidity benefit have largely focused on ventricular chamber mechanics and energetics[48, 49]. However, very little is known about the effects of CRT on the molecular changes that occur in DHF. In this study, the authors used a novel canine model of DHF to study the effects of CRT on the molecular abnormalities that arise in DHF.

Methods and results

A model of DHF was used, whereby 22 mongrel dogs were subjected to left-bundle branch radiofrequency ablation to induce dyssynchronous ventricular activation and then subjected to three weeks of right atrial tachypacing to induce heart failure. After three weeks, half these dogs were then switched to biventricular pacing (i.e. CRT) whilst the other half continued atrial pacing (DHF group). At six weeks, the CRT dogs had marginally better LV ejection fractions compared with the DHF group (30.9 ± 3.3% vs. 25.6 ± 3.7%, p = 0.02), though both groups still had significant systolic dysfunction.

The authors then studied the expression of multiple stress-response proteins using immunoblotting. In DHF hearts, p38 MAP kinase (MAPK), CaMKII, and tumour-necrosis factor (TNF) alpha were increased in the late-contracting lateral wall, but this rise in stress-response proteins was reduced and homogenized by CRT. The adverse molecular changes induced by DHF were not limited to regional changes in the late-activating part of the ventricles, but there was also a global increase in apoptosis as evidenced by increased terminal deoxynucleotidyl transferase dUTP nick end labelling (TUNEL) staining and increased caspase 3 activity, both widely accepted markers of apoptosis. Again, this increased apoptosis seen in DHF was significantly reduced by CRT. The authors also showed that CRT likely reduced apoptosis by enhancing a prominent cell-survival pathway linked to phosphorylated Akt kinase.

Conclusions and clinical implications

The authors demonstrate for the first time that cardiac resynchronization does not merely improve ventricular chamber mechano-energetics, but also has significant effects at the molecular level. Specifically, these changes include reducing the expression of multiple stress-related proteins in the late-activating ventricular wall, reducing apoptosis throughout the ventricles, and enhancing cell-survival pathways.

This important study is the first to provide evidence that cardiac resynchronization can reverse the molecular remodelling seen in DHF and highlight novel benefits of CRT. The increase in cell-survival signalling and reversal of abnormal regional stress responses in resynchronized hearts are likely to contribute to the improved outcomes seen in CRT clinical trials. Subsequent studies have shown that CRT also reverses the electrical remodelling[50] and the changes in regional gene expression[51] in dyssynchronous heart failure. These results propose a new paradigm, where the benefits of CRT are not solely due to improved chamber mechano-energetics, but also in part due to reverse molecular remodelling.

Further reading

- CRT reverses electrophysiological consequences of dyssnchronous HF:
  Aiba T, Hesketh GG, Barth AS, *et al.* Electrophysiological consequences of dyssynchronous heart failure and its restoration by resynchronization therapy. *Circulation* 2009; 119: 1220–30.
- CRT reverses changes in gene expression in dyssnchronous HF:
  Barth AS, Aiba T, Halperin V, *et al.* Cardiac resynchronization therapy corrects dyssynchrony-induced regional gene expression changes on a genomic level. *Circ Cardiovasc Genet* 2009; 2: 371–8.

Genetic basis of inherited cardiac arrhythmia syndromes

Wang Q, Shen J, Splawski I, Atkinson D, Li Z, Robinson JL, Moss AJ, Towbin JA, Keating MT. SCN5A mutations associated with an inherited cardiac arrhythmia, long QT syndrome. *Cell* 1995; 80: 805–11.

Background

The existence of inherited disorders that can cause sudden cardiac death from arrhythmias is well known. By the early 1990s, inherited syndromes such as long QT syndrome and Brugada syndrome were well-described clinically. However, the genetic basis and the molecular and electrophysiological mechanisms that underlie these disorders remained elusive.

By the mid-1990s, the positions of three long QT loci (LQT1, LQT2, and LQT3) had been mapped[52, 53]. In the case of long QT3, the locus was mapped to chromosome 3p21–24[53]. Although positional information was now available, the specific genes responsible were yet to be identified. In this study, the authors attempted to identify specific genetic polymorphisms associated with LQT3.

Methods and results

First, the authors used a candidate gene approach to identify the gene responsible for LQT3. Candidate genes were selected based on pre-existing knowledge of the pathophysiology of LQT3 and also the position of the LQT3 locus. The prolongation of the QT interval suggests that LQT syndrome is a disorder of cardiac repolarization, and thus genes encoding for ion channels are suitable candidate genes. The sodium channel gene SCN5A had then just recently been mapped to chromosome 3p21[53], which also happened to be the position of the LQT3 locus, thus the authors selected this as their candidate gene. Once the polymorphisms within the SCN5A gene

were identified, linkage analyses in chromosome 3-linked families with LQT syndrome were then performed. These linkage analyses showed that LQT3 and specific SCN5A polymorphisms were tightly linked in all families studied.

Next, the authors went on to identify the specific intragenic deletion in SCN5A that was present in LQT families, but not in over 500 control individuals. DNA sequencing experiments revealed the presence of a nine base pair deletion at the beginning of nucleotide 4661, which disrupted the coding sequence, resulting in the deletion of three amino acids in the cytoplasmic linker of the sodium channel (a region of known importance for sodium channel inactivation). This identical deletion was then also found in two apparently unrelated LQT families.

Conclusions and clinical implications

Taken together, the results above strongly suggest that mutations in the sodium channel-encoding gene SCN5A are responsible for LQT3. By affecting a region of the sodium channel thought to be important in regulating its inactivation, these deletions are thought to delay sodium channel inactivation, prolong repolarization, and lead to the long QT phenotype.

Results from this study (together with a parallel study from the same group showing the association between the potassium channel gene HERG and LQTS[54]), were the first descriptions of specific genetic mutations responsible for the long QT phenotype. Since then, many more mutations in the sodium and potassium channel-encoding genes have been described.

This landmark study paved the way for the routine use of genetic testing in clinical practice in families with inherited arrhythmic syndromes such as long QT syndrome. Genetic testing is now used not only to confirm the presence or absence of disease, but also to help risk stratify patients and guide therapy, as we now know that the severity of disease and response to therapy in individuals with LQTS vary with the genetic loci involved[55].

Learning points

♦ Mutations of SCN5A are responsible for LQT3.
♦ Specific deletions in SCN5A were identified, which result in the deletion of three amino acids

---

in a region of the sodium channel that is known to be important in regulating sodium channel inactivation.
♦ These deletions are thought to delay sodium channel inactivation, prolong repolarization and lead to the long QT phenotype.

Further reading

● HERG mutations and long QT syndrome
Curran ME, Splawski I, Timothy KW, Vincent GM, Green ED, Keating MT. A molecular basis for cardiac arrhythmia: HERG mutations cause long QT syndrome. *Cell* 1995; 80: 795–803.
● Genetic testing in long QT syndrome.
Napolitano C, Priori SG, Schwartz PJ, *et al*. Genetic testing in the long QT syndrome: development and validation of an efficient approach to genotyping in clinical practice. *JAMA* 2005; 294: 2975–80.

Genome-wide association studies (GWAS) in cardiac electrophysiology

Gudbjartsson DF, Arnar DO, Helgadottir A, Gretarsdottir S, Holm H, Sigurdsson A, Jonasdottir A, Baker A, Thorleifsson G, Kristjansson K, Palsson A, Blondal T, Sulem P, Backman VM, Hardarson GA, Palsdottir E, Helgason A, Sigurjonsdottir R, Sverrisson JT, Kostulas K, Ng MCY, Baum L, So WY, Wong KS, Chan JCN, Furie KL, Greenberg SM, Sale M, Kelly P, MacRae CA, Smith EE, Rosand J, Hillert J, Ma RCW, Ellinor PT, Thorgeirsson G, Gulcher JR, Kong A, Thorsteinsdottir U, Stefansson S. Variants conferring risk of atrial fibrillation on chromosome 4q25. *Nature* 2007; 448: 353–7.

Background

The previous landmark paper by Wang *et al.*[7] described the identification of specific single-gene mutations that are responsible for arrhythmia syndromes. However, most arrhythmias are multifactorial in aetiology, of which genetic predisposition may be one of many aetiological factors. One new approach to identify genetic polymorphisms that are associated with an increased risk of disease is to use genome-wide association studies (GWAS)[56]. These are generally 'hypothesis-free' studies whereby the frequencies of all known single nucleotide polymorphisms (SNPs) are compared between individuals with and without a disease to identify disease-associated SNPs.

Within the field of cardiac electrophysiology, one major GWAS was the study by Gudbjartsson *et al.*, looking for SNPs associated with atrial fibrillation in three European populations and one Chinese population.

Methods and results

First, a genome-wide association study was carried out in an Icelandic population with or without atrial fibrillation (AF) or atrial flutter (AFl) (550 patients and 4476 controls). A total of 316,515 SNPs were tested for association with AF and AFl. Three SNPs were found to be strongly correlated to AF, all located within a single linkage disequilibrium block on chromosome 4q25. The SNP rs2200733 T carried an odds ratio of 1.75 of developing AF (p = 1.9 x 10^{-10}). A further study of SNPs in that vicinity identified a further SNP (rs10033464 T) associated with AF (OR = 1.42, p = 0.0024).

Subsequently, the authors went on to replicate their original discovery from the Icelandic population by testing these variants for association with AF in three other populations, two of European ancestry and one Han Chinese population. The association of rs2200733 was replicated in the Swedish (OR = 2.07, p = 0.00027) and

American populations (OR = 1.84, p = 9.8x10⁻¹⁰). The association for rs10033464 was weaker but also replicated in the Swedish populations (OR = 1.65, p = 0.0087). As for the Hong Kong population, again there was a strong association between rs2200733 and AF (OR = 1.42, p = 0.00064).

Conclusions and clinical implications

The authors of this landmark study identified two sequence variants on chromosome 4q25 that are associated with atrial fibrillation. These two variants (rs2200733 T and rs10033464 T) are not uncommon in European populations (35% of individuals of European descent have one or more of these variants), and they lead to a 1.72 and 1.39-fold increase in the risk of developing atrial fibrillation, respectively. The association is even stronger in Chinese populations, where 75% of individuals carry the stronger variant.

Genome-wide association studies are excellent for identifying common variants which increase the risk of disease modestly (as opposed to uncommon variants that confer significant risk)[56]. In terms of the implications of this landmark study, it not only provides a way of identifying individuals predisposed to AF, but it also provides valuable insight into the pathogenesis of AF.

We know that the triggers of AF arise from the pulmonary vein myocardial sleeves and current ablative therapy is directed towards isolating the pulmonary veins. The genetic sequence variants identified in this study are adjacent to the PITX2 gene, which is involved in left-right symmetry of the heart[57]. Intriguingly, the PITX2 gene was also recently shown to be important in the formation of pulmonary vein myocardium as PITX2c-deficient mice do not develop pulmonary vein myocardial sleeves[58], thus providing a putative explanation for the association between these genetic variants and AF.

Learning points

♦ Two genetic sequence variants on chromosome 4q25 were identified to be associated with AF.
♦ These variants increase the risk of AF by 1.72 and 1.39-fold, respectively.
♦ These sequence variants are adjacent to the PITX2 gene. PITX2 plays an important role in normal development of pulmonary vein myocardium, which is a site for triggers of AF.

Further reading

• Review of genome-wide association studies (GWAS): Manolio TA. Genome-wide association studies and assessment of the risk of disease. *N Engl J Med*. 2010; 363: 166–76.
• Role of PITX2 in formation of pulmonary myocardium: Mommersteeg MT, Brown NA, Prall OW, *et al.* Pitx2c and Nkx2–5 are required for the formation and identity of the pulmonary myocardium. *Circ Res* 2007; 101: 902–9.

Mathematical modelling of cardiac electrophysiology

Luo CH, Rudy Y. A Dynamic Model of the Cardiac Ventricular Action Potential I. Simulations of Ionic Currents and Concentration Changes. *Circ Res* 1994; 74: 1071–96.

Background

Although experimental cardiac electrophysiology has flourished over the past three decades due in no small part to the advent of novel research tools referred to in the introduction, there remain limits to the questions that experimental science can pose and answer. This relates in part to the difficulties in setting up appropriate biological experiments to study complex electrophysiological phenomena such as fibrillation.

To improve the understanding of processes that underlie arrhythmogenesis in humans, one approach is to use mathematical or computational models (as opposed to cell, tissue, or animal models) to study the electrophysiological mechanisms of cardiac arrhythmias. Computational electrophysiology models have evolved over the past few decades[59, 60], but many of these models are based on, and incorporate, early work on simulating cardiac action potentials [9, 61, 62].

One much-cited landmark paper in the field of computational modelling of cardiac electrophysiology is that by Luo and Rudy, who described a dynamic model of cardiac ventricular action potential.

Methods and results

This study built on the previous iteration of the Luo-Rudy model[62], which was a passive model of the ventricular action potential. The original model included ionic currents through gated channels in the sarcolemma, but did not incorporate other processes, such as ionic pumps and exchangers and Ca^{2+} release from the sarcoplasmic reticulum (SR), that contribute to ionic changes in the myocyte. This new dynamic Luo-Rudy model incorporated multiple new processes, amongst others the Na^+-K^+ pump, the Na^+-Ca^{2+} exchanger, buffering of Ca^{2+} ions and the release and uptake of Ca^{2+} by the SR.

In order to generate a model that is faithful to real-life biology, the authors used experimental data from guinea pig ventricular myocytes to guide their simulations and modelling. Realistic cell dimensions and ionic concentrations were used for the modelling, and individual processes in this model (e.g. ionic currents) were formulated quantitatively based on experimental data. This approach resulted in a model that incorporated the multiple subcellular processes that contribute to the ionic changes in a cardiomyocyte and accurately reproduced the ventricular action potential.

Conclusions and clinical implications

This landmark paper established a dynamic mathematical model of the cardiac ventricular action potential, and provided the basis for the study of arrhythmogenic activity in the single myocyte, including early and delayed after-depolarizations. Subsequent computational models have built on the work by Luo and Rudy to produce models for two and three-dimensional tissue.

The advance in mathematical modelling of cardiac excitation and conduction in the past few decades has two important implications. First, computational models provide researchers with additional tools to study mechanisms of arrhythmogenesis[63], for example in situations where physical experiments are unsuitable or not possible. Second, there are potential clinical implications from the improvement in computational modelling techniques. There are now attempts to integrate computational models with anatomical data from imaging techniques, such as MRI, to provide predictive modelling of cardiac electrophysiology[59], in an attempt to guide clinical management and therapies.

Learning points

- The Luo-Rudy model is a dynamic model of the cardiac action potential based on experimental data from the guinea pig ventricular myocyte.
- The Luo-Rudy model allowed for the study of arrhythmogenic factors at the single myocyte level.

Further reading

- Predictive modelling of cardiac electrophysiology:
  Vigmond E, Vadakkumpadan F, Gurev V, *et al.* Towards predictive modelling of the electrophysiology of the heart. *Exp Physiol* 2009; 94: 563–77.
- Part 2 of Luo-Rudy dynamic model:
  Luo CH, Rudy Y. A dynamic model of the cardiac ventricular action potential. II. Afterdepolarizations, triggered activity, and potentiation. *Circ Res* 1994; 74: 1097–113.

Epidemiology of atrial fibrillation and stroke

Wolf PA, Dawber TR, Thomas HE Jr, Kannel WB. Epidemiologic assessment of chronic atrial fibrillation and risk of stroke: the Framingham study. *Neurology* 1978; 28: 973–7.

Background

The Framingham Heart Study is a long-term cardiovascular study first started in 1948 to help improve understanding of the epidemiology of cardiovascular disease[64]. This study initially followed the 5209 adults who lived in the town of Framingham, Massachusetts, and is now on its third generation of participants, with recruitment of

second and third-generation participants occurring in 1971 and 2002 respectively.

The epidemiological data acquired over the decades from Framingham have helped to inform and change clinical practice. Within cardiac electrophysiology, perhaps the most significant paper to emerge from the Framingham Heart Study was that by Wolf *et al.* in the late

1970s, which reported for the very first time the association between AF and stroke.

Methods and results

The authors followed 5184 individuals from the Framingham Heart Study over a 24-year period and documented the incidence of strokes. Individuals enrolled in this study were examined every two years. Follow-up was good and less than 5% of the original cohort was lost to follow-up. The incidence of strokes was recorded by daily monitoring of all admissions to the only general hospital in Framingham. The incidences of strokes in individuals with and without chronic AF were compared.

Over the 24 years of follow-up, 168 strokes occurred in men and 177 in women. Chronic AF in the absence of rheumatic heart disease was associated with more than a 5.6-fold increase in stroke incidence (p <0.01), while AF with rheumatic heart disease demonstrated a 17-fold increase. The incidence of strokes increased as duration of AF increased, with no obvious vulnerable period. Chronic AF was shown to be an important independent risk factor and precursor of cerebral embolism.

Conclusions and clinical implications

This study showed that individuals with AF, with or without rheumatic heart disease, are at greatly increased risk of stroke. Occurrence of strokes increased as the duration of AF increased.

This landmark epidemiological study highlighted for the first time the association between AF and stroke, and is a classic example of epidemiological research transforming clinical practice. The authors' remark that 'controlled trials of anticoagulants . . . in persons with chronic

AF may demonstrate if strokes can be prevented in this highly susceptible group' has since been proven true and the use of anticoagulants to prevent strokes is now routine clinical practice and incorporated into all major clinical guidelines[65, 66]. The practice of reducing stroke risk in AF has progressed in the past few years, and alternatives to conventional warfarin, such as novel direct thrombin inhibitors[67], direct factor Xa inhibitors[68], and percutaneous atrial appendage closure devices[69] are now clinically available.

Learning points

- ◆ Chronic AF in the absence of rheumatic heart disease is associated with more than a five-fold increase in stroke incidence.
- ◆ Atrial fibrillation with rheumatic heart disease is associated with a 17-fold increase in stroke incidence.

Further reading

- Epidemiology of AF:
  Kannel WB, Abbott RD, Savage DD, McNamara PM. Epidemiologic features of chronic atrial fibrillation: the Framingham study. *N Engl J Med* 1982; 306: 1018–22.
- Oral anticoagulants prevent strokes in AF:
  Aguilar MI, Hart R. Oral anticoagulants for preventing stroke in patients with non-valvular atrial fibrillation and no previous history of stroke or transient ischemic attacks. *Cochrane Database Syst Rev.* 2005; 3: CD001927.

Epidemiology of post-myocardial infarction sudden cardiac death

Adabag AS, Therneau TM, Gersh BJ, Weston SA, Roger VL. Sudden death after myocardial infarction. *JAMA* 2008; 300: 2022–9.

Background

Sudden cardiac death (SCD), due to cardiac arrhythmia, is a well-known complication of myocardial infarction (MI)[70]. Individuals who survive myocardial infarction are at increased risk of SCD. However, our knowledge of the incidence of SCD and the natural history post-myocardial infarction was predominantly from studies in

the 1970s and 1980s[71, 72]. These long-term follow-up studies were performed in an age before revascularization therapy and before evidence-based therapies such as beta blockers, statins, and ACE inhibitors were widely used in these patients. There was also little community-based data to reflect contemporary risk of SCD post-myocardial infarction.

Adabag *et al.* carried out a population-based surveillance study to address this question, and also specifically to evaluate the impact of intercurrent events such as recurrent ischaemia and heart failure on SCD.

Methods and results

This epidemiological study was carried out in Olmsted County, Minnesota, a county that is relatively isolated from other urban centres. Lists of patients discharged from hospital were assessed to identify all patients with a diagnosis of myocardial infarction between 1979 and 2005. Baseline demographic and clinical characteristics were documented and intercurrent episodes of recurrent ischaemia and heart failure were also recorded. All patients were followed up until death or the last date of follow-up.

A total of 3296 patients with a diagnosis of acute MI were identified and median follow-up for this cohort was 4.7 years (25–75th percentiles: 1.6–7.1 years). A total of 1160 deaths occurred during follow-up, of which 24% were attributed to SCD. The incidence of SCD post-MI had been steadily decreasing over the 27-year period between 1979 and 2005.

The risk of SCD was greatest in the first 30 days post-myocardial infarction (4.18 times that of the general population), and this risk reduced progressively over the next four years. Intercurrent events occurred frequently over the period of follow-up: 842 patients had recurrent ischaemia alone, 365 had heart failure alone, and 873 had both. The occurrence of heart failure during follow-up was associated with a 4.2-fold increase in the hazard ratio for SCD (95% CI: 3.1–5.7, p <0.01).

Conclusions and clinical implications

The authors of this important epidemiological study reported contemporary community-based data on the incidence of SCD post-MI. This provided a timely update to existing epidemiology data on SCD post-MI which were mainly acquired a couple of decades ago. Specifically, compared with older epidemiological data, they demonstrated a steady decline in the risk of SCD between 1979 and 2005.

They identified a high-risk period of SCD in the first month post-MI, which is a period during which ICDs fail to confer a mortality benefit[73, 74]. They also showed that the occurrence of heart failure at any time during the follow-up period dramatically increased the risk of SCD. This underlines the fact that risk stratification for ICDs in the post-infarction population must be of a dynamic nature and take into account any intercurrent events.

Learning points

- The incidence of SCD post-MI has steadily decreased between 1979 and 2005, presumably due to new evidence-based therapies.
- The risk of SCD is greatest during the first 30 days post-myocardial infarction.
- The occurrence of heart failure at any time during the post-infarction period increased the risk of SCD by over four-fold, stressing the importance of continued surveillance and the dynamic nature of risk stratification.

Further reading

- Long-term recording of post-myocardial infarction arrhythmias:
  Bloch Thomsen PE, Jons C, Raatikainen MJ, *et al.*; Cardiac Arrhythmias and Risk Stratification After Acute Myocardial Infarction (CARISMA) Study Group. Long-term recording of cardiac arrhythmias with an implantable cardiac monitor in patients with reduced ejection fraction after acute myocardial infarction: the Cardiac Arrhythmias and Risk Stratification After Acute Myocardial Infarction (CARISMA) study. *Circulation* 2010; 122: 1258–64.
- Pathogenesis of sudden cardiac death post-myocardial infarction:
  Pouleur AC, Barkoudah E, Uno H, *et al.*; VALIANT Investigators. Pathogenesis of sudden unexpected death in a clinical trial of patients with myocardial infarction and left ventricular dysfunction, heart failure, or both. *Circulation* 2010; 122: 597–602.

Conclusion: the future

Unprecedented progress has been made in the fields of basic science and epidemiology of cardiac electrophysiology in the past three to four decades, as evidenced by the breakthroughs described in the landmark papers above. Looking to the future, discoveries in basic science and epidemiology of cardiac electrophysiology can be expected to grow exponentially in the near future.

Molecular biology and genetic research techniques will continue to develop, allowing us to probe deeper into the causes of arrhythmias. Physiological techniques such as optical mapping will develop ever more sophistication, with greater spatial and temporal resolution. We will have a greater variety of disease models, including genetic knockout models, to answer disease-specific questions. And where experimental science has reached its limits, computational and mathematical modelling will provide novel tools to study arrhythmia mechanisms.

In terms of potential new therapies, there are many on the horizon. Biological therapies, such as gene therapy for arrhythmias, are promising candidates. There are also potentially novel pharmaceutical agents that have targets distinct from the ion channel targeted by conventional anti-arrhythmics, such as cellular coupling and calcium handling.

Although it would be foolish to attempt to predict the future, we can confidently say that it is a near certainty that the advances in cardiac electrophysiology over the next four decades will outstrip and surpass those of the previous four.

References

1. Wijffels MC, Kirchhof CJ, Dorland R, Allessie MA. Atrial fibrillation begets atrial fibrillation. A study in awake chronically instrumented goats. *Circulation* 1995; 92: 1954–68.
2. de Bakker J, van Capelle F, Janse M, *et al*. Re-entry as a cause of ventricular tachycardia in patients with chronic ischemic heart disease: electrophysiologic and anatomic correlation. *Circulation* 1988; 77: 589–606.
3. Peters NS, Coromilas J, Severs NJ, Wit AL. Disturbed connexin43 gap junction distribution correlates with the location of re-entrant circuits in the epicardial border zone of healing canine infarcts that cause ventricular tachycardia. *Circulation* 1997; 95: 988–96.
4. Watanabe H, Chopra N, Laver D, *et al*. Flecainide prevents catecholaminergic polymorphic ventricular tachycardia in mice and humans. *Nat Med* 2009; 15: 380–3.
5. Brown HF, DiFrancesco D, Noble SJ. How does adrenaline accelerate the heart? *Nature* 1979; 280: 235–6.
6. Chakir K, Daya SK, Tunin RS, *et al*. Reversal of global apoptosis and regional stress kinase activation by cardiac resynchronization. *Circulation* 2008; 117: 1369–77.
7. Wang Q, Shen J, Splawski I, *et al*. SCN5A mutations associated with an inherited cardiac arrhythmia, long QT syndrome. *Cell* 1995; 80: 805–11.
8. Gudbjartsson DF, Arnar DO, Helgadottir A, *et al*. Variants conferring risk of atrial fibrillation on chromosome 4q25. *Nature* 2007; 448: 353–7.
9. Luo C, Rudy Y. A dynamic model of the cardiac ventricular action potential. I. Simulations of ionic currents and concentration changes. *Circ Res* 1994; 74: 1071–96.
10. Wolf PA, Dawber TR, Thomas HE, Jr., Kannel WB. Epidemiologic assessment of chronic atrial fibrillation and risk of stroke: the Framingham study. *Neurology* 1978; 28: 973–7.
11. Adabag A, Therneau T, Gersh B, Weston S, Roger V. Sudden death after myocardial infarction. *JAMA* 2008; 300: 2022–9.
12. Marmont G. Studies on the axon membrane; a new method. *J Cell Physiol* 1949; 34: 351–82.
13. Hodgkin AL, Huxley AF, Katz B. Measurement of current-voltage relations in the membrane of the giant axon of Loligo. *J Physiol* 1952; 116: 424–48.
14. Beeler GW, Jr., Reuter H. Voltage clamp experiments on ventricular myocarial fibres. *J Physiol* 1970; 207: 165–90.
15. Spear JF, Michelson EL, Moore EN. The use of animal models in the study of the electrophysiology of sudden coronary deaths. *Ann N Y Acad Sci* 1982; 382: 78–89.
16. David D, Michelson EL, Dreifus LS. The role of animal models in electrophysiologic studies of life-threatening arrhythmias. *Pacing Clin Electrophysiol* 1986; 9: 896–907.
17. Efimov IR, Nikolski VP, Salama G. Optical imaging of the heart. *Circulation Research* 2004; 95: 21–33.
18. Ding C, Gepstein L, Nguyen DT, *et al*. High-resolution optical mapping of ventricular tachycardia in rats with chronic myocardial infarction. *Pacing Clin Electrophysiol* 2010; 33: 687–95.
19. Knollmann BC, Roden DM. A genetic framework for improving arrhythmia therapy. *Nature* 2008; 451: 929–36.
20. Litovsky SH, Antzelevitch C. Transient outward current prominent in canine ventricular epicardium but not endocardium. *Circ Res* 1988; 62: 116–26.
21. Sicouri S, Antzelevitch C. A subpopulation of cells with unique electrophysiological properties in the deep subepicardium of the canine ventricle. The M cell. *Circ Res* 1991; 68: 1729–41.
22. Rohr S, Kucera J, Fast V, Kleber A. Paradoxical improvement of impulse conduction in cardiac tissue by partial cellular uncoupling. *Science* 1997; 275: 841–4.
23. Kopecky SL, Gersh BJ, McGoon MD, *et al*. The natural history of lone atrial fibrillation. A population-based study over three decades. *N Engl J Med* 1987; 317: 669–74.

24. Brand FN, Abbott RD, Kannel WB, Wolf PA. Characteristics and prognosis of lone atrial fibrillation. 30-year follow-up in the Framingham Study. *JAMA* 1985; 254: 3449–53.

25. Suttorp MJ, Kingma JH, Koomen EM, van 't Hof A, Tijssen JG, Lie KI. Recurrence of paroxysmal atrial fibrillation or flutter after successful cardioversion in patients with normal left ventricular function. *Am J Cardiol* 1993; 71: 710–3.

26. Haissaguerre M, Jais P, Shah DC, *et al.* Spontaneous initiation of atrial fibrillation by ectopic beats originating in the pulmonary veins. *N Engl J Med* 1998; 339: 659–66.

27. Smelley MP, Knight BP. Approaches to catheter ablation of persistent atrial fibrillation. *Heart Rhythm* 2009; 6: S33–8.

28. Yap YG, Duong T, Bland M, *et al.* Temporal trends on the risk of arrhythmic vs. non-arrhythmic deaths in high-risk patients after myocardial infarction: a combined analysis from multicentre trials. *Eur Heart J* 2005; 26: 1385–93.

29. Wellens HJ, Duren DR, Lie KI. Observations on mechanisms of ventricular tachycardia in man. *Circulation* 1976; 54: 237–44.

30. Horowitz LN, Josephson ME, Harken AH. Epicardial and endocardial activation during sustained ventricular tachycardia in man. *Circulation* 1980; 61: 1227–38.

31. Stevenson WG, Soejima K. Catheter ablation for ventricular tachycardia. *Circulation* 2007; 115: 2750–60.

32. Severs NJ, Bruce AF, Dupont E, Rothery S. Remodelling of gap junctions and connexin expression in diseased myocardium. *Cardiovasc Res* 2008; 80: 9–19.

33. Smith JH, Green CR, Peters NS, Rothery S, Severs NJ. Altered patterns of gap junction distribution in ischemic heart disease. An immunohistochemical study of human myocardium using laser scanning confocal microscopy. *Am J Pathol* 1991; 139: 801–21.

34. Cabo C, Yao J, Boyden PA, *et al.* Heterogeneous gap junction remodeling in re-entrant circuits in the epicardial border zone of the healing canine infarct. *Cardiovasc Res* 2006; 72: 241–9.

35. Dhein S, Hagen A, Jozwiak J, *et al.* Improving cardiac gap junction communication as a new antiarrhythmic mechanism: the action of antiarrhythmic peptides. *Naunyn Schmiedebergs Arch Pharmacol* 2010; 381: 221–34.

36. Lau DH, Clausen C, Sosunov EA, *et al.* Epicardial border zone overexpression of skeletal muscle sodium channel SkM1 normalizes activation, preserves conduction, and suppresses ventricular arrhythmia: an in silico, in vivo, in vitro study. *Circulation* 2009; 119: 19–27.

37. Leenhardt A, Lucet V, Denjoy I, Grau F, Ngoc DD, Coumel P. Catecholaminergic polymorphic ventricular tachycardia in children. A 7-year follow-up of 21 patients. *Circulation* 1995; 91: 1512–9.

38. Priori SG, Napolitano C, Tiso N, *et al.* Mutations in the cardiac ryanodine receptor gene (hRyR2) underlie catecholaminergic polymorphic ventricular tachycardia. *Circulation* 2001; 103: 196–200.

39. Wehrens XHT, Lehnart SE, Reiken SR, *et al.* Protection from cardiac arrhythmia through ryanodine receptor-stabilizing protein calstabin2. *Science* 2004; 304: 292–6.

40. Wehrens XH, Lehnart SE, Marks AR. Ryanodine receptor-targeted anti-arrhythmic therapy. *Ann N Y Acad Sci* 2005; 1047: 366–75.

41. Katz AM, Messineo FC, Herbette L. Ion channels in membranes. *Circulation* 1982; 65: I2–10.

42. DiFrancesco D. The role of the funny current in pacemaker activity. *Circ Res* 2010; 106: 434–46.

43. Fox K, Ford I, Steg PG, Tendera M, Ferrari R. Ivabradine for patients with stable coronary artery disease and left-ventricular systolic dysfunction (BEAUTIFUL): a randomised, double-blind, placebo-controlled trial. *Lancet* 2008; 372: 807–16.

44. Fox K, Ford I, Steg PG, Tendera M, Robertson M, Ferrari R. Heart rate as a prognostic risk factor in patients with coronary artery disease and left-ventricular systolic dysfunction (BEAUTIFUL): a subgroup analysis of a randomised controlled trial. *Lancet* 2008; 372: 817–21.

45. Swedberg K, Komajda M, Bohm M, *et al.* Ivabradine and outcomes in chronic heart failure (SHIFT): a randomised placebo-controlled study. *Lancet* 2010; 376: 875–85.

46. Bristow MR, Saxon LA, Boehmer J, *et al.* Cardiac-resynchronization therapy with or without an implantable defibrillator in advanced chronic heart failure. *N Engl J Med* 2004; 350: 2140–50.

47. Cleland JG, Daubert JC, Erdmann E, *et al.* The effect of cardiac resynchronization on morbidity and mortality in heart failure. *N Engl J Med* 2005; 352: 1539–49.

48. Nelson GS, Berger RD, Fetics BJ, *et al.* Left ventricular or biventricular pacing improves cardiac function at diminished energy cost in patients with dilated cardiomyopathy and left bundle-branch block. *Circulation* 2000; 102: 3053–9.

49. Nowak B, Sinha AM, Schaefer WM, *et al.* Cardiac resynchronization therapy homogenizes myocardial glucose metabolism and perfusion in dilated cardiomyopathy and left bundle branch block. *J Am Coll Cardiol* 2003; 41: 1523–8.

50. Aiba T, Hesketh GG, Barth AS, *et al.* Electrophysiological consequences of dyssynchronous heart failure and its restoration by resynchronization therapy. *Circulation* 2009; 119: 1220–30.

51. Barth AS, Aiba T, Halperin V, *et al.* Cardiac resynchronization therapy corrects dyssynchrony-induced regional gene expression changes on a genomic level. *Circ Cardiovasc Genet* 2009; 2: 371–8.

52. Keating M, Atkinson D, Dunn C, Timothy K, Vincent GM, Leppert M. Linkage of a cardiac arrhythmia, the long QT syndrome, and the Harvey ras-1 gene. *Science* 1991; 252: 704–6.

53. Jiang C, Atkinson D, Towbin JA, *et al.* Two long QT syndrome loci map to chromosomes 3 and 7 with evidence for further heterogeneity. *Nat Genet* 1994; 8: 141–7.

54. Curran ME, Splawski I, Timothy KW, Vincent GM, Green ED, Keating MT. A molecular basis for cardiac arrhythmia: HERG mutations cause long QT syndrome. *Cell* 1995; 80: 795–803.

55. Napolitano C, Priori SG, Schwartz PJ, *et al.* Genetic testing in the long QT syndrome: development and validation of an efficient approach to genotyping in clinical practice. *JAMA* 2005; 294: 2975–80.

56. Manolio TA. Genomewide association studies and assessment of the risk of disease. *N Engl J Med* 2010; 363: 166–76.

57. Franco D, Campione M. The role of Pitx2 during cardiac development. Linking left-right signaling and congenital heart diseases. *Trends Cardiovasc Med* 2003; 13: 157–63.

58. Mommersteeg MTM, Brown NA, Prall OWJ, *et al.* Pitx2c and Nkx2–5 are required for the formation and identity of the pulmonary myocardium. *Circ Res* 2007; 101: 902–9.

59. Vigmond E, Vadakkumpadan F, Gurev V, *et al.* Towards predictive modelling of the electrophysiology of the heart. *Experimental Physiology* 2009; 94: 563–77.

60. Winslow RL, Scollan DF, Holmes A, Yung CK, Zhang J, Jafri MS. Electrophysiological modeling of cardiac ventricular function: from cell to organ. *Annu Rev Biomed Eng* 2000; 2: 119–55.

61. DiFrancesco D, Noble D. A model of cardiac electrical activity incorporating ionic pumps and concentration changes. *Philos Trans R Soc Lond B Biol Sci* 1985; 307: 353–98.

62. Luo CH, Rudy Y. A model of the ventricular cardiac action potential. Depolarization, repolarization, and their interaction. *Circ Res* 1991; 68: 1501–26.

63. Sachse FB, Moreno AP, Seemann G, Abildskov JA. A model of electrical conduction in cardiac tissue including fibroblasts. *Ann Biomed Eng* 2009; 37: 874–89.

64. Dawber TR, Meadors GF, Moore FE, Jr. Epidemiological approaches to heart disease: the Framingham Study. *Am J Public Health Nations Health* 1951; 41: 279–81.

65. Camm AJ, Kirchhof P, Lip GY, *et al.* Guidelines for the management of atrial fibrillation: the Task Force for the Management of Atrial Fibrillation of the European Society of Cardiology (ESC). *Eur Heart J* 2010; 31: 2369–429.

66. Estes NA, 3rd, Halperin JL, Calkins H, *et al.* ACC/AHA/Physician Consortium 2008 clinical performance measures for adults with nonvalvular atrial fibrillation or atrial flutter: a report of the American College of Cardiology/American Heart Association Task Force on Performance Measures and the Physician Consortium for Performance Improvement (Writing Committee to Develop Clinical Performance Measures for Atrial Fibrillation): developed in collaboration with the Heart Rhythm Society. *Circulation* 2008; 117: 1101–20.

67. Schulman S, Kearon C, Kakkar AK, *et al.* Dabigatran versus warfarin in the treatment of acute venous thromboembolism. *N Engl J Med* 2009; 361: 2342–52.

68. ROCKET AF Study Investigators. Rivaroxaban-once daily, oral, direct factor Xa inhibition compared with vitamin K antagonism for prevention of stroke and Embolism Trial in Atrial Fibrillation: rationale and design of the ROCKET AF study. *Am Heart J* 2010; 159: 340–7 e1.

69. Bayard YL, Omran H, Neuzil P, *et al.* PLAATO (Percutaneous Left Atrial Appendage Transcatheter Occlusion) for prevention of cardioembolic stroke in non-anticoagulation eligible atrial fibrillation patients: results from the European PLAATO study. *EuroIntervention* 2010; 6: 220–6.

70. Zipes DP, Wellens HJ. Sudden cardiac death. *Circulation* 1998; 98: 2334–51.

71. Kannel WB, Sorlie P, McNamara PM. Prognosis after initial myocardial infarction: the Framingham study. *Am J Cardiol* 1979; 44: 53–9.

72. Mukharji J, Rude RE, Poole WK, *et al.* Risk factors for sudden death after acute myocardial infarction: two-year follow-up. *Am J Cardiol* 1984; 54: 31–6.

73. Hohnloser SH, Kuck KH, Dorian P, *et al.* Prophylactic use of an implantable cardioverter-defibrillator after acute myocardial infarction. *N Engl J Med* 2004; 351: 2481–8.

74. Steinbeck G, Andresen D, Seidl K, *et al.* Defibrillator implantation early after myocardial infarction. *N Engl J Med* 2009; 361: 1427–36.

Chapter 9

Atrial fibrillation

Dr Luke Tapp and Professor Gregory Lip

Introduction

Atrial fibrillation (AF) is the most common sustained cardiac arrhythmia affecting 1–2% of the UK population. Prevalence increases with advancing age, indicating its significance as the global demographic leans towards a more elderly population. Consequently, prevalence is predicted to double in the next 50 years. However, the increasing prevalence of AF is multifactorial, and not solely related to an ageing population. Atrial fibrillation accounts for 1% of overall healthcare expenditure in the UK and is therefore an increasingly important public health issue.

Atrial fibrillation is associated with substantial morbidity and mortality. Far from being a benign arrhythmia, the risk of death is doubled by AF, which is independent of other cardiovascular risk factors. Additionally, AF can also decrease quality of life, with multiple debilitating symptoms, including shortness of breath, palpitations,

fatigue, and often frequent hospital admissions. The most devastating complication of AF is the association with an increased risk of stroke. Strokes secondary to AF are more likely to be fatal, result in more severe disability, and be recurrent.

Great advances have been made in our understanding and management of AF in recent times. Identification of risk factors for stroke and development of risk stratification tools has promoted higher uptake of warfarin in patient groups, with clear evidence of benefit, especially in the elderly. Conversely, the recent identification of a user-friendly scoring system to assess the risk of haemorrhagic complications from anticoagulation has refined yet further the indications for warfarin. There have been great leaps forward recently in drug development, with novel antithrombotic agents and a safer antiarrhythmic drug. Perhaps most importantly, the wait for a warfarin substitute, which has been the gold-standard drug for stroke risk reduction for over 50 years, is now over.

The advancements in our understanding and management of AF have been underpinned by several pivotal papers which are discussed in this chapter. They include papers describing important epidemiological advances, novel medications, and management concepts. These 'landmark' papers have been chosen as they have clearly made an impact on our understanding of the disease and/or changed our clinical management.

Atrial Fibrillation as an Independent Risk Factor for Stroke: The Framingham Study

Wolf PA, Abbott RD, Kannel WB. *Stroke* 1991; 22: 983–8.

Background

Several risk factors associated with an increased risk of stroke had been identified, including AF, hypertension, heart failure, coronary artery disease, and advancing age. These conditions commonly co-exist, and the relative contribution each makes to the overall risk of stroke was unclear. A better understanding of the risk factors for ischaemic stroke was vital to guide appropriate management of AF.

Methods

Wolf and colleagues investigated the relative impacts of non-rheumatic AF, hypertension, coronary artery disease, and heart failure on the incidence of stroke in 5070 participants free of cardiovascular disease at enrolment in the Framingham study. This cohort had been followed up for 34 years. The development of symptoms and signs of neurological disease suggestive of stroke were assessed at each biennial study visit, as was the presence of AF. A neurologist evaluated suspected acute strokes. Computed tomography (CT) scanning contributed to assessment of possible strokes when it became available in 1981. Hypertension was defined as a systolic or diastolic blood pressure reading >160 and >95 mmHg, respectively.

Results

The prevalence of hypertension, coronary artery disease, heart failure, and AF all increased significantly with age. In comparison with subjects free of these conditions, the age-adjusted incidence of stroke more than doubled in the setting of coronary artery disease (p <0.001) and more than trebled in the presence of hypertension (p <0.001). There was a more than four-fold increased incidence of stroke in subjects with heart failure (p <0.001) and a near five-fold increase with AF (p <0.001). The excess stroke risk in women was statistically significant (p <0.01).

With advancing age the effects of hypertension, coronary artery disease, and heart failure on stroke risk became progressively weaker (p <0.05). Conversely, advancing age amplified the impact of AF upon risk of stroke. In subjects aged 80–89 years, AF was the sole cardiovascular condition to exert an independent effect on stroke incidence (p <0.001). The attributable risk of stroke for all cardiovascular contributors decreased with age except for AF, for which the attributable risk increased significantly (p <0.01), rising dramatically from 1.5% in those aged 50–59 years to 23.5% in those aged 80–89 years.

Limitations

The diagnosis of stroke prior to the availability of CT scanning may have been less robust. Similarly, a diagnosis of heart failure was largely on clinical grounds, which correlates less strongly with stroke risk than proven left ventricular systolic impairment on an echocardiogram. The definition of hypertension has changed dramatically since the Framingham study began. Hence, the impact of this risk factor may have been under-estimated.

Conclusions

This seminal study identified AF as being an independent risk factor for stroke. Furthermore, other cardiovascular risk factors for stroke were shown to become less powerful with advancing age, whereas the influence of AF became stronger.

Learning points

- Atrial fibrillation is an independent risk factor for stroke.
- Advancing age amplifies the impact of AF on risk of stroke.

Further reading

- Phillips SJ. Is atrial fibrillation an independent risk factor for stroke? *Can J Neurol Sci* 1990; 17(2): 163–8.

- Wolf PA, Abbott RD, Kannel WB. Atrial Fibrillation: a major contributor to stroke in the elderly. The Framingham Study. *Arch Int Med* 1987; 147(9): 1561–4.

Risk factors for stroke and efficacy of antithrombotic medication in atrial fibrillation: analysis of pooled data from randomized controlled trials

Atrial Fibrillation Investigators. *Arch Intern Med* 1994; 154: 1449–57.

Background

The association between AF and an increased risk of ischaemic stroke had become established. Five randomized-controlled trials (RCTs) had convincingly demonstrated the efficacy of warfarin for the primary prevention of stroke in AF patients. Indeed, four trials had been stopped earlier than planned due to overwhelming evidence of benefit from warfarin. The fifth was also stopped early, when the results of the other four trials were published. The relatively small numbers of patients enrolled in each of these trials, the truncated duration of follow-up, and consequently the small number of outcome events had limited their individual power to reach definitive conclusions. To address these shortcomings, the AF investigators pooled data from all five trials to facilitate a deeper analysis of the results and thereby address several important clinical questions: first, to identify factors predictive of a high or low risk of ischaemic stroke; second, to evaluate the efficacy and safety of antithrombotic therapy in reducing the incidence of stroke in AF; finally, to assess the efficacy of antithrombotic therapy in major patient subgroups, especially women who had historically been under-represented in anticoagulation trials.

Methods

Each of the five original study authors provided data to the coordinating centre. Data on a total of 4253 patients was pooled from the five RCTs comparing warfarin (all studies) or aspirin (two studies) with control groups in patients with AF. The dose of aspirin was either 75 mg or 325 mg daily. The therapeutic effect of warfarin was monitored using prothrombin time ratios in three studies and the international normalized ratio (INR) in two studies. The lowest target intensity of anticoagulation was a prothrombin time ratio of 1.2 to 1.5 and the highest target intensity was an INR of 2.8 to 4.2. The primary end points were ischaemic stroke and major haemorrhage, as assessed by each study. Average follow-up ranged from 1.2 to 2.3 years. A multivariate analysis was used to identify factors predictive of stroke.

Results

Mean age was 69 years and 26% were female. Mean blood pressure was 142/82 mmHg; 46% of patients had a history of hypertension, 6% had a previous transient ischemic attack (TIA) or stroke, and 14% had diabetes. The independent risk factors that predicted ischaemic stroke in control patients were increasing age, history of hypertension, previous TIA or stroke, and diabetes. Neither the category (paroxysmal or permanent) nor duration of AF affected the rate of stroke. The annual rate of stroke in non-anticoagulated patients ranged from 1.0% (95% confidence interval [CI] 0.3–3.0%) in patients aged <65 years with no risk factors (15% of all patients) to 8.1% (95% CI, 4.7– 13.9%) in patients aged >75 years with ≥1 risk factor. Warfarin reduced the risk of stroke in all subgroups except those aged <65 years with no risk factors. This effect was consistent among the five trials. Overall, warfarin reduced the incidence of stroke by 68% (95% CI, 50–79%; p <0.001). Additionally, the rate of stroke causing a permanent neurological deficit was reduced by 68% (95% CI, 39–83%, p <0.001). Warfarin reduced the rate of death by 33% (95% CI, 9–51%, p = 0.01). In women, warfarin decreased the risk of stroke by 84% (95% CI, 55–95%, p <0.001) compared with 60% (95% CI, 35–76%, p <0.001) in men.

The efficacy of aspirin in reducing stroke risk was not as consistent as that seen with warfarin; only one of the two studies reached statistical significance. When both studies were combined, aspirin reduced stroke risk by 36% (95% CI, 4–57%; p = 0.03), but there was no significant impact on death or disabling stroke.

The annual rate of major haemorrhage (intracranial bleeding or a bleed requiring hospitalization or a two-unit blood transfusion) was 1% for the control group, 1% for the aspirin group, and 1.3% for the warfarin group.

Limitations

There were inevitable variations in definitions of clinical events, including stroke between trials and inconsistencies in the target intensity of anticoagulation and how this was monitored. However, there was enough uniformity to allow meaningful conclusions to be drawn.

Conclusions

The AF investigators showed that collaboration between research groups with pooling of results allows powerful examination of a disease and the possibility of addressing fundamentally important clinical questions not achievable by a single trial. Thus, a number of pivotal findings were described. Independent risk factors for stroke in AF patients were identified (increasing age, previous stroke or TIA, hypertension, and diabetes), which now form the backbone of all stroke risk stratification schemes. A dramatic benefit from warfarin in stroke risk reduction was demonstrated. This was particularly marked in females, a cohort previously neglected in clinical trials. There was no increase in major haemorrhage with warfarin. A large number of older patients were included (20% aged >75 years), suggesting that the findings are applicable to this important group of patients with AF. Importantly, a group was identified (age <65 years with no risk factors) in whom warfarin did not reduce the risk of stroke, introducing the concept that some patients do not require anticoagulation.

Learning points

- Advancing age, prior stroke or TIA, hypertension, and diabetes are independent risk factors for stroke in the setting of AF.
- Warfarin is associated with a dramatic reduction in stroke risk in patients with AF.
- Anticoagulation with warfarin is not associated with an increase in major haemorrhagic complications.

Further reading

- Connolly SJ, Laupacis A, Gent M, Roberts RS, Cairns JA, Joyner C. Canadian Atrial Fibrillation Anticoagulation (CAFA) study. *J Am Coll Cardiol* 1991; 18: 349–55.
- Ezekowitz MD, Bridgers SL, James KE *et al*. Warfarin in the prevention of stroke associated with non-rheumatic atrial fibrillation. *N Engl J Med* 1992; 327: 1406–12.
- Petersen P, Boysen G, Godtfredsen J, Andersen E. Placebo-controlled, randomised trial of warfarin and aspirin for prevention of thromboembolic complications in chronic atrial fibrillation: the Copenhagen AFASAK study. *Lancet* 1989; 1: 175–8.
- Stroke Prevention in Atrial Fibrillation Investigators. Stroke Prevention in Atrial Fibrillation Study: final results. *Circulation* 1991; 84: 527–39.
- The Boston Area Anticoagulation Trial for Atrial Fibrillation Investigators. The effect of low-dose warfarin on the risk of stroke in patients with non-rheumatic atrial fibrillation. *N Engl J Med* 1990; 323: 1505–11.

Validation of clinical classification schemes for predicting stroke risk: results from the National Registry of Atrial Fibrillation

Gage BF, Waterman AD, Shannon W, Boechler M, Rich MW, Radford MJ. *JAMA* 2001; 285: 2864–70.

Background

Atrial fibrillation had been shown to be associated with an increased incidence of ischaemic stroke at the population level. However, an individual's absolute risk of stroke depends on their age and associated comorbidities. Concurrently, the absolute benefit gain from anticoagulant drugs correlates with the individual's stroke risk. It is therefore of fundamental importance to be able to accurately predict the patient-specific risk of stroke to allow individualization of therapy. This requires a robust, user-friendly, validated risk-stratification tool. Two classification schemes, the Atrial Fibrillation Investigators (AFI) and the

Stroke Prevention and Atrial Fibrillation (SPAF) scores had been proposed, but several disadvantages were apparent. Low-risk patients according to one scheme could be classified as moderate or high risk by the other. Appropriate classification of successfully treated hypertensives was uncertain. The average age of trial participants used to create the schemes was 69 years and therefore utility in the large elderly population with AF was unproven. Validation of the two existing schemes in an independent cohort would be a fundamental step in assessing their utility. Merging the schemes into a single unifying model may optimize appropriate delivery of anticoagulation.

Methods

Gage and colleagues assessed the predictive value of the AFI and SPAF classification schemes in an independent sample cohort. The AFI and SPAF schemes were subsequently combined into a new stroke-risk scoring system with the acronym CHADS$_2$. The CVD–Heart Attack–Diabetes (CHADS$_2$) score is evaluated by assigning one point each for the presence of congestive heart failure, history of hypertension, age ≥75 years, and diabetes, and two points for history of stroke or TIA (summarized in Table 9.1).

The predictive accuracy of the AFI, SPAF, and CHADS$_2$ schemes was assessed using data from a National Registry of Atrial Fibrillation (NRAF) cohort comprising 1733 Medicare patients aged 65–95 years with AF who were not prescribed warfarin. This cohort contained more female and elderly subjects than the AF populations used to derive the AFI and SPAF scores, and had a higher prevalence of risk factors for stroke. The mean duration of follow-up was 1.2 years. The study outcome was hospitalization for ischaemic stroke, which was identified from Medicare claims data. The predictive accuracy of the three models was quantified using the c statistic to test the hypothesis that the classification schemes performed better than chance.

Results

The mean CHADS$_2$ score was 2.1 for participants not taking antithrombotic therapy and 2.3 for those on aspirin. During 2121 patient years of follow-up, 94 patients were admitted to hospital due to an ischaemic stroke (stroke rate, 4.4 per 100 patient years). Of these, 27% died within 30 days of admission. As indicated by a c statistic >0.5, the two existing classification schemes predicted stroke better than chance: c statistic of 0.68 (95% confidence interval [CI], 0.65–0.71) for AFI and c statistic of 0.74 (95% CI, 0.71–0.76) for SPAF. However, the CHADS$_2$ index was the most accurate predictor of stroke, with a c statistic of 0.82 (95% CI, 0.80–0.84). The stroke rate per 100 patient-years

without antithrombotic therapy increased by a factor of 1.5 (95% CI, 1.3–1.7) for each one-point increase in the CHADS$_2$ score (p <0.001). The adjusted stroke rate associated with the CHADS$_2$ score is summarized in Table 9.2. Post-hoc analysis confirmed that the superiority of CHADS$_2$ was independent of aspirin usage.

Limitations

There are inevitable limitations with trying to artificially compartmentalize patients into risk strata when stroke risk is actually a continuum. The CHADS$_2$ scheme classifies up to 60% of patients as moderate risk (CHADS$_2$ score of one or two). Many guidelines suggest either aspirin or warfarin for these patients rather than dichotomizing between therapies. This may confuse clinicians further and also lead to favouring of aspirin due to ease of use. Additionally, prior stroke or TIA as the only risk factor would give a CHADS$_2$ score of two, suggesting only moderate risk, whereas such patients are clearly at high risk and should receive warfarin. In these situations, identifying additional stroke risk factors such as female gender and vascular disease or echocardiography, looking for features associated with stroke risk such as left ventricular systolic dysfunction, may aid clinical decision making. These limitations illustrate that risk stratification tools should be used judiciously in combination with sound clinical judgement.

Conclusions

An accurate, objective, and validated stroke risk stratification scheme is crucial in guiding appropriate antithrombotic prescription in patients with AF. This study validated the AFI and SPAF stroke-risk classification schemes and also a third novel scheme it proposed,

Table 9.2 Adjusted stroke rate associated with CHADS$_2$ scores

CHADS$_2$ score	Patients (total = 1733)	Adjusted stroke risk %/year (95% confidence interval)
0	120	1.9 (1.2–3.0)
1	463	2.8 (2.0–3.8)
2	523	4.0 (3.1–5.1)
3	337	5.9 (4.6–7.3)
4	220	8.5 (6.3–11.1)
5	65	12.5 (8.2–17.5)
6	5	18.2 (10.5–27.4)

CHADS$_2$ score 0 = low risk, 1–2 = moderate risk, >2 = high risk

Table 9.1 Composition of the CHADS$_2$ score

	Clinical feature	Points awarded (maximum score = 6)
C	Congestive heart failure	1
H	Hypertension	1
A	Age >75 years	1
D	Diabetes	1
S$_2$	Stroke or TIA	2

named $CHADS_2$. The $CHADS_2$ score had greater predictive accuracy of ischaemic stroke than either the AFI or SPAF schemes. $CHADS_2$ is simple to remember and used in everyday clinical practice. It does not incorporate echocardiographic parameters or biomarkers. The $CHADS_2$ score is applicable to elderly patients with AF who are often excluded from clinical trials.

Learning points

- A validated stroke risk stratification scheme is important in identifying AF patients who can potentially benefit from anticoagulation.
- The $CHADS_2$ tool is simple and has fairly good predictive accuracy for stratifying stroke risk in patients with AF.

Further reading

- Atrial Fibrillation Investigators. Risk factors for stroke and efficacy of antithrombotic therapy in atrial fibrillation. *Arch Intern Med* 1994; 154: 1449–57.
- Lip GYH, Nieuwlaat R, Pisters R, Lane DA, Crijns HJGM. Refining Clinical Risk Stratification for Predicting Stroke and Thromboembolism in Atrial Fibrillation Using a Novel Risk Factor-Based Approach. The Euro Heart Survey. *Chest* 2010; 137: 263–72.
- Stroke Prevention in Atrial Fibrillation Investigators. Risk factors for thromboembolism during aspirin therapy in patients with atrial fibrillation: The Stroke Prevention in Atrial Fibrillation study. *J Stroke Cerebrovasc Dis* 1995; 5: 147–57.

A comparison of rate control with rhythm control in patients with recurrent persistent atrial fibrillation

Van Gelder IC, Hagens VE, Bosker HA, Kingma JH, Kamp O, Kingma T, Said SA, Darmanata JI, Timmermans AJ, Tijssen JG, Crijns HJ. *N Engl J Med* 2002; 347: 1834–40.

Background

Broadly speaking, two strategies for managing the arrhythmia in patients with atrial AF had emerged, 'rhythm control' and 'rate control'. Rhythm control had historically been favoured due to a perceived potential for reducing symptoms and the risk of ischaemic stroke, improving survival and quality of life, and possibly to enable withdrawal of anticoagulation. However, there was no data to support these perhaps reasonable assumptions. Both approaches have their advantages and disadvantages. Rate control avoids the requirement for antiarrhythmic drugs, which are often poorly tolerated. Rhythm control may resolve the symptoms associated with AF, including palpitations, breathlessness, and fatigue.

The Atrial Fibrillation Follow-up Investigation of Rhythm Management (AFFIRM) study addressed this conundrum by investigating whether a rhythm control (cardioversion and use of antiarrhythmic drugs to maintain sinus rhythm—SR) strategy conferred advantages (including a mortality benefit) over a rate control (use of rate-limiting drugs whilst allowing AF to persist) strategy in patients with AF.

Methods

Patients with AF were eligible if aged >65 years or if they had other risk factors for stoke and death (70.8% had hypertension, 38.2% coronary artery disease). Their AF was felt clinically likely to be recurrent, and there had to be no contraindication to anticoagulation. Mean age was 69.7 years, 61.7% were men and 11.4% were from an ethnic minority. A group of 4060 patients were randomly assigned to a rhythm control or rate control strategy. The choice of rhythm control drug was at the discretion of the clinician. Most commonly used drugs were permissible (except class I antiarrhythmic drugs). Electrical cardioversion could be utilized. After failure of ≥2 rhythm control drugs, non-pharmacological approaches could be employed, including percutaneous and surgical ablation and pacing strategies. In the rate control group, the target heart rate was ≤80 beats per minute at rest and ≤110 beats per minute during a six-minute walk test. In both groups, the target INR was 2.0–3.0. In the rhythm control group anticoagulation could be withdrawn at the physician's discretion if SR persisted for four, but preferably twelve weeks, whereas continuous anticoagulation was mandatory in the rate control group. Mean duration of follow-up was 3.5 years, maximum 6 years. The primary end point was overall mortality, with a secondary composite end point of death, disabling stroke, disabling anoxic encephalopathy, major bleeding, and cardiac arrest. Secondary analyses evaluated outcomes amongst pre-specified subgroups including age, sex, rhythm at randomization, duration of AF, and presence or absence of heart failure, coronary artery disease, or hypertension.

Results

Digoxin (48.5%) and beta blockers (46.8%) were the most commonly used drugs for initial rate control. The eventual use of combinations of drugs was common and >80% achieved the targets for satisfactory rate control, with 34.6% remaining in SR at five years. In the rhythm control group, amiodarone (37.5%) and sotalol (31.2%) were the most commonly employed first-line drugs. Changes in therapy were frequent: 62.8% had received amiodarone by the end of the study; 37.8% patients had had at least one attempt at electrical cardioversion; and 62.6% were in SR at five years. Some (37.5%) crossed over to a rate control strategy, largely due to inability to maintain SR and drug intolerances. In the rate control group, 85% patients remained on warfarin. There was a gradual decline in the use of warfarin in the rhythm control group, although this remained above 70%; 62.3% of INRs were in the therapeutic range.

None of the presumed advantages of rhythm control were demonstrated in the AFFIRM study, with the overall balance of benefit favouring rate control. There were significantly more hospitalizations (p <0.001) and adverse drug events (p <0.001) in the rhythm control group. There was a strong trend towards more deaths (p = 0.08) in the rhythm control group, and although this did not achieve statistical significance, the survival curves continued to diverge at five years of follow-up. The secondary end point was similar in the two groups (p = 0.33). There was no difference in ischaemic or haemorrhagic stroke. The majority of strokes in both groups occurred in those whose anticoagulation was discontinued or INRs were subtherapeutic. All comparisons in pre-specified subgroups showed either no significant difference or a benefit favouring rate control.

Limitations

A choice between rhythm and rate control is often lifelong. Therefore, longer duration of follow-up may have been more informative. This may have allowed continuing divergence of the mortality curves and achievement of statistical significance for the primary end point favouring rate control, which would have had even more profound implications. Unrestricted use of antiarrhythmic drugs may have rendered this even more of a 'real-world' study, allowing more clinicians to relate the results to their own practice.

These results cannot be generalized to patients younger than 65 years with no risk factors for stroke, and are obviously not applicable to those with intolerable symptoms due to AF as these patients were excluded.

Conclusions

The population studied is a good representation of the general population with AF, including a decent proportion of female participants. Follow-up was for a reasonable length of time. An aggressive approach to rhythm control resulted in twice as many subjects maintaining SR at five-year follow-up than rate control. However, the AFFIRM study is the most robust demonstration in the literature that contradicts the long-held belief that maintenance of SR confers a survival advantage. This is perhaps a surprising finding given the severe complications associated with AF. The absence of benefit for a rhythm control strategy may be related to the cardiac and non-cardiac side effects of antiarrhythmic drugs.

Control of the ventricular rate and anticoagulation to reduce the risk of stroke has consequently become established as an acceptable initial approach in the majority of patients with AF. This strategy avoids the need for antiarrhythmic drugs which are often toxic and poorly tolerated. In the AFFIRM subgroup analysis, rhythm control appeared superior to rate control in patients aged <65 years or with heart failure and may be beneficial in patients who remain symptomatic despite optimal rate control. The findings of AFFIRM also support the concept that warfarin should not be discontinued even if SR is restored.

Learning points

- A rate control and anticoagulation approach is an acceptable management strategy in patients with AF.
- There is no clinical benefit from attempting restoration and maintenance of sinus rhythm in asymptomatic patients with AF.
- Warfarin should not be discontinued if sinus rhythm is restored.

Further reading

- Carlsson J, Miketic S, Windeler J, *et al.*, and the STAF Investigators. Randomized trial of rate-control versus rhythm control in persistent atrial fibrillation. *J Am Coll Cardiol* 2003; 41: 1690–6.
- Hohnloser SH, Kuck KH, Lilienthal J. Rhythm or rate control in atrial fibrillation - Pharmacological Intervention in Atrial Fibrillation (PIAF): a randomised trial. *Lancet* 2000; 356: 1789–94.
- Ogawa S, Yamashita T, Yamazaki T, *et al.* Optimal treatment strategy for patients with paroxysmal atrial fibrillation: J-RHYTHM Study. *Circ J* 2009; 73: 242–8.
- Opolski G, Torbicki A, Kosior DA, *et al.* Rate control vs. rhythm control in patients with nonvalvular persistent atrial fibrillation: the results of the Polish How to Treat Chronic Atrial Fibrillation (HOT CAFE) Study. *Chest* 2004; 126: 476–86.
- Roy D, Talajic M, Nattel S, *et al.* Rhythm control versus rate control for atrial fibrillation and heart failure. *N Engl J Med* 2008; 358: 2667–77.

Warfarin versus aspirin for stroke prevention in an elderly community population with atrial fibrillation (the Birmingham Atrial Fibrillation Treatment of the Aged Study, BAFTA): a randomized controlled trial

Mant J, Hobbs FD, Fletcher K, Roalfe A, Fitzmaurice D, Lip GY, Murray E. *Lancet* 2007; 370: 493–503.

Background

An increasing body of evidence had demonstrated that oral anticoagulant drugs were more efficacious than antiplatelet agents at reducing stroke risk in patients with AF, and that the benefits outweighed the increased risk of haemorrhagic complications. However, whether this overall benefit could be extrapolated into the large cohort of elderly patients with AF was unknown, as elderly patients had been under-represented in many anticoagulation in AF trials. This was a particularly pertinent clinical question, as the incidence of AF, stroke, and haemorrhage all increase with advancing age. Uncertainty had consequently translated into under-prescribing of warfarin in the older patient. The BAFTA investigators assessed whether warfarin reduced risk of major stroke, arterial embolism, or other intracranial haemorrhage compared with aspirin in elderly patients in the primary care setting.

Methods

The BAFTA study was a prospective randomized open-label trial with blinded assessment of end points. A group of 973 patients was recruited from 260 primary care practices in England and Wales. Patients were randomly assigned to dose-adjusted warfarin (target INR 2.5, acceptable range 2.0–3.0) or aspirin (75 mg daily). No patients were prescribed both drugs. Inclusion criteria were age ≥75 years, with AF or atrial flutter on ECG within the previous two years. Exclusion criteria included rheumatic heart disease, major non-traumatic haemorrhage within the previous five years, intracranial haemorrhage, proven peptic ulcer disease within one year, oesophageal varices, blood pressure >180/110 mmHg. Patients were also excluded if their primary care physician (PCP) felt there was already a strong indication or contraindication for warfarin based on the individual's risk factor profile for stroke and haemorrhage. Therefore, patients were only randomized if there was clinical uncertainty as to the optimal antithrombotic strategy. The primary end point was the first occurrence of fatal or disabling stroke (ischaemic or haemorrhagic), intracranial haemorrhage, or clinically significant arterial embolism. Secondary end points were the frequency of major extracranial haemorrhage, hospital admission for haemorrhage, hospital admission or death due to a non-stroke vascular event, and all-cause mortality. Follow-up was for a mean of 2.7 years and was terminated as planned at the end of the research funding period.

Results

Mean patient age was 81.5 years; 28% patients had a $CHADS_2$ score of ≥3 and 30% patients were identified via the opportunistic finding of an irregular pulse at a planned PCP visit. Some 54.4% of eligible patients were excluded based on the PCP's judgement that one treatment would clearly be more beneficial (of which 79% were prescribed warfarin, 21% aspirin). A group of 67% patients allocated to warfarin remained on treatment throughout the study and 67% of INR values were within the therapeutic range (mean INR 2.4).

There were 24 primary events (21 strokes, two other intracranial haemorrhages, one systemic embolus) in the warfarin group, and 48 primary events (44 strokes, one other intracranial haemorrhage, three systemic emboli) in the aspirin group (yearly risk 1.8% vs. 3.8%, relative risk 0.48, 95% CI 0.28–0.80, p = 0.003; absolute yearly risk reduction 2%, 95% CI 0.7–3.2). Warfarin was as effective in patients aged ≥85 years as it was in younger patients. The composite outcome of major vascular event (stroke, myocardial infarction, pulmonary embolism, vascular death) was lower for warfarin compared with aspirin (5.9% vs. 8.1%; p <0.03). There was no difference in all-cause mortality. Importantly, the yearly risk of extracranial haemorrhage was similar for the two therapies; 1.4% with warfarin and 1.6% with aspirin (relative risk 0.87, CI 0.43–1.73; absolute risk reduction 0.2%, -0.7–1.2).

Limitations

There is an inevitable element of selection bias in the BAFTA trial. First, it was felt unethical to deny warfarin to patients felt to have a clear clinical indication on the basis of their PCP's clinical judgement. Second, those considered (rightly or wrongly) to have unacceptably high risk of bleeding may have been excluded. Third, the majority of patients enrolled were already taking an anti-thrombotic drug and were therefore known to tolerate such therapy, rather than being treatment naive. Overall, only 21% of patients identified entered the trial. Hence, participation was restricted, and this cannot perhaps be considered a truly 'all-comers' trial. However, the commonest reason for exclusion was the PCP's preference for warfarin, suggesting that the benefit of warfarin in those subsequently randomized may have been underestimated. These restrictions may partly explain why there was a lower prevalence of risk factors and a lower rate of thrombotic and bleeding events in BAFTA compared to other trials. These low rates reduce the absolute risk reduction of warfarin over aspirin to 2% per year. However, this suggests that warfarin is superior to aspirin

even in a low stroke-risk elderly group. The wide confidence limits for the risk of major haemorrhage suggest that the trial may have been underpowered to detect a genuine increase in bleeding with warfarin.

Conclusions

The dose of aspirin used (75 mg) and target INR (2.5) directly reflect current UK practice. The pivotal BAFTA trial gave the first evidence of benefit for warfarin in thromboprophylaxis in a large cohort of elderly AF patients, a hitherto neglected yet vitally important patient group. Moreover, it also demonstrated that there was no significant increase in major bleeding or haemorrhagic stroke with warfarin compared to aspirin, disproving a popular myth. The BAFTA trial has increased the utilization of anticoagulation in this patient group, who are at highest risk of stroke and therefore have the most to gain. The modern paradigm subsequently suggests that elderly patients should be prescribed warfarin unless there is a very compelling reason not to.

> ### Learning points
>
> - Elderly patients with AF benefit from anticoagulation with warfarin.
> - Aspirin is not associated with less major haemorrhagic complications (or intracranial haemorrhage) than warfarin.

Further reading

- Lane DA, Lip GY. Anticoagulation intensity for elderly atrial fibrillation patients: Should we use a conventional INR target (2.0 to 3.0) or a lower range. *Thromb Haemost* 2010; 103: 254–6.

Independent predictors of stroke in patients with atrial fibrillation: a systematic review

The Stroke Risk in Atrial Fibrillation Working Group. *Neurology* 2007; 69: 546–54.

Background

The absolute risk of stroke had been seen to vary widely amongst patients with AF. This appeared to be related to the presence or absence of a variety of features, many of which co-existed, especially in older patients. It was felt

important to be able to estimate an individual's absolute risk of stroke, to fully inform clinical decisions when considering long-term anticoagulation and the balance between benefit versus risk of bleeding.

Methods

The Stroke Risk in AF Working Group undertook a systematic review of the contemporary data to unravel this problem. The primary aim was to identify independent risk factors for ischaemic stroke in non-anticoagulated patients, and second to quantify the absolute rate of stroke associated with each risk factor. Multivariate regression techniques were used to identify independent risk factors. A summary estimate of the relative risk associated with each risk factor was calculated using a maximum likelihood method.

Results

Seven studies meeting the inclusion criteria were identified. This comprised six entirely independent cohorts, and a seventh that had partial patient overlap between two studies. The six patient cohorts were from two randomized-controlled trials, two prospective clinical cohorts, one epidemiological study, and one case-control study. The overall mean age was 71 years and 40% were female. A mean of 30% had paroxysmal AF.

Eight clinical features associated with stroke were identified, of which four were consistently independently predictive of stroke. Prior stroke or TIA was the strongest independent risk factor for future stroke, with a relative risk of 2.5 (95%, CI 1.8–3.5). Advancing age was associated with a relative risk of 1.5 per decade (95% CI 1.3–1.7). A history of hypertension (relative risk 2.0, 95% CI 1.6–2.5) or diabetes (relative risk 1.7, 95% CI 1.4–2.0) were also consistently stroke predictors (summarized in Table 9.3).

Heart failure was not a consistent independent predictor of stroke, although the definition of this condition varied widely from purely clinical grounds to a variety of echocardiographic criteria. Coronary artery disease had various definitions, including prior myocardial infarction, and angina with or without revascularization, and was not independently predictive of stroke. Female sex was not independently associated with stroke risk.

Observed absolute stroke rates for non-anticoagulated patients with a single independent risk factor ranged from 6–9% per year for prior stroke or TIA, 1.5–3% per year for history of hypertension, 1.5–3% per year for age >75 years, and 2.0–3.5% per year for diabetes.

Limitations

Quantitative pooling of event rates from several studies may lead to inaccuracies due to variation in definitions of events such as stroke. The varying prevalence of background factors such as prior stroke or TIA and concomitant antiplatelet drug use limits comparisons between studies. Calculations regarding stroke risk can only be made based on those risk factors included in each study. For example, the presence of atherosclerotic disease was not examined, as trial datasets do not consistently include this information. However, many stroke patients with AF have significant carotid disease and both coronary and peripheral arterial disease are associated with an increased mortality in AF patients. Additionally, complex plaque in the descending aorta is an independent risk factor for ischaemic stroke.

Identifying risk factors based purely on a clinical history (such as heart failure) is less effective than an objective assessment (such as by quantifying left ventricular ejection fraction by echocardiography). This may explain why heart failure was not found to be a consistent predictor of stroke in this analysis.

The severity and duration of diabetes and hypertension and the success of their treatment may be confounding factors on the absolute stroke rate associated with these conditions.

Conclusions

Determining which patients with AF are at risk of stroke is of fundamental importance in everyday clinical practice. The Stroke Risk in Atrial Fibrillation Working Group was able to identify four independent predictors of stroke in AF. These are easily and rapidly identifiable and can be used to guide clinical decisions when considering anticoagulation.

Table 9.3 Independent risk factors for stroke, their prevalence and associated relative risk

Risk factor	Prevalence	Relative risk (95% CI)
Prior stroke or TIA	7%	2.5 (1.8 to 3.5)
Hypertension	48%	2.0 (1.6 to 2.5)
Diabetes	15%	1.7 (1.4 to 2.0)
Advancing age	—	1.5 per decade (1.3–1.7)

Learning points

♦ Prior stroke or TIA, advancing age, diabetes, and hypertension are independent risk factors for stroke in patients with AF.
♦ Prior stroke or TIA is the most powerful predictor of future stroke in patients with AF.

Further reading

- Conway DS, Lip GY. Comparison of outcomes of patients with symptomatic peripheral artery disease with and without atrial fibrillation (the West Birmingham Atrial Fibrillation Project). *Am J Cardiol* 2004; 93: 1422–5.

- Lane D, Lip GY. Female gender is a risk factor for stroke and thromboembolism in atrial fibrillation patients. *Thromb Haemost* 2009; 101: 802–5.

Comparison of 12 Risk Stratification Schemes to Predict Stroke in Patents With Nonvalvular Atrial Fibrillation

Stroke Risk in Atrial Fibrillation Working Group. *Stroke* 2008; 39: 1901–10.

Background

Amongst patients with AF, an individual's absolute risk of ischaemic stroke had been shown to be dependent upon their age and associated comorbidities. An accurate assessment of stroke risk is vital in evaluating whether the benefits of oral anticoagulation (OAC) outweigh the associated risks, principally haemorrhagic complications. Several schemes for stratifying stroke risk in patients with nonvalvular AF had been published, comprising a variety of clinical and echocardiographic parameters. However, differences between these schemes had led to variations in estimation of stroke risk and therefore inconsistent prescription of anticoagulant drugs. Determining the most robust method of stroke risk stratification would increase the number of patients appropriately recommended OAC. Concurrently, a smaller but significant group of patients may not require OAC if their stroke risk is genuinely low.

Methods

The Stroke Risk in Atrial Fibrillation Working Group analysed twelve schemes which stratified for stroke risk and made recommendations for anticoagulation in patients with nonvalvular AF not currently receiving OAC. Each stratification scheme was applied to a sample of 1000 patients from the Stroke Prevention in Atrial Fibrillation III trial. Observed stroke rates in independent test cohorts were compared with predicted risk status.

Results

Of the twelve schemes, seven were based directly on event-rate analyses, whereas five resulted from expert panel consensus. Four considered only clinical features, whereas seven schemes also incorporated echocardiographic parameters. One scheme included the result of a CT brain scan in identifying strokes. The number of variables in the scheme ranged from four to eight (median, six). The most frequently included components were previous stroke or TIA (100% of schemes), patient age (83%), hypertension (83%), and diabetes (83%). Combinations of eight additional variables were included in the other schemes. It was possible to identify eleven independent test cohorts for eight of the twelve schemes. The composition of these eleven cohorts varied in terms of mean age (between 72 and 81 years) and prevalence of previous stroke (between 8 and 25%). Two cohorts were limited to primary prevention only. Mean duration of follow-up ranged from 1.2 to 5.3 years (median 2 years). All eight schemes tested successfully stratified stroke risk, but the absolute stroke rates attributed to each stratum varied widely. Stroke rates for those categorized as low risk ranged from 0% to 2.3% per year and those categorized as high risk ranged from 2.5% to 7.9% per year. When applied to a common test cohort, the proportion of patients categorized by the different schemes as low risk varied from 12% (0.1% annual stroke rate) to 37% (0.9% annual stroke rate) and those categorized as high-risk varied from 16% (4% annual stroke risk) to 80% (2.5% annual stroke risk).

Limitations

Several of the schemes included in this analysis had not been tested to validate their predictive accuracy. The short duration of follow-up limits the predictive accuracy of longitudinal risk. The severity, duration, and success in treatment of hypertension and diabetes is likely to confound the stroke risk attributable to these conditions. Prior stroke or TIA is the most powerful predictor of future stroke, and is included in most risk assessment schemes. The utility of these schemes in the more relevant primary prevention setting is therefore uncertain.

Conclusions

The Stroke Risk in Atrial Fibrillation Working Group highlights the important issue of the substantial clinically relevant differences amongst stroke risk stratification schemes. The wide ranges in classification of patients into risk groups illustrates the variation in stroke risk as determined by different schemes. Dividing stroke risk which is a continuous variable into compartmentalized strata of risk will inevitably lead to imprecision. This suggests that the current methods of utilizing risk stratification schema can be improved upon.

Learning points

- Risk of stroke in patients with AF is a continuous variable.

- Stroke risk schemes artificially compartmentalize stroke risk into discrete low/moderate/high strata, which have poor predictive value.
- Stroke risk stratification schemes should be used in conjunction with sound clinical judgement to guide appropriate prescription of anticoagulants.

Further reading

- Nieuwlaat R, Capucci A, Lip GYH, *et al.* on behalf of the Euro Heart Survey Investigators. Antithrombotic treatment in real-life atrial fibrillation patients: a report from the Euro Heart Study Survey on Atrial Fibrillation. *Eur Heart J* 2006; 27: 3018–28.
- Thomson R, McElroy H, Sudlow M. Guidelines on anticoagulant treatment in atrial fibrillation in Great Britain: variation in content and implications for treatment. *BMJ* 1998; 316: 509–513.

Effect of dronedarone on cardiovascular events in atrial fibrillation

Hohnloser SH, Crijns HJ, van Eickels M, Gaudin C, Page RL, Torp-Pedersen C, Connolly SJ. *N Engl J Med* 2009; 360: 668–78.

Background

Medical management of non-permanent AF has been limited by the modest efficacy of available antiarrhythmic drugs and their significant side effects. These include pro-arrhythmia, especially in patients with structural heart disease, which represents a substantial proportion of the AF population. Amiodarone has become established as the most efficacious drug for maintenance of SR in patients with AF. However, its clinical utility is limited by commonly occurring and significant side effects. Moreover, amiodarone and other anti-arrhythmic drugs have only modest efficacy in maintenance of SR and may be paradoxically pro-arrhythmogenic, especially in the setting of structural heart disease. Hospitalizations for AF are becoming an increasing healthcare burden. Costs associated with hospitalization have spiralled to consume over 50% of the overall healthcare expenditure on AF. No antiarrhythmic drug has been proven to reduce the rate of hospitalization in patients with AF.

There is clearly a need for alternative antiarrhythmic drugs. Dronedarone is a novel antiarrhythmic drug, derived from the amiodarone molecule with adaptations including removal of the iodine component designed to reduce the incidence of thyroid and pulmonary-related adverse effects. These modifications also reduce lipophilicity, which shortens the half-life to approximately 24 hours and reduces tissue accumulation. Dronedarone has an electro-pharmacological profile similar to amiodarone, including anti-adrenergic properties and inhibition of potassium, sodium, and calcium channels. Previous randomized controlled trials had shown that dronedarone was more effective than placebo at maintaining SR and at controlling ventricular rate in AF patients. However, dronedarone was associated with an excess risk of death compared to placebo in patients with severe heart failure.

A Placebo-Controlled, Double-Blind, Parallel Arm Trial to Assess the Efficacy of Dronedarone 400 mg bid for the Prevention of Cardiovascular Hospitalization or Death from Any Cause in Patients with Atrial Fibrillation/Atrial Flutter ATP (Adeonsine Tri-Phosphate) (ATHENA) trial was designed to test the hypothesis that dronedarone would reduce the rate of hospitalization due to cardiovascular events or death in patients with AF.

Methods

The ATHENA trail was a randomized, double-blind, placebo-controlled trial at 551 centres in 37 countries.

A group of 4628 patients were randomly assigned to receive dronedarone 400 mg twice daily or placebo. Patients eligible had paroxysmal or persistent AF or atrial flutter (assessed by ECG documentation of both AF and SR in the preceding six months), with at least one of the following criteria: age ≥70 years, hypertension requiring ≥2 antihypertensive drugs, diabetes, previous stroke, TIA or systemic embolism, left atrial diameter >50 mm or left ventricular ejection fraction ≤40%. Due to lower than anticipated mortality rates in the trial, the inclusion criteria were expanded to include patients aged >75 years without any of the above factors. Exclusion criteria included permanent AF, haemodynamically unstable cardiac disease, New York Heart Association class IV heart failure symptoms, myocarditis, heart rate <50 beats per minute and PR interval >280 msec. The primary efficacy outcome was the first hospitalization due to cardiovascular events or death from any cause. Secondary outcomes were death from any cause, death from cardiovascular causes, and first hospitalization due to cardiovascular events.

Results

Mean patient age was 71.6 years and 46.9% were female. At randomization, 25% had AF, 60.2% were currently taking oral anticoagulant, and 70.6% were on a beta blocker. The mean follow-up period was 21 ± 5 months. The primary outcome was significantly lower in the dronedarone group (31.9%) compared to the placebo group (39.4%), with a hazard ratio for dronedarone of 0.76 (95% CI 0.69–0.84; p <0.001). This was mainly driven by a significant reduction in hospitalization for AF with dronedarone (14.6%) compared to placebo (21.9%, p <0.001). There was no significant difference in the rate of death from any cause, or in hospitalization for other cardiovascular events. There were 63 deaths from cardiovascular causes (2.7%) in the dronedarone group and 90 (3.9%) in the placebo group (hazard ratio, 0.71; 95% CI, 0.51–0.98; p = 0.03), largely due to a reduction in the rate of death from arrhythmia with dronedarone.

Premature discontinuation of study drugs was very high; 30.2% in patients receiving dronedarone and 30.8% in patients receiving placebo. Discontinuation due to adverse events was significantly higher in the dronedarone group (12.7% vs. 8.1%, p <0.001), including significantly more gastrointestinal side effects, prolongation of the QT-interval, bradycardia, and elevation of serum creatinine; the latter is attributed to a reduction in creatinine clearance rather than an effect on glomerular filtration rate. Importantly, rates of thyroid and pulmonary disorders were not significantly different between the two groups.

Limitations

There is a clear trade-off with dronedarone between better safety but reduced efficacy. It may have been clinically more meaningful to compare both efficacy and safety of dronedarone with active treatment, specifically amiodarone, the 'gold-standard' drug. However, comparison against placebo is the standard trial design in this setting. Longer follow-up than the average of 21 months in ATHENA may be necessary to detect certain side effects associated with amiodarone, such as pulmonary fibrosis. Long-term safety is clearly a key issue in evaluating drugs derived from amiodarone, which is yet to be addressed.

The patients enrolled in ATHENA were not necessarily symptomatic from paroxysmal AF. There was no measure of symptom relief or quality of life, and therefore greater patient satisfaction correlated with reduced frequency of hospitalizations can only be assumed.

The main driver of benefit from dronedarone in ATHENA is reduced hospitalization for cardiovascular cause, yet no detail is given about the nature of these hospital admissions. There were more women in the dronedarone group than placebo group (p = 0.002), which may have influenced the results. The rate of adverse events was significantly higher in the dronedarone group compared to placebo, which may have led to its premature discontinuation.

Conclusions

The ATHENA study is the largest antiarrhythmic drug trial ever conducted. Women were well represented; 46.9% of participants were female. The very high rate of hospitalization during follow-up demonstrates that ATHENA addressed an important aspect of management of patients with AF. The ATHENA study assessed a meaningful hard clinical outcome (hospitalization) which reflects and informs clinical practice better than time to AF recurrence. The benefit of dronedarone in terms of reduction in this end point suggests the need for a re-appraisal of the rate versus rhythm control debate. In terms of efficacy (compared to amiodarone), dronedarone does not represent an advancement. However, the results of ATHENA have prompted a re-evaluation in management strategy for patients with AF. A reduction in recurrent hospitalizations may be more important to patients compared with maintaining SR, and potentially represents an important health-economic benefit.

Further reading

● Camm AJ, Kirchhof P, Lip GY, *et al*. Guidelines for the management of atrial fibrillation: the Task Force for the Management of Atrial Fibrillation of the European Society of Cardiology. *Eur Heart J* 2010; 31: 2369–429.

● Køber L, Torp-Pedersen C, McMurray JJV, *et al*.; for the Dronedarone Study Group. Increased mortality after dronedarone therapy for severe heart failure. *N Eng J Med* 2008; 358: 2678–87.

● Le Heuzey J, De Ferrari GM, Radzik D, Santini M, Zhu J, Davy JM. A Short-Term, Randomized, Double-Blind, Parallel-Group Study to Evaluate the Efficacy and Safety of Dronedarone versus Amiodarone in Patients with Persistent Atrial Fibrillation: The DIONYSOS Study. *J Cardiovasc Electrophysiol* 2010; 21: 597–605.

● Singh BN, Connolly SJ, Crijns HJGM, *et al*.; for the EURIDIS and ADONIS Investigators. Dronedarone for maintenance of sinus rhythm in atrial fibrillation or flutter. *New Eng J Med* 2007; 357: 987–99.

Dabigatran versus warfarin in patients with atrial fibrillation

Connolly SJ, Ezekowitz MD, Yusuf S, Eikelboom J, Oldgren J, Parekh A, Pogue J, Reilly PA, Themeles E, Varrone J, Wang S, Alings M, Xavier D, Zhu J, Diaz R, Lewis BS, Darius H, Diener HC, Joyner CD, Wallentin L; RE-LY Steering Committee and Investigators. *N Engl J Med* 2009; 361: 1139–51.

Background

Warfarin had long been established as the gold-standard oral anticoagulant drug in patients with AF, with clear evidence of major benefit in reducing the risk of stroke. However, warfarin has several unfavourable characteristics. It increases the risk of haemorrhagic events, has a narrow therapeutic range, has multiple common drug and dietary interactions, and requires close monitoring with its associated costs and inconvenience. These factors promoted both patient and physician dissatisfaction and had contributed to the under-utilization of warfarin in patient groups with clear evidence of benefit. Therefore, the search for a novel anticoagulant drug to replace warfarin had become the focus of intense research.

Dabigatran is an oral direct thrombin inhibitor, which produces predictable dose-dependent anticoagulation and does not require monitoring or dose adjustment. It has limited drug and dietary interactions. Connolly and colleagues conducted the Randomized Evaluation of Long Term Anticoagulant Therapy (RE-LY) study to examine the efficacy and safety of dabigatran compared to warfarin in patients with AF.

Methods

The RE-LY study was designed as a non-inferiority trial for two doses of dabigatran compared with warfarin. Inclusion criteria were AF at randomization or during the previous six months and at least one risk factor for stroke (previous stroke or transient ischaemic attack – TIA), left ventricular ejection fraction <40%, New York Heart Association heart failure symptoms of at least class II, age >75years or age 65–74 years with diabetes, hypertension, or coronary artery disease. Exclusion criteria were severe valvular heart disease, stroke within the previous 14 days, severe stroke within the previous six months, conditions predisposing to haemorrhage, creatinine clearance <30 ml per minute, active liver disease and pregnancy. A group of 18,113 patients were blindly assigned to one of two fixed doses of dabigatran (110 mg or 150 mg twice daily—bid) or unblinded, open-label, dose-adjusted warfarin, with a target INR of 2.0–3.0. Concomitant antiplatelet therapy was permitted. The primary efficacy outcome was systemic embolism or stroke (including haemorrhagic stroke). The primary safety outcome was major haemorrhage. Secondary efficacy outcomes were stroke, systemic embolism, death, myocardial infarction, pulmonary embolism, TIA, and hospitalization. The primary net clinical benefit outcome was the composite of stroke, systemic embolism, pulmonary embolism, myocardial infarction, death, or major haemorrhage.

Results

The mean age was 71 years and 63.6% were men. In the group, 50.4% were warfarin-naive. The mean CHADS$_2$

score was 2.1. The mean time within the therapeutic INR range was 64% for patients in the warfarin group. This is similar to that seen in other contemporary warfarin trials. Median duration of follow-up was 2.0 years. Non-inferiority was demonstrated for dabigatran 110 mg bid versus warfarin. Rates of the primary outcome (expressed as percentage per year) were 1.69% in the warfarin group compared to 1.53% for dabigatran 110 mg bid (relative risk for dabigatran 0.91; 95% CI 0.74–1.11; p <0.001 for non-inferiority). Moreover, *superiority* was demonstrated for dabigatran 150 mg bid versus warfarin, where the rate for the primary outcome was 1.11% (relative risk, 0.66; 95% CI 0.53–0.82; p <0.001 for superiority). This benefit was largely driven by a reduction in ischaemic stroke.

The rate for major bleeding was 3.36% in the warfarin group, 2.71% in the dabigatran 110 mg bid group (relative risk with dabigatran, 0.80; 95% CI, 0.69–0.93; p = 0.003) and 3.11% in the dabigatran 150 mg bid group (relative risk, 0.93; 95% CI, 0.81–1.07; p = 0.31). Rates of life-threatening bleeding, intracranial bleeding, and major or minor bleeding were higher with warfarin (1.80%, 0.74%, and 18.15%, respectively) than with either dabigatran 110 mg bid (1.22%, 0.23%, and 14.62%, respectively) or dabigatran 150 mg (1.45%, 0.30%, and 16.42%, respectively, p <0.05 for all comparisons of dabigatran with warfarin). There was a significantly higher rate of major gastrointestinal bleeding with dabigatran 150 mg bid than with warfarin. The rate of haemorrhagic stroke, the most feared complication of anticoagulation was, however, lower, with both doses of dabigatran: 0.38% in the warfarin group, 0.12% for dabigatran 110 mg bid (p <0.001) and 0.10% with dabigatran 150 mg bid (p <0.001). The mortality rate was 4.13% in the warfarin group, 3.75% with dabigatran 110 mg bid (p = 0.13) and 3.64% with dabigatran 150 mg bid (p = 0.051).

The rate of the pre-specified net clinical benefit outcome was 7.64% with warfarin, 7.09% with dabigatran 110 mg bid (relative risk, 0.92; 95% CI, 0.84–1.02; p = 0.10) and 6.91% with dabigatran 150 mg bid (relative risk, 0.91; 95% CI, 0.82–1.00; p = 0.04). Importantly, there was no excess of hepatotoxicity in the dabigatran groups, which was seen previously with the direct thrombin inhibitor ximelagatran. Interestingly, there was a higher rate of myocardial infarction with dabigatran 150 mg bid (0.74%, p = 0.048) and dabigatran 110 mg bid (0.72%, p = 0.07) compared to warfarin (0.53%).

Limitations

The main limitation of the RE-LY trial was the comparison with open-label warfarin, which introduces the possibility of reporting and adjudication bias. However, this bias is reduced in prospective, randomized, open-label, blinded end point (PROBE design) trials, such as RE-LY, by the blinded evaluation of outcome events. The duration of follow-up is relatively short for a drug designed for long-term use, although this is being addressed in the Long Term Multi-center Extension of Dabigatran Treatment in Patients With Atrial Fibrillation Who Completed RE-LY Trial (RELY-ABLE study). The higher withdrawal rate of dabigatran, especially related to dyspepsia, raises concerns, although this may be related to the open-label design.

Conclusions

The search for a safe and effective alternative to warfarin ended with the landmark RE-LY study, which has changed the anticoagulation landscape forever. It is the first trial to demonstrate non-inferiority and even *superiority* of a novel oral anticoagulant drug in AF with similar or even lower bleeding risk compared to warfarin. The simplicity of taking dabigatran compared to warfarin may improve access to anticoagulation for patients hitherto not anticoagulated for logistical reasons. The high prevalence of AF suggests that this drug may be beneficial to millions of people around the world.

Learning points

- Dabigatran produces predictable dose-dependent anticoagulation and does not require monitoring or dose adjustment.
- Dabigatran is a safe and effective alternative to warfarin for anticoagulation in patients with AF.

Further reading

- Roskell NS, Lip GY, Noack H, Clemens A, Plumb JM. Treatments for stroke prevention in atrial fibrillation: a network meta-analysis and indirect comparisons versus dabigatran etexilate. *Thromb Haemost* 2010; 104(6): 1106–15.
- Schulman S, Kearon C, Kakkar AK, *et al.* for the RE-COVER Study Group. Dabigatran versus warfarin in the treatment of acute venous thromboembolism. *N Engl J Med* 2009; 361: 2342–52.
- Wolowacz SE, Roskell NS, Plumb JM, Caprini JA, Eriksson BI. Efficacy and safety of dabigatran etexilate for the prevention of venous thromboembolism following total hip or knee arthroplasty. A meta-analysis. *Thromb Haemost* 2009; 101: 77–85.

A novel user-friendly score (HAS-BLED) to assess one-year risk of major bleeding in atrial fibrillation patients: The Euro Heart Survey

Pisters R, Lane DA, Nieuwlaat R, de Vos CB, Crijns HJ, Lip GY. *Chest* 2010; 188: 1093–1100.

Background

Atrial fibrillation is clearly associated with a substantial increase in risk of ischaemic stroke. Overwhelming evidence has established that this risk is reduced significantly by OAC. However, stroke and haemorrhage share many common risk factors, including advancing age and diabetes. The risk of bleeding is inevitably exacerbated by OAC. Many risk factors for anticoagulation-associated bleeding are also indications for anticoagulation. An assessment of both stroke risk and bleeding risk is vital at the individual level, to fully inform clinical decisions about the balance of benefit and risk of OAC in patients with AF. Although tools for stroke risk-stratification (most notably CHADS$_2$) in AF have become established, there was not a validated, practical stratification scheme for the risk of bleeding. This situation had perhaps contributed to the under-utilization of OAC in groups with clear evidence of benefit, particularly older patients, where there had been major concerns about the potential for major bleeding. Pisters and colleagues sought to address this vital need and developed a user-friendly score to estimate the one-year risk for major bleeding in a contemporary cohort of 'real world' AF patients.

Methods

A group of 5333 patients with AF from the Euro Heart Survey on AF database were studied. Inclusion criteria included any patient aged ≥18 years with AF proven by ECG or ambulatory monitoring in the preceding year. A one-year follow-up assessed survival and major adverse cardiovascular events. Major bleeding was defined as either intracranial, causing hospitalization, causing a haemoglobin drop >2 g/L and/or requiring blood transfusion.

All potential risk factors for bleeding identified from a univariate analysis of the cohort with a p value <0.10 (age >65 years, female gender, diabetes, heart failure, chronic obstructive pulmonary disease, valvular heart disease, renal failure, prior major bleeding episode, and clopidogrel use) were entered into a multivariate logistic regression analysis model together with established bleeding risk factors (OAC use, alcohol use, and hypertension). Variables less strongly-linked to bleeding were sequentially removed from the model when the p value was >0.10.

Those variables with p <0.05 in the final model were considered to be significant contributors.

A novel bleeding risk score was derived with the acronym HAS-BLED (Hypertension, Abnormal Renal/Liver Function, Stroke, Bleeding History or Predisposition, Labile INR, Elderly, Drugs/Alcohol Concomitantly score). The components of the HAS-BLED scoring system are summarized in Table 9.4. A score of ≥3 suggests 'high risk' of bleeding, and a cautious approach to prescribing OAC with regular review is indicated.

The predictive accuracy of HAS-BLED was compared with another bleeding risk scoring tool named HEMOR-2RHAGES (Hepatic or renal disease, Ethanol abuse, Malignancy, Older age (>75 years), Rebleeding, Reduced platelet count or function, Hypertension (uncontrolled), Anemia, Genetic factors, Excessive fall risk, and Stroke).

Table 9.4 Components of the HAS-BLED scheme

	Clinical feature	Points awarded (maximum score 9 points)
H	**H**ypertension	1
A	**A**bnormal liver or renal function (1 point each)	1 or 2
S	**S**troke	1
B	**B**leeding	1
L	**L**abile INRs	1
E	**E**lderly (age >65)	1
D	**D**rugs or alcohol (1 point each)	1 or 2

Definitions:

Hypertension: systolic BP >160 mmHg.

Abnormal liver function: chronic liver disease or significant abnormality of LFTs (e.g. bilirubin >2x upper limit normal with AST/ALT/ALP >3x upper limit normal).

Abnormal renal function: serum creatinine >200 µmol/L, on dialysis or renal transplantation.

Stroke: history of stroke.

Bleeding: history of or predisposition to bleeding (e.g. anaemia, clotting disorder).

Labile INRs: time within therapeutic range <60% or high INRs.

Drugs or alcohol: concomitant use of drugs predisposing to bleeding (e.g. NSAIDs, antiplatelet agents), alcohol consumption ≥8 units/week.

Results

A group of 3456 patients in the EuroHeart Survey on AF with complete follow-up were evaluated. The mean age was 66.8 (standard deviation 12.8) years, 59% were male. 64.8% were on OAC, 12.8% of whom were also on antiplatelet therapy, 24% received antiplatelet therapy alone, and 10.2% no antithrombotic therapy. A small number (1.5%) experienced a major bleed during one year follow-up. The annual bleeding rate rose with an increasing number of risk factors. The HAS-BLED schema demonstrated good predictive accuracy (c-statistic 0.72) of bleeding risk in AF patients. HAS-BLED substantially improved the predictive accuracy of bleeding risk in AF patients receiving antiplatelet therapy alone (c-statistic 0.91) or in those not on antithrombotic therapy (c-statistic 0.85). This suggests it has everyday clinical utility in decision making about OAC in a newly diagnosed AF patient or those on concomitant antiplatelet therapy such as in the case of co-existing coronary artery disease. Combined assessment of stroke and bleeding risk with the CHADS$_2$ and HAS-BLED scores respectively would have resulted in withholding of OAC in 12% of patients who experienced major bleeding, and initiation of OAC in 95% patients at high stroke risk not taking OAC who subsequently suffered a stroke within one year.

Limitations

One of the factors in the HAS-BLED score (labile INRs) cannot be assessed at the time when an anticoagulant is first considered. However, the risk of bleeding (and indeed the risk of stroke) changes with time, and should be regularly re-evaluated. Stability of the INR can be assessed at these time points.

A large number of patients were lost to follow-up, which may predispose to an underestimation of rates of bleeding. The number of major bleeds was quite small, and follow-up was relatively short, which increases the possibility of not identifying some risk factors for bleeding.

There was a relatively small number of elderly patients in this study, which limits the applicability of the findings to this population. This is particularly important as the prevalence of AF and the risk of bleeding both increase with advancing age, leading to treatment dilemmas in this cohort. It would be pertinent to validate the HAS-BLED score in a large cohort of older patients with AF.

Conclusion

Pisters and colleagues describe a novel user-friendly risk scoring system to estimate the one-year risk of major bleeding in patients on OAC. The HAS-BLED score is simple to use, with similar predictive accuracy to other bleeding schemes (or greater in some subgroups). In comparison, the HEMOR2RHAGES scoring system is cumbersome due to the number of components and incorporation of laboratory parameters and genetic factors which are not routinely evaluated. The HAS-BLED scoring system was assessed in a 'real-world' registry setting, rendering it particularly applicable to everyday clinical practice when contemplating initiation of OAC or aspirin.

An assessment of bleeding risk may help the clinician choose between anticoagulation strategies, such as between the two doses of dabigatran in the RE-LY study. The HAS-BLED score has been recommended in the new 2010 European Society of Cardiology and 2010 Canadian guidelines on AF management.

Learning points

◆ Recommendation of anticoagulation for a patient with AF should take into account stroke risk and the risk of haemorrhagic complications.
◆ The HAS-BLED score is a validated, accurate, user-friendly tool for estimating the risk of haemorrhagic complications associated with warfarin.

Further reading

- Beyth RJ, Quinn LM, Landefeld CS. Prospective evaluation of an index for predicting the risk of major bleeding in outpatients treated with warfarin. *Am J Med*. 1998; 105: 91–9.
- Gage BF, Yan Y, Milligan PE, *et al*. Clinical classification schemes for predicting haemorrhage: results form the National Registry of Atrial Fibrillation (NRAF). *Am Heart J* 2006; 151: 713–9.
- Kuijer PM, Hutten BA, Prins MH, Buller HR. Prediction of the risk of bleeding during anticoagulant treatment for venous thromboembolism. *Arch Intern Med* 1999; 159: 457–60.
- Lip GY, Frison L, Halperin JL, Lane D. Comparative Validation of a Novel Risk Score for Predicting Bleeding Risk in Anticoagulated Patients With Atrial Fibrillation. The HAS-BLED (Hypertension, Abnormal Renal/Liver Function, Stroke, Bleeding History or Predisposition, Labile INR, Elderly, Drugs/Alcohol Concomitantly) Score. *J Am Coll Cardiol* 2010. (Epub 24 Nov 2010) PubMed PMID: 21111555.
- Shireman TI, Howard PA, Kresowik TF, Ellerbeck EF. Combined anticoagulant-antiplatelet use and major bleeding events in elderly atrial fibrillation patients. *Stroke* 2004; 35: 2362–7.

Conclusion

Major advances have been made in the management of patients with AF in recent years, as illustrated by the landmark papers we have discussed. The modern clinician is now able to confidently identify independent risk factors for stroke and haemorrhagic complications in individual patients and tailor therapy accordingly, safe in the knowledge that a rate control strategy is perfectly valid.

The immediate challenge is to implement the current evidence to confidently advise appropriate patients that anticoagulation with warfarin is of definite benefit. This message must be spread to hitherto neglected groups of patients, particularly the elderly. The now disproven belief that aspirin is a safer yet effective alternative to warfarin must be resolutely abandoned.

The future challenge will be to embrace the potential of the new drugs available for management of atrial fibrillation, in concert with complementary strategies, including ablation and atrial appendage occlusion devices. A range of novel anticoagulant drugs are likely to enter the arena in the next few years, with the potential to confine warfarin to the history books.

Chapter 10

Interventional electrophysiology

Dr James Harrison, Dr Nick Linton, Dr Matthew Wright, and Dr Mark O'Neill

Introduction

One challenge in compiling a chapter of this nature is to achieve a fair balance between the inclusion and exclusion of studies with equally valid claims to be landmarks in the field. Interventional electrophysiology is rich with important contributions, certainly far more than can be included in a shortlist of ten. The last 30 years have seen a shift from an almost exclusively diagnostic specialty, with electrocardiography and pharmacological management the mainstays of the field, to an interventional subspecialty which has grown exponentially in the last decade, and which offers a curative option for many common cardiac arrhythmias.

The earlier years of the specialty were of necessity dominated by critical contributions to the understanding of arrhythmia mechanisms, including, among very many other great names, Langendorf, Moe, Wellens, Coumel, and Josephson. Through observations gleaned from meticulous examination of the 12 lead electrocardiogram, the development of intracardiac recording techniques

opened the door to the first therapies for cardiac arrhythmias. For contemporary trainees, it is difficult to visualize an era where open chest cardiac surgery offered the only chance of cure for the Wolff-Parkinson-White syndrome, when today it can usually be treated percutaneously with minimal risk, often in less than one hour using only local anaesthesia.

A landmark is an event, discovery, or change, marking an important stage or turning point in something. Each of the papers included in this chapter fulfils this definition, all in slightly different ways. In the spirit of cardiac electrophysiology, we have included studies (2–4, 6, and 8) almost entirely devoted to the elucidation of arrhythmia mechanism as, without this understanding, there is no basis for interventional arrhythmia management. Contributions to the understanding and treatment of atrial (4–7), AV node-dependent (1–3), and ventricular arrhythmias (8 and 9) are included. The chapter concludes with a description of transpericardial epicardial mapping, a technique used increasingly frequently, and one which means no part of the heart is now inaccessible to the interventional electrophysiologist.

Treatment of supraventricular tachycardia due to atrioventricular nodal reentry by radiofrequency catheter ablation of slow-pathway conduction

Jackman WM, Beckman KJ, McClelland JH, Wang X, Friday KJ, Roman CA, Moulton KP, Twidale N, Hazlitt HA, Prior MI, Oren J, Overholt ED, Lazzara R. *N Eng J Med* 1992; 327: 313–8.

Background

Atrioventricular nodal re-entry tachycardia (AVNRT) can be successfully treated surgically by interrupting connections between the AV node and the atrium, and by catheter ablation directed towards the atrial insertion of the fast pathway. However, both of these approaches have a high rate of complete heart block (between 3% and 10%) requiring permanent pacing. In this study, the operators carefully mapped the atrial insertion of the slow pathway and delivered radiofrequency energy at this point. They were able to demonstrate convincingly that the slow and fast pathways were anatomically separate and that there were distinct potentials to guide ablation both in sinus rhythm and in tachycardia. The authors demonstrated for the first time that ablation targeted towards the atrial insertion of the slow pathway is effective in curing patients of AVNRT and that this can be done safely with a low risk of complete heart block.

Methods

A group of 80 patients with confirmed AVNRT were enrolled into the study. The area of the atrial insertion of the slow pathway was carefully mapped either in fast-slow AVNRT, with single echo beats utilizing the slow pathway for retrograde conduction or with ventricular pacing with fast pathway block. This region was also investigated antegradely in sinus rhythm, and, if the atrial insertion of the slow pathway could not be found retrogradely, slow pathway potentials seen in sinus rhythm were used to guide ablation.

Results

Patients enrolled into this study were intensively monitored for 48 hours following ablation as an in-patient, with the vast majority of patients undergoing a transoesophageal echocardiogram in addition to ambulatory ECG.

No patients had a recurrence of AVNRT during a mean follow-up of over a year, and 40% underwent a repeat EP study to assess the properties of the slow and fast pathway and to check for inducibility of AVNRT.

The atrial insertion of the slow pathway could be mapped during retrograde conduction in 41% of patients, and the earliest atrial activation was seen to change from the anterior septum, close to the bundle of His, to posterior, either between the coronary sinus ostium and the tricuspid annulus or in the coronary sinus. The characteristic low voltage atrial electrogram either before or following a high frequency, large amplitude electrogram in sinus rhythm or during retrograde conduction of the slow pathway was recorded in all patients (there was a mean interval of 24 msec between the two potentials in sinus rhythm). Although some conduction of the slow pathway was detectable after ablation in 65% of patients, this was not sufficient to maintain sustained tachycardia in any, with only single echo beats on isoprenaline.

Complications arising from ablation targeted at the slow pathway were rare, with a 1.3% incidence of complete heart block requiring pacing, and this was due to inadvertent right bundle branch block due to catheter manipulation in a patient with pre-existing left bundle branch block.

Conclusions

This manuscript led to the now common ablation strategy of targeting the slow pathway for treatment of AVNRT. This has a low risk of complete heart block requiring permanent pacemaker implantation compared with surgical treatment or catheter ablation of the fast pathway. The findings of two disparate sites for the atrial insertion of the slow and fast pathways suggested that the mechanism of the arrhythmia was not completely intranodal.

Further reading

● Calkins H, Yong P, Miller JM, *et al.* Catheter ablation of accessory pathways, atrioventricular nodal reentrant tachycardia, and the atrioventricular junction: final results of a prospective, multicenter clinical trial. *Circulation* 1999; 99: 262–70.
● Kalbfleisch SJ, Strickberger SA, Williamson B, *et al.* Randomized comparison of anatomic and electrogram mapping approaches to ablation of the slow pathway of atrioventricular node reentrant tachycardia. *J Am Coll Cardiol* 1994; 23: 716–23.

A new method for differentiating retrograde conduction over an accessory AV pathway from conduction over the AV node

Hirao K, Otomo K, Wang X, Beckman KJ, McClelland JH, Widman L, Gonzalez MD, Arruda M, Nakagawa H, Lazzara R, Jackman WM. Para-hisian pacing. *Circulation* 1996; 94: 1027–35.

Background

When patients undergo ablation procedures for SVT, the success of the procedure is dependent upon correct identification of the tachycardia mechanism as well as achievement of the appropriate end points. This can be particularly challenging in patients with accessory pathways that are near the AV node. In particular, the atrial activation pattern following retrograde conduction through the pathway may be almost identical to the pattern following retrograde conduction through the node. At the time of this study, very few publications had systematically evaluated manoeuvres to help distinguish accessory pathway mediated tachycardias from atypical AV nodal re-entrant tachycardia (AVNRT).

Concept

The para-Hisian pacing site is unique because it is anatomically close but electrically far from the His bundle. Para-Hisian pacing is performed with a catheter close to the His bundle, or proximal right bundle, and another catheter measuring atrial activation. With changes in pacing output (or small movements of the catheter relative to the His bundle) the volume and location of tissue that is captured by pacing is altered. This results in a change between beats where (1) both ventricular myocardium and His tissue are captured by pacing, and (2) only ventricular myocardium is captured and not His tissue. The surface ECG will change allowing recognition of the change in capture. If only ventricular tissue is captured in the normal heart, then activation must pass from

the base towards the apex in order to enter Purkinje tissue, returning to the His bundle in order to conduct retrogradely through the AV node. This will cause a change in the time between stimulation and the onset of atrial activation. However, if an accessory pathway is present, which conducts from ventricle to atrium more rapidly than the AV node and is close to the AV node, then the fastest conduction from the pacing site to the atrium will always be via the pathway: the VA conduction time will be independent of His capture. Using more advanced analysis, it is also possible to determine fusion between conduction via the AV node and conduction via a pathway.

Methods

The new method—para-Hisian pacing—was tested in 149 patients with an accessory pathway and 53 patients with AVNRT. In 2 of 202 patients, the manoeuvre could not be performed because of proximal right bundle branch block.

Results

Para-Hisian pacing correctly identified the presence of a retrogradely conducting accessory pathway in all 104 patients with a rapidly conducting right-sided or septal accessory pathway. The technique was less sensitive for left lateral pathways (25/34 patients) and for patients with persistent junctional reciprocating tachycardia (i.e. slowly conducting pathways), due to the long conduction time taken to conduct from the ventricular septum to the atrial septum via the pathway.

After accessory pathway ablation, retrograde conduction was present in 104 of 147 patients. In all of these patients, para-Hisian pacing produced an AV-nodal atrial retrograde atrial activation pattern that was independent of His capture.

Implications

Techniques for identifying accessory pathways involve the use of entrainment manoeuvres or the identification of abnormal activation patterns. Before the description of para-Hisian pacing, detection of abnormal retrograde atrial activation was not possible for pathways near to the AV node. This method provided a simple way to detect abnormal retrograde atrial activation, albeit indirectly. This is particularly useful in difficult cases when the results of entrainment manoeuvres are equivocal. Additionally, para-Hisian pacing provides a simple way to assess the effects of ablation.

Conclusion

Para-Hisian pacing is now a standard technique and comprises a complementary diagnostic approach to the detection of accessory pathways near to the septum.

Learning points

◆ Para-Hisian pacing involves pacing near to the His bundle, such that the pacing captures both ventricle and His tissue, or just ventricular tissue alone. If a rapidly conducting septal pathway is present, then the conduction time to the atrium will not change during this manoeuvre.

◆ Para-Hisian pacing is most useful when combined with other diagnostic information gained during an EP study.

Further reading

● Michaud GF, Tada H, Chough S, *et al.* Differentiation of atypical atrioventricular node re-entrant tachycardia from orthodromic reciprocating tachycardia using a septal accessory pathway by the response to ventricular pacing. *J Am Coll Cardiol* 2001; 38: 1163–7.

● Segal OR, Gula LJ, Skanes AC, Krahn AD, Yee R, Klein GJ. Differential ventricular entrainment: a maneuver to differentiate AV node reentrant tachycardia from orthodromic reciprocating tachycardia. *Heart Rhythm* 2009; 6: 493–500.

Diagnostic value of tachycardia features and pacing maneuvers during paroxysmal supraventricular tachycardia

Knight BP, Ebinger M, Oral H, Kim MH, Sticherling C, Pelosi F, Michaud GF, Strickberger SA, Morady F. *J Am Coll Cardiol* 2000; 36: 574–82.

Background

When patients present with SVT there are a number of individual features both of the tachycardia and the response to various pacing manoeuvres that support or refute a specific diagnosis. Although there is no 'standard' routine that is employed throughout all electrophysiology (EP) laboratories, this manuscript systematically examined a number of features and pacing manoeuvres to quantitate their individual diagnostic value. In doing so, as well as achieving the aim of the manuscript it also acts as a reference for a 'standard' EP study.

Methods

Patients were recruited into the study if they had paroxysmal SVT and underwent invasive EP study. A group of 196 patients (with a total of 200 inducible tachycardias) were enrolled into the study.

The baseline parameters and tachycardia features examined were:

◆ Ventricular pre-excitation
◆ Dual AV nodal physiology
◆ VA block cycle length (CL) at >600 msec at baseline
◆ Extranodal response to para-Hisian pacing during sinus rhythm
◆ Induction dependent on a critical atrial-His (AH) interval
◆ Isoproterenol required to sustain tachycardia
◆ Tachycardia cycle length (CL) ≥500 msec
◆ Septal VA interval >70 msec
◆ Eccentric atrial activation
◆ Spontaneous AV block during tachycardia
◆ Spontaneous termination with AV block
◆ Development of bundle branch block
◆ Effect of bundle branch block on VA time

The pacing manoeuvres used were:

- Atrial pacing during SVT at CL 10–40 msec <SVT CL
- Atrial pacing during SVT at AV block CL
- Ventricular pacing during SVT at CL <10–40 msec <SVT CL
- Ventricular pacing during SVT at 200–250 msec for 3–6 beats
- Scan diastole with a premature ventricular stimulus

Results

Of the 200 tachycardias, 56.5% were due to atrioventricular nodal re-entry (AVNRT), 31% orthodromic reciprocating tachycardia (ORT), and 12.5% due to atrial tachycardia (AT).

Atrioventricular nodal re-entrant tachycardia (AVNRT)

The only feature diagnostic of typical AVNRT was a septal ventriculoarterial (VA) time of ≤70 msec. The features that were strongly predictive of AVNRT were dual AV nodal physiology, induction of tachycardia dependent upon a critical AH interval, and concentric activation. Eccentric activation excluded AVNRT, and occurred in 31% of tachycardias. An increase in the VA interval ≥20 msec with bundle branch block also excluded AVNRT and was present in 7%.

No pacing manoeuvres confirmed AVNRT, but it could be excluded with a different atrial activation sequence during entrainment from the ventricle, an A-A-V response on cessation of entrainment from the ventricle, or if the tachycardia terminated with a ventricular extrastimulus when the His bundle was refractory.

Orthodromic reciprocating tachycardia (ORT)

An increase in the VA interval with development of ipsilateral bundle branch block was diagnostic for ORT. Ventricular pre-excitation had a positive predictive value (PPV) of 86% for ORT, and other features that had a high PPV for ORT were an extranodal response to para-Hisian pacing and the development of left bundle branch block with tachycardia. Although absence of VA conduction at baseline was rare in patients with ORT, it did not completely rule out the diagnosis.

Pacing manoeuvres were able to completely rule in or out the diagnosis of ORT; however, these occurred rarely. Termination of tachycardia with a ventricular extrastimulus during His bundle refractoriness without atrial depolarization was diagnostic of ORT, but only occurred in 10% of tachycardias. Other responses that ruled out ORT in the study included a different atrial activation sequence with entrainment of the tachycardia from the ventricle, an A-A-V response on cessation of entrainment from the ventricle, an inability to entrain the atrium from the ventricle because the VA block cycle length (CL) was longer than the tachycardia CL, and dissociation of the ventricle from the atrium during ongoing tachycardia.

Atrial tachycardia (AT)

There was no tachycardia feature that had a significant PPV for AT. However, the presence of an A-A-V response following cessation of entrainment from the ventricle and a different atrial activation sequence during entrainment from the ventricle were diagnostic of AT. Any effect of a ventricular extrastimulus during His bundle refractoriness excluded AT. Another useful feature was the inability to entrain the tachycardia from the ventricle due to a VA block length greater than tachycardia CL, having a PPV of 80%.

Conclusions

Although no simple algorithm could be generated to guarantee successful diagnosis for all SVTs, the combination of assessing the septal VA interval, the retrograde atrial activation sequence, and the response after ventricular entrainment were able to provide a diagnosis for 65% of SVTs in the study, and exclude a tachycardia mechanism in 27% of cases.

Learning points

- It is uncommon to diagnose an SVT with a single observation or manoeuvre.
- A combination of the septal VA interval, atrial activation during ventricular pacing, and the response on cessation of ventricular entrainment can give the diagnosis in the majority of cases.

Further reading

- Knight BP, Zivin A, Souza J, *et al.* A technique for the rapid diagnosis of atrial tachycardia in the electrophysiology laboratory. *J Am Coll Cardiol* 1999; 33: 775–81.
- Veenhuyzen GD, Coverett K, Quinn FR, *et al.* Single diagnostic pacing maneuver for supraventricular tachycardia. *Heart Rhythm* 2008; 5: 1152–8.

Entrainment and interruption of atrial flutter with atrial pacing: studies in man following open heart surgery

Waldo AL, MacLean WA, Karp RB, Kouchoukos NT, James TN. *Circulation* 1977; 56: 737–45.

Background

Atrial flutter had been studied in animal models and could be induced reproducibly after creating a crush lesion between the superior vena cava (SVC) and the inferior vena cava (IVC) in the canine heart. Limited, sequential mapping of this arrhythmia model had demonstrated an activation pattern consistent with re-entry around the caval veins and crush lesion. However, in the late 1970s there was still controversy over the mechanism: an automatic focus near to the septum, with conduction blocked at the CTI, could produce the same activation pattern as re-entry around the tricuspid annulus. Additionally, there was interest in the therapeutic use of pacing as a means to terminate tachycardias, which was the primary aim of this study. However, the lasting impact of the study was due to the electrophysiological observations made by the investigators—both at the time of this study and in the following years.

Methods

Thirty patients with atrial flutter following cardiac surgery were studied. All patients had temporary electrodes implanted on the right atrial epicardium as part of their routine care. Bipolar atrial pacing was initiated at a rate of about 10 beats/min faster than the tachycardia rate and continued for at least 30 seconds. The atrial pacing rate was then manipulated with various pre-defined protocols in an attempt to terminate the arrhythmia.

Results

The investigators found that in order to terminate atrial flutter, the pacing rate had to be above a 'critical' rate and the duration of pacing had to be longer than a 'critical' duration (these could not be prospectively assessed). However, they also reported key observations relating to the mechanism of atrial flutter. The morphology of the flutter waves was modified by overdrive pacing (fusion) and if flutter terminated, then the morphology suddenly changed to the fully paced p-wave morphology.

Implications

This was the first systematic study of entrainment in humans. Although fusion was noted during this study, the full implications were not realized at the time. However, it set a precedent for further systematic studies, which were performed in the setting of atrial flutter as well as atrioventricular reciprocating tachycardia and VT. Over the next few years, specific criteria for entrainment were developed and included the observation of fusion during overdrive pacing. These criteria were applied to assist with diagnosis during the invasive electrophysiology procedures. They are also critical to the conceptual understanding of re-entry circuits.

The first criterion of entrainment is observed when the surface ECG during entrainment has an intermediate morphology that is between the tachycardia morphology and the paced morphology. This was observed in this study (see Results). Entrainment as a tool for terminating arrhythmias remains important, mainly in the context of ICDs. All ICDs have the capability for 'anti-tachycardia pacing', which is frequently used in an attempt to terminate ventricular tachycardia before delivering shock therapy if termination does not occur.

Conclusions

This was the first systematic study of entrainment and became the first of a series of studies relating to entrainment. Criteria for entrainment were developed, on the basis of observation and insight into the underlying mechanism: these are now fundamental to the practice of electrophysiology.

Learning points

- Re-entrant arrhythmias can be entrained by pacing.
- Termination of re-entrant arrhythmias using pacing only occurs if the pacing rate is fast enough and the duration of pacing is long enough.

Further reading

- Stevenson WG, Sager PT, Friedman PL. Entrainment techniques for mapping atrial and ventricular tachycardias. *J Cardiovasc Electrophysiol* 1995; 6: 201–16.
- A general review.
- Waldo AL. From bedside to bench: entrainment and other stories. *Heart Rhythm* 2004; 1: 94–106.
  An unusual review from the founder of entrainment—the history and thinking of the time is juxtaposed with a detailed description of the mechanism of entrainment.

Radiofrequency ablation of the inferior vena cava-tricuspid valve isthmus in common atrial flutter

Cosio FG, Lopez-Gil M, Goicolea A, Arribas F, Barroso JL. *Am J Cardiol* 1993; 71: 705–9.

Background

In the 15 years following the first description of entrainment, the re-entrant circuit involved in common atrial flutter was extensively studied. There was a consensus that activation exited from the cavotricuspid isthmus (CTI) with caudocranial activation of the septum, followed by craniocaudal activation of the lateral right atrial wall. There was also interest in using ablation therapy to modify the circuit by targeting tissue near the exit from the CTI: open heart cryoablation, direct current (DC) ablation and radiofrequency (RF) ablation had all been utilized. However, Cosio *et al.* were the first to employ a 'line' of ablation in order to create electrical block across the anatomically defined cavotricuspid isthmus. They used intracardiac catheters with RF ablation, and this formed the basis for a procedure that is now first-line treatment for common atrial flutter. Additionally, this concept is now applied to the treatment of all other atrial macro-re-entrant tachycardias.

Methods

Nine consecutive patients with persistent (n = 7) or paroxysmal (n = 2) atrial flutter were studied. All patients had undergone cardioversion and were refractory to at least two antiarrhythmic drugs. The procedure was performed under conscious sedation. If the patient was not in flutter, then the arrhythmia was induced by paced stimulation. A catheter with a 4 mm tip electrode was then placed into the right ventricle and slowly withdrawn across the cavotricuspid isthmus to the inferior vena cava. Where atrial electrograms were identified, ablation was performed at multiple points (25–30 W for 30–60 s). This was continued until the arrhythmia terminated and could no longer be re-induced. If arrhythmia remained inducible, then the investigators ablated 3–4 lines parallel to the initial line and then advanced the catheter to the heart via the SVC in an attempt to improve catheter contact forces.

Results

Ablation interrupted tachycardia in all patients by causing a failure of conduction at the CTI, as demonstrated by multiple endocardial recordings. Atrial flutter was non-inducible in seven patients after 1–4 ablation sessions. Flutter free periods of 2–18 months were observed, without arrhythmic drug therapy. At repeat ablation sessions, it was noted that gaps in the line of block were frequently located at either end, that is, close to the IVC or to the tricuspid annulus. It was also noted that at gaps there were sharper, higher amplitude electrograms than at other parts of the line.

Limitations

Since the initial descriptions of CTI ablation for typical flutter, success rates have been improved by the use of large tip (8–10 mm) or irrigated ablation catheters, and by confirming that bidirectional conduction block persists for at least 20 minutes after ablation. Currently, acute success rates are approximately 95%, with long-term recurrence rates of 7–10%. Complication rates are approximately 3%, many of which relate to femoral access. Despite success in preventing atrial flutter, the development of atrial fibrillation is common in this group of patients—more than 50% within five years.

Conclusions

This study described a new approach for the ablation of typical flutter that interrupted the macro-re-entrant path, based upon an anatomically defined circuit. The authors described the technique of slowly withdrawing the ablation catheter along the isthmus from the tricuspid annulus to the IVC. Additionally, they described findings at repeat procedures when further ablation was necessary to block the line—high amplitude, non-fragmented electrograms.

The principles used in this study for the ablation of typical flutter have since been applied to other macro-re-entrant atrial tachycardias. For example, lines may be ablated in the left atrium in order to prevent re-entrant tachycardias during ablation for persistent AF. Additionally, re-entrant circuits around right atriotomy scars can be treated by ablation from the scar to the IVC (usually in combination with a CTI line).

Further reading

● Asirvatham SJ. Correlative anatomy and electrophysiology for the interventional electrophysiologist: Right atrial flutter. *J Cardiovasc Electrophysiol* 2009; 20: 113–22. A comprehensive discussion of the anatomical features and possible pitfalls for the electrophysiologist.
● Gerstenfeld EP, Marchlinski FE. Mapping and ablation of left atrial tachycardias occurring after atrial fibrillation ablation. *Heart Rhythm* 2007; 4: S65–72. This review describes linear ablation in the left atrium for macro-re-entrant tachycardias.
● Perez FJ, Schubert CM, Parvez B, Pathak V, Ellenbogen KA, Wood MA. Long-term outcomes after catheter ablation of cavo-tricuspid isthmus dependent atrial flutter: A meta-analysis. *Circ Arrhythm Electrophysiol* 2009; 2: 393–401. A large meta-analysis giving the most comprehensive analysis of success rates and complications from CTI ablation.

Spontaneous initiation of atrial fibrillation by ectopic beats originating in the pulmonary veins

Haissaguerre M, Jais P, Shah DC, Takahashi A, Hocini M, Quiniou G, Garrigue S, Le Mouroux A, Le Metayer P, Clementy J. *N Engl J Med* 1998; 339: 659–66.

Background

In recent years, catheter ablation has emerged as an effective and curative approach for patients with symptomatic paroxysmal and persistent atrial fibrillation (AF), who have failed drug therapy. The demonstration in this study that paroxysmal AF is frequently triggered by pulmonary vein (PV) ectopy has led to the emergence of PV isolation as a widely practiced therapy for this arrhythmia and even as a first-line therapy in selected patients. In the early days of AF ablation, only spontaneously firing PVs were ablated. However, high recurrence rates, the increasing recognition that all PVs can initiate AF and technological developments now mean that it is routine practice to isolate all four PVs.

Methods

A group of 45 patients with frequent AF (occurring at least once every two days) were entered into the study. They had to be resistant to more than two drugs, on anticoagulation and to have frequent isolated atrial ectopic beats.

During the electrophysiological study, a roving mapping/ablation catheter was introduced transvenously and multielectrode catheters were placed in the right atrial appendage and coronary sinus to act as references for timing during mapping. The initial phase of the study mapped isolated atrial ectopic beats. The site of the ectopic focus was determined by finding the point of earliest atrial activation. If there was no clear atrial signal in the right atrium >10 msec before the onset of the ectopic P-wave, the focus was deemed to be left atrial and mapping of the left atrium and PVs was performed (either via a patent foramen ovale or transeptal puncture).

Under sedation, radiofrequency ablation was performed at the site of earliest atrial activation. Intravenous heparin was given if this was found to be in the left atrium. The patients were anticoagulated for three months, but received no antiarrhythmic drugs. They were followed up with Holter recordings and clinical assessment every three months.

Results

Effective mapping in these patients was often problematic, as spontaneous ectopic beats and paroxysms of AF occurred unpredictably. Equally, sustained AF required either waiting for spontaneous cardioversion or electrical cardioversion.

One ectopic focus was found in 29 patients, 2 were identified in 9 patients, 3 were identified in 6 patients and 4 were identified in 1 patient, making a total of 69 ectopic foci. In this group 65 of these 69 ectopic foci (94%) were found to originate in the PVs (31 in the left superior PV, 17 in the right superior, 11 in the left inferior, and 6 in the right inferior).

The earliest site of atrial activity was 2–4 cm within the main PV or one of its proximal branches, preceding the ectopic P-wave by 106 ± 24 msec. Spontaneous initiation of AF was recorded in 36 patients, with initiation preceded by a single ectopic focal discharge in 3 patients and by a burst of two or more repetitive focal discharges in 40 patients. The mean rate of these repetitive discharges was 340 per minute. In the other 9 patients, there was no spontaneous initiation of AF, but all had frequent isolated atrial ectopics originating from a single PV or atrial focus.

Successful ablation of ectopic foci was achieved in 38 patients; 25 of these required 2 ablation procedures and 6 patients required 3 procedures, with almost all recurrences occurring within a few days of the initial procedure. There were no significant complications during the study. In-hospital Holter recordings in these patients showed a reduction in atrial ectopic beats from 4377 ± 3629 to 98 ± 91 per 24 hours.

During a follow-up period of 8 ± 6 months, 28 patients remained free of AF without antiarrhythmic drug therapy, whilst 17 had a recurrence of AF.

Conclusions

This study demonstrated that most atrial ectopic beats that initiate frequent paroxysms of AF are located in the PVs. Atrial fibrillation is triggered following a repetitive burst of ectopic activity. These ectopic foci can be treated by radiofrequency ablation, which forms the basis of current catheter ablation for AF.

Learning points

- In patients with frequent paroxysms of AF, the most common origin of atrial ectopics is in the pulmonary veins.
- Rapid repetitive firing of these ectopic foci can trigger AF in these patients.
- These ectopic foci can be treated with radiofrequency ablation.

Further reading

- Scherlag BJ, Yamanashi W, Patel U, Lazzara R, Jackman WM. Autonomically induced conversion of pulmonary vein focal firing into atrial fibrillation. *J Am Coll Cardiol* 2005; 7: 1878–86.
- Weerasooriya R, Khairy P, Litalien J, *et al.* Catheter ablation for atrial fibrillation: are results maintained at 5 years of follow-up? *J Am Coll Cardiol* 2011; 57: 160–6.

Catheter ablation of long-lasting persistent atrial fibrillation: critical structures for termination

Haissaguerre M, Sanders P, Hocini M, Takahashi Y, Rotter M, Sacher F, Rostock T, Hsu L-F, Bordachar P, Reuter S, Roudaut R, Clementy J, Jais P. *J Cardiovasc Electrophysiol* 2005; 16: 1125–37.

Background

Whilst catheter ablation is an effective treatment for patients with symptomatic paroxysmal atrial fibrillation (AF), the success rates for persistent (particularly long-standing) AF are more modest. A number of different ablation strategies have been suggested for persistent AF in addition to pulmonary vein isolation (PVI), including linear lesions to interrupt re-entrant wavelets, posterior left atrial ablation, and ablation of fractionated potentials or sites of short cycle length.

Atrial fibrillation cycle length (AFCL) is seen to gradually prolong in the course of a catheter ablation procedure prior to arrhythmia termination. This study prospectively investigated the relative contribution of different atrial regions in sustaining AF, by evaluating the effect of regional ablation on AFCL and the development of organized atrial arrhythmias.

Methods

A group of 60 patients undergoing catheter ablation for symptomatic persistent (mean duration 17 ± 27 months) AF were entered into the study. Left atrial (LA) ablation involved up to four steps:

(1) Pulmonary vein isolation.
(2) Superior vena cava (SVC) and coronary sinus (CS) isolation.
(3) Atrial ablation at sites with continuous electrical activity, complex fractionated electrograms, a gradient

of activation or a cycle length shorter than in the left atrial appendage (LAA).

(4) Linear ablation (cavotricuspid isthmus line, LA roof line and left inferior pulmonary vein to lateral mitral annulus line).

The sequence for the first three steps was randomized, but linear ablation was always the last step (as sinus rhythm (SR) was required to demonstrate its completion with bidirectional conduction block).

The effect of each stage was measured by the effect on AFCL (measured in the CS, LAA, and right atrial appendage, averaged over 30 consecutive cycles) and the termination of AF (transition directly to sinus rhythm or conversion to atrial tachycardia (AT)). When AF converted to an AT, activation mapping and entrainment manoeuvres were used to define its location and mechanism.

Results

Atrial fibrillation terminated in 52 of the 60 patients (87%), directly to SR in 7 or via an intermediate AT in 45 patients. This termination was preceded in all patients by an increase in the AFCL (from 151 ± 22 msec to 190 ± 21 msec). Three structures had the greatest influence on AFCL prolongation—the anterior LA, CS, and the pulmonary veins (PVs). In this group 44% of the intermediate atrial tachycardias were focal and the remaining 56% were macro-re-entrant (involving the LA roof or mitral/tricuspid isthmus). The 8 patients without AF termination

displayed shorter AFCL at baseline (130 ± 14 msec vs. 156 ± 23 msec; p = 0.002).

Conclusions

This study showed that termination of persistent AF by catheter ablation can be achieved in a significant majority of patients and that three sites—the anterior LA/LAA, CS, and PVs—have the greatest impact on the maintenance of persistent AF.

Learning points

- Persistent AF can often be terminated by catheter ablation.
- This is preceded by prolongation of AFCL and often a sequence of organized atrial arrhythmias.
- The anterior LA/LAA, CS, and PVs are the most important sites in the maintenance of persistent AF.

Further reading

- Cappato R. Calkins H, Chen SA, *et al*. Updated worldwide survey on the methods, efficacy, and safety of catheter ablation for human atrial fibrillation. *Circ Arrhythm Electrophysiol* 2010; 3: 32–8.
- Wijffels MC, Kirchhof CJ, Dorland R, Allessie MA. Atrial fibrillation begets atrial fibrillation. A study in awake chronically instrumented goats. *Circulation* 1995; 92: 1954–68.

Identification of reentry circuit sites during catheter mapping and radiofrequency ablation of ventricular tachycardia late after myocardial infarction

Stevenson WG, Khan H, Sager P, Saxon LA, Middlekauff HR, Natterson PD, Wiener I. *Circulation* 1993; 88: 1647–70.

Background

Ablation of ischaemic VT is challenging, in part due to the many areas of damaged myocardium capable of disordered electrical activation. It is difficult to differentiate between zones of slow conduction that are essential to the mechanism of the tachycardia, and 'bystander' sites which are not part of the tachycardia circuit. This study involved computer modelling of human VT and mapping and ablation of clinical VT in 15 patients.

Methods

Computer modelling was used to explore entrainment of a typical 'figure of eight' VT circuit, with conduction through a common isthmus located between two 'islands' of scar. The model included bystander pathways and slow conduction in the isthmus. The relationship between pacing site and the following features was assessed:

- QRS morphology

- Stimulus-to-QRS time compared to electrogram-to-QRS time
- Effect of pacing: single stimuli scanning the tachycardia and trains of stimuli
- Post-pacing interval

Results

Entrainment with concealed fusion

When entrainment is performed from the common isthmus, an orthodromic wavefront travels out of the isthmus to activate the ventricle with the same pattern as tachycardia. The antidromic wavefront collides with the wavefront from the previous beat. If this collision occurs within the common isthmus then it will not have any effect on the surface ECG. Therefore there will be concealed fusion, that is, the surface ECG morphology will be the same as during tachycardia, but accelerated to the rate of pacing.

Stimulus to QRS onset

Although entrainment with concealed fusion is predictive of a successful RF ablation site, there are exceptions. If there is a 'blind alley' connecting to the common isthmus, then pacing from within it will result in concealed fusion. However, the change in the path of excitation that occurs with pacing will cause a change in the timing relationship between activation at the electrode and the QRS. If the stimulus-QRS time during pacing is the same as electrogram-QRS time during tachycardia, then this suggests that the catheter is on a critical part of the circuit. In this situation, the time from stimulus-QRS allows the position within the common isthmus to be inferred: a time of zero implying that the pacing position is at the exit site, whereas a time of >60 msec suggests the pacing electrode is deeper within the isthmus.

Post-pacing interval

The post-pacing interval is the time between the last pacing stimulus and the first beat of tachycardia at the pacing site. If entrainment is performed from a site within the tachycardia circuit, then the post-pacing interval should be near zero.

Electrogram duration

The final observation was electrogram duration, a marker of slow conduction. However, there was no relation between electrogram duration and termination of tachycardia.

Predictors of termination by ablation

Univariate logistic regression analysis demonstrated that a combination of entrainment with concealed fusion, a post-pacing interval that was within 30 msec of the VT cycle length, and a stimulus to QRS onset of >60 msec but <70% of the VT cycle length was associated with a 36% chance of successful termination of VT at that site. If none of these features was present then likelihood of successful termination was less than 4%. With multivariate analysis, all factors except entrainment with concealed fusion were independent predictors of successful RF ablation sites, and if the post-pacing interval was removed from the model, entrainment with concealed fusion was also independently predictive of a successful site.

Conclusions

Although no single observation guarantees successful ablation sites for VT, the tools to help find sites that are likely to be involved in the tachycardia mechanism were identified. When ablation is directed using these observations and is acutely successful the outcome was good, albeit in this small number of patients.

Learning points

- The substrate for ischaemic VT is complex, and sites that are optimal for ablation have a number of features, including entrainment with concealed fusion, a post-pacing interval that is within 30 msec of the tachycardia cycle length and a stimulus to QRS time that is the same as the local electrogram time to QRS recorded during VT.
- Zones of slow conduction within the common isthmus are promising sites for ablation.
- Even at sites that display all of these features ablation is not guaranteed to terminate VT if the isthmus is broad.
- The post-pacing interval is a key measurement to avoid ablating bystander pathways, which are poor sites to target.

Further reading

- Soejima K, Suzuki M, Maisel WH, *et al.* Catheter ablation in patients with multiple and unstable ventricular tachycardias after myocardial infarction: short ablation lines guided by reentry circuit isthmuses and sinus rhythm mapping. *Circulation* 2001; 104: 664–9.
- Stevenson WG, Friedman PL, Kocovic D, *et al.* Radiofrequency catheter ablation of ventricular tachycardia after myocardial infarction. *Circulation* 1998; 98: 308–14.

Prophylactic catheter ablation for the prevention of defibrillator therapy

Reddy VY, Reynolds MR, Neuzil P, Richardson AW, Taborsky M, Jongnarangsin K, Kralovec S, Sediva L, Ruskin JN, Josephson ME. *N Engl J Med* 2007; 357: 2657–65.

Background

In patients with a history of myocardial infarction (MI), who have survived an episode of ventricular arrhythmia, implantable cardioverter-defibrillators (ICDs) reduce the risk of sudden death from ventricular fibrillation (VF) or ventricular tachycardia (VT). However, ICDs do not treat the underlying arrhythmogenic substrate and ICD shocks are painful and associated with significant psychological distress.

The Substrate Mapping and Ablation in Sinus Rhythm to Halt Ventricular Tachycardia (SMASH-VT) study was a prospective, multicentre (two hospitals in the United States and one in the Czech Republic), unblinded, randomized controlled trial to assess whether catheter ablation aimed at eradicating VT could reduce ICD shocks.

Methods

Between 2000 and 2004, 128 patients with previous MI and an ICD implanted for VF, haemodynamically unstable VT, or syncope with inducible VT at electrophysiological study were entered into the study and randomly assigned to either a control group (no additional therapy; n = 64) or adjunctive substrate-based VT ablation while in sinus rhythm (n = 64). After the study had commenced, enrolment was extended to include patients who received an ICD for primary prevention and received a single episode of appropriate ICD therapy.

Patients were excluded if they were taking class I or III antiarrhythmic drugs, if the ventricular arrhythmia was not thought to be due to MI, if there was active and ongoing ischaemia, or if incessant ventricular arrhythmias necessitated immediate treatment.

Nearly all patients were receiving aspirin, beta blockers, and angiotensin converting enzyme inhibitors/angiotensin receptor blockers (ACEi/ARB). Patients treated with VT ablation additionally received warfarin for 4–6 weeks following ablation (unless <5 ablation lesions had been made, in which case aspirin alone was deemed sufficient).

Patients were followed up for two years at 3, 6, 9, 12, 18, and 24 months with ICD interrogation. The primary end point was survival, free from appropriate ICD therapy (defined as shocks or anti-tachycardia pacing). Secondary end points included freedom from ICD shocks and mortality.

Results

Results were analysed on an intention to treat basis and three patients assigned to the VT ablation group did not undergo the procedure (one death, two lost to follow-up).

In the control group 21 (33%) patients received at least one appropriate ICD therapy (shocks or anti-tachycardia pacing), compared with 8 (12%) in the VT ablation group (p = 0.007). Of these patients, 20 (31%) received shocks (without anti-tachycardia pacing) in the control group, compared with 6 (9%) in the VT ablation group (p = 0.003). There was no significant difference in mortality between the two groups (11 (17%) in the control group vs. 6 (9%) in the VT ablation group; p = 0.29). There was no 30-day mortality following VT ablation.

Conclusions

This relatively small randomized study of post-MI patients who received an ICD after a first arrhythmic event has shown that substrate-based catheter ablation can be performed to reduce the incidence of ICD therapies.

Learning points

- Patients with previous MI, who survive a ventricular arrhythmia, are at high risk of sudden death. This is reduced, although not abolished, by ICD implantation.
- Implantable cardioverter defibrillators do not treat the underlying arrhythmogenic substrate and ICD shocks are associated with significant morbidity.
- Prophylactic VT ablation can reduce the incidence of ICD therapy in these patients, but does not impact mortality.

Further reading

- Aliot EM, Stevenson WG, Almendral-Garrote JM, *et al.* EHRA/HRS Expert Consensus on Catheter Ablation of Ventricular Arrhythmias. *Europace* 2009; 11: 771–817.
- Kuck KH, Schaumann A, Eckardt L, *et al.* Catheter ablation of stable ventricular tachycardia before defibrillator implantation in patients with coronary heart disease (VTACH): a multicentre randomised controlled trial. *Lancet* 2010; 375: 31–40.

A new technique to perform epicardial mapping in the electrophysiology laboratory

Sosa E, Scanavacca M, D'Avila A, Pilleggi F. *J Cardiovasc Electrophysiol* 1996; 7: 531–6.

Background

Before the development of endocardial catheter ablation, surgical epicardial approaches were used to treat refractory arrhythmias, including VT and supraventricular tachycardia (SVT). While the majority of monomorphic VTs probably originate from a re-entrant circuit within the subendocardium, some may involve epicardial circuits inaccessible via standard transvenous routes, a potential reason for procedural failure in VT ablation. This study was the first description of epicardial mapping performed through a percutaneous pericardial puncture in three patients with Chagas disease and recurrent VT. This technique, combined with radiofrequency ablation, has since been described in larger series of patients.

Methods

Under deep sedation, quadripolar catheters were placed transvenously in the right ventricular (RV) apex and coronary sinus and a steerable catheter placed in the left ventricular (LV) lateral wall via the right femoral artery. Pericardial puncture was performed with the patient lying horizontally using a standard subxiphoid approach, with contrast injection to confirm position of the needle tip. Using the Seldinger technique, a 7-French steerable catheter was introduced into the pericardial space and moved to map the entire surface of the LV and RV. Mapping was performed during sinus rhythm and after VT induction by programmed stimulation. The LV and epicardial catheters were placed at the earliest activation site on the endocardium and epicardium, respectively.

As the aim of the study was to assess safety and feasibility of epicardial mapping alone, radiofrequency ablation was not used during the procedure.

Results

In all three patients, the pericardial space was entered without complications. The epicardial catheter was easily moved within the pericardial sac, and the majority of the LV and RV epicardial surfaces were covered. In one of the three patients, epicardial activation was earlier than endocardial activation, following the induction of VT. In this patient, it was easier to induce VT by epicardial stimulation than by endocardial stimulation. There were no post-procedural complications and echocardiography showed no pericardial effusions.

Conclusions

Failure of endocardial catheter ablation for VT may reflect the presence of an epicardial arrhythmia substrate. This study demonstrated that epicardial instrumentation via a transpericardial approach was safe and feasible. Subsequent studies have extended this technique to larger patient cohorts and included successful radiofrequency ablation.

Learning points

- Ventricular tachycardia may involve an epicardial circuit, which is not accessible with standard transvenous catheter techniques.
- Transpericardial instrumentation for epicardial mapping and radiofrequency ablation is safe and feasible and may be suitable in patients in whom a previous VT ablation has been unsuccessful.

Further reading

- Lachman N, Syed FF, Habib A, *et al.* Correlative anatomy for the electrophysiologist, part I: the pericardial space, oblique sinus, transverse sinus. *J Cardiovasc Electrophysiol* 2010; 21: 1421–6.
- Schweikert RA, Saliba WI, Tomassoni G, *et al.* Percutaneous pericardial instrumentation for endo-epicardial mapping of previously failed ablations. *Circulation* 2003; 108: 1329–35.
- Sosa E, Scanavacca M, D'Avila A, Antônio J, Ramires F. Nonsurgical transthoracic epicardial approach in patients with ventricular tachycardia and previous cardiac surgery. *J Interv Card Electrophysiol* 2004; 10: 281–8.

Conclusion

Interventional cardiac electrophysiology has advanced rapidly during the last three decades. The papers presented in this chapter span that development, from the purely mechanistic investigational work by Waldo and colleagues, laying the basis for our understanding of re-entrant arrhythmias in the human heart, to the high technology interventional techniques being used today for the cure of arrhythmias, which previously could only be treated suboptimally using medication.

While technological advances have played a large role in the maturation of this exciting specialty, the core of electrophysiology remains an understanding of the arrhythmia mechanism at work in an individual patient at any given time. The constant development of new interventional tools and improvements in already well established ones can, at times, divert the attention of trainees away from this principle. The continued partnership of deductive and inquisitive clinicians with responsible and innovative technology development is likely to lead to further important advances in the coming years.

Just as cardiac surgery for the Wolff-Parkinson-White syndrome seems alien to the generation of cardiac electrophysiologists beginning their practice today, perhaps in a further three decades, it will be possible to diagnose and treat cardiac arrhythmias with close to 100% success, totally non-invasively, and with a vanishingly low risk of complications. Whatever the future may bring, it will be founded on mechanism-informed intervention and it is certain that all of the papers and investigators in this chapter will have played some role in that process.

Chapter 11

Anti-arrhythmic drug therapy

Dr Boon Lim and Dr Pier Lambiase

Introduction

The definition of a 'landmark paper' is multi-factorial as a paper can only be measured ultimately by its impact on clinical practice, whether positively, that is, by demonstrating the application of a specific therapy which has a significant and sustained clinical effect, or negatively, by informing the physician that therapy is not efficacious, or even dangerous. The technical criteria for such a publication should include the fact that the trial of therapy was randomized and double-blinded to avoid bias and the end points assessed should be unequivocal. The population recruited into the trial should reflect the target population treated by the physician such that it is relevant to contemporary practice. Therefore, any evaluation of landmark clinical trials of anti-arrhythmic drug therapy should begin with high quality randomized placebo controlled trials in large populations looking at key unequivocal

primary end points which impact both on the individual patient and the management of populations in terms of mortality and cost-efficacy. In the anti-arrhythmic therapy field there are numerous small studies which demonstrate efficacy, but frequently the groups studied are too small to allow application to the wider population. The effects of these agents are often not pure or achieved through a single target. Figure 11.1 summarizes the main anti-arrhythmic classes, modulators of arrhythmia, and key therapeutic targets based upon arrhythmia mechanisms.

In this series of ten papers we have aimed to highlight the studies that have significantly changed or informed practice with the highest level of evidence. The series can be divided into trials of agents to prevent lethal arrhythmia and sudden death, atrial anti-arrhythmic

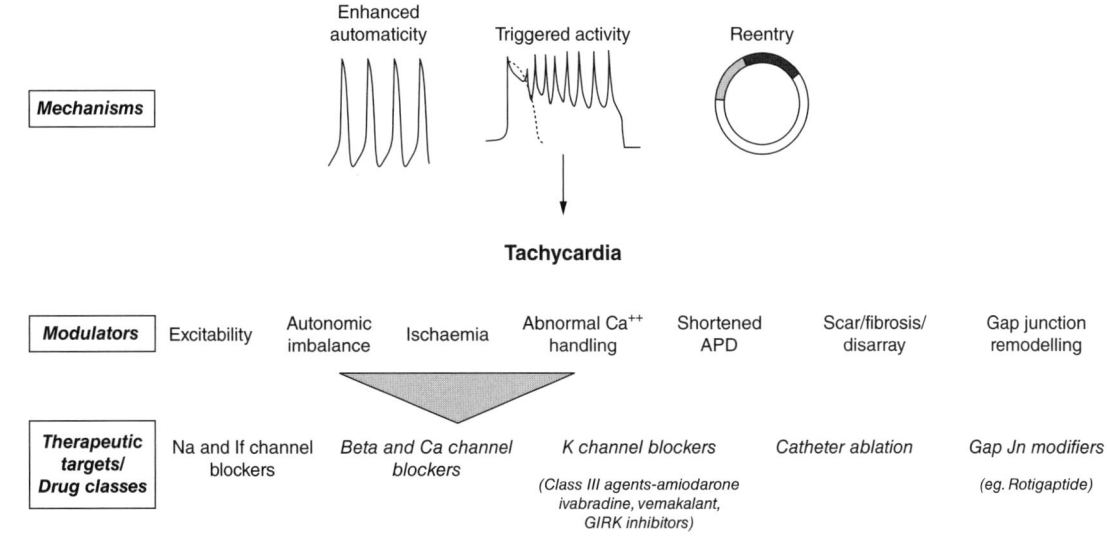

Figure 11.1 Mechanisms, modulators, and potential therapeutic targets for arrhythmia prevention. These mechanisms and modulators are not mutually exclusive.

agents (reflecting the high burden of atrial fibrillation (AF) in the community), and those trials which were important negatives, showing the detrimental effects of certain agents in specific patient populations.

First International Study of Infarct Survival Collaborative Group

The ISIS Investigators. Randomised trial of intravenous atenolol among 16,027 cases of suspected acute myocardial infarction: ISIS-1. *Lancet* 1986; 328: 57–66.

Background

The ISIS-1 set out to address the fundamental question as to whether a beta blocker (atenolol) administered early in the course of acute myocardial infarction (AMI) reduces mortality. This trial stands today as an example of efficient recruitment and randomization through the use of a simple computer based randomization process requiring physician input of easily accessible information in the emergency department.

This trial changed practice and initiated the standardization of an evidence-based approach to AMI which is now firmly embedded in our healthcare system and contributed significantly to the reduction in mortality from MI we see today—a foundation built upon by other randomized trials in the series of ISIS studies involving aspirin and thrombolysis that have stood the test of time and changed practice.

Methods

Between 1981 and 1985, 16,027 patients entering 245 coronary care units at a mean of five hours after the onset of suspected AMI were randomized either to a control group or to a group receiving intravenous (IV) atenolol (5–10 mg immediately, followed by 100 mg/day orally for seven days). The study was intended to be of patients with suspected MI, who were thought by the responsible physician to be within 12 hours of the onset of symptoms, not already on beta-blockers or verapamil, and with no clear indication for, or contraindication to, beta blockade (e.g. heart rate persistently below 50 beats/min, systolic blood pressure <100 mmHg, heart block, severe heart failure, or bronchospasm).

Results

During the treatment period (days 0–7) there were 313 (3.9%) vascular deaths in the atenolol group compared with 365 (4.6%) in the control group. This 15% lower vascular mortality in the atenolol group is conventionally significant (2p <0.04), but the 95% confidence interval is wide, ranging from 1% to 27%. Treatment was most effective when given early—in patients randomized within two hours from the onset of pain, the difference in vascular mortality during the treatment period was larger than the overall reduction of 15% (17/531 atenolol vs. 38/555 control). There were 189 cardiac arrests in the atenolol arm versus 198 in the placebo control in Metoprolol In Acute Myocardial Infarction (MIAMI) (48/2877 metoprolol vs. 52/2901 control), and in all other IV beta blocker studies (available data, 69/2862 vs. 105/2815). These suggest that early IV beta blocker treatment might produce a reduction of about 15% (standard deviation 7%; 2p <0.05) in the odds of cardiac arrest. Data on re-infarction in hospital were available for the later three-quarters of ISIS-1 (148/5807 atenolol vs. 161/5834 control re-infarctions), for MIAMI (85 metoprolol vs. 111 control), and for the other IV trials (available data, 75/2341 vs. 99/2331). Overall, these suggest a reduction of about 18% (standard deviation 7%; 2p <0.02) in the odds of early re-infarction.

Limitations

The trial was primarily designed to detect a significant difference in survival between beta blockade and control in the acute phase of MI. It was not designed to look specifically for arrhythmic event rates, although ventricular fibrillation/ventricular tachycardia (VF/VT) arrests were captured in the acute phase. Also, detailed echocardiographic or Holter data were not collected to assess effects of beta blockade on left ventricular remodelling or arrhythmic events during follow-up.

Conclusions

Taken together with other studies of IV beta blockade for AMI, ISIS-1 demonstrated that treatment reduces mortality in the first week by about 15%, but with a rather less extreme effect in days 0–1 than was observed in ISIS-1 alone. It also provides highly significant (2p <0.0002) evidence of an effect on the combined end point of death, arrest, or re-infarction, suggesting that treatment of about 200 patients would lead to the avoidance of one re-infarction, one arrest, and one death during days 0–7. The ISIS-1 suggests these early gains persist in the year post-infarction.

Learning points

♦ Immediate treatment with beta blockade in the early phases of AMI reduces mortality, achieving reductions in infarct size, re-infarction and the development of lethal ventricular arrhythmias. Initiation of beta blockers is mandatory in the post MI period.

Further reading

- The MIAMI Trial Research Group. Metoprolol in acute myocardial infarction (MIAMI). A randomised placebo-controlled international trial. *Eur Heart J* 1985; 6 (3): 199–226.
- Rossi R, Yusuf S, Ramsdale D, Furze L and Sleight P, Reduction of ventricular arrhythmias by early intravenous atenolol in suspected acute myocardial infarction. *Br Med J* 1986; 286 (6364): 506–10.
- Yusuf S, Sleight P, Rossi P, *et al.* Reduction in infarct size, arrhythmias, chest pain and morbidity by early intravenous beta-blockade in suspected acute myocardial infarction. *Circulation* 1983; 67: 32–41.

The Cardiac Arrhyhmia Suppression Trial (CAST)

Echt DS, Liebson PR, Mitchell LB, Peters RW, Obias-Manno D, Barker AH, Arensberg D, Baker A, Friedman L, Green HL, Huther ML, Richardson DW, and the CAST Investigators. Mortality and morbidity in patients receiving encainide, flecainide, or placebo. *N Engl J Med* 1991; 324: 781–8.

Background

Ventricular premature depolarizations are a recognized risk factor for sudden and non-sudden cardiac death after MI. Ventricular arrhythmia and left ventricular dysfunction are independent predictors of mortality. The Cardiac Arrhythmia Pilot Study (CAPS) had shown that class IC drugs suppressed arrhythmias adequately in patients up to one year following a myocardial infarct.

The Cardiac Arrhythmia Suppression Trial (CAST) was therefore designed as a multi-centre trial to test whether suppression of ventricular arrhythmia with anti-arrhythmic drug therapy post-MI would reduce the risk of arrhythmic death. The class IC agents tested were flecainide, encainide, and moricizine. However, the trial was stopped prematurely due to the excess mortality in the flecainide and encainide arms; the moricizine drug study was continued and later on reported in the CAST II study, which showed the similar finding of increased mortality in the moricizine arm.

Methods

Patients presenting with MI between six days to two years prior to enrolment were eligible if they had an average of six or more ventricular premature depolarizations per hour on ambulatory electrocardiographic monitoring of at least 18 hours' duration, and no runs of VT of 15 or more beats at a rate of >120 bpm. Patients were required to have an ejection fraction (EF) of 55% or less if recruited within 90 days of the MI, or 40% or less if recruited 90 days or more after the MI.

This was an open-labelled drug study, in which patients with ectopy were initially assigned to a class IC agent to see if this resulted in reduction of ectopy burden. Patients in whom arrhythmias were suppressed were then enrolled into the main study and randomly assigned to receive either the effective drug or corresponding placebo. Flecainide was not given to any patient with an EF <30%.

The primary end point of the trial was death or cardiac arrest due to arrhythmia. Secondary end points included all death, death from cardiac causes, VT (15 consecutive ventricular beats >120 bpm), MI, syncope, permanent pacemaker implantation, congestive heart failure, angina, and coronary artery revascularization.

Results

This trial was terminated early after interim analysis of 1498 patients assigned to treatment showed increased all-cause mortality or cardiac arrest in the flecainide or encainide arm (63 patients, 8.3%) compared to 26 patients (3.4%) in the placebo arm. A significantly greater number of deaths and cardiac arrests due to arrhythmia (pre-specified primary end point) occurred in the active drug arm (relative risk 2.64, 95% CI, 1.60–4.36). These findings were similar in subgroup analyses of patients with EF of <30%.

In 62 of the 89 patients who died, the cardiac rhythm was documented electrocardiographically. More deaths due to arrhythmia in which asystole was the documented rhythm occurred in the active-treatment groups. There was a trend for more of the patients receiving active drug to have VT or VT degenerating into VF.

The incidence of non-lethal, cardiac secondary end points was similar in the active-drug and placebo groups. The incidence of adverse effects requiring discontinuation of the study drug was similar in the active drug and placebo groups. In particular, non-fatal pro-arrhythmia was not detected in the patients receiving active drug.

Limitations

The design of CAST was based on CAPS, a focused study that showed a suppression of arrhythmias in post-MI patients. Although the major increase in adverse outcomes was attributed primarily to unforeseen death or cardiac arrest due to arrhythmia in the active drug arm, there was not a correspondingly higher incidence of non-lethal events involving arrhythmia, such as VT, syncope, or need for permanent pacemaker. This inability to detect non-lethal effects may be due to lack of continuous monitoring during the study.

Conclusions

The class IC agents flecainide and encainide are associated with increased mortality in patients with ventricular arrhythmia following MI.

> ### Learning points
>
> - There is no role for the class IC agents flecainide or encainide in patients with arrhythmias following MI.
> - The increased mortality with flecainide and encainide is mainly attributable to increased lethal arrhythmic risk, regardless of EF.

Further reading

- Furberg DC. Effect of Anti-arrhythmic drugs on mortality after myocardial infarction. *Am J Cardiol* 1983; 52: 32C–6C.
- The Cardiac Arrhythmia Pilot Study (CAPS) Investigators. Effects of encainide, flecainide, imipramine and moricizine on ventricular arrhythmias during the year after acute myocardial infarction: The CAPS. *Am J Cardiol* 1988; 321: 406–12.
- The Cardiac Arrhythmia Suppression Trial II Investigators. Effect of the Anti-arrhythmic agent moricizine on survival after myocardial infarction. *N Engl J Med.* 1992; 327: 227–33.

Effect of d-sotalol on mortality in patients with left ventricular dysfunction after recent and remote myocardial infarction

Waldo AL, Camm AJ, deRuyter H, Friedman PL, MacNeil DJ, Pauls JF, Pitt B, Pratt CM, Schwartz PJ, Veltri EP; for the SWORD investigators. *Lancet* 1996; 348: 7–12.

Background

Left ventricular dysfunction after MI is associated with an increased risk of sudden cardiac death. Results from previous trials investigating class I drugs (CAST) showed that these were associated with increased all-cause mortality. However, amiodarone, which has some potassium-channel blocking action, has been previously shown to be safe following MI.

Among available potassium channel blockers, d-sotalol, an I_{Kr} blocker, was the most widely used at the time of the SWORD trial. The Survival With ORal D-sotalol (SWORD) trial was a multi-centre study that tested the hypothesis that d-sotalol reduces all cause mortality in patients with previous MI and left ventricular dysfunction.

Methods

The SWORD study was a multinational, multi-centre, placebo-controlled, randomized, double-blind trial conducted at 546 centres. Inclusion criteria were men or women >18 years, with left ventricular EF <40% and either a recent (6–42 days) or a remote (>42 days) MI with overt heart failure (New York Heart Association class II or III).

Major exclusion criteria were: unstable angina, sustained ventricular tachycardia/fibrillation or cardiac arrest unrelated to a MI, history of sick sinus syndrome or high-grade atrioventricular block untreated by permanent pacemaker, history of recent (within 14 days) coronary angioplasty or coronary artery bypass grafting, severe electrolyte abnormalities, corrected QT interval (QTc) >460 msec, use of concomitant anti-arrhythmic drugs (except beta blockers, calcium channel blockers, or digoxin), or drugs that prolong the QT intervals.

Patients who qualified were randomized to either oral d-sotalol 100 mg twice daily or matching placebo for one week. If this dose was tolerated with a QTc of less than 520 msec, the dose was increased to 200 mg or matching placebo for a further week. If tolerated with a QTc of less than 560 msec, this dose was given for the duration of the study.

The primary end point was all-cause mortality. Secondary end point was cardiac mortality. Tertiary end points were cardiovascular mortality, presumed arrhythmic death, non-fatal severe arrhythmic events, hospital admission for cardiovascular causes, and composites of these.

Results

The SWORD study was terminated early after recruiting 3121 patients with a mean follow-up of 148 days, due to increased mortality in the patients assigned d-sotalol. At the time of study termination, there were 30 excess deaths in the d-sotalol group compared with placebo (78/1549 [5.0%] vs. 46/1572 [3.1%]: relative risk 1.65 [95% CI: 1.15–2.36], p = 0.006). The increased mortality was accounted for by a significantly greater number of cardiac and arrhythmic deaths. Rates of non-fatal cardiac events were similar in both groups.

Subgroup analyses showed that d-sotalol increased mortality risk irrespective of age, sex, time from index infarction, left ventricular EF, or concomitant therapy with beta blockers, diurectics, or calcium channel blockers. This risk was more pronounced in patients with better ventricular function (31–40%) than those with a lower EF.

Limitations

The SWORD study was published five years after CAST, which demonstrated an increased mortality following MI with the class I agents flecainide and encainide. The SWORD trial was designed to test the hypothesis that a pure potassium channel blocking drug reduces all cause mortality in patients with previous MI and left ventricular dysfunction. However, extrapolation of pure potassium channel blockade may be unwarranted on the basis of safety from trials of amiodarone following MI. Amiodarone has potassium blocking effects, but has other ion channel effects, including sodium channel and calcium channel blockade, and non-competitive alpha-adrenergic and beta-adrenergic blockade.

This trial was conducted between 1992 and 1994, during which time use of what we now regard as standard drug therapy post-MI was less than ideal. Only 31% of patients received a beta blocker, 63% received aspirin, and 70% received an ACE-inhibitor. This might partly explain the somewhat surprising findings that d-sotalol increased mortality risk in patients with higher ejection fractions (31–40%) compared to patients with EF ≤30%. This is because the clinical impact of Anti-arrhythmic drug therapy depends on the efficacy of the drug in preventing VF, balanced against the risk that the drug itself will cause a lethal arrhythmia that would not have occurred in the drug's absence. In the low EF group with relatively high VF rates, the potential reduction in rates of VF with d-sotalol was counteracted by the increased risk of torsades de pointes, with the overall effect that neither benefit nor harm was demonstrated in this group. However, the group with a higher EF (with a lower inherent risk of VF) had little more to gain from the anti-fibrillatory effect of d-sotalol, so the proarrhythmic effect of d-sotalol predominated, leading to an increased all-cause mortality.

Conclusions

The use of d-sotalol in patients with left ventricular dysfunction following MI is associated with an increased mortality, particularly in patients with relatively preserved ejection fractions.

Learning points

◆ The use of d-sotalol is associated with an increased risk of all-cause mortality.
◆ The findings from SWORD cannot be extrapolated to other potassium blocking agents, as d-sotalol is a pure I_{Kr} blocker. Other drugs which block different components of the potassium current might be associated with different anti-arrhythmic profiles.

Further reading

● Singh SN, Fletcher RD, Gross-Fisher S, *et al.* Amiodarone in patients with congestive heart failure and asymptomatic ventricular arrhythmia. *N Engl J Med* 1995; 333: 77–82.

Randomized trial of effect of amiodarone on mortality in patients with left-ventricular dysfunction after recent myocardial infarction: EMIAT

Julian DG, Camm AJ, Frangin G, Janse MJ, Munoz A, Schwartz PJ, Simon P; for the European Myocardial Infarct Amiodarone Trial Investigators. *Lancet* 1997; 349: 667–75.

Background

The European Myocardial Infarct Amiodarone Trial (EMIAT) followed a number of trials, including CAST, which showed that traditional sodium channel blocking anti-arrhythmic drugs were detrimental in post-MI patients. Apart from beta blockers, the only other drug to have shown any promise in this group of patients at this time was amiodarone. The EMIAT trial was a multi-centre study to test the hypothesis that amiodarone reduces mortality in patients with impaired ventricular function following MI.

Methods

The EMIAT study was a randomized, double-blind, placebo-controlled, multi-centre, European trial that recruited patients following MI aged 18–75 years who had ejection fractions of <40%. Patients were excluded if they were amiodarone intolerant, or had had amiodarone in the previous six months, documented bradycardia or heart block, clinically significant hepatic or thyroid disease, long QT syndrome, severe angina, or a need for anti-arrhythmic therapy other than beta blockers.

Eligible patients were randomly assigned amiodarone or placebo, and followed up between one and two years. Patients were assessed at baseline, two weeks, two months, and then every four months up to two years, with Holter monitoring performed at baseline, two weeks and four months.

The primary end point was all-cause mortality and the secondary end points were cardiac mortality, arrhythmic death, and arrhythmic death and resuscitated cardiac arrest.

Results

A total of 1486 patients were recruited after a mean of 15 days following the index MI and were randomized to receive amiodarone (743 patients) or placebo (743 patients).

There was no difference in all-cause mortality, or cardiac mortality between the two groups, even after patients were grouped according to EF. However, there was a significant 35% risk reduction in arrhythmic deaths, but an increase in non-arrhythmic cardiac and non-cardiac deaths in the amiodarone-treated patients. Forty per cent of the trial population had documented arrhythmias at baseline: amiodarone treatment significantly reduced the combined end point of arrhythmic death and resuscitated cardiac deaths in this group compared to the placebo.

A history of prior MI significantly increased the risk of death, regardless of amiodarone use. A strong tendency towards favourable interaction between use of beta blockers and cardiac mortality was shown, independently of left ventricular function.

Limitations

There were differences in the patient populations between the amiodarone and placebo groups, including EF, New York Heart Associated Functional Class, and particularly, history of previous MI (26% of placebo group vs. 32% amiodarone group), which may have skewed results against the benefit of amiodarone.

The finding that there was significant reduction in arrhythmic deaths and resuscitated cardiac arrests in the amiodarone group suggests that any possible pro-arrhythmic effects of amiodarone do not outweigh its anti-arrhythmic benefit. However, the reduction in arrhythmic deaths was balanced by non-cardiac and non-arrhythmic cardiac deaths, including three deaths caused by pulmonary fibrosis, with the end result being no difference in all-cause mortality between the two groups. This finding is similar to that demonstrated in CAMIAT (the Canadian Amiodarone Myocardial Infarction Trial Investigators), which showed no difference in all-cause mortality in 1202 myocardial infarct survivors with repetitive ventricular premature depolarizations randomized to amiodarone or placebo. In CAMIAT, just as in EMIAT, there was a significant reduction in arrhythmic deaths or resuscitated cardiac arrest.

A post-hoc analysis of EMIAT and CAMIAT showed that the effect of amiodarone was greater in patients who received beta blockers, which strongly suggests that amiodarone should not replace beta blocker therapy.

Conclusions

The EMIAT and CAMIAT trials do not support the routine use of amiodarone in patients following MI. However, the significant reduction in arrhythmic deaths and resuscitated cardiac arrests in the amiodarone-treated groups suggests that amiodarone can be considered in individual patients based on underlying risk factors and arrhythmic risk.

Learning points

♦ Amiodarone should not be used routinely following MI, but may be considered in individual patients with high risk.
♦ The lack of overall survival benefit with amiodarone (or any other anti-arrhythmic drug apart from beta blockers) post-MI subsequently spurred an era of the development of non-pharmacological treatment (implantable defibrillators) to improve overall mortality in the late 1990s and early 2000s. It provides evidence to treat ICD recipients with a high burden of ventricular arrhythmia to reduce shock frequency.

Further reading

- Boutitie F, Boissel JP, Connolly SJ, *et al.* Amiodarone interaction with beta blockers: Analysis of the merged EMIAT and CAMIAT Databases. *Circulation* 1999; 99: 2268–75.
- Cairns JA, Connolly SJ, Roberts R, Gent M, for the Canadian Amiodarone Myocardial Infarction Arrhythmia Trial Investigators. Randomised trial of outcome after MI in patients with frequent or repetitive ventricular premature depolarisations: CAMIAT. *Lancet* 1997; 249: 675–82.

A comparison of antiarrhythmic-drug therapy with implantable defibrillators in patients resuscitated from near-fatal ventricular arrhythmias

The Antiarrhythmics Versus Implantable Defibrillators (AVID) Investigators. *N Engl J Med* 1997; 337: 1576–83.

Background

Survivors of VF or symptomatic VT have a high risk of arrhythmia recurrence, which is often fatal. The AVID trial investigated whether implantable cardioverter-defibrillator (ICD) or anti-arrhythmic drug therapy was more effective in reducing mortality in patients successfully resuscitated from VF or sustained VT with haemodynamic compromise.

Methods

The AVID study was a multi-centre, randomized comparison of the two treatment strategies for successfully resuscitated patients. Amiodarone and sotalol were considered best contemporary treatments at the time of this trial, and if the patients could tolerate either drug, they were then randomized to either amiodarone or sotalol at the physician's discretion. The patients in the ICD arm received this intervention only. The primary end point was overall mortality. Secondary end points were cost and quality of life.

Results

A total of 1016 well-matched patients were randomly assigned to ICD or drug therapy. The mean age was 65 years and 79% of patients were male. A total of 455 patients had VF, and 561 had VT. The mean EF was 32% in the ICD group and 31% in the drug group.

The ICD group consisted of 507 patients, with 93% having a transvenous system, 5% receiving an epicardial system, with no ICD implanted in a further 2%. Of the 509 patients in the drug group, amiodarone was assigned in 356 patients immediately. A further 153 patients in the drug group were randomly assigned to amiodarone (79 patients) or sotalol (74 patients). However, only 13 of the 74 patients on sotalol had adequate suppression of arrhythmia. Of the remaining 61 patients, 58 were given amiodarone, one received another anti-arrhythmic drug, and two received an ICD. More patients were taking beta blockers in the ICD group compared to the drug group at two years follow-up (39% vs. 10%, p <0.001).

Fewer deaths occurred in the ICD group (80 deaths) compared to the drug group (122 deaths). Over a mean follow-up of 18 months, the death rates were 16% in the ICD group compared to 24% in the drug group. Implantable cardioverter-defibrillator therapies were more common among patients who had VT (81% patients receiving therapy at two years) rather than VF (53% patients receiving therapy at two years) as the index arrhythmia.

Multivariate analysis showed the beneficial effect of ICD after adjusting for other factors including age, beta blocker use, VT, congestive heart failure, and revascularization at index event.

Limitations

Although recognized now as an important gold-standard therapy, the use of beta blockers in AVID was particularly low (10% in the drug group and 39% in the ICD group). This was because many physicians at the time felt that addition of a beta blocker to either amiodarone or sotalol was not necessary, might aggravate bradyarrhythmias, or complicate treatment regimens. Furthermore, beta blockers are often given to control the ventricular rate in AF, thus preventing inappropriate ICD therapy. Adjustment of this imbalance in beta blocker use slightly reduced the estimated survival benefit (unadjusted hazard ratio 0.62, adjusted hazard ratio 0.67).

The AVID trial design enrolled patients into the ICD arm only if they did not have a need for concurrent anti-arrhythmic drug therapy. Greater prevalence of anti-arrhythmic therapy in clinical practice is likely, especially as clinicians attempt to limit painful shocks, which might explain the crossover rate of 26% from the ICD to drug group (compared with a 19% crossover from the drug to ICD group) at two years.

Conclusions

The AVID trial demonstrated that ICD use was superior to anti-arrhythmic drug therapy in prolonging survival among patients resuscitated after symptomatic sustained VT or VF.

Learning points

- Patients successfully resuscitated after VF or sustained symptomatic VT should be offered an ICD.
- The use of ICD for secondary prevention, particularly following sustained symptomatic VT, is associated with a high rate of ICD therapies. Anti-arrhythmic drugs appear to minimize the risk of recurrent ICD therapies.
- Subsequent ICD trials such as Multi-centre Automatic Defibrillator Implantation Trial II (MADIT II) have demonstrated mortality benefit in primary prevention against sudden cardiac death in patients with reduced EF (<30%).

Further reading

- Moss AJ, Hall WJ, Cannom DS, *et al.* Improved survival with an implanted defibrillator in patients with coronary disease at high risk for ventricular arrhythmia. Multi-centre Automatic Defibrillator Implantation Trial Investigators. *N Engl J Med* 1996; 26: 1933–40.
- Moss AJ, Zareba W, Hall WJ, *et al.*; for the Multi-centre Automatic Defibrillator Implantation Trial (MADIT) II Investigators. Prophylactic implantation of a defibrillator in patients with myocardial infarction and reduced ejection fraction. *N Engl J Med* 2002; 346: 877–83.

Amiodarone as compared with lidocaine for shock-resistant ventricular fibrillation (ALIVE)

Dorian P, Cass D, Schwartz, Cooper R, Zelaznikas R, Barr A. *N Engl J Med* 2002; 346: 884–90.

Background

Ventricular fibrillation is the most common cause of out-of-hospital cardiac arrest. Anti-arrhythmic therapy is often administered to patients with VF, with lidocaine being the traditional drug of choice in the setting of resuscitation. However, no randomized clinical trial has demonstrated the efficacy of lidocaine for these indications.

The Amiodarone versus Lidocaine in Prehospital Ventricular Fibrillation Evaluation (ALIVE) was a double-blind clinical trial comparing amiodarone with lidocaine in patients with out-of-hospital VF in Toronto.

Methods

Patients were eligible if they were adults with out-of-hospital VF that was not due to trauma, documented on electrocardiogram. The VF had to have been resistant to three shocks from an external defibrillator, with at least one dose of intravenous epinephrine, and a fourth defibrillator shock administered. Patients had to have continued to have VF or had recurrent VF after successful initial defibrillation.

Drug kits containing either active amiodarone (5 mg/kg body weight) with lidocaine placebo, or active lidocaine (1.5 mg/kg body weight) with amiodarone placebo were given in a randomized order to ambulance crews to be administered rapidly in a peripheral vein during a cardiac arrest. A further dose of the active drug was administered if VF persisted.

The primary end point was survival to admission to the hospital intensive care unit; patients who died in the emergency department were not considered to have been admitted. Secondary end points included survival to discharge, and adverse events, defined as the need to administer atropine or dopamine after administration of the study drug.

Results

Between 1995 and 2001, 347 patients with a mean age of 67 years were randomly assigned to receive amiodarone (180 patients) or lidocaine (167 patients). All patients had VF or pulseless VT at some stage of the cardiac arrest. The mean interval between dispatch of paramedics to arrival at the scene was 7 ± 3 minutes, and the mean interval between dispatch to time of drug administration was 25 ± 8 minutes.

The following clinical variables predicted survival: shorter intervals between dispatch of the crew to the administration of study drug, cardiac arrest due to VF (rather than asystole or pulseless electrical activity), and transient return of spontaneous circulation at the time of the primary cardiac arrest. However, among patients whose initial rhythm was VF, the interval between the first shock to the administration of the drug was a significant predictor of survival (odds ratio for each minute of delay, 0.87; 95% CI, 0.80–0.96, p = 0.003).

Forty-one patients (23%) in the amiodarone group survived to hospital admission, as compared with 20 patients (12%) in the lidocaine group (p = 0.009). The only factors that significantly influenced the primary outcome were the study drug assignment, the length of time to the administration of the drug, and the presence or absence of a transient return of spontaneous circulation before the administration of the study drug. The adjusted odds ratio for survival to hospital admission in amiodarone recipients compared to lidocaine recipients was 2.49 (95% CI, 1.28–4.85, p = 0.007). The proportion of patients in whom asystole occurred after administration of the initial study drug was significantly higher in the lidocaine group (41 of 142 patients, 29%) than in the amiodarone group (28 of 52 patients, 18%, p = 0.04).

Among the 41 patients who survived to hospital admission after receiving amiodarone, 9 (5% of entire group) survived to hospital discharge, compared to 5 of the 20 initial survivors in the lidocaine group (3% of entire group). The initial rhythm was VF in all long-term survivors.

Limitations

Although there was a statistically significant relative risk reduction in survival to hospital admission in the amiodarone limb compared to the lidocaine group, there was only a trend in favour of amiodarone increasing the number of hospital discharges due to the relatively small numbers of patients who survived to discharge. It remains to be seen whether amiodarone administration earlier in the course of cardiac resuscitation improves survival to discharge.

Conclusions

This trial has clearly demonstrated the superiority of amiodarone over lidocaine. The consistency of outcome data between the Amiodarone for Resuscitation after Out-of-Hospital Cardiac Arrest Due to Ventricular Fibrillation (ARREST, please refer to Further reading) and ALIVE trials has broad implications for the treatment and prevention of VF and VT.

Learning points

- Amiodarone is the drug of choice in shock-resistant VF or VT.
- The use of amiodarone should also be considered in cardiac arrests in the emergency department and intensive care units.
- Current advance life support algorithms (Resuscitation Council UK 2010) support the use of amiodarone in VF or VT. Lidocaine may be administered in the absence of amiodarone, but not if amiodarone has already been administered.

Further reading

- Kudenchuk PJ, Cobb LA, Compass MK, *et al.* Amiodarone for resuscitation after out-of-hospital cardiac arrests due to ventricular fibrillation. *N Eng J Med* 1999; 341: 871–8.

A comparison of rate control with rhythm control in patients with recurrent persistent atrial fibrillation

Wyse DG, Waldo AL, DiMarco JP, Domanski MJ, Rosenberg Y, Schron EB, Kellen JC, Greene HL, Mickel MC, Dalquist JE and Corley SD; for the Atrial Fibrillation Follow-up Investigation of Rhythm Management (AFFIRM) Investigators. *N Engl J Med* 2002; 347: 1825–33.

Background

A strategy of maintaining sinus rhythm (SR) remains the therapeutic goal in patients with persistent AF. However, frequent recurrences of AF and side effects of anti-arrhythmic drugs mitigate the potential benefits of a strategy of maintaining SR through electrical cardioversion in persistent AF patients. The rate-control approach may simplify therapy for AF, avoiding the use of more less toxic drugs. The AFFIRM study compared the effects of long-term treatment of the rate-control and rhythm-control strategy.

Methods

This multi-centre study recruited patients >65 years with persistent AF, who had other risk factors for stroke or death, in whom anticoagulation was not contraindicated.

Rate control was achieved with digoxin, a calcium-channel blocker, a beta blocker, or a combination of these drugs, to achieve a resting heart rate of <80 bpm, and six-minute walk test <110 bpm. In the rhythm-control group, mainly class I and III anti-arrhythmics were used. Attempts to maintain SR included cardioversion as necessary. After failure of at least two drugs in either arm, patients could be considered for non-pharmacological therapy, including radiofrequency ablation, a maze surgical procedure, or pacing strategies.

Anticoagulation was mandatory in the rate-control group, whereas in the rhythm-control group, anticoagulation could be stopped at the treating physician's discretion if SR had been maintained for at least four weeks. The primary outcome was overall mortality. A composite secondary end point comprised death, disabling stroke, disabling anoxic encephalopathy, major bleeding, and cardiac arrest. Secondary analyses evaluated results within pre-specified subgroups including age, sex, rhythm at randomization, AF duration, and the presence or absence of hypertension, congestive heart failure or coronary artery disease.

Results

A total of 4060 well-matched patients were randomly assigned to receive rate-control (2027) or rhythm-control (2033). The mean age was 70 ± 9 years, mean EF 55 ± 14%, and over 50% of patients had hypertension. Over 80% of patients in the rate-control arm achieved satisfactory rate control, with 35% of patients remaining in SR at five years. Fifteen per cent of patients had crossed over into the rhythm-control group. The most commonly used drugs in this group were digoxin (49%) and beta blockers (47%). In the rhythm-control group, amiodarone (38%) and sotalol (31%) were the most commonly used first-line drugs. A total of 63% of patients in the rhythm-control group were in SR at five years, although 38% of patients crossed over to the rate-control strategy, mainly due to inability to maintain SR or drug intolerance. Eighty-five per cent of patients in the rate-control group remained on wafarin, compared with 70% of patients in the rhythm-control group.

There was no difference in all-cause mortality, or the composite secondary outcomes, between both treatment groups. There were significantly more hospitalizations and adverse drug events in the rhythm control group (p <0.001). There was no difference in ischaemic or haemorrhagic stroke. The majority of strokes occurred in patients who had stopped anticoagulation or whose INRs were subtherapeutic.

Limitations

A major limitation of AFFIRM was the high cross-over (and subsequent return to the original strategy) rate between treatment strategies. Primary analysis was conducted on an intention-to-treat basis, which was appropriate for a randomized study like AFFIRM. However, subsequent modelling studies evaluating outcomes based on actual treatment received showed that the presence of SR, and warfarin use, was associated with a lower risk of death (SR was also shown to improve survival in the Danish Investigations of Arrhythmia and Mortality on Dofetilide [DIAMOND] trial).

Anti-arrhythmic drugs have been shown to increase mortality from several large trials (CAST II, SWORD). The AFFIRM study did not specifically look at the relationship of mortality to the use of anti-arrhythmic drugs. However, subsequent on-treatment analyses of AFFIRM showed anti-arrhythmic drugs were associated with increased mortality, only after adjustment for presence or absence of SR. When models were run without adjustment for SR, then anti-arrhythmic drugs were no longer associated with adverse outcomes. One potential explanation for this finding is that the beneficial effect of these drugs (e.g. maintenance of SR), was offset by the adverse effects (e.g. toxicity, morbidity, and mortality). This suggests that if an effective method for maintaining SR with fewer adverse effects were available, it might improve survival.

Conclusion

Overall, none of the presumed benefits of rhythm control were demonstrated in the AFFIRM study. A rhythm-control strategy resulted in twice as many patients maintaining SR at five years compared to a rate control strategy. The absence of a clear survival benefit for a rhythm control strategy may be related to the detrimental effects of anti-arrhythmic drugs, or the higher rate of warfarin discontinuation in the rhythm control group, which might have increased mortality due to strokes.

The data from AFFIRM clearly demonstrate the beneficial effects of continued anticoagulation use, even when SR is restored.

Learning points

- Anticoagulation should be continued in patients with AF with risk factors for stroke, even if SR is restored.
- There appears to be no survival benefit in using anti-arrhythmic drugs to maintain SR in asymptomatic patients over 65 years with AF.

Further reading

- Corley SD, Epstein AE, DiMarco JP, *et al.* Relationships between sinus rhythm, treatment, and survival in the Atrial Fibrillation Follow-Up Investigation of Rhythm Management (AFFIRM) Study. *Circulation* 2004; 109: 1509–13.
- Echt DS, Liebson PR, Mitchell LB, *et al.*, and the CAST Investigators. Mortality and morbidity in patients receiving encainide, flecainide, or placebo. The Cardiac Arrhyhmia Suppression Trial (CAST). *N Engl J Med* 1991; 324: 781–8.
- Hohnloser SH, Kuck KH, Lilienthal J. Rhythm or rate control in atrial fibrillation- Pharmacological Intervention in Atrial Fibrillation (PIAF): a randomised trial. *Lancet* 2000; 356: 1789–94.
- Pederson OD, Bagger H, Keller N, *et al.* Efficacy of dofetilide in the treatment of atrial fibrillation-flutter in patients with reduced left ventricular function. A Danish Investigations of Arrhythmia and Mortality ON Dofetilide (DIAMOND) Substudy. *Circulation* 2001; 104: 292–6.
- Roy D, Talajic M, Nattel S, *et al.* Rhythm control versus rate control for atrial fibrillation and heart failure. *N Engl J Med* 2008; 358: 2667–77.
- The Cardiac Arrhythmia Suppression Trial II Investigators. Effect of the Anti-arrhythmic agent moricizine on survival after myocardial infarction. *N Engl J Med.* 1992; 327: 227–33.
- Waldo AL, Camm AJ, deRuyter H, *et al.*; for the SWORD investigators. Effect of d-sotalol on mortality in patients with left ventricular dysfunction after recent and remote myocardial infarction. *Lancet* 1996; 348: 7–12.

Dronedarone for maintenance of sinus rhythm in atrial fibrillation or flutter

Singh BH, Connolly SJ, Crijns HJGM, Roy D, Kowey PR, Capucci A, Radzik D, Aliot EM, Hohnloser SH; for the EURIDIS and ADONIS Investigators. *N Engl J Med* 2007; 357: 987–99.

Background

Management of AF is aimed at reducing thromboembolic risk, and reducing arrhythmia-related symptoms. Sinus rhythm is associated with an improvement in quality of life and exercise capacity, therefore restoration of SR is a major therapeutic goal for patients with AF.

Amiodarone is the most efficacious drug for maintenance of SR, but it induces potentially serious side effects. Dronedarone is a benzofuran derivative which closely resembles amiodarone in electropharmacological profile, but structural differences prevent the thyroid or lung complications associated with amiodarone use. The half life of dronedarone is 1–2 days, compared with the 30–55 days for amiodarone.

This multi-centre trial, a combination of a European Trial in Atrial Fibrillation or Flutter Patients Receiving Dronedarone for the Maintenance of Sinus Rhythm (EURIDIS) and a non-European trial—American-Australian-African Trial with Dronedarone in Atrial Fibrillation or Flutter Patients for the Maintenance of Sinus Rhythm (ADONIS) evaluated the efficacy of dronedarone in maintaining SR in patients with AF or atrial flutter.

Methods

This multi-centre, double-blind, randomized study was conducted in 17 countries. A total of 1237 matched patients were randomly assigned to receive in a 2:1 ratio either dronedarone 400 mg twice daily or placebo. Qualifying criteria for enrolment was age >21 years, >1 episode of AF documented on electrocardiogram in the preceding three months, and SR at least one hour before randomization. Excluded from the study were patients with: permanent AF, sinus bradycardia or AV block, New York Heart Association class III or IV heart failure, severe electrolyte abnormalities or hepatic, pulmonary, endocrine dysfunction, or patients taking class I drugs.

Rhythm was monitored by frequent trans-telephonic monitoring during a 12-month period. The primary end point was the time to the first documented recurrence of AF (lasting >10 minutes). The main secondary end points were symptomatic AF and the mean ventricular rate during first recurrence.

Results

Mean age of all patients was 63 years (69% male). Eleven per cent of patients had atrial flutter. Eighteen per cent of patients taking dronedarone and 15% of patients taking placebo prematurely discontinued taking the drug.

The first documented episode of AF was 116 days in the dronedarone group and 53 days in the placebo group. At 12 months, the rate of recurrence was 64.1% in the dronedarone group and 75.2% in the placebo group, (across subgroups including those with hypertension, heart failure, and structural heart disease). Symptomatic recurrences occurred in 37.7% of patients in the dronedarone group and 46.0% in the placebo group. The majority of documented first recurrences were symptomatic, and the patterns of symptoms did not differ between groups.

The ventricular rate during AF in the dronedarone group at first recurrence was 103 bpm compared with 117 bpm in the placebo group. The rate of death or hospitalizations was 22.8% in the dronedarone group compared with 30.9% in the placebo group. There was no significant difference in death from any cause between the two groups. Dronedarone did not have a worse side effect profile compared to placebo, apart from mildly elevated creatinine levels.

Limitations

The major limitation of this trial (and other large trials of dronedarone, including ATHENA) is that dronedarone was compared to placebo, and not an active drug. The follow-up period was short, lasting only 12 months, which limits the ability to demonstrate long-term avoidance of side effects. However, the Short-Term, Randomized, Double-Blind, Parallel-Group Study to Evaluate the Efficacy and Safety of Dronedarone versus Amiodarone in Patients with Persistent Atrial Fibrillation (DIONYSOS trial), which directly compared amiodarone to dronedarone in 504 patients with AF demonstrated that dronedarone was less efficacious, but better tolerated than amiodarone at one year follow-up.

Conclusions

This multi-centre trial incorporating two major trials (EURIDIS and ADONIS) showed that the rates of the first recurrence of AF and of the first symptomatic recurrence at one year were significantly reduced with dronedarone, as compared with placebo. Dronedarone also reduced the ventricular rate in AF during recurrence of arrhythmia.

Learning points

- Dronedarone reduces the rate of first symptomatic recurrence of AF compared to placebo.
- Dronedarone reduces the ventricular rate in AF during recurrences.

Further reading

- Hohnloser SH, Crijns HJ, van Eickels M, *et al*. Effect of dronedarone on cardiovascular events in atrial fibrillation. *N Engl J Med* 2009; 360: 668–78.
- Le Heuzey JY, De Ferrari GM, Radzik D, Santini M, Zhu J, Davy JM. A short-term, randomized, double-blind, parallel-group study to evaluate the efficacy and safety of dronedarone versus amiodarone in patients with persistent atrial fibrillation: the DIONYSOS study. *J Cardiovasc Electrophysiol* 2010; 21: 597–605.

Catheter ablation versus antiarrhythmic drugs for atrial fibrillation

Jais P, Cauchemez B, Macle L, Daoud E, Khairy P, Subbiah R, Hocini M, Extramiana F, Sacher F, Bordachar P, Klein G, Weerasooriya R, Clementy J and Haissaguerre M. The A4 Study. *Circulation* 2008; 118: 2498–505.

Background

The mainstay of treatment for AF has traditionally been pharmacological. However, success rates from catheter ablation for paroxysmal AF have improved, raising the possibility of using catheter ablation earlier in management of AF.

The A4 trial was therefore designed as a multi-centre trial comparing a strategy of using additional anti-arrhythmic drugs with catheter ablation for patients with paroxysmal AF who had failed with at least one anti-arrhythmic drug.

Methods

A total of 112 patients were enrolled into this trial. Inclusion criteria were patients >18 years of age with symptomatic, documented paroxysmal AF over a span of >6 months with at least two episodes in the preceding month. Exclusion criteria were; contraindication to more than two anti-arrhythmic drugs or oral anticoagulants, prior AF ablation, intracardiac thrombus, AF from a reversible cause, pregnancy, or contraindication to the discontinuation of oral anticoagulation.

A 90-day blanking period after randomization allowed for up to three ablation procedures and various changes in anti-arrhythmic drugs, individually or in combination. Formal follow-up commenced from day 91 to day 365. The catheter ablation strategy included electrical isolation of all pulmonary veins, and other lesions at the operator's discretion.

Recurrent AF lasting >3 minutes, whether documented by electrocardiogram or reported by the patient as AF, occurring after the blanking period was considered a treatment failure, after which crossover to the alternative therapy was offered.

At the first day of randomization, an electrocardiogram, Short Form-36 quality-of-life questionnaire, AF symptom frequency and severity checklist, and a 24-hour Holter was performed. Further 24-hour Holter recording was performed at 3, 6, and 12 months. Transthoracic echocardiography and an exercise treadmill test were also performed at baseline and at day 365.

The primary end point of the study was the proportion of patients free of recurrent AF between months 3 and 12. Secondary end points were time to recurrent AF, complications, and adverse effects, change in left heart dimensions and function, quality of life, exercise capacity, AF burden, and efficacy of amiodarone when used for the first time during the study.

Results

A total of 112 patients, with a mean age of 51 years were enrolled from eight centres. Patients had experienced a median of 12 episodes of AF per month lasting 5.5 hours before randomization and had failed two class I or III anti-arrhythmic drugs.

Catheter ablation was performed in 52 patients who underwent a mean of 1.8 procedures. Forty-six (89%) patients who underwent ablation were free of arrhythmias without anti-arrhythmic drugs at one year. Five (9%) patients crossed over and were treated with anti-arrhythmic drugs. Fifty-nine patients were randomized to anti-arrhythmic drugs, with a total of 147 drugs used, with a mean of 2.5 ± 1.0 per patient. At least one combination of drugs was attempted in all patients, which included amiodarone in 35 patients. At one year, 13 (23%) patients remained free of atrial arrhythmias. Thirty-seven (63%) patients crossed over to ablation at 192 ± 80 days.

Atrial fibrillation burden, AF symptom score, and exercise capacity were significantly improved in patients who underwent catheter ablation compared to anti-arrhythmic drug therapy.

Predictors of successful ablation outcome included: shorter AF duration, higher baseline EF, and fewer direct current cardioversions. At one year follow-up, no significant difference was found in left atrial size or left ventricular EF between the ablation and anti-arrhythmic drug groups.

There were two episodes of cardiac tamponade, two groin haematomas, and one pulmonary vein stenosis amongst the 155 ablation procedures performed, with a favourable outcome in all. One case of hyperthyroidism was observed in the anti-arrhythmic drug group.

Limitations

This study has a small sample size with a short follow-up period. The primary outcome of AF recurrence was defined as AF >3 minutes either documented by electrocardiography or by patients reporting symptoms of AF. There is a possibility of a placebo effect in this context, with the possibility of patients over-reporting symptoms in the drug arm, particularly as a crossover to the catheter ablation arm was permitted in the event of AF recurrence. As with all AF trials, there is a possibility of asymptomatic AF recurrence which would only be detected by continuous long-term monitoring.

Lastly, catheter ablation for AF is a complex and time-consuming procedure, requiring intensive training and is only available in specialized cardiac centres. Repeat ablation procedures were required in a sizeable number of patients, and complications were observed. These findings underscore the need for careful patient selection, focusing on those most affected by debilitating symptoms.

Conclusions

Catheter ablation is superior to anti-arrhythmic drug therapy in patients with paroxysmal AF previously refractory to anti-arrhythmic drugs.

Learning points

- Catheter ablation for paroxysmal AF may be used in symptomatic patients refractory to anti-arrhythmic drugs.
- Catheter ablation is an invasive, complex, and time-consuming procedure that may require repeat procedures.
- The decision to offer a catheter ablation procedure should take into account the symptom burden of patients, and the likely procedural success rate, based on known predictors of success, including left atrial size and duration of AF in persistent cases.

Further reading

- McCready JW, Smedley T, Lambiase PD, *et al.* Predictors of recurrence following radiofrequency ablation for persistent atrial fibrillation. *Europace* 2011; 13(3): 355–61.
- The Antiarrhythmics Versus Implantable Defibrillators (AVID) Investigators. A comparison of antiarrhythmic-drug therapy with implantable defibrillators in patients resuscitated from near-fatal ventricular arrhythmias. *N Engl J Med* 1997; 337: 1576–83.
- Wazni OM, Marrouche NF, Martin DO, *et al.* Radiofrequency ablation vs. antiarrhythmic drugs as first-line treatment of symptomatic atrial fibrillation: a randomized trial. *JAMA* 2005; 293: 2634–40.
- Wilber DJ, Pappone C, Neuzil P, *et al.* Comparison of Anti-arrhythmic Drug Therapy and Radiofrequency Catheter Ablation in Patients With Paroxysmal Atrial Fibrillation. A Randomized Controlled Trial. *JAMA* 2010; 303 (4): 333–40.

Heart rate as a risk factor in chronic heart failure (SHIFT): the association between heart rate and outcomes in a randomized placebo-controlled trial

Bohm M, Swedberg K, Komajda M, Borer JS, Ford I, Dubost-Brama A, Lerebours G, Tavazzi L; on behalf of the SHIFT investigators. *Lancet* 2010; 376: 886–94.

Background

Resting heart rate is a predictor of cardiovascular mortality. Previous evidence suggests that heart-rate reduction improves contractility, and energy supply while reducing expenditure. The Systolic Heart failure treatment with IF inhibitor ivabradine Trial (SHIFT) was designed to test the hypothesis that heart-rate reduction per se could improve cardiovascular outcomes in heart failure.

Methods

The SHIFT study was a randomized, double-blind, multinational trial of ivabradine versus placebo in 6505 patients with symptomatic chronic heart failure (EF <35%) in SR with heart rates >70 bpm. Mean age was 60.4 years, 76% were men, and there was an equal distribution of patients with New York Heart Association class II, and III or IV heart failure. All patients received recommended background treatment in accordance with heart failure guidelines. Heart rate was determined by electrocardiogram at baseline, and at one month, and every four months thereafter. Heart rate reduction was achieved with ivabradine, an I_f inhibitor, which was titrated to achieve a resting heart rate of <70 bpm in the first month of the study.

The primary end point was a composite of cardiovascular mortality and hospital admission for worsening heart failure. The pre-specified secondary end points were all-cause mortality, cardiovascular mortality, and death from heart failure, all-cause hospital admission, hospital admission for worsening heart failure, any cardiovascular hospital admission, and non-fatal MI.

Results

The 6505 well-matched patients were divided into quintiles of pre-treatment heart rates as follows: 70–<72, 72–<75, 75–<80, 80–<87, and >87 bpm. The rates of concurrent heart failure therapy were as follows: beta blockers (>82%), ACE inhibitors (>75%), aldosterone antagonists (>56%), diuretics (>81%), cardiac glycosides (>18%). Over 50% of patients had a previous myocardial infarct, over 62% patients had hypertension, and over 26% of patients were diabetic, with over 7% of patients with a history of either AF or atrial flutter. Median follow-up duration was 23 months.

Patients in the higher heart rate quintiles were younger and more likely to smoke, have lower ejection fractions, higher NYHA classes, and more likely to have non-ischaemic heart failure. Higher heart rates were also associated with lower use of beta blockers. When the placebo group was divided by baseline heart rate quintiles, the incidence of the primary composite end point was greatest in patients with high heart rates (greater than two-fold risk for primary end point in the >87 bpm group compared to 70–<72 bpm group). Similar results were shown to all major secondary end points. In the placebo group, analysis with heart rate as a continuous variable showed that for every beat increase in heart rate, risk of a primary composite end point increased by 3%.

Treatment with ivabradine led to improved primary end point outcomes, particularly in patients with raised heart rates at baseline, who also had the greatest reductions in resting heart rate during treatment with ivabradine.

Analysis of resting heart rates following treatment showed that patients given ivabradine were more likely to be in the two lowest quintiles (<60 bpm, and 60–<65 bpm). Patients with the lowest heart rate (<60 bpm) had fewer primary composite end point events during the study compared to patients with higher heart rates.

Limitations

Patients with primary end points during the first 28 days were excluded from analysis, which could have possibly skewed results. The heart rate at 28 days was used as the on-treatment heart rate for subsequent analyses, although it is possible that heart rate continued to vary throughout the trial. Lastly, the lowest on-treatment heart rate quintile was <60 bpm, which was associated with improved outcomes. However, as further heart rate groups were not defined below this, it was not possible to state an ideal target heart rate that predicts best outcome.

Conclusions

Meta-analysis of previous beta blocker trials, including Metoprolol CR/XL Randomized Intervention Trial in congestive Heart Failure (MERIT-HF), the Carvedilol Or Metoprolol European Trial (COMET), and CIBIS-II: the Cardiac Insufficiency Bisoprolol Study II (CIBIS II) showed a benefit on mortality related to the heart-rate reduction achieved in each trial. However, it has not been possible to separate the effects of heart rate reduction from those of other potentially important actions of beta blockers, such as anti-arrhythmic effects, and direct beta-adrenergic effects.

The SHIFT study is therefore an important trial that addresses the importance of heart rate lowering alone in

improving mortality and cardiovascular outcomes in patients with heart failure. These findings suggest that heart rates of <60 bpm should be pursued if it can be achieved and tolerated in patients with chronic heart failure.

Learning points

- High resting heart rate is an adverse risk factor in heart failure.
- Selective lowering of heart rates improves cardiovascular outcomes, and should be an important target for the treatment of heart failure.
- Ivabradine, which selectively lowers heart rate, improves cardiovascular outcomes in heart failure.

Further reading

- Gullestad L, Wikstrand J, Deedwania P, *et al*. What resting heart rate should one aim for when treating patients with heart failure with a beta blocker? Experiences from the Metoprolol Controlled Release/Extended Release Randomized Intervention Trial in Chronic Heart Failure (MERIT-HF). *J Am Coll Cardiol* 2005; 45: 252–9.
- Lechat P, Hulot JS, Escolano S, *et al*. Heart rate and cardiac rhythm relationships with bisprolol benefit in chronic heart failure in CIBIS II trial. *Circulation* 2001; 103: 1428–33.
- Metra M, Torp-Pederson C, Swedberg K, *et al*. Influence of heart rate, blood pressure, and beta-blocker dose on outcome and the differences in outcome between carvedilol and metoprolol tartrate in patients with chronic heart failure: results from the COMET trial. *Eur Heart J* 2005; 26; 2259–68.

Final conclusions

The future of arrhythmia therapy is at a crossroads as the treatments beyond the realm of pharmacology are beginning to emerge and establish themselves in the field. These newer therapies have the advantage that they are based on the engineering principles designed to treat an output, for example defibrillation for VF or compartmentalizing the fibrillating atrium using ablation. Although technologically impressive, such therapies only treat the final common pathways of complex biological processes. Trials of anti-arrhythmics to prevent ventricular arrhythmia are high risk for any pharmaceutical

company as CAST and SWORD have demonstrated. For pharmacological therapies to re-establish themselves to prevent arrhythmias with superior efficacy, some fundamental changes need to be made. Certainly, the combination of statins and anti-hypertensives have impacted upon MI rates, hence reducing the number of patients with myocardium at risk of ischaemia related arrhythmias. More sophisticated approaches to upstream determinants of myocardial fibrosis, triggered activity and myocardial conduction need to be developed to create a stable myocardial substrate less susceptible to primarily re-entrant arrhythmias. Such agents are beginning to emerge targeting G protein subunits, hence modulating receptor function or up-regulating gap junction conductance (e.g. rotigaptide) to improve myocardial conduction, reducing the excitable gap needed to maintain re-entry. In the field of AF, novel drug targets include Kv1.5, GIRK, SK (Ca^{++} activated potassium) channels facilitating action potential prolongation. The CaM II Kinase inhibitors modulating ryanodine receptor phosphorylation, and hence reducing cytosolic calcium to reduce triggered activity, may also begin to appear with some of the GIRK channel inhibitors currently in phase II trials. Choosing a single agent which is likely to emerge as revolutionary and likely to change practice is challenging, as illustrated by ivabradine which one wouldn't necessarily have expected to have had significant prognostically important effects. It is this unpredictability which constantly challenges our understanding but also opens up new lines of investigation and therapeutic opportunities. As Nils Bohr once stated: 'prediction is very difficult, especially if it's about the future'.

Part III

Heart failure

Chapter 12

Epidemiology

Dr Kaushik Guha and Professor Theresa McDonagh

Introduction

Heart failure is a well recognized and documented disease entity. Over the last four decades developments have been made in its diagnosis, treatment, management, and epidemiology. However despite the transformation in its management and outcomes, it remains a widely prevalent disease with high levels of mortality. Due to the burden of disease it also carries economic consequences for healthcare systems. Heart failure, four decades ago, carried an extremely poor prognosis, with the medical profession as bystanders. Treatment was with mercurial diuretics and digoxin. Forty years on the modern heart failure patient is treated with a sophisticated algorithm of neuro-hormonal and sympathetic antagonists. Device therapy is also established for patients with heart failure; cardiac resynchronization therapy and implantable cardioverting defibrillators are now commonly implanted and have significantly impacted on morbidity and mortality. Complex health management systems are now the norm, including a variety of multi-disciplinary team members to deal with the medical, electrical, psychological, and social issues which challenge the care of patients with heart failure.

The cornerstone of understanding any disease process is its epidemiology. This is defined as the study of patterns of health and associated factors at the population level. Only once the fundamental patterns of disease have been ascertained can developments be made in terms of therapeutics and selective targeting of aetiologies. Whereas once the epidemiology of heart failure was relatively scarce, there has been much work in this area over the last four decades. There is now a more mature literature resource which is able to guide not only therapeutics but also the deployment of care and the best care models.

However, epidemiology, like all other branches of medicine, has to generate scientifically accurate and robust studies. There are some noteworthy problems with epidemiology, including the methodology of 'case definition', the methods of obtaining the data, and the temporal setting of the study. Due to the changes in management, one cannot compare contemporaneous data with historical data. Hence the epidemiology of heart failure has and will continue to evolve. Though much is now known with regards to left ventricular systolic dysfunction, there are still areas which lack a depth and breadth of knowledge. In an increasingly globalized community, it is now becoming evident that some of the traditional risk factors identified from previous work in the West are now applicable to cohorts within the developing world. It should also be remembered that with globalization and the ease of movement, aetiologies of heart failure which are long forgotten in the West may well reappear.

This chapter will focus on ten key papers within the field and highlight their importance, but also their contribution. The chapter is not intended to be an up-to-the-minute review and, if interested, readers are urged to delve into the literature. The papers were chosen because in the authors' beliefs they were landmark papers which transformed previously held concepts. A landmark paper should be considered a seminal piece of work which both increased understanding of the mechanism of disease, but also conclusively proved an alternative hypothesis. This has led to a constant revision of the best models of care. It is meant to be a summary of heart failure epidemiology and not an overview of heart failure. Therefore in terms of subject areas, it will stay focused on the epidemiology.

The original Framingham study

McKee PA, Castelli WP, McNamara PM, Kannel WB. The natural history of congestive heart failure: the Framingham study. *N Engl J Med* 1971; 285(26): 1441–6.[1]

Following the Second World War a growing realization that cardiovascular disease was starting to become the predominant source of mortality drove the field of cardiovascular epidemiology. Henceforth the Framingham cohort was created, with 5209 participants identified in the town of Framingham, Massachusetts, United States. This was then analysed in a classical longitudinal prospective format. All participants at enrolment were aged 30–62 years of age. Participants underwent biennial physical examinations and basic biochemistry, radiology, and electrocardiography.

The original Framingham and heart failure study was published in 1971. This remains the landmark paper in heart failure epidemiology. William Kannel and authors demonstrated several key facts within heart failure epidemiology which subsequently have been corroborated in

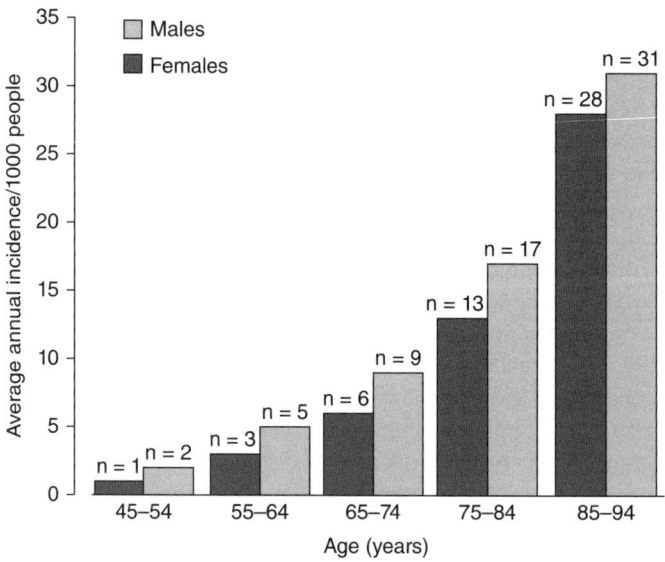

Figure 12.1 Incidence of heart failure within the Framingham cohort.

other cohorts. Using available techniques (the paper preceded widespread usage of echocardiography) the authors noted an increasing incidence of heart failure with advancing age (see Figure 12.1). Within males, the incidence rose from 0.4/1000 at the age of 40–44 years to 8.7/1000 at the age of 70–74. This was also reflected amongst the female population, with a rise in incidence between similar age groups from 0.6/1000 to 3.0/1000. The commonest aetiology was hypertension, where it was felt that it was responsible in three quarters of the population. Lastly, Framingham demonstrated for the first time the very high mortality associated with heart failure. Men within the cohort with heart failure had a less than 50% chance of survival beyond five years.

The publication of this paper drove the need for therapeutics and further developments in heart failure care. However, the diagnosis of heart failure was based predominately on clinical criteria. This may have resulted in both 'false positive' and 'false negative' index cases, which ultimately could disrupt analysis. Ultimately this is the first major heart failure epidemiology study and hence

stimulated interest and a desire to further investigate this condition with such morbidity and mortality. It should be remembered that the mainstays of treatment for heart failure were mercurial diuretics and digoxin. Hence the mortality rates quoted within the study are not directly comparable to modern studies. Also, the setting of the study meant that all initial recruits were Caucasian. Hence the results could not necessarily be extrapolated to more ethnically diverse populations. The original Framingham study used classical epidemiological techniques on a scale not previously witnessed. It remains, with the further generational follow-up, almost unique in terms of longitudinal epidemiology.

Learning points

♦ The Framingham Study was the first study to denote the prevalence and incidence of heart failure, using a clinical definition based on symptoms and signs.

'The men born in 1913'

Eriksson H, Svardsudd K, Larsson B, Ohlson LO, Tibblin G, Welin L, Wilhelmsen L. Risk factors for heart failure in the general population: the study of men born in 1913. *Eur Heart J* 1989; 10(7): 647–56.[2]

Heart failure remained a difficult and dangerous condition to have throughout the 1970s and early 1980s. After anecdotal reports and much pre-clinical science, the Cooperative North Scandinavian Enalapril Survival Study (CONSENSUS) was published in 1987[3]. It showed, that enalapril, an ACE inhibitor, could reduce heart failure mortality. The positive findings were so marked that the trial was discontinued early. However, despite its success, the patients enrolled within this trial had advanced disease (New York Heart Association class IV). This category of patients was still uncommon within the wider community and hence there was a need for contemporaneous heart failure epidemiology.

'The men born in 1913' was one such study. The study was based in Gothenburg, Sweden. Random sampling methods identified a cohort aged 50 in 1963. The cohort was then repeatedly examined at approximate seven yearly intervals. Apart from physical history and examination, blood pressures, blood chemistry, and spirometry were recorded. The presence of heart failure was documented with the population cohort aged 67. Cases were

diagnosed using a combination of clinical scoring system and basic echocardiography. The prevalence of heart failure within the population aged 67 years old was 13%. If all possible cases identified were included within the ultimate figure, the calculated prevalence of heart failure was 23%. The underlying risk factors were found to be hypertension, smoking, and obesity. The diagnosis of heart failure was once again clinical; however, the findings mirrored those of the Framingham study approximately a decade previously.

Similar criticisms of the study exist. The robustness of the diagnosis can be questioned. Again the majority of those labelled with heart failure, were diagnosed by clinical methods. At this point in time, however, there was no universal definition of heart failure. Nonetheless the fact remains this trial was the first large prospective study in Europe. It demonstrated similar findings and again the high mortality associated with heart failure. Due to the nature and geographical location of the trial, it focused on white Scandinavian males. Hence the trial results, though corroborating the Framingham results, could not be extrapolated to all populations. The study was reliant on a different clinical scoring system to that used in the Framingham heart study. However, the dependence on a non-imaging technique may have either under or over-estimated the prevalence. Certain patient symptoms are recognized as well-known heart failure mimics, for example shortness of breath, and the study may have over-diagnosed the actual prevalence of heart failure.

> **Learning points**
>
> ◆ This was the first European study of the prevalence of heart failure in the population, which also included a description of the major risk factors.

The First National Health and Nutrition Survey—NHANES I

Schocken DD, Arrieta MI, Leaverton PE, Ross EA. Prevalence and mortality rate of congestive heart failure in the United States. *J Am Coll Cardiol* 1992; 20(2): 301–6.[4]

The National Health and Nutrition Survey (NHANES) was conceived by the US government. Following the National Health Survey Act in 1956, the US government recognized the desire for further epidemiological investigation of the burden of several chronic diseases. Previous epidemiological studies had used isolated populations (e.g. Framingham) or had used heterogeneous methodology to identify cases of heart failure. Several had concentrated on hospitalized patients, with a combination of retrospective analyses of hospital admission codes, death certificates, or medical records. Hence prior epidemiology was subject to the criticisms of being unrepresentative of the general population, including the elderly or ethnic minorities, or being subject to biases.

The first cycle of NHANES collected prospective data for 14,407 adults aged between 1971 and 1975. Fifteen districts across the continental United States were included in the survey. The survey deliberately chose a random sample of males and females, young and elderly, and ethnic minorities. The cohort was assessed at regular intervals, including full physical histories and examinations, biochemical analyses, chest radiographs, and electrocardiograms. Follow-up data was collected at two further time points, 10 and 15 years post the initial study period. Two definitions of heart failure were used within the study. First, a questionnaire-based survey of physician-labelled heart failure was used. Second, a modified Framingham clinical criteria scoring was used. This included patient-orientated symptoms, physical signs, and radiographic changes consistent with pulmonary congestion and oedema. Deaths were analysed by means of relative interviews, or interrogation of death certificates.

The prevalence of heart failure, when using a combination of the above methodologies, was 1.6% within females aged 25–54. However, at the age group of 65–74 years the calculated prevalence was 7.5%. Similar prevalences were found in the male population, with a trend to an increasing prevalence with age. Mortality rates differed slightly in terms of the actual method used to diagnose heart failure in the first instance. At the age of 65–74 years, the ten-year mortality was 59.6% for the group scored by the clinical scoring system and 65.4% for the group scored by the self-reported methods. Heart failure was thought to affect up to two million persons, which approximated to 2% of all non-institutionalized adults within the US.

This was a landmark study in the field because for the first time it revealed the scale of the problem on a national level. The study was also remarkable for encompassing segments of the population not covered within other studies. Heart failure once again had been shown to increase its prevalence with age. Once again it had been demonstrated to have high levels of mortality. This also highlighted the need for further investigation and the urgent need to investigate novel therapies.

However, despite the scale of the study and ambition, there are some notable criticisms. The study initiated recruitment in the 1970s. Again, using self-reporting and clinical criteria may have misrepresented the actual number of cases of heart failure. The era of recruitment preceded the widespread availability of transthoracic echocardiography. Also, questionnaires and medical and hospital records are subject to retrospective bias. The authors state that by relying on different methods they wanted to ensure a higher degree of accuracy. Lastly, the ten-year period for which heart failure mortality data was collected, was a period where modern heart failure treatments had yet to be evaluated. Hence the documented mortality is not comparable to contemporary rates.

The Hillingdon heart failure study

Cowie MR, Wood DA, Coats AJ, Thompson SG, Poole-Wilson PA, Suresh V, Sutton GC. Incidence and aetiology of heart failure; a population-based study. *Eur Heart J* 1999; 20(6): 421–8.[5]

The Hillingdon heart failure study was conceived and executed by Philip Poole Wilson's group. Hillingdon is a district located within west London. The growing realization that heart failure was making a significant impact on healthcare resources meant that studies of heart failure incidence were necessary. The bulk of economic costs were driven by an increasing trend towards hospitalization. The historic trials as discussed above represented a different temporal period in which the diagnosis of heart failure was predominately based on clinical criteria. They were also subject to the limitations as previously

discussed. Heart failure treatment had advanced, with the first neuro-hormonal antagonists (ACE inhibitors) becoming widely used. However, a consensual definition of heart failure was still absent; hence the need for further studies of heart failure incidence and prevalence using more robust diagnostic criteria.

The study design remains unique. A specialist heart failure referral service was created for the local district general hospital within Hillingdon. All new cases identified during the study period were referred to the clinic, from primary care. Hospitalized cases were identified by

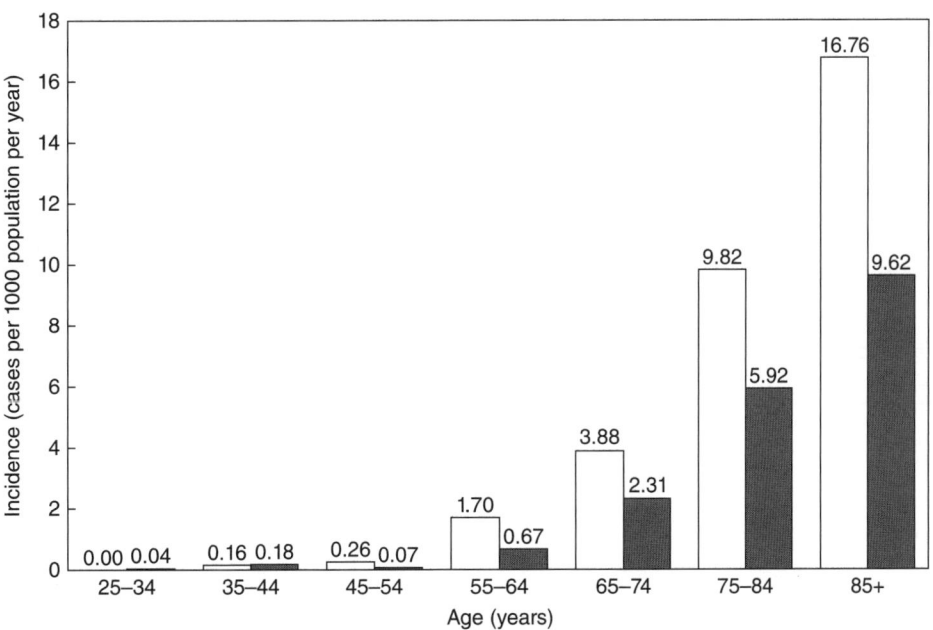

Figure 12.2 Incidence of heart failure by sex and age group in the Hillingdon Heart Failure Study.

Reproduced from Cowie MR *et al.*, Incidence and aetiology of heart failure; a population-based study. *Eur Heart J* 1999; 20: 421–8, with permission from Oxford University Press.

daily data surveillance. Cases were defined by symptoms, signs, response to therapy, and, importantly, an abnormality of cardiac structure or function. All relevant data was presented to a panel of three experienced cardiologists who ultimately decided as to whether the information presented was decisive to diagnose heart failure. In this study 99% of the cohort had an electrocardiogram, 98% had a chest radiograph and 91% had a transthoracic echocardiogram to a prespecified protocol. Reproducibility and reliability of data was checked and the methodology was found to be both reproducible and accurate at the identification of local cases of heart failure.

Over the 20-month study period, 220 new cases of heart failure were ascertained. The age range of cases was between 29–95 years. The incidence steadily rose from 0.02/1000 in the 25–34 age group to 11.6/1000 in the over-85 years age group (see Figure 12.2). The median age at presentation was 76 years of age.

The paper remains seminal in the field. For the first time a reliable method of diagnosis had been used to identify incident cases of heart failure in a multicultural geographical area. The two most important messages being the median age represented an elderly population, often excluded from clinical trials and that incidence rose swiftly with age. These findings have been subsequently corroborated by others and led to a deeper understanding of not just heart failure prevalence but also incidence. The study can be criticized for not using further diagnostic aids such as cardiac biomarkers, for example B type natriuretic peptide. The other main limitation was that case ascertainment on internal validation was 90%. Hence, theoretically, cases of heart failure may have been missed; however, due to the progressive nature of heart failure; it remains unlikely that over 20 months, numerous cases were omitted from the process of data capture.

Learning point

◆ This was the first study to define the incidence of heart failure using an acceptable modern definition.

The MONICA project and symptomatic and asymptomatic left ventricular systolic dysfunction

McDonagh TA, Morrison CE, Lawrence A, Ford I, Tunstall-Pedoe H, McMurray JJ, Dargie HJ. Symptomatic and asymptomatic left-ventricular systolic dysfunction in an urban population. *Lancet* 1997; 350(9081): 829–33.[6]

The advances in heart failure epidemiology and treatment led to a shift in focus. Increasing hospitalization rates had been documented throughout the Western hemisphere in the 1990s. The emphasis moved from that of the hospitalized cohorts with high levels of mortality to that of case ascertainment within the community. Widespread introduction of echocardiography enabled a more robust identification of systolic dysfunction.

The Multinational Monitoring of Cardiovascular Disease Project (MONICA) is a World Health Organization survey of cardiovascular disease and its risk factors. There are 32 centres in 21 countries. Dr Dargie's group chose to examine the North Glasgow centre cohort in further detail. North Glasgow was originally chosen as a participating centre due to the large burden of ischaemic heart disease.

A group of 2000 people who had participated within the third MONICA Glasgow survey in 1992 were invited to enter into this study, and 1640 of those invited subsequently took part. All those recruited had a questionnaire detailing medical co-morbidities, including ischaemic heart disease, electrocardiograms, blood pressure recordings, and serum lipids measured. Crucially, every participant underwent routine transthoracic echocardiography with subsequent calculation of an ejection fraction via Biplane Simpson's methodology.

In the study, 1467 participants had a technically adequate study in which LVEF could be measured. The LVEF could not be measured in 173 recruits. Across all age groups the mean LVEF was 47.3 ± 6.5%. Confirmed left ventricular systolic dysfunction (LVEF <30%) was documented in 43 subjects. Symptomatic left ventricular systolic dysfunction was present in 1.5% of the cohort and asymptomatic left ventricular systolic dysfunction was present in 1.4% of the cohort. The levels of systolic dysfunction rose with age and were more predominate amongst males. Within targeted subgroups of those with prior ischaemic heart disease and/or those with pre-existent hypertension, the rates of systolic dysfunction (both symptomatic and asymptomatic) were higher.

The study demonstrated for the first time the realization that there was a large burden of patients within the community with significant but asymptomatic left ventricular dysfunction. This created several further issues, with the notion that targeted screening of the highest risk groups may reveal levels of systolic dysfunction which had not been previously suspected. The LVEF cutoff point of 30% was a decisive one. The study was published in 1997, in an era which preceded that of widespread device therapy. An LVEF of 30% is one of the selection criteria in all contemporaneous device guidelines. Hence it is even more noteworthy that 2.9% of the population studied had marked systolic dysfunction; 50% of these were asymptomatic, which also raises the possibility that if these individuals were selectively targeted, screened, and correctly identified, then they could become candidates for the complete spectrum of heart failure therapies. The backdrop of this study was the trend for improving acute coronary care, combined with increased awareness and understanding of heart failure therapies. The ACE inhibitor trials had been published within the late 1980s and early 1990s, but the major beta blocker trials were published from the late 1990s onwards.

The main limitations of the trial emanated from the dependence on echocardiography. Echocardiography was performed by the lead researcher and was cross checked against a secondary observer. The inter-observer variability was 10%. Ejection fraction is a notoriously irreproducible variable and subject to change due to a variety of intra- and extra-cardiac conditions, for example atrial fibrillation. There is no comment on the prevalence of these conditions within the study. Also, 173 patients did not possess suitable acoustic windows for echocardiography. No other imaging modality was used to investigate these further; it is possible that if an alternative imaging modality such as radionuclide ventriculography had been used the levels of symptomatic and asymptomatic dysfunction may have been higher.

This study and its sister study using the same group of patients confirmed the levels of systolic dysfunction in an unselected community with high background rates of coronary artery disease. The subsequent study with natriuretic peptides performed by the same group demonstrated that natriuretic peptides and especially B-type natriuretic peptides (BNP) are robust methods to identify those with systolic dysfunction[7]. The encouraging results of these studies allied with further work by others has now become incorporated both into national and international guidelines[8,9]. The gold standard method of investigating putative cases of heart failure is to use a combined clinical, imaging and biochemical model.

Learning points

◆ The study was the first on the prevalence of systolic dysfunction in the population and the first to document the burden of asymptomatic left ventricular systolic dysfunction (LVSD). The second study proved that LVSD could be detected by natriuretic peptides.

Temporal trends in heart failure epidemiology

Senni M, Tribouilloy CM, Rodeheffer RJ, Jacobsen SJ, Evans JM, Bailey KR, Redfield MM. Congestive heart failure in the community: a study of all incident cases in Olmsted County, Minnesota, in 1991. *Circulation* 1998; 98(21): 2282–9.[10]

Thus far the incidence and prevalence of heart failure both within the community and hospitalized cohorts had been investigated. However, the temporal settings of these studies predated advances in cardiovascular disease care. Within heart failure this was the discovery of the beneficial effects of ACE inhibition. In the intervening decades, acute care of myocardial infarction had been transformed with the creation of coronary care units and thrombolysis. Due to the evidence-based changes, there was a need to perform a comparative temporal study.

By the 1990s, heart failure epidemiology and the impact on healthcare systems was apparent. In 1985 it was estimated that up to 2.3 million Americans were affected by heart failure[11]. Approximately 400,000 incident cases were occurring year on year and 274,000 deaths were attributed to heart failure.

To investigate the impact of other therapies on the burden of heart failure, this study was devised. This was a retrospective longitudinal study based within Olmsted County, Minnesota, US. Olmsted County is the local district allied to the Mayo Clinic based within Rochester, Minnesota. The Olmsted County epidemiology project was created to investigate chronic diseases. Two time points were chosen at 1981 and 1991. Retrospective interrogation of medical records identified cases by scoring against the Framingham Heart Study criteria. In this way 107 incident cases were identified in 1981 and 141 incident cases in 1991. The total population incidence remained unchanged at 2.8 per 1000 person years. The five-year mortality for both cohorts at respective time points was 66% and 67%. This made heart failure more lethal than many solid organ malignancies. It also revealed that over three decades there had been little impact on morbidity and mortality.

Amendments in cardiovascular care had not translated into a reduction in heart failure cases. This study, along with others, stimulated further investigational work into pharmacotherapeutics and device therapy. The publication of the first Randomized ALdactone Evaluation Study (RALES) in the same year and the large beta blocker trials published at the start of this century are testament to the impact of epidemiological studies[12].

The limitations are similar to those noted previously, with a reliance on a retrospective clinical scoring system. Due to the nature of medical records they are also subject to the possibility that the attendant physician did not accurately record the actual physical signs and symptoms. The authors also only noted the date of death. No effort was made to investigate the actual modality of death, which raises the possibility of patients with heart failure dying from concomitant causes. Rochester is a small town within Minnesota. The main employer within the area is the Mayo Clinic Consortium. Therefore the population over the study period contained very few elderly residents. Ethnically there was a strong white male preponderance, so the study results may not be generalizable to other populations.

The authors explain their lack of change in either incidence or mortality over the ten-year period, via several mechanisms. First, there was a greater burden of elderly patients within the cohort in 1991. Though cardiovascular intervention was available during the study period, it was still not widely available. There may have been a reticence to initiating elderly patients on ACE inhibitors due to the lack of randomized controlled trial evidence. Only 40% of the cohort was on an ACE inhibitor in 1991, despite commercial availability since 1983. The authors also suppose that any cardiovascular disease modification may not manifest its effects within a ten-year period. It was also suggested that there was under-utilization of a proven heart failure treatment with clear mortality benefit. Unfortunately, this has been subsequently corroborated with current surveys and registries. Despite the availability of rennin-angiotensin inhibition via either ACE inhibitors or angiotensin II receptor blockers, or via aldosterone antagonists and sympathetic inhibition via beta blockade, rates of medication usage, though improving, remain suboptimal. It is not uncommon to find elderly patients who though on core agents, are on suboptimal non-target doses[13]. The authors make an important point within the paper that the mortality rate of heart failure may have been reduced if more of the population had been on an ACE inhibitor and had achieved target dosages.

Learning points

◆ The incidence and mortality of heart failure had not fallen in this study over a ten-year period; this highlighted the need for more action.

The first heart failure epidemiology study within the elderly—the Cardiovascular Health Study

Gottdiener JS, Arnold AM, Aurigemma GP, Polak JF, Tracy RP, Kitzman DW, Gardin JM, Rutledge JE, Boineau RC. Predictors of congestive heart failure in the elderly: the Cardiovascular Health Study. *J Am Coll Cardiol* 2000; 35(6): 1628–37.[14]

By the start of the twenty-first century, heart failure epidemiology had evolved. Whereas once there had been a scanty evidence base, it was recognized that heart failure was widely prevalent; incidence varied geographically, but uniformly rose with age. Several studies had also demonstrated a rise in incidence in heart failure cases associated with male gender.

The Cardiovascular Health Study was designed to test those concepts in more detail. It was one of the first prospective epidemiological analyses of heart failure within an elderly (>65 years) population. A group of 5888 participants were recruited in four geographical locations within the US. The age range was 65–100 years and the mean age was 73 years of age. The study deliberately included a significant minority of African Americans. The four areas were deliberately chosen to illustrate differing areas of social affluence and deprivation (Forsyth County, NC; Sacramento County, CA; Allegheny County, PA; and Washington County, MD). The mean length of follow-up was 5.5 years. All participants underwent full physical histories and examinations at baseline along with both baseline and repeat echocardiography. The diagnosis of a case of heart failure was made with a self-reported physician diagnosis and that the patient was on heart failure treatment. Cases were divided into probable and definite. Cases where heart failure was mentioned on the death certificate were further interrogated to provide the underlying aetiology.

Within the cohort there were 597 incident cases of heart failure, resulting in a calculated incidence rate of heart failure of 19.3/1000 person years. Males had almost double the incidence rate of females. The incidence of heart failure increased from 10.6/1000 person years in the group aged 60–69 years of age to 42.5/1000 person years in those aged ≥80 years. There were no racial differences in the incidence of heart failure. With men, there was an association with incident heart failure and reduced left ventricular systolic function at baseline and prevalent coronary artery disease. With both genders there was also a finding of incident heart failure, but with preserved left ventricular systolic function (heart failure with normal ejection fraction—HeFNEF). Atherosclerotic disease

and diabetes also had an association with the development of heart failure. The leading predictors were prevalent coronary artery disease, poorly controlled systolic blood pressure, and a raised C-reactive protein.

The findings of the study supported what had been documented approximately three decades earlier in the Framingham study. Heart failure incidence rose steeply with age, affected males more so than females, and was associated with coronary artery disease, diabetes, atherosclerotic disease, and hypertension. The study is a landmark paper because it specifically evaluated an elderly population. These individuals are conventionally excluded from most randomized clinical trials due to the high prevalence of co-morbidities and selection bias. To date there has only been one specific trial evaluating heart failure pharmacotherapy in an elderly population[15]. However, it is a subtle but important point that with the progressive ageing of Western populations the bulk of the disease burden lies within cohorts who are beyond the remit of the evidence base. It is strongly suggestive that heart failure within elderly cohorts should be more closely studied.

The main limitation of the study is the method of case ascertainment. Physician diagnoses of heart failure and clinical criteria lead once again to the possibility of misrepresentation of the actual number of cases of heart failure. Dyspnoea is a multifactorial symptom and may have correlated with other aetiologies, for example chronic obstructive airways disease. Also, by studying a population aged above 65 years, there may have been inherent selection bias with those with the susceptibility to develop heart failure excluded from the analysis. Lastly, in terms of ethnicity, the study may have been underpowered to reliably assess incident rates within differing populations.

Learning points

- Heart failure is mainly a disease of the elderly—this has importance consequences for healthcare management.

The aetiology of heart failure

Fox KF, Cowie MR, Wood DA, Coats AJ, Gibbs JS, Underwood SR, Turner RM, Poole-Wilson PA, Davies SW, Sutton GC. Coronary artery disease as the cause of incident heart failure in the population. *Eur Heart J* 2001; 22(3): 228–36.[16]

The start of the twenty-first century had seen significant improvements in the understanding and treatment of heart failure. Epidemiology had now proved that it was a common disease which remained lethal. Hospitalizations were common and the disease particularly affected the elderly.

However, the underlying aetiology was still unclear. The early clinical score-based studies of Framingham and Gothenburg had identified hypertension as the principal causative agent. However, neither undertook invasive coronary angiography to delineate actual coronary anatomy. Subsequently further, more recent, studies had concluded that ischaemic heart disease was the leading aetiological factor. However, their conclusions were founded on retrospective documentary evidence rather than prospective appropriate investigatory evidence.

To evaluate the underlying aetiology in a *de novo* population of heart failure, this study was performed. The study group included both Philip Poole Wilson and Martin Cowie amongst others. The chosen location was Bromley, a district in south-east London. It contained 292,000 people within its borders at the time of the study. All new cases of putative heart failure were referred to a specialist clinic based within the local hospital. All hospital admissions were under daily surveillance by one of the research team. Cases underwent a full physical history and examination, electrocardiogram, chest radiograph, and echocardiogram. All patients were diagnosed with heart failure in conjunction with the available guidelines of the time. This was the presence of symptoms and signs in the context of abnormal cardiac function. Aetiology was assessed by a variety of methods. Coronary artery disease was identified as an aetiology only in the context of an acute ischaemic episode or stable angina and a positive exercise test or myocardial perfusion scan. All patients who had not had a previous coronary angiogram underwent coronary angiography and ventriculography. The images were reported by two consultant cardiologists. A proportion of these went on to have a myocardial perfusion scan. The upper age cutoff was 75 years. This was chosen as a balance between ethics and research, but with the previously described median age of 76 years. The final decision for the underlying aetiology was decided by a panel of three senior experienced

cardiologists. Heart failure was only ascribed to ischaemia in the presence of regional wall motion abnormalities, ischaemic valvular dysfunction, or an abnormal myocardial perfusion scan.

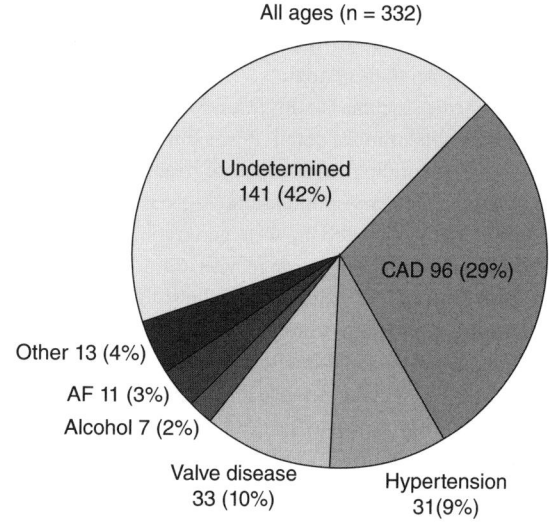

All ages (n = 332)

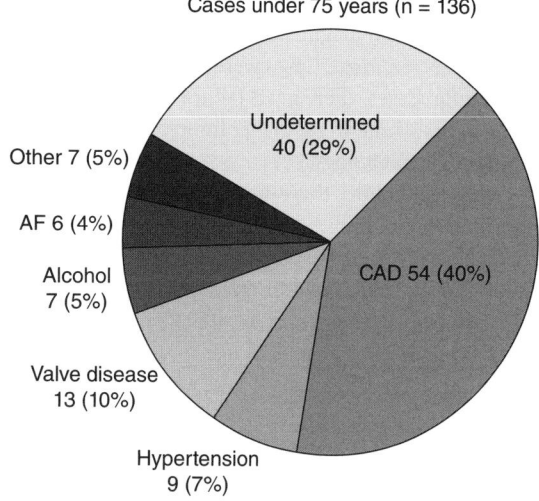

Cases under 75 years (n = 136)

Figure 12.3 Aetiology of the 332 cases of heart failure.

Reproduced from Fox KF *et al.*, Coronary artery disease as the cause of incident heart failure in the population. *Eur Heart J* 2001; 22: 228–36, with permission from Oxford University Press.

Over a 15-month study period 332 incident cases were identified (see Figure 12.3). The median age at presentation was 76 years of age. The incidence for men was higher in all age groups as compared to women. The incidence rose from 0.036 cases/1000 population per year in males aged 35–44 to 10.44 cases/1000 population per year in the cohort aged above 85. An audit of local general practitioner records estimated that the study failed to capture 12% of patients below the age of 75 years with heart failure within the district. In the group, 99 cases proceeded to angiography and significant coronary disease was identified in two-thirds of this cohort. Ultimately in the <75 years of age group, ischaemia was felt to be the aetiology in 52% of cases. Only 4.4% of this cohort was felt to have hypertension as the major contributing factor to the heart failure presentation.

The findings from this study are important in the discussion of whether ischaemia induces ventricular hibernation and subsequent heart failure. Over half of the population with heart failure below the age of 75, were shown to have significant coronary artery disease.

The total figure may be a conservative estimate as not all of this sample underwent invasive testing. However, in addition to the documented rates of incidence, this tellingly demonstrated that a proportion of patients who present with heart failure do have significant coronary disease. The need for myocardial revascularization strategies was also raised by the study. This is currently under further investigation via a large multi-centre, randomized controlled trial, which is due to report initial findings in the next few years[17]. The substantial presence of coronary disease also meant that these patients would be candidates for secondary prevention. This included lipid lowering therapy, smoking cessation, and optimal concomitant medical therapy.

Learning points

◆ Over the last 20 years there has been a shift in the aetiology of heart failure from hypertension to coronary artery disease.

Revisiting the Framingham cohort—the lifetime risk of developing heart failure

Ho KK, Anderson KM, Kannel WB, Grossman W, Levy D. Survival after the onset of congestive heart failure in Framingham Heart Study subjects. *Circulation* 1993; 88(1): 107–15.[18]

As the literature progressed, the changes in incidence and prevalence have been well documented. Different methodologies and differing settings had confounded the issues with regards to incidence and prevalence. However, the most recent studies as above had clarified the actual incidence rate. The aetiology had also clearly been demonstrated in a younger population to be predominately ischaemic heart disease. However, the background changes in demographics and care had also changed. Hypertension had reliable definitions, novel treatments, and better medical awareness. The survival after myocardial infarction was vastly increased by the widespread availability of thrombolysis and primary percutaneous intervention. Healthcare models had also been revised and adjusted to incorporate triage and facilitate acute treatment.

In terms of heart failure what was unclear was the individual's lifetime risk of developing the disease. This study was a landmark one due to the fact that ambitiously it set out to investigate the lifetime risk of developing

heart failure. Daniel Levy and others returned to revisit the data from the Framingham cohort. Lifetime risk is defined as the absolute cumulative risk of an individual developing a given disease during his or her remaining lifetime.

At the time of the original study, Framingham had been ongoing for 23 years. Since that publication the cohort had been maintained and a second cycle recruited (the offspring of the original cohort and spouses of offspring of the original cohort) in 1971. Both arms of the study were included in the present study. All recruits had an examination between 1971 and 1996 and were aged between 40 and 94 years. Cases were discovered by reviewing hospital records, examinations, electrocardiograms, and chest radiograph reports. All identifiable events were approved for inclusion by a panel of three senior experienced cardiologists.

In this study, 8229 participants (3757 men, 4472 women) were followed up from 1971 to 1996. This created a total follow-up period of 124,262 person-years.

During the study period 583 cases of incident heart failure were recorded. The absolute lifetime risk for both men and women was 20% or one in five. This was the same at both age 40 and 80. The lifetime risk was doubled for all participants with a blood pressure >160/100 mmHg as compared to those with a reading of <140/90 mmHg. Prior myocardial infarction in men raised the lifetime risk from one in nine in those without to one in five.

Once again the key culprits for the development for heart failure were shown to be hypertension and prior myocardial infarction. However, previous studies had not demonstrated a gender difference with regards to the aetiologies. Interestingly, the lifetime risk of heart failure was maintained throughout all age groups. This is indicative of the raised incidence in the more elderly, which outweighs the increasing mortality from other causes. Similar to the original Framingham heart study, the main limitation is the actual study cohort. Framing-

ham, even with the second cycle, remains a predominantly white, middle-class town. Hence, results are not representative of the general population. Also, due to the recurrent nature of follow-up examinations, volunteers within the cohort may have amended their health behaviour.

Nevertheless the study illustrated that the lifetime risk of heart failure is high and despite changes in cardiovascular care, remained so. In terms of hypothesis generation, it would be interesting to see whether improved lifestyle modification and focused interventions on the highest risk populations could modify lifetime risk.

Learning points

◆ The lifetime risk of developing heart failure was defined and the benefits of treating hypertension and MI underscored.

Heart failure hospitalizations

Jhund PS, Macintyre K, Simpson CR, Lewsey JD, Stewart S, Redpath A, Chalmers JW, Capewell S, McMurray JJ. Long-term trends in first hospitalization for heart failure and subsequent survival between 1986 and 2003: a population study of 5.1 million people. *Circulation* 2009; 119(4): 515–23.[19]

The much described 'epidemic' of heart failure had not been demonstrated. A true epidemic is defined by a rise in incidence, which has not recently been shown. However, over the intervening decades, increasingly ageing cohorts have equated to increased prevalence and an added fiscal burden. Hospitalization is the principal driver for healthcare costs due to heart failure. To minimize hospitalizations, much has been done with the creation of disease management programmes. This is allied to a dispersion of the message that widespread usage of evidence-based heart failure therapies minimizes mortality and morbidity, and ultimately hospitalization.

Recent work from the US, revealed a trend toward increased hospitalization over the time period of 1979–2004[20]. However, US healthcare services are configured differently to those within publicly funded healthcare systems. The method of funding healthcare for elderly patients within the US may have also influenced the trend towards hospital admission.

Within Europe, Scotland offered a unique opportunity. It had a population of 5.1 million people. Data capture

was facilitated by the National Health Service records. The study period covered the entirety of Scotland between 1986 and 2003. Every patient with a first episode of heart failure was logged and followed up until death or the end of 2004. To ensure data integrity, hospital admissions were analysed. A heart failure hospitalization was classified only when an appropriate heart failure International Classification of Disease code was in the primary position. All patients had a primary care practitioner who could be accessed. Throughout Scotland there are free prescriptions for the elderly. All prescriptions resulting from a heart failure consultation were revealed by interrogating Read codes.

In the study, 116,556 individual patients were identified over the time period: 55,173 of these were men and 61,383 were women. The mean age at presentation rose from 70.7 years at the start of the period to 72.4 years at 2003 in men, and 76 to 77.3 years in women. In both men and women the peak of incident heart failure hospitalization was reached in 1994; subsequently the trend reversed. However, the trend for repeat admissions

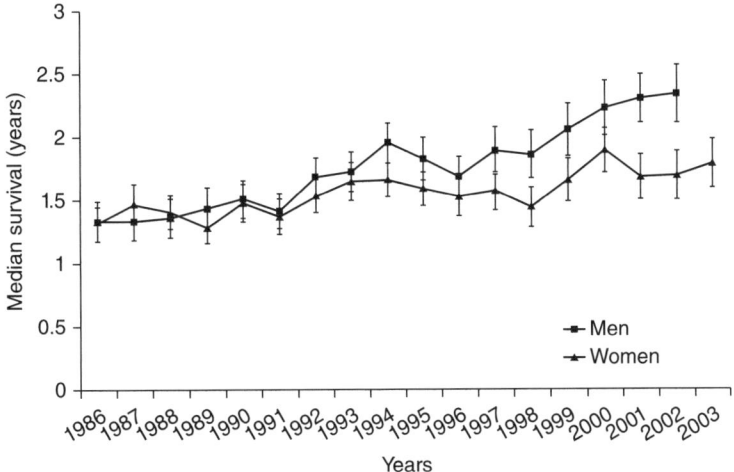

Figure 12.4 Trends in median survival in Scotland from 1986 until 2003.

Reproduced from Jhund PS *et al.*, Long term trends in first hospitalization for heart failure and subsequent survival between 1986 and 2003: A study of 5.1 million people. *Circulation* 2009; 119: 515–23, with permission from Wolters Kluwer Health.

increased throughout the study period. Co-morbidities were increasingly prevalent, bar the incidence of myocardial infarction, which actually fell during the time period. Median survival post initial heart failure hospitalization increased from 1.3 years in 1986 to 2.34 years in 2002 in men, this was replicated in women (see Figure 12.4). Thirty-day survival also increased steadily throughout the temporal period. Prescription rates for beta blockers, ACE inhibitors, and aldosterone antagonists rose throughout the period.

This study confirmed the earlier findings from Scotland, Sweden, and the Netherlands. Heart failure hospitalizations within Europe seemed to have reached a peak within the mid-1990s. Subsequently they have declined and the rate of decline has been maintained. Within the study the rates of appropriate medication usage rose, which may have impacted on the number of hospitalizations. There was no method of analysing medication adherence within the study. The main limitation within the study is the primary focus on heart failure hospitalizations, there is little comment on the epidemiology within the community during the time period. Though coding was checked to ensure accuracy, hospital coding is notoriously subject to misclassification, which may have biased statistical analysis. Prescription rates were encouraging, but there was no echocardiographic data,

hence the inclusion of HeFNEF may have skewed results. If the HeFNEF cohort is excluded it is probable that the dosages of appropriate heart failure medication remain suboptimal. There was also no individual data available for hospitalizations.

The trend for a reduction in incidental hospitalization is positive and has been corroborated with other European data. The prescription rates of evidence-based medication indicate a population effect similar to that demonstrated in ischaemic heart disease. Though encouraging, the results of the study should be viewed as an impetus for further improvements in care. The temporal background of the study also preceded widespread device therapy for heart failure; it would be most interesting to repeat the study in a further decade's time to review further impact on heart failure morbidity and mortality.

Learning points

♦ Heart failure mortality is improving; first hospitalizations are falling, but we need to beware as repeat hospitalizations are on the increase and the population is ageing. Therefore the prevalence is rising. This will place an increasing burden on healthcare systems.

Conclusions

These key landmark papers have given an overview of heart failure epidemiology. Whereas once there was a dearth of information, there is now an abundance. The facts gleaned from the epidemiology are that heart failure is not an 'epidemic' but has an increasing prevalence. It has a predilection for the elderly, with a median age at presentation within the seventies. The main aetiological factors are consistently coronary artery disease and hypertension. Outside of these studies, heart failure care has been transformed over the last three decades, with large randomized controlled trials providing support for numerous pharmacotherapies alongside device therapy. It remains to be seen what the impact of these further adjustments will bring. Despite the success, there is still much to be done. Further investigative work reminiscent of forty years ago, needs to be performed in patients with HeFNEF. Currently there are no evidence-based therapies for this condition, yet it has a similar mortality rate to that of systolic dysfunction. The usage of appropriate therapies remains suboptimal. More sophisticated healthcare systems need to be created to ensure high levels of care for all patients with heart failure and access to specialist knowledge and treatment. This will be the biggest challenge for the next few decades in Westernized countries, where the burden of elderly individuals and hence disease will continue to increase. In transitional countries, little is known. The epidemiological changes within the once 'Third world' countries are vast. Little is known about the burden of disease or aetiology and in the twenty-first century this will certainly need to be investigated further.

It is hoped that the reader has found the chapter both enlightening and interesting. The chapter was intended as a highlight of the historical key papers in heart failure epidemiology, not as a definitive text. If the reader's appetite has been stimulated, it is recommended that they consult the reading list below for further material.

Further reading

- One of the first epidemiology reviews overviewing the historical literature:
  Cowie MR, Mosterd A, Wood DA *et al*. The epidemiology of heart failure. *Eur Heart J* 1997; 18(2): 208–25.
- A more modern review of heart failure epidemiology:
  Mosterd A, Hoes AW. Clinical epidemiology of heart failure. *Heart* 2007; 93(9): 1137–46.

References

1. McKee PA, Castelli WP, McNamara PM, Kannel WB. The natural history of congestive heart failure: the Framingham study. *N Engl J Med* 1971; 285(26): 1441–6.
2. Eriksson H, Svardsudd K, Larsson B *et al*. Risk factors for heart failure in the general population: the study of men born in 1913. *Eur Heart J* 1989; 10(7): 647–56.
3. Swedberg K, Kjekshus J. Effects of enalapril on mortality in severe congestive heart failure: results of the Cooperative North Scandinavian Enalapril Survival Study (CONSENSUS). *Am J Cardiol* 1988; 62(2): 60A–6A.
4. Schocken DD, Arrieta MI, Leaverton PE, Ross EA. Prevalence and mortality rate of congestive heart failure in the United States. *J Am Coll Cardiol* 1992; 20(2): 301–6.
5. Cowie MR, Wood DA, Coats AJ *et al*. Incidence and aetiology of heart failure; a population-based study. *Eur Heart J* 1999; 20(6): 421–8.
6. McDonagh TA, Morrison CE, Lawrence A *et al*. Symptomatic and asymptomatic left-ventricular systolic dysfunction in an urban population. *Lancet* 1997; 350(9081): 829–33.
7. McDonagh TA, Robb SD, Murdoch DR *et al*. Biochemical detection of left-ventricular systolic dysfunction. *Lancet* 1998; 351(9095): 9–13.
8. Al-Mohammad A, Mant J, Laramee P, Swain S. Diagnosis and management of adults with chronic heart failure: summary of updated NICE guidance. *BMJ* 2010; 341: c4130.
9. Dickstein K, Cohen-Solal A, Filippatos G *et al*. ESC Guidelines for the diagnosis and treatment of acute and chronic heart failure 2008: the Task Force for the Diagnosis and Treatment of Acute and Chronic Heart Failure 2008 of the European Society of Cardiology. Developed in collaboration with the Heart Failure Association of the ESC (HFA) and endorsed by the European Society of Intensive Care Medicine (ESICM). *Eur Heart J* 2008; 29(19): 2388–442.
10. Senni M, Tribouilloy CM, Rodeheffer RJ *et al*. Congestive heart failure in the community: a study of all incident cases in Olmsted County, Minnesota, in 1991. *Circulation* 1998; 98(21): 2282–9.

11. Smith WM. Epidemiology of congestive heart failure. *Am J Cardiol* 1985; 55(2): 3A–8A.

12. Pitt B, Zannad F, Remme WJ *et al.* The effect of spironolactone on morbidity and mortality in patients with severe heart failure. Randomized Aldactone Evaluation Study Investigators. *N Engl J Med* 1999; 341(10): 709–17.

13. Castelino RL, Chen TF, Guddattu V, Bajorek BV. Use of evidence-based therapy for the prevention of cardiovascular events among older people. *Eval Health Prof* 2010; 33(3): 276–301.

14. Gottdiener JS, Arnold AM, Aurigemma GP *et al.* Predictors of congestive heart failure in the elderly: the Cardiovascular Health Study. *J Am Coll Cardiol* 2000; 35(6): 1628–37.

15. Flather MD, Shibata MC, Coats AJ *et al.* Randomized trial to determine the effect of nebivolol on mortality and cardiovascular hospital admission in elderly patients with heart failure (SENIORS). *Eur Heart J* 2005; 26(3): 215–25.

16. Fox KF, Cowie MR, Wood DA *et al.* Coronary artery disease as the cause of incident heart failure in the population. *Eur Heart J* 2001; 22(3): 228–36.

17. Velazquez EJ, Lee KL, O'Connor CM *et al.* The rationale and design of the Surgical Treatment for Ischemic Heart Failure (STICH) trial. *J Thorac Cardiovasc Surg* 2007; 134(6): 1540–7.

18. Ho KK, Anderson KM, Kannel WB, Grossman W, Levy D. Survival after the onset of congestive heart failure in Framingham Heart Study subjects. *Circulation* 1993; 88(1): 107–15.

19. Jhund PS, Macintyre K, Simpson CR *et al.* Long-term trends in first hospitalization for heart failure and subsequent survival between 1986 and 2003: a population study of 5.1 million people. *Circulation* 2009; 119(4): 515–23.

20. Fang J, Mensah GA, Croft JB, Keenan NL. Heart failure-related hospitalization in the US, 1979 to 2004. *J Am Coll Cardiol* 2008; 52(6): 428–34.

21. Cowie MR, Mosterd A, Wood DA *et al.* The epidemiology of heart failure. *Eur Heart J* 1997; 18(2): 208–225.

22. Mosterd A, Hoes AW. Clinical epidemiology of heart failure. *Heart* 2007; 93(9): 1137–46.

Chapter 13

Medical management

Dr Jamal Khan, Dr Tania Pawade, and Professor John Cleland

Introduction

Heart failure is common and may afflict people at any age, but the great majority of patients in developed countries are aged >60 years[1,2]. At least one in five people will develop heart failure at some time in their life[3], but this might be a serious under-estimate due to inadequate case ascertainment and frequent failure to identify heart failure as a complication of other cardiac problems[4,5]. Many people with high blood pressure and most people who have a heart attack or develop atrial fibrillation will first develop heart failure before they die[6,7]. Good treatment of predisposing conditions will delay the onset of heart failure but may not prevent it.

The life-time risk of developing heart failure may be high, but the prevalence is modest and probably at most 3% of adults or about 2% of the entire population[8]. The disparity between incidence and prevalence reflects the high mortality[9], which ranges from about 5% per year in stable, well-treated patients with mild disease to more than 30% in patients who have new-onset heart failure or who have experienced a recent hospitalization for worsening symptoms[10,11,12]. As survival rates for heart failure improve, its prevalence will rise. Heart failure is often a terminal process with prognosis measured in days, weeks, or months rather than years. However, expert care can restore many patients to a good quality of life for prolonged periods.

Effective management of hypertension and coronary artery and valve disease will delay the onset of heart failure and reduce its incidence in younger people[13,14]. However, as life expectancy increases and the proportion of the population aged >70 years rises, the prevalence of heart failure will rise inexorably[8]. Patients who previously would have died of a myocardial infarction will now survive longer, which may fuel a further increase in heart failure. Moreover, contemporary pharmacological therapy may have tripled life expectancy and, therefore, provided the patient can be stabilized on therapy, the prevalence of heart failure will rise[15].

Heart failure is a complex, multidimensional problem. The pathophysiology is diverse[1,2,16,17,18]. Some treatments, such as diuretics, may be applied generically to all forms of heart failure, but most are directed at specific subgroups such as valve disease, electrical disturbances, or left ventricular systolic dysfunction. Although heart failure is common, only a small proportion may be suitable for a particular therapy. Moreover, some patients will respond very well to specific therapies, for instance valve repair, and may not need the full panoply of heart failure therapy. Other patients have disease or multiple cardiac and non-cardiac co-morbidities that are so severe that it renders palliative care the preferred management strategy rather than trying to prolong life[19, 20, 21]. Good patient management requires in-depth knowledge of the disease and its treatment as well as a more holistic assessment of the patients' needs.

The following section focuses on patients with *chronic* heart failure due primarily to left ventricular systolic or diastolic dysfunction. Several treatments have been shown to be highly effective at improving symptoms and prognosis in patients with left ventricular systolic function and, in some cases, this has been associated with an improvement in cardiac structure (reverse remodelling) and function suggesting modification of the underlying disease. The cumulative effect of these treatments may have reduced the annual mortality of patients with moderately severe disease from more than 30% to less than 10%[15]. Few other cardiovascular conditions have yielded so much to innovations in treatment over the last 25 years. The impact is much larger than, for instance, coronary artery bypass surgery for three vessel coronary disease[22]. The search for treatments for patients with primarily diastolic dysfunction has been less successful and there is no evidence that treatment has improved the outcome of patients with acute heart failure at all in the last 25 years[23, 24, 25, 26]. In other words, we have made a useful start to tackling the problem of heart failure but the war is not yet half won and, indeed, may turn out only to have been, so far, a successful rearguard action.

Management of systolic heart failure

ACE inhibitors (ACEi)

Consensus

The CONSENSUS Trial Study Group. Effects of enalapril on mortality in severe congestive heart failure. Results of the Cooperative North Scandinavian Enalapril Survival Study. *N Eng J Med* 1987; 316(23): 1429–35.

Background

When this study was planned, the mortality of patients who required hospitalization for severe heart failure was exceedingly high (about 50% at one year) and no treatment was known to be effective in improving outcome.

Methods and results

The trial recruited patients hospitalized with severe congestive cardiac failure (NYHA class IV), many of whom did not have an echocardiogram done. Left ventricular ejection fraction was not an entry criterion. Patients were randomly assigned to placebo or enalapril (target dose 20 mg twice daily) in addition to background therapy. Primary end points were six-month mortality and cause of death. The study was terminated ahead of schedule for benefit. By this stage, 247 patients had been enrolled (127 to enalapril, 120 to placebo). Six-month mortality was 44% in the placebo group versus 26% in the enalapril group (p = 0.002). Mortality at 12 months was also reduced (36% and 52% in the enalapril and placebo groups, respectively, p = 0.001) primarily due to a reduction in mortality from progressive heart failure (p <0.001).

Enalapril was generally well tolerated, but the average dose achieved was only 9.2 mg bd, indicating that most patients achieved 5 mg bd or less, whilst the 'dose' of placebo was 13.7 mg bd. Enalapril associated hypotension, hyperkalaemia, or renal dysfunction appears to have substantially limited the dose given.

Strengths and limitations

This trial only included patients with severe heart failure. Further studies were advocated to clarify the role of enalapril in more stable patients with milder or no symptoms.

Learning points

- ◆ Enalapril reduced mortality in patients with heart failure and severe symptoms (NYHA class IV) requiring hospital admission.

Further reading

- Furberg CD, Yusuf S. Effect of vasodilators on survival in chronic congestive heart failure. *Am J Cardiol* 1985; 55: 1110–3.
- The Task Force on ACE-inhibitors of the European Society of Cardiology. Expert consensus document on angiotensin converting enzyme inhibitors in cardiovascular disease. *European Heart J.* 2004; 25(16): 1454–70.

Studies of Left Ventricular Dysfunction (SOLVD) trials

The SOLVD Investigators. Effect of enalapril on survival in patients with reduced left ventricular ejection fractions and congestive cardiac failure (for the SOLVD Investigators). *N Eng J Med* 1991; 325(5): 293–302. (The 'Treatment' Trial)

The SOLVD Investigators. Effect of Enalapril on Mortality and the Development of Heart Failure in Asymptomatic Patients with Reduced Left Ventricular Ejection Fraction. *N Eng J Med* 1992; 327(10): 685–91. (The 'Prevention' Trial)

Background

The CONSENSUS trial had established that enalapril could reduce mortality in patients with severe heart failure. The SOLVD investigators set out to find out whether it worked in mild heart failure. To reduce diagnostic uncertainty, a low LVEF was required due to uncertainty about the accuracy of clinical diagnosis alone and because patients with LVSD were known to have an increased mortality even if they were asymptomatic.

Methods

Patients with LVEF ≤35% were divided into two randomized, double-blind, placebo-controlled, component trials. The 2569 patients with 'overt congestive cardiac failure' were enrolled into the 'treatment' arm, of whom 90% had NHYA class II–III symptoms and 75% of whom were treated with loop diuretics. Average follow-up was 41.4 months. The 4228 'asymptomatic' patients were entered into the 'prevention' arm (67% and 33% were NHYA classes I and II respectively and only 7% were treated with loop diuretics). Average follow-up was 37.4 months. Patients were randomized to receive enalapril (target dose 10 mg twice daily) or placebo. The primary end point was all-cause mortality. Secondary end points included hospitalization for heart failure, specific causes of mortality, and the composite of mortality and morbidity.

Results: 'treatment' trial

Of patients assigned to enalapril, about 49% achieved target dose. However, only 49% of patients assigned to placebo achieved target dose suggesting that factors unrelated to drug effects was responsible for failing to achieve target. All-cause mortality was reduced in the enalapril group (452 deaths vs. 510 with placebo, RR 16%, CI 5–26%, p = 0.0036). This was driven primarily by a reduction in sudden death amongst patients who also had evidence of worsening heart failure. All the benefit occurred in this group, a post-hoc decision never fully explained by the investigators at the time. Mortality rates due to non-cardiovascular causes were similar in each group. There was a reduction in the number of patients reaching the combined end point of death or hospitalization for cardiovascular causes with 736 (57%) patients in the placebo group versus 613 (48%) in the enalapril group (p <0.001). There was also a reduction in all cause hospitalizations, driven by a reduction in cardiovascular hospitalizations: 810 (64%) patients in the placebo group versus 729 (57%) in the enalapril group (p <0.001).

Results: 'prevention' trial

The event rate was substantially lower in the prevention compared to treatment arm of the study. All-cause mortality was similar in patients assigned to placebo (n = 334) and enalapril (n = 313; p = 0.3). Fewer patients reached the combined end point of death and heart failure in the enalapril group (818 [39%] vs. 630 [30%] in the placebo group, RR 29%, CI 21–36%, p <0.001). There were also fewer hospitalizations for heart failure (306 on enalapril vs. 454 with placebo). The median time to heart failure doubled from 13.2 months in those assigned to placebo to 27.8 months in those assigned to enalapril. In a 12-year follow-up analysis, many years after study completion, at which time patients stopped their assigned study treatment, patients who had originally been assigned to enalapril had a lower long-term mortality.

Strengths and limitations

More than 55% of patients in the 'treatment' study were NYHA class II. Although reduction in mortality was clearly significant the absolute and relative reduction was modest. Patients aged >80 years were excluded. Nonetheless these trials were pivotal in the management of heart failure patients.

Learning points

- Enalapril reduced mortality and hospitalizations in patients with symptomatic heart failure.
- In 'asymptomatic' patients, enalapril did not reduce mortality but did reduce the incidence of heart failure and hospitalizations.
- Symptoms or signs of heart failure requiring treatment with a loop diuretic indicate a poor prognosis.

Further reading

- Exner DV, Dries DL, Domanski MJ, Cohn JN. Lesser response to angiotensin-converting-enzyme inhibitor therapy in black as compared with white patients with left ventricular dysfunction. *NEJM*. 200; 344(18): 1351–7.

- Jong P, Yusuf S, Rousseau MF, Ahn SA, Bangdiwala SI. Effect of enalapril on 12-year survival and life expectancy in patients with left ventricular systolic dysfunction: a follow-up study. *Lancet*. 2003; 361(9372): 1843–8.

Assessment of Treatment with Lisinopril And Survival (ATLAS)

The ATLAS Investigators. Comparative effects of low and high doses of the angiotensin-converting enzyme inhibitor, lisinopril, on morbidity and mortality in chronic heart failure. *Circulation* 1999; 100(23): 2312–8.

Background

Many patients in the CONSENSUS and SOLVD trials received treatment at much lower than target doses and this also occurred in clinical practice. The concept that side effects were dose related but perhaps that therapeutic efficacy might be as high or higher with low doses of ACE inhibitors was raised.

The NETWORK investigators first studied whether a dose-dependent relationship existed between enalapril and clinical outcome in heart failure patients. A group of 1532 patients enrolled from primary and secondary care with symptomatic heart failure were randomized to one of three doses of enalapril (2.5 mg, 5 mg, and 10 mg bd) and followed up for six months. The primary end point was a composite of all-cause mortality, heart failure related hospitalization or worsening heart failure. Outcomes in the three groups were similar (62 patients (12.3%) reached the end point in those assigned 2.5 mg bd, 66 patients (12.9%) amongst those assigned 5 mg bd, and 76 patients (14.7%) amongst those assigned 10 mg bd). However, NETWORK lacked robustness, since it treated patients for only six months, included patients with a clinical diagnosis of heart failure regardless of LVEF, and reported too few deaths and hospitalizations. The ATLAS study, comparing low and high doses of lisinopril, was much larger and focused on heart failure due to LVSD.

Methods and results

This randomized trial recruited 3164 patients with heart failure symptoms requiring treatment with a diuretic and with a left ventricular ejection fraction (LVEF) of <30%. Patients were randomized to either low (2.5–5 mg OD, n = 1596) or high-dose lisinopril (32.5–35 mg OD, n = 1568) and followed up for at least three years. Following randomization, target doses were achieved by 92.7% in the low-dose cohort and 91.3% in the high-dose cohort.

Trends towards a lower mortality in the high-dose group did not achieve statistical significance. Patients on high-dose lisinopril had a slightly lower risk of reaching the prioritized secondary end point of all-cause mortality and hospitalization for any reason (1250 (80%) patients on high-dose vs. 1338 (84%) patients on low-dose, RR 0.88, CI 0.82–0.96, p = 0.002). The former also experienced 13% fewer all-cause hospitalizations (p = 0.021), 16% fewer cardiovascular hospitalizations (p = 0.05), and 24% fewer heart failure hospitalizations (p = 0.002). Benefits of high-doses may have been greater in patients with milder symptoms who were more likely to remain on their assigned dose. Maintaining differences in dose in sicker patients was confounded by the perceived clinical needs of the patient.

Strengths and limitations

The study lacked a placebo group and therefore the effect of low-dose lisinopril on outcome cannot be evaluated. However, assuming that high-dose lisinopril was effective, lower doses were associated, at worst, with only a modest disadvantage. The ATLAS strategy was to increase the risk of potential events compared to the SOLVD study entry criteria, especially limiting the number of patients in NYHA class II that could be enrolled, but this may have had an effect contrary to expectations. Clinical trialists should remember that it is essential to include patients with modifiable risk rather than just high risk. Patients who have mild and very severe disease have little opportunity to respond to therapy.

Learning points

- Uncertainty exists, but on balance, patients with HF and LVSD should be prescribed ACEi at substantial doses when tolerated, to reduce morbidity. This may apply particularly to patients with few symptoms on low doses of diuretic.
- Target doses of lisinopril are generally well tolerated.

Further reading

- The Network Investigators: Clinical outcome with enalapril in symptomatic chronic heart failure; a dose comparison. The NETWORK Investigators. *Eur Heart J* 1998; 19: 481–9.

- Pacher R, Stanek B, Globits B, *et al.* Effects of two different enalapril dosages on clinical, haemodynamic and neurohumoral response of patients with severe congestive heart failure. Eur Heart J 1996; 17: 1223–32.

Angiotensin-receptor blockers (ARBs)

VALHeFT

Valsartan Heart Failure Trial Investigators. A randomized trial of the angiotensin-receptor blocker valsartan in chronic heart failure. *N Eng J Med* 2001; 345: 1667–75.

Background

Pathophysiologically, levels of angiotensin-II may persist despite treatment with an ACE inhibitor. The effects of angiotensin-II on the AT-1 receptor may be attenuated by angiotensin receptor blockade (ARB).

Methods and results

This randomized, placebo-controlled, double-blind trial recruited 5010 patients with symptomatic heart failure and LVEF <40%. Patients were stratified according to whether they were on beta blocker therapy before randomization. In the study, 2511 patients were randomly assigned to receive valsartan (target dose 160 mg twice daily) and 2499 to placebo. Follow-up was for 23 months. The co-primary end points were all-cause mortality, which was unaffected and the composite of mortality and morbidity (defined as cardiac arrest requiring resuscitation, hospitalization for heart failure or intravenous therapy for heart failure), which was 13% lower with valsartan than with placebo (RR 0.87, CI 0.77–0.97, p = 0.009). There was a reduction in the rate of hospitalizations for worsening heart failure as a first event from 18% (455 patients) in those receiving placebo to 14% (346 patients) in those receiving valsartan (p <0.001). Hospitalizations for other causes were unaffected. Small improvements in LVEF, symptoms, and quality of life were noted amongst patients assigned to valsartan.

Subgroup analysis suggested that patients receiving both ACE inhibitors and beta blockers had an adverse outcome if also assigned to valsartan. In the 366 patients who were not receiving ACEi, being assigned to valsartan reduced the primary composite end point by 44% (RR 0.56, CI 0.39–0.81) and all-cause mortality by 33% (RR 0.67, CI 0.42–1.06).

Strengths and limitations

Subgroup analyses are often over-interpreted as was the case in Val-HeFT. The greater effect of valsartan in patients who were not taking ACEi is plausible but throws doubt on whether there was benefit in addition to an ACEi. The subgroup analysis otherwise appears to have been misleading in the light of further research.

> **Learning points**
>
> - Valsartan reduced heart failure related hospitalization in patients with symptomatic heart failure and LVEF <40%, but not mortality.
> - Valsartan improved survival and reduced hospitalizations in patients not receiving an ACEi, suggesting its role as an alternative therapy in ACEi intolerant patients.
> - The adverse effect of valsartan observed in patients already on ACEi and beta blockers has since been refuted by the CHARM series.

Further reading

- Baruch L, Anand I, Cohen IS, *et al.* Augmented short and long-term haemodynamic and hormonal effects of an angiotensin receptor blocker added to angiotensin converting enzyme inhibitor therapy in patients with heart failure. *Circulation* 1999; 99: 2658–64.
- Pitt B, Poole-Wilson PA, Segal R, on behalf of the ELITE II investigators. Effect of losartan compared with captopril on mortality in patients with symptomatic heart failure: randomised trial—the Losartan Heart Failure Survival Study ELITE II. *Lancet* 2000; 355: 1582–7.

Candesartan in Heart Failure Assessment of Reduction in Mortality and Morbidity (CHARM)

Pfeffer MA, Swedberg K, Granger CB, Held P, McMurray JJ, Michelson EL, Olofsson B, Ostergren J, Yusuf S, Pocock S; CHARM Investigators and Committees. Effects of candesartan on mortality and morbidity in patients with chronic heart failure: the CHARM-Overall programme. *Lancet* 2003; 362(9386): 767–71.

Yusuf S, Pfeffer MA, Swedberg K, Granger CB, Held P, McMurray JJ, Michelson EL, Olofsson B, Ostergren J; CHARM Investigators and Committees. Effects of candesartan in patients with chronic heart failure and preserved left-ventricular ejection fraction: the CHARM-Preserved Trial. *Lancet* 2003; 362(9386): 777–81.

Background

The Val-HeFT study showed inconclusive evidence of a benefit from adding an ARB to an ACEi in patients with HF and LVSD. The subgroup of patients who were ACEi naive was small. The possibility that ARBs (or ACEi) might also improve outcome in patients with heart failure with a preserved ejection fraction (HF-PEF) remained unexplored.

Candesartan in Heart Failure Assessment of Reduction in Mortality and Morbidity (CHARM)

The CHARM programme investigated the effects of candesartan (target dose 32 mg daily) on cardiovascular death and morbidity in patients with symptomatic heart failure. It consisted of three component trials (total 7601 patients). The primary end point in each was the composite of cardiovascular death or hospitalization for heart failure. The primary outcome of the overall programme was all-cause mortality.

CHARM-Alternative: patients intolerant of ACEi

This component trial investigated the effects of candesartan in patients with LVSD who were intolerant of ACEi. Patients were randomized to receive candesartan (n = 1013) or placebo (n = 1015) and followed up for an average of 33.7 months. Of patients assigned to placebo, 40% reached the composite end point compared to 33% on candesartan (23% relative risk reduction; p = 0.004). This was driven by a reduction in hospitalization for heart failure in patients assigned to candesartan rather than placebo (20.4% vs. 28.2%; OR 0.68, CI 0.62–0.85, p <0.001). After adjustment for co-variates, there was also a reduction in all-cause and cardiovascular mortality.

CHARM-Added: patients already established on ACEi

This component trial investigated the effects of candesartan in patients with LVSD who were taking ACEi for at least 30 days prior to enrolment. Patients were randomized to candesartan (n = 1278) or placebo (n = 1272) and followed up for an average of 41 months; 96% were on target doses of ACEi.

Of patients assigned to placebo, 42% reached the composite end point compared to 38% on candesartan (15% relative risk reduction; p = 0.01) with similar effects on each component of the primary end point. All-cause mortality was not reduced.

CHARM-Preserved: patients with 'preserved' LVEF (>40%) who may or may not have received ACEi

This component trial investigated the effects of candesartan in patients with HF-PEF, some of whom were taking an ACEi. Patients were randomized to candesartan (n = 1514) or placebo (n = 1509) and followed up for an average of 36.6 months. A similar proportion of patients in each group reached the primary end point (333 (22%) of those assigned to candesartan and 366 (24%) in those assigned to placebo (OR 0.89, CI 0.77–1.03, p = 0.118)). Fewer patients were hospitalized for heart failure in those assigned to candesartan than placebo (230 vs. 279 patients/402 vs. 566 events, p = 0.017). New onset diabetes mellitus was 40% lower in patients assigned to candesartan (p = 0.005).

CHARM summary

Combined analysis of the component trials revealed that candesartan conferred a 9% reduction in mortality, which approached statistical significance (OR 0.91, CI 0.83–1.0, p = 0.055), and a reduction in hospitalization for worsening heart failure.

Strengths and limitations

This was a large, well-powered study. Patients in the CHARM-added trial were adequately treated with ACEi, making the conclusions robust. This was the first major trial investigating patients with preserved LVEF. However, the mortality rate in both arms of CHARM-Preserved was lower than expected and the trial may have been unable to detect small differences. Combined analysis with Val-HeFT suggest that ARBs are an effective alternative to ACEi but may have little or no benefit when added to them.

Learning points

◆ Candesartan may reduce morbidity and mortality when added to ACEi and beta blockers.
◆ Hyperkalaemia may preclude use in addition to ACEi and ARA and there is no compelling evidence of benefit amongst patients taking both of these classes of agent.
◆ Candesartan can be used as an alternative to ACEi in patients who are intolerant of ACEi.

Further reading

● Preiss D, Zetterstrand S, McMurray JJ, *et al.* Predictors of development of diabetes in patients with chronic heart failure in the Candesartan in Heart Failure Assessment of Reduction in Mortality and Morbidity (CHARM) program. *Diabetes Care* 2009; 32(5): 915–20.
● Shah RV, Desai AS, Givertz MM. The effect of renin-angiotensin system inhibitors on mortality and heart failure hospitalization in patients with heart failure and preserved ejection fraction: a systematic review and meta-analysis. *J Card Fail* 2010; 16(3): 260–7.

Heart failure Endpoint evaluation of Angiotensin II Antagonists Losartan trial (HEAAL)

HEAAL Investigators. Effects of high-dose versus low-dose losartan on clinical outcomes in patients with heart failure (HEAAL study): a randomised, double-blind trial. *Lancet* 2009; 374: 1840–8.

Background

Trials of ARBs suggested that they might be less effective than ACEi. Larger doses of ARBs might be more effective and equivalent in effect to an ACEi.

Methods and results

This double-blind, randomized trial recruited 3846 patients with symptomatic heart failure and an LVEF ≤40% who were intolerant of ACEi. Patients were stratified according to use of beta blockers before randomization to losartan 150 mg daily (n = 1927) or 50 mg daily (n = 1919). Median follow-up was 4.7 years. The primary composite end point of death or admission for heart failure was lower in patients assigned to 150 mg/day (43% vs. 46%; HR 0.90; 95% CI 0.82–0.99; p = 0·027). This was primarily driven by a reduction in heart failure hospitalization (450 patients with high and 503 on lower doses; OR 0.87, CI 0.76–0.98, p = 0.025). Mortality was similar in each group. Discontinuation of treatment was similar in the high and low dose groups.

Strengths and limitations

These findings can only be applied to ACEi-intolerant patients as there is no evidence to suggest that the benefits achieved from up-titration of losartan could not be achieved or surpassed by an ACEi. Furthermore, as the study was not placebo controlled the magnitude of benefit from increased dose losartan could not be truly ascertained.

Learning points

◆ Losartan at a dose of 150 mg daily significantly reduced hospitalization for heart failure compared to 50 mg daily.
◆ Although the increased dose is well tolerated it is important to be vigilant for adverse effects.

Further reading

● Krum H. Optimizing management of chronic heart failure. *Lancet* 2009; 6736(9): 6192–9.

Beta blockers

Cardiac Insufficiency Bisoprolol Study II (CIBIS-II)

The Cardiac Insufficiency Bisoprolol Study II: a randomised trial (CIBIS-II). *Lancet* 1999; 353: 9–13.

Background

For decades doctors had been taught, based on scant evidence, that beta blockers should not be used or should be withdrawn in patients with heart failure. By 1999, meta-analyses of series of inadequately powered placebo-controlled trials, including a trial of bisoprolol called CIBIS, had suggested that beta blockers reduced morbidity and mortality in patients with LVSD. However, evidence from adequately powered trials was required to change guidelines and clinical practice. When this study was planned, the mortality of patients who required hospitalization for severe heart failure was exceedingly high (about 50% at one year) and no treatment was known to be effective in improving outcome.

Methods and results

This multinational, randomized, double-blind trial recruited 2647 patients with stable heart failure with moderate to severe symptoms (NYHA III–IV) and LVEF ≤35% on background treatment with an ACEi, diuretic ± digoxin or vasodilators. Patients were randomized to bisoprolol (n = 1327) or placebo (n =1320). Bisoprolol was commenced at 1.25 mg daily and up-titrated to 2.5 mg/day and 3.75 mg/day at one-week intervals with further titration every four weeks to a target of 10 mg/day. Most patients achieved 10 mg daily. All-cause mortality, the primary outcome, was lower in those assigned to bisoprolol (156 [11.8%] vs. 228 [17.3%], OR 0.66 [CI 0.54–0.81] p <0.0001; annual mortality 8.8% vs. 13.2%). Secondary outcomes were all-cause hospitalization (lower with bisoprolol, p = 0.005), cardiovascular mortality (lower with bisoprolol, p = 0.0006), cardiovascular hospitalizations (lower with bisoprolol, p = 0.0004), and treatment withdrawals (similar, 15% in each group).

Strengths and limitations

This was the first adequately powered randomized-controlled trial to investigate the effects of beta blockers on morbidity and mortality in patients with heart failure. It included a wide age range and spectrum of aetiologies, and 96% of patients were on appropriate background therapy. Encouragingly, most patients were titrated to appropriate doses (≥7.5 mg daily). However, only patients with severe heart failure (NYHA III–IV) were studied and patients were substantially younger than in clinical practice.

Learning points

- In patients with heart failure, LVSD, and moderate to severe symptoms, bisoprolol reduced all-cause mortality (by 34%), all-cause hospitalization, cardiovascular mortality, and hospitalization.
- Bisoprolol was well tolerated when started at a low-dose and titrated up over a period of months. However, evidence of a dose-related response is lacking.

Further reading

- CIBIS investigators and committees. A randomized trial of β-blockade in heart failure: the Cardiac Insufficiency Bisoprolol Study (CIBIS). *Circulation* 1994; 90: 1765–73.
- Lechat P, Packer M, Chalon S, *et al.* Beta-blockers in heart failure: meta-analysis of randomized trials. *Circulation* 1998; 98: 1184–91.

Metoprolol CR/XL Randomized Intervention Trial in congestive Heart Failure (MERIT-HF)

Hjalmarson Å, Goldstein S, Fagerberg B, Wedel H, Waagstein F, Kjekshus J, Wikstrand J, El Allaf D, Vítovec J, Aldershvile J, Halinen M, Dietz R, Neuhaus KL, Jánosi A, Thorgeirsson G, Dunselman PH, Gullestad L, Kuch J, Herlitz J, Rickenbacher P, Ball S, Gottlieb S, Deedwania P. Effects of controlled-release metoprolol on total mortality, hospitalizations and well-being in patients with heart failure: The metoprolol CR/XL randomized intervention trial in congestive heart failure (for the MERIT-HF Investigators). *JAMA* 2000; 283(10): 1295–302.

Background

This study was initiated before the results of CIBIS-II were known. It provided an opportunity to confirm the CIBIS-II result and to discover whether the benefits of beta blockers reflected a class effect.

Methods and results

This double-blind, randomized-controlled trial recruited 3991 patients with heart failure, NYHA class II–IV, and LVEF ≤40%, who were stabilized on appropriate background medical therapy (ACEi (or vasodilator) + diuretic). Patients were randomized to metoprolol CR/XL (n = 1990) or placebo (n = 2001). Metoprolol was commenced at 25 mg daily and up-titrated every two weeks to the target dose of 200 mg OD. All-cause mortality, the primary outcome, was 34% lower in patients assigned to metoprolol CR/XL (11.0% vs. 7.2% annualized risk; relative risk 0.66 [95% CI 0.53–0.81]; p = 0.00009) as was the composite end point of total mortality or all-cause hospitalization (439 vs. 311 events, RR 31% [20–40]). The number of heart failure hospitalizations, NYHA class and McMaster Overall Treatment Evaluation score (quality of life) all improved in those assigned to metoprolol CR/XL arm.

Strengths and limitations

This study reinforced the results of CIBIS-II, provided further evidence of a class-effect of beta blockers and extended evidence of benefit to patients with less severe LVSD and/or symptoms. However, as with most heart failure trials at this time, the mean age of patients (63 years) was lower than the average observed in common clinical practice. Also, less than 25% of patients were women. However, it should be noted that although half of patients with heart failure in clinical practice are women, most of these have heart failure with preserved ejection fraction (HF-PEF). Studies of LVSD should not expect >30% of patients enrolled to be women if they reflect clinical practice.

Learning points

♦ Metoprolol CR/XL reinforced and extended the results of CIBIS-II to a broader group of patients with LVSD.
♦ Metoprolol CR/XL improved NYHA class and quality of life, and reduced hospitalization.
♦ These results should not be extended to other formulations of metoprolol that have short durations of action. Metoprolol CR/XL is not available in the UK.

Further reading

• The Cardiac Insufficiency Bisoprolol Study II: a randomised trial (for the CIBIS-II investigators). *Lancet.* 1999. 353: 9–13.

Carvedilol Prospective Randomized Cumulative Survival (COPERNICUS)

The Carvedilol Prospective Randomized Cumulative Survival Study Group. Effect of Carvedilol on Survival in Severe Chronic Heart Failure. *N Engl J Med* 2001; 344: 1651–8.

Background

Trials of beta blockers suggested benefit in stable patients with mild or moderate symptoms, but uncertainty persisted over the wisdom of starting therapy on patients with severe heart failure.

Methods and results

This was a randomized, double-blind trial comparing carvedilol titrated to 25 mg bd and placebo in 2289 patients with severe chronic heart failure, LVEF <25%, and symptoms at rest or on minimal exertion despite appropriate conventional therapy for heart failure. Patients had to be clinically euvolemic. All-cause mortality was reduced by 35% with the annual hazard rate, dropping from 19.7% on placebo to 12.8% on carvedilol (p <0.001). The composite outcomes of death and heart failure and death or all-cause hospitalization were also reduced. Benefit appeared early and persisted.

Strengths and limitations

This study confirmed the benefits of beta blockers in severe heart failure. The study was stopped prematurely by its DSMB due to the large benefit observed, which meant that long-term effects could not be assessed. Premature closure of studies create uncertainty about the true magnitude of benefit, although clearly this was substantial in this case.

Learning points

♦ Beta blockers are beneficial in severe heart failure.
♦ Patients with severe heart failure derive substantial benefit from anti-adrenergic therapy in terms of both mortality and morbidity.

Further reading

- Bristow MR. β-adrenergic receptor blockade in chornic heart failure. *Circulation* 2000; 101: 558–69.
- Packer M, Fowler MB, Roecker EB, *et al.* Effect of carvedilol on the morbidity of patients with severe chronic heart failure: results of the Carvedilol Prospective Randomized Cumulative Survival (COPERNICUS) study. *Circulation* 2002; 106: 2194–87.
- Wollert KC, Drexler H. Carvedilol prospective randomized cumulative survival (COPERNICUS) trial. Carvedilol as the sun and center of the β-blocker world. *Circulation* 2002; 106: 2164–6.

Carvidelol Hibernating Reversible ISchaemia Trial: Marker of Success (CHRISTMAS)

CHRISTMAS investigators. Myocardial viability as a determinant of the ejection fraction response to carvedilol in patients with heart failure: randomised controlled trial (CHRISTMAS investigators). *Lancet* 2003; 362: 14–21.

Background

Long term beta blocker use reduced left ventricular volumes and increased LVEF in heart failure; however, the mechanisms underlying this were unclear. The improvement in LVEF was more consistent in those with idiopathic dilated rather than ischaemic cardiomyopathy. This was thought to be a result of the varied myocardial substrate in the latter, including myocardium, which was scarred, hibernating, stunned, and well-remodelled with good systolic function. It was postulated that the improvement in LVEF with carvedilol in patients with ischaemic cardiomyopathy was dependent upon the volume of hibernating myocardium (viable with contractile failure).

Methods and results

This randomized, double-blind, multinational trial recruited 387 patients ≥40 years old with stable chronic heart failure in NYHA classes I–III; 193 received carvedilol, and 194 received placebo. Echocardiography, myocardial perfusion imaging (MPI) and radionuclide angiography (MUGA—multi-gated acquisition scan) were performed to measure wall-motion, hibernation, and LVEF, respectively. Patients were subdivided into 'hibernators' (>2 severely hypokinetic segments on MPI with over 60% uptake of sestamibi tracer) and 'non-hibernators' within the carvedilol and placebo groups. The primary outcome was change in LVEF on MUGA in patients designated as 'hibernators' and 'non-hibernators' on placebo versus carvedilol. Left ventricular ejection fraction did not change in either group on placebo. However, LVEF increased with carvedilol similarly in 'hibernators' and 'non-hibernators' (+2.5% [SE 0.9] and + 3.2% [SE 0.8] respectively, p <0.0001). However, a statistically significant linear trend was observed between volume of hibernating or ischaemic myocardium and the increase in LVEF on carvedilol (p <0.01).

Strengths and limitations

This was the first randomized trial to study the interaction between the myocardial substrate and a therapy to improve left ventricular remodelling. The measure of LVEF was MUGA, which is generally more accurate than echocardiography alone, as employed in other heart failure trials at the time. Most patients were receiving contemporary appropriate medical therapy (87% on ACEi). However, the study population is unlikely to be truly generalizable, with 90% of subjects being white, Caucasian men. The mean duration of treatment was 189 days, and a longer study duration may have demonstrated more significant differences between 'hibernators' and 'non-hibernators'. More accurate methods of identifying viable but dysfunctional myocardium may have improved the result.

Learning points

- Carvedilol increased LVEF in patients with stable systolic left ventricular ischaemic dysfunction.
- Although the primary end point was not reached, the study provides strong evidence that the volume of ischaemic/hibernating myocardium is an important determinant of the LV response to beta blockers.

Further reading

- Unverferth DV, Magorien RD, Lewis RP, *et al.* The role of subendocardial ischemia in perpetuating myocardial failure in patients with non-ischemic congestive cardiomyopathy. *Am Heart J* 1983; 105: 176–9.

The Carvedilol Or Metoprolol European Trial (COMET)

Carvedilol Or Metoprolol European Trial Investigators. Comparison of carvedilol and metoprolol on clinical outcomes in patients with chronic heart failure in the Carvedilol Or Metoprolol European randomised controlled Trial (COMET). *Lancet* 2003; 362(5): 7–13.

Background

The beneficial effect of beta blockers on heart failure outcomes is not a simple class effect. Bucindolol demonstrated no mortality benefit, and a meta-analysis comparing beta blockers suggested a greater increase in LVEF with carvedilol. This could be explained by differences in pharmacology. Carvedilol blocks a wider range of adrenergic receptors (α1, β1, β2) than metoprolol and bisoprolol (β1), increases insulin sensitivity, and its antioxidant properties may be cardioprotective.

Methods and results

This multi-centre, randomized, double-blind trial recruited patients with stable symptomatic heart failure (NYHA II–IV) and LVEF ≤35% on background treatment (ACE inhibitor ± digoxin, vasodilator or diuretic, n = 3029). Patients were randomized to carvedilol (target 25 mg BD, n = 1511) or metoprolol (target 50 mg BD, n = 1518). The co-primary outcomes were all-cause mortality, which was lower on carvedilol (512 vs. 600, CI 0.74–0.93, p = 0.0017) and the composite of all-cause mortality or all-cause hospitalization, which was not different between groups as the rates of hospitalizations were similar (0.97 (CI 0.89–1.05, p = 0.45).

Strengths and limitations

This was the first trial to compare the effects of two beta blockers on mortality and morbidity in systolic heart failure. Most patients were on appropriate background therapy (~98% on ACEi or ARBs). Features precluding the generalizability of the study include the fact that 99% of subjects were white Caucasian and 80% were men, and that the formulation of metoprolol was not the same as that approved for use in systolic heart failure (MERIT-HF). In addition, the target dose of metoprolol (100 mg daily) was less than that in the MERIT-HF trial (200 mg daily). The difference in benefit between carvedilol and metoprolol may have been less significant had larger doses of metoprolol been used in this trial. However, carvedilol 50 mg bd has been proposed as a target dose for patients who weigh >85 kg. Also, there is very little evidence that dose of beta blocker is an important determinant of survival. Achieved heart rate seems more important.

Learning points

- Carvedilol extended survival when compared with metoprolol in patients with stable systolic heart failure and LVEF ≤35% on appropriate background treatment.
- This may be due to the more comprehensive adrenergic blockade, antioxidant properties, and insulin sensitization associated with carvedilol.
- The incidence of all-cause hospitalization, side-effects, and drug withdrawals did not differ between the two beta blockers.

Further reading

- Packer M, Antonopoulos GV, Berlin JA, *et al.* Comparative effects of carvedilol and metoprolol on left ventricular ejection fraction in heart failure: results of a meta-analysis. *Am Heart J* 2001; 141: 899–907.
- The Beta-Blocker Evaluation of Survival Trial Investigators. A trial of the beta-blocker, bucindolol in patients with advanced chronic heart failure. *N Eng J Med* 2001; 344: 1659–67.

Mineralocorticoid (Aldosterone) Receptor Antagonists

RALES

Randomized ALdactone Evaluation Study Investigators. The effect of spironolactone on morbidity and mortality in patients with severe heart failure. *N Eng J Med* 1999; 341(10): 709–17.

Background

The renin-angiotensin-aldosterone pathway appears important in the pathophysiology of heart failure. Aldosterone is known to promote sodium retention, potassium loss, sympathetic activation, and perhaps myocardial and vascular fibrosis. It was known that ACEi would only partially suppress aldosterone formation. Moreover, hepatic aldosterone degradation is an important determinant of plasma concentrations that is not dependent on secretion rate. It was feared that combining an ACEi and aldosterone-receptor blocker could cause serious hyperkalaemia. Mineralo-corticoid antagonists (MRAs) were thus rarely used in heart failure.

Methods and results

This double-blind randomized trial enrolled heart failure patients with NYHA class III or IV symptoms, LVEF ≤35%, who were on an ACEi and diuretic. In the study, 822 patients received spironolactone in doses ranging from 12.5 mg to 50 mg/day (mostly 25 mg/day) and 841 received placebo. Patients with a serum potassium of >5 mmol/l were excluded. The trial was stopped early for benefit by its Data and Safety Monitoring Board (DSMB). Spironolactone reduced the primary end point, all-cause mortality, by 30% (35% vs. 46% deaths with placebo, OR 0.7, CI 0.6–0.82, p <0.001). Spironolactone also reduced cardiac deaths (31% reduction, 27% vs. 37%, CI 0.58–0.8, p <0.01) and cardiac hospitalization (35% reduction, CI 0.54–0.77, p <0.001) and improved NYHA class (41% vs. 33% on placebo, p <0.001). The benefits persisted at 24 months. Spironolactone increased serum potassium concentration by a mean of 0.3 mmol/L (p <0.001), but the incidence of serious hyperkalaemia (>6 mmol/L) was low (2%) and not different from that observed on placebo.

Strengths and limitations

This trial was the first to demonstrate the effects of adding MRAs to standard contemporary therapy on morbidity and mortality amongst patients with severe heart failure. The incidence of dangerous hyperkalaemia may be greater in clinical practice. Feminizing side effects, especially gynaecomasta were reported in 10% of men, although the true incidence may be higher as many patients think that breast enlargement is just due to heart failure or age. The study excluded patients with less severe symptoms (NYHA I–II) and thus the efficacy of MRAs in such patients was uncertain. The ideal serum potassium may be 4.0–4.5 mmol/L; mortality rises when serum potassium falls below 4.0 mmol/L or rises above 5.0 mmol/L.

> ## Learning points
>
> - In patients with severe heart failure, spironolactone reduces total and cardiac mortality, hospitalizations for cardiac causes, and improves symptoms and functional class.
> - The increase in serum potassium with spironolactone at 25 mg/day (average dose) is small (0.3 mmol/L), despite concomitant ACEi use.
> - Spironolactone is thought to reduce progressive heart failure by inhibiting sodium retention and perhaps myocardial fibrosis, and to prevent sudden cardiac death by preventing hypokalaemia and increasing myocardial norepinephrine uptake.
> - The evidence for spironolactone is limited to those with NYHA III–IV heart failure but recent evidence indicates that eplerenone reduces morbidity and mortality in patients with heart failure in NYHA class II and severe LVSD (refer to the Eplerenone in Mild Patients Hospitalization And SurvIval Study in Heart Failure (EMPHASIS-HF) trial).

Further reading

- Barr CS, Lang CC, Hanson J, *et al.* Effects of adding spironolactone to an angiotensin-converting enzyme inhibitor in chronic heart failure secondary to CAD. *Am J Card* 1995; 76: 1259–65.
- Pitt B, Remme W, Zannad F, *et al.* Eplerenone, a selective aldosterone blocker, in patients with left ventricular dysfunction after myocardial infarction (EPHESUS trial). *N Eng J Med* 2003; 348: 1309–21.
- Zannad F, McMurray JJV, Krum H, *et al.* for the EMPHASIS-HF Study Group. Eplerenone in patients with systolic heart failure and mild symptoms. *N Engl J Med* 2011; 364: 11–21.

Digoxin

DIG TRIAL

The Digitalis Investigation Group. The effect of digoxin on mortality and morbidity in patients with heart failure. *N Eng J Med* 1997; 336: 525–33.

Background

Digoxin has diverse effects, including a weak positive inotropic actions on cardiac myocytes and a parasympathomimetic action that slows heart rate. At high plasma concentrations, especially in the presence of hypokalaemia it may be arrhythmogenic. Digoxin has few side effects at plasma concentrations that are within what is believed to be its therapeutic window but this range is narrow. In the mid-1990s, a number of randomized trials demonstrated that withdrawal of digoxin led to worsening symptoms, exercise capacity, and LVEF in patients with heart failure and LVSD. Its effects on hospitalization for heart failure and mortality were uncertain.

Methods and results

This randomized, double-blind, multi-centre trial recruited patients with heart failure who were in sinus rhythm. The main study included only patients with LVEF ≤45% and an ancillary trial of patients with HF-PEF. Patients received digoxin (n = 3397) or placebo (n = 3403). Doses from 125 mcg to 500 mcg were used (>70% received 250 mcg). All-cause mortality, the primary outcome, was similar in each group both amongst those with LVEF <45% (1181 deaths [34.8%] with digoxin vs. 1194 [35.1%] with placebo, CI 0.91–1.07, p = 0.8) and in those with LVEF >45%. Rates for cardiovascular deaths were also similar (1016 [29.9%] with digoxin vs. 1004 [29.5%] with placebo). There was trend to fewer deaths from worsening heart failure (394 with digoxin vs. 449 with placebo, CI 0.77–1.01, p = 0.06) but a trend to an increase in sudden death. Digoxin reduced all-cause hospitalization, an effect that appeared to be driven entirely by a reduction in hospitalizations for heart failure (910 [26.8%] vs. 1180 [34.7%], p <0.001). The effect on heart failure hospitalization was similar in patients with HF-PEF. There was a small increase in hospitalization due to suspected digoxin toxicity in the digoxin group (67 [2%] vs. 31 [0.9%], CI 1.4–3.3, p <0.001).

Strengths and limitations

This is the largest trial studying the role of digoxin in patients with heart failure. It included a broad spectrum of patients. Although over 94% of patients were on appropriate contemporary medical therapy (ACEi ± diuretics), this included few patients on beta blockers or MRAs. Digoxin might be safer in the presence of these agents, but if heart rate reduction is an important mechanism of its benefit it may be less effective. Further research is required after more than 200 years of use. Patients taking

digoxin could be included and so the trial was a mixture of digoxin withdrawal, continuation, or withdrawal. However, this does not appear to have biased the result. The effect of digoxin in patients with atrial fibrillation and systolic heart failure cannot be inferred from this trial.

Learning points

◆ In patients with heart failure in sinus rhythm, digoxin reduced hospitalization for heart failure and deaths from worsening heart failure, but this was counter-balanced by a slight increase in sudden death.

◆ Most patients were prescribed 250 mcg digoxin, which was well tolerated. However, further analysis suggests that lower doses (125 mcg/day) may be associated with more favourable effects.

◆ The efficacy and safety of digoxin in conjunction with current medical therapy (including beta blockers) is unknown.

Further reading

- Ahmed A, Rich MW, Love TE, *et al*. Digoxin and reduction in mortality and hospitalization in heart failure: a comprehensive post hoc analysis of the DIG trial. *Eur Heart J* 2006; 27(2): 178–86.
- Packer M, Gheorghiade M, Young JB, *et al*. Withdrawal of digoxin from patients with chronic heart failure treated with angiotensin-converting-enzyme inhibitors. *N Eng J Med* 1993; 329: 1–7.
- Uretsky BF, Young JB, Shahidi FE, *et al*. Randomized study assessing effect of digoxin withdrawal in patients with mild-moderate chronic congestive heart failure: PROVED Trial. *J Am Coll Cardiol* 1993; 22: 955–62.

Vasodilators

V-HEFT-I

Cohn JN, Archibald DG, Ziesche S, Franciosa JA, Harston WE, Tristani FE, Dunkman WB, Jacobs W, Francis GS, Flohr KH, Goldman S, Cobb FR, Shah PM, Saunders R, Fletcher RD, Loeb HS, Hughes VC, Baker B. Effect of vasodilator therapy on mortality in chronic congestive heart failure: Results of a Veterans Administration Cooperative Study (V-HEFT-I). *N Eng J Med* 1986; 314: 1547–52.

Background

Vasodilators can reduce preload and afterload that may be of benefit in heart failure. The V-HeFT-1 was the first

trial to attempt to show that treatment could alter disease progression in heart failure and reduce mortality.

Methods and results

This multi-centre, randomized double-blind trial recruited 642 men with a clinical diagnosis of heart failure, reduced exercise tolerance who had either cardiomegaly on the chest X-ray or LVSD on an imaging test, and who were taking digoxin and a diuretic. Patients were randomly assigned to placebo, prazosin (target dose 20 mg daily), or the combination of hydralazine (target dose 300 mg daily) and isosorbide dinitrate (target dose

160 mg/day) (Hyd-Iso). Follow-up averaged 2.3 years. Over the entire follow-up period (5.7 years) mortality was slightly lower in patients assigned to Hyd-Iso (p = 0.093). At two-years, a pre-specified analysis showed a significant 34% reduction in mortality (26% vs. 34% with placebo, p = 0.028). There was a greater increase in LVEF at one year on Iso-Hyd (by 4.2%; p <0.001). Outcomes in the prazosin arm were similar to those with placebo, although prazosin exerted the greatest reduction in blood pressure. Hyd-Iso was split into four doses, but side effects were common and few patients tolerated the target dose. Further analysis suggested that most of the benefit occurred in patients of African-American origin.

Strengths and limitations

The study was underpowered but was the first real attempt at an outcomes clinical trial. Generalizability of the study is reduced by the small sample size in which only men (US Veterans) were recruited and the fact that patients were not on modern background therapy (ACEi, ARB, beta blockers). Treatment was not well tolerated.

Learning points

- Hyd-Iso, added to diuretics and digoxin, improved LVEF in men with heart failure, mostly due to LVSD and may have improved prognosis.
- The use of nitrates in heart failure is supported by evidence only for the dinitrate form.
- Another vasodilator, prazosin, that blocks alpha-adrenergic receptors did not improve cardiac function or outcomes and may have caused fluid retention and weight gain. All vasodilators are not similarly effective.

Further reading

- Captopril Multicenter Research Group. A placebo-controlled trial of captopril in refractory chronic congestive heart failure. *JACC.* 1983; 2: 755–63.
- Cohn JN, Franciosa JA. Vasodilator therapy of cardiac failure. *NEJM.* 1977; 297: 27–31, 254-8.

V-HEFT-II

V-HEFT-II Investigators. A comparison of enalapril with hydralazine-isosorbide dinitrate in the treatment of chronic congestive heart failure (V-HEFT-II). *N Eng J Med* 1991; 325(5): 303–10.

Background

The study V-HEFT-I suggested that Iso-Hyd could reduce mortality in patients with heart failure. Shortly afterwards, CONSENSUS and SOLVD showed that ACE inhibitors could also reduce mortality. Would benefits be similar or would one treatment strategy be superior?

Methods and results

This multi-centre, randomized trial recruited 804 men aged 18–75 with a clinical diagnosis of heart failure, reduced exercise tolerance who had either cardiomegaly on the chest X-ray or LVSD on an imaging test, and who were taking digoxin and a diuretic. Patients were randomized to hydralazine plus isosorbide dinitrate (Hyd-Iso, n = 401) in the same target doses as V-HeFT-1, or enalapril at a target dose of 10 mg bd (n = 403). At two-year follow-up, mortality, the primary outcome, was lower in those assigned to enalapril (132 [33%] died vs. 153 [38%] in Hyd-Iso group, p = 0.016), but thereafter survival curves converged resulting in no overall difference in mortality. Left ventricular ejection fraction increased to a greater extent with Hyd-Iso (p = 0.026). Patients assigned to enalapril had a lower rate of sudden death, perhaps reflecting reduction in hypokalaemia, improved autonomic function, fewer vascular events, and additional metabolic and/or effects on myocardial tissues.

Strengths and limitations

This was a relatively small study, but unique in that it compared two vasodilator regimens that were thought to reduce mortality. Most patients were titrated to target doses in both groups (average doses were 199 mg Hyd + 100 mg Iso, or 15 mg enalapril). On balance, the study suggested an advantage to ACEi in terms of outcome, tolerability, convenience, and weight of evidence. Further analyses of both V-HeFT-I and II indicate that African-Americans, who have less renin-angiotensin-aldosterone (RAA) system activation, may gain greater benefits from Hyd-Iso than other groups of patients. Again, as in V-HEFT-I, generalizability is reduced by the fact that only men were recruited and that patients were not on modern background therapy.

Learning points

◆ Enalapril may reduce mortality more than Hyd-Iso in patients with heart failure, possibly by reducing sudden death, which may be due to the prevention of hypokalaemia or other effects.

◆ In contemporary clinical practice Hyd-Iso retains a role in managing patients who are unable to tolerate ACEi or ARB due to renal dysfunction.

◆ Unfortunately, hydralazine is no longer available in many countries.

Further reading

● Cohn JN, Archibald DG, Ziesche S, *et al*. Effect of vasodilator therapy on mortality in chronic congestive heart failure: Results of a Veterans Administration Cooperative Study (V-HEFT-I). *N Eng J Med* 1986; 314: 1547–52.

● The CONSENSUS Trial Study Group. Effects of enalapril on mortality in severe congestive heart failure: results of the Cooperative North Scandinavian Enalapril Survival Study. *N Eng J Med* 1987; 316: 1429–35.

● Yusuf S, Pepine CJ, Garces C, et al. Effect of enalapril on myocardial infarction and unstable angina in patients with low ejection fractions. Lancet 1992; 340: 1173–8.

African-American HEart Failure Trial (A-HEFT)

Taylor AL, Ziesche S, Yancy C, Carson P, D'Agostino R Jr, Ferdinand K, Taylor M, Adams K, Sabolinski M, Worcel M, Cohn JN; African-American Heart Failure Trial Investigators. Combination of isosorbide dinitrate and hydralazine in blacks with heart failure. *N Eng J Med* 2004; 351: 2049–57.

Background

The two studies V-HEFT-I and V-HEFT-II demonstrated survival benefits from the combination of the antioxidant arterial vasodilator hydralazine and the nitric oxide donor isosorbide dinitrate (Hyd-Iso). Post-hoc analysis in Val-HEFT supported the notion that black patients have a less active renin-angiotensin system. The V-HeFT studies suggested that African-Americans had a greater response to Hyd-Iso. A prospective study to investigate this was needed.

Methods and results

This multi-centre, placebo-controlled, randomized trial recruited 1050 patients who identified themselves as black (African descent) with stable NYHA class III–IV heart failure and LVEF ≤35% (or ≤45% if the left ventricle was dilated) on standard background therapy which included beta blockers and MRAs for many patients. In the group, 518 received Hyd-Iso and 532 received placebo. The primary outcome was a composite score comprised of weighted values for all-cause mortality, heart failure hospitalization, and change in quality of life (significantly better with Hyd-Iso, p = 0.01). Secondary outcomes included individual components of the composite score and change in LVEF (all significantly better in Hyd-Iso group). The trial was stopped early due to a reduction in mortality in the Hyd-Iso group (6.2% mortality vs. 10.2% with placebo, p = 0.02).

Strengths and limitations

This well-powered study was the first randomized, placebo-controlled study to investigate the effects of therapy exclusively in African-American patients with heart failure. Approximately 40% were women and more than 68% achieved the target dose (Hyd 225 mg + Iso 120 mg daily). The patients were well-treated on appropriate background therapy (>70% on beta blockers, ACEi, ARB, diuretics). The key limitation of the study was that patients with mild to moderate heart failure (NYHA I–II) were excluded. Whether similar benefits would accrue in other racial groups is uncertain.

Learning points

◆ The addition of Hyd-Iso to standard therapy in black patients with moderate-severe heart failure (NYHA III-IV) reduced morbidity and mortality.

◆ This combination was well-tolerated with the majority reaching target doses.

◆ Evidence that Hyd-Iso has greater effects in the AA population than other racial groups is lacking.

Further reading

● Cardillo C, Kilcoyne CM, Cannon RO, Panza JA. Racial differences in nitric oxide-mediated vasodilator response to mental stress in the forearm circulation. *Hypertension* 1998; 31: 1235–9.

● Cohn JN, Tognoni G. A randomised trial of the angiotensin-receptor blocker valsartan in chronic heart failure (VAL-HEFT). *N Eng J Med* 2001; 345: 1667–75.

Diuretics

Furosemide

Davidov M, Kavaviatos N, Finnerty FA. Intravenous Administration of Furosemide in Heart Failure. *JAMA* 1967; 200(10): 824–9.

Background

The utility of intravenous furosemide as a diuretic was demonstrated in this study.

Methods

Fifty-two patients with refractory generalized oedema, 41 of whom had heart failure, were administered intravenous furosemide. The starting dose was 40 mg, which was up-titrated until it was sufficient to induce a 500 ml diuresis in an hour. Patients would then continue this daily dose until their oedema had resolved. With intravenous furosemide, significant diuresis began within a minute and was maximal after 25 minutes. All patients experienced complete clearing of their oedema within 4–6 days with an average daily dose of 107 mg ± 21 mg.

In five heart failure patients, total plasma volume was measured using radio-labelled albumin. In six patients relative changes in the cardiac output were calculated using a dye dilution method. Intravenous administration of furosemide resulted in a 25% decrease in plasma volume, an 18% increase in cardiac output, and a 22% decrease in total peripheral resistance two hours after administration.

In a group of ten patients, intravenous furosemide (n = 5) was found to be only slightly more potent than oral (n = 5, 5 ± 3%) as ascertained by urinary output at two hours.

Strengths and limitations

This small study demonstrated the rapidity and effectiveness of intravenous furosemide. However no comparison was made of the time to onset of diuresis between oral and intravenous furosemide, which is of importance in emergency settings such as acute pulmonary oedema. More recently the Diuretic Optimization Strategies Evaluation (DOSE) trial suggested that high-dose IV bolus furosemide was somewhat superior to lower doses or infusions for the management of decompensated heart failure.

> ### Learning points
>
> ◆ Furosemide is an effective diuretic in oedematous patients.
> ◆ It has a rapid onset of action when administered intravenously.

Further reading

- Felker GM, Lee KL, Redfield MM; for the NHLBI Heart Failure Clinical Research Network. Diuretic strategies in patients with acute decompensated heart failure. *N Engl J Med* 2011; 364: 797–805.
- Godwin TF, Gunton RW. Clinical trial of a new diuretic, furosemide: comparison with hydrochlorothiazide and mercaptomerin. *Can Med Assoc J* 1965; 93(25): 1296–300.

Ivabradine

SHIFT

Swedberg K, Komajda M, Bohm M; on behalf of the SHIFT Investigators. Ivabradine and outcomes in chronic heart failure: a randomised placebo-controlled study (Systolic Heart Failure Treatment with the I$_f$-inhibitor Ivabradine (SHIFT)). *Lancet* 2010; 376: 875–85.

Background

People with low physiological heart rates live longer. Beta blockers reduce mortality but the mechanism of effect is uncertain. It had been assumed that blockade of adrenergic receptors were their key mechanism of action, but analyses suggested that heart rate reduction rather than dose was key to their actions. There is little evidence of a

dose-related reduction in morbidity and mortality, but side effects are dose-related. Ivabradine is a selective inhibitor of the sinoatrial I$_f$-channel. Unlike beta blockers, it reduces heart rate, with no effect on myocardial contractility. The SHIFT trial evaluated the effect of ivabradine in addition to standard heart failure treatment.

Methods and results

This multinational, randomized, placebo-controlled trial recruited patients with symptomatic heart failure and LVEF ≤35%, who were in sinus rhythm with heart rate ≥70 bpm, and on stable background treatment including a beta blocker if tolerated. In the group, 3241 received ivabradine (2.5 mg bd to 7.5 mg bd) and 3264 placebo, with a median follow-up of 23 months. The primary outcome was the composite of cardiovascular deaths or hospitalizations for heart failure. This was lower in patients assigned to ivabradine (793 [24%] vs. 937 [29%], OR 0.82, CI 0.75–0.9, p <0.001), mainly due to reduced hospitalization for heart failure (514 [16%] vs. 672 [21%], OR 0.74, CI 0.66–0.83, p <0.001). The number needed to treat to prevent one primary outcome was 26. Cardiovascular deaths were not reduced significantly but heart failure deaths were (OR 0.74, CI 0.58–0.94, p = 0.014). Further analyses suggested greater effects in those with a baseline heart rate ≥77/minute and that patients who achieved a resting heart rate of 50–60 bpm on treatment had the best outcome. Ivabradine was well-tolerated, with fewer serious adverse events than on placebo. Symptomatic bradycardia and visual effects were commoner on ivabradine (5% vs. 1%, and 3% vs. 1% respectively, p <0.001).

Strengths and limitations

This trial was the first to evaluate the effects of a specific heart-rate lowering agent in patients with LVSD and heart failure. It included a broad spectrum of patients. However, the proportion of elderly patients was low (average age 60 in both groups), and thus the results cannot be generalized to the overall CHF population. In addition, the trial excluded two important groups in CHF: those not in sinus rhythm and those with devices (CRT, ICD, and conventional pacemakers) pacing ≥40% of the day. Many patients were not receiving target doses of beta blockers (26% in the ivabradine group and 26% in the placebo group were at target dose of beta blocker). If patients were genuinely intolerant of target doses this does not matter, but if they could have been titrated further this might have reduced the number of available patients with heart rate >70 bpm and may have reduced the impact of ivabradine. Ivabradine appeared most effective in the small subgroup of patients who were not

taking beta blockers. Ivabradine also had favourable effects on quality of life and on ventricular function.

Learning points

- In patients with heart failure and LVEF ≤35%, with resting heart rate ≥70 in sinus rhythm, ivabdradine reduced heart rate and heart failure morbidity and mortality.
- Ivabradine is well-tolerated, including in those already on beta blockers.
- Reducing resting heart rate to 50–60 bpm improves outcomes in patients with LVSD and heart failure.
- Similar benefits might be achieved with higher doses of beta blocker alone, if they are tolerated.

Further reading

- Ekman I, Chassany O, Komajda M, *et al*. Heart rate reduction with ivabradine and health related quality of life in patients with chronic heart failure: results from the SHIFT study. *Eur Heart J* 2011; 32(19): 2395–404. (Epub 29 Aug 2011).
- Flannery G, Gehrig-Mills R, Billah B, *et al*. Analysis of RCTs on the effect of magnitude of heart rate reduction on clinical outcomes in patients with systolic chronic heart failure receiving β-blockers. *Am J Card* 2008; 1010: 865–9.
- Tardif JC, Berry C. From coronary artery disease to heart failure: potential benefits of ivabradine. *Eur Heart J Suppl* 2006; 8 (suppl D): D24–D29.
- Tardif JC, O'Meara E, Komajda M, *et al*. for the SHIFT Investigators. Effects of selective heart rate reduction with ivabradine on left ventricular remodelling and function: results from the SHIFT echocardiography substudy. Heart rate reduction with ivabradine and health related quality of life in patients with chronic heart failure: results from the SHIFT study. *Eur Heart J* 2011; 32(20): 2507–15. (Epub 29 Aug 2011).

Statins

CORONA

Kjekshus J, Apetrei E, Barrios V, Böhm M, Cleland JG, Cornel JH, Dunselman P, Fonseca C, Goudev A, Grande P, Gullestad L, Hjalmarson A, Hradec J, Jánosi A, Kamenský G, Komajda M, Korewicki J, Kuusi T, Mach F, Mareev V, McMurray JJ, Ranjith N, Schaufelberger M, Vanhaecke J, van Veldhuisen DJ, Waagstein F, Wedel H, Wikstrand J; CORONA Group. Rosuvastatin in older patients with systolic heart failure. *N Eng J Med* 2007; 357(22): 2248–61.

Background

Autopsy studies suggest that acute coronary syndromes (ACS) are common causes of death in patients with HF. This observation, combined with the low rate of myocardial infarction in patients with heart failure, suggested that sudden death may be a common presentation of ACS in this population. Statins reduce cholesterol and have anti-inflammatory actions that should reduce vascular events and might improve myocardial and endothelial function. However, patients with heart failure and high cholesterol have a bad prognosis, which might reflect loss of a protective effect of cholesterol against endotoxins. Also, statins reduce plasma concentrations of antioxidants such as coenzyme-Q10 and selenoproteins. The benefit/risk ratio of statins in heart failure was uncertain.

Methods and results

This multinational, randomized, placebo-controlled trial enrolled 5011 patients aged >60years with stable NYHA II–IV heart failure and LVEF ≤35%, who were on standard treatments for heart failure. Patients were randomly assigned to receive rosuvastatin 10 mg at night or placebo. Plasma LDL cholesterol fell from 3.5 mmol/L to 2.0 mmol/L at three months with this dose of rosuvastatin. The primary end point was the composite of cardiovascular death, non-fatal myocardial infarction, and non-fatal stroke. There was no difference in the primary outcome (692 patients on rosuvastatin vs. 723 on placebo, OR 0.92, CI 0.83–1.02, p = 0.12). All-cause mortality (728 on rosuvastatin vs. 759 on placebo, CI 0.86–1.05, p = 0.3), any coronary event (554 on rosuvastatin vs. 588 on placebo, CI 0.82–1.04, p = 0.18), and cardiovascular death were similar in each group. Treatment effects were similarly neutral, regardless of baseline plasma LDL concentration. However, there were fewer cardiovascular hospitalizations on rosuvastatin (1104 [22.9%] vs. 1164 [25%], CI 0.85–0.99, p = 0.04). About half of this effect was due to fewer hospitalizations with heart failure. No difference in overall safety was observed. Further analysis suggested that patients with milder heart failure, with NT-proBNP <103 pmol/L *may* benefit from rosuvastatin (refer to Further reading list below), but that patients with more advanced HF derived no benefit.

Strengths and limitations

This was the largest trial investigating the role of statins in heart failure. The study investigated older patients with LVSD, IHD, and moderate to severe symptoms of heart failure, and the results should be extrapolated to other groups with care.

Learning points

- Rosuvastatin did not reduce mortality, non-fatal myocardial infarction, or non-fatal stroke in older patients with IHD and moderate-to-severe symptoms of heart failure receiving standard treatment. These data suggest that athero-thrombotic events are either unimportant contributors to sudden death and HF progression or that statins do not reduce such events in this population (a composite outcome of fatal and non-fatal MI and stroke events was reduced by rosuvastatin).
- Rosuvastatin reduced cardiovascular hospitalizations.
- Patients with mild heart failure may have benefited from rosuvastatin.

Further reading

- Cleland JG, McMurray JJ, Kjekshus J, *et al*. Plasma concentration of amino-terminal pro-brain natriuretic peptide in chronic heart failure: prediction of cardiovascular events and interaction with the effects of rosuvastatin: a report from CORONA (Controlled Rosuvastatin Multinational Trial in Heart Failure). *J Am Coll Cardiol* 2009; 54: 1850–9.
- Kjekshus J, Apetrei E, Barrios V, *et al*. Rosuvastatin in older patients with systolic heart failure. *NEJM*. 2007 357; 22: 2248–61.
- Shepherd J, Blauw GJ, Murphy MB, *et al*. Pravastatin in elderly individuals at risk of vascular disease (PROSPER): a randomised controlled trial. *Lancet* 2002; 360: 1623–30.

Anticoagulants

WASH

The Warfarin/Aspirin Study in Heart failure (WASH). A randomized trial comparing antithrombotic strategies for patients with heart failure. *Am Heart J* 2004; 148(1): 157–64.

Background

Patients with heart failure in sinus rhythm may be at an increased risk of thromboembolic and coronary ischaemic events, thereby suggesting a potentially protective role for antithrombotic agents. A post-hoc analysis of the SOLVD trial suggested that aspirin negated the benefits of ACE inhibitors, but that there might be a beneficial effect of anticoagulation in this population.

Methods and results

The WASH trial was a pilot study investigating antithrombotic therapy in heart failure patients. It was an open-label, randomized, controlled trial recruiting 279 patients with heart failure and left ventricular systolic dysfunction requiring diuretic therapy. Ninety-nine patients were assigned to receive no antithrombotic therapy, 91 patients received aspirin (300 mg daily), and 89 patients received warfarin (target INR 2.5). Average follow-up was 27 months.

There was no significant difference in the primary outcome of death, non-fatal myocardial infarction, or non-fatal stroke between the groups. Of those enrolled, 26 (26%), 29 (32%), and 23 (26%) patients randomized to no antithrombotic treatment, aspirin, and warfarin, respectively, reached the primary outcome. More patients randomized to aspirin were hospitalized for cardiovascular reasons, especially worsening heart failure (p = 0.044).

These findings suggest that aspirin has the potential to exacerbate heart failure in these patients, possibly due to its effect on prostaglandin synthesis and may not have a major impact on cardiovascular events in patients with heart failure.

Strengths and limitations

This was the first study investigating the effects of antithrombotic therapy in heart failure. However, it failed to detect any significant differences between the three treatment arms. It was underpowered. However, re-examination of the aspirin literature identifies remarkably little evidence of any long-term benefit for patients with cardiovascular disease. The landmark study that established aspirin's benefit after myocardial infarction lasted only five weeks. Despite discontinuation of aspirin in most patients, the benefits of short-term aspirin therapy after an MI persisted for many years. Long-term therapy with aspirin in CV disease may be unnecessary.

Learning points

◆ This study raises concerns about the benefit/risk ratio of aspirin in patients with heart failure.

Further reading

- Dagenais GR, Pogue J, Fox K, Simoons ML, Yusuf S. Angiotensin-converting-enzyme inhibitors in stable vascular disease without left ventricular systolic dysfunction or heart failure: a combined analysis of three trials. *Lancet* 2006; 368: 581–8.
- The SOLVD Investigators. Effect of Enalapril on Survival in Patients with Reduced Left Ventricular Ejection Fractions and Congestive Cardiac Failure (for the SOLVD Investigators). *N Eng J Med* 1992; 327(10): 685–91 (prevention); *N Eng J Med* 1991; 325(5): 293–302 (treatment).

WATCH

Massie BM, Collins JF, Ammon SE, Armstrong PW, Cleland JG, Ezekowitz M, Jafri SM, Krol WF, O'Connor CM, Schulman KA, Teo K, Warren SR; WATCH Trial Investigators; for the WATCH Trial Investigators. Randomized trial of warfarin, aspirin and clopidogrel in patients with chronic heart failure. The Warfarin and Antiplatelet Therapy in Chronic Heart Failure (WATCH) Trial. *Circulation* 2009; 119: 1616–24.

Background

This trial sought to extend the observations of WASH and included a clopidogrel treatment arm as an antiplatelet agent that did not interfere with the prostaglandin system.

Methods and results

This randomized, controlled trial recruited 1587 patients with symptomatic heart failure, in sinus rhythm and a LVEF <35%. In the study, 540 patients were randomized to open-label warfarin (INR 2–3), 523 to double-blind aspirin (162 mg daily), and 524 to double-blind clopidogrel (75 mg daily). Follow-up was 1.9 years. The primary composite end point of all-cause mortality, non-fatal MI, and non-fatal stroke was similar across all three groups. However, there was a reduction in the risk of non-fatal stroke in those assigned to warfarin compared to aspirin and clopidogrel (p <0.01), although total numbers were small (1, 9, and 11 respectively). The number of patients hospitalized for heart failure was higher in those assigned to aspirin (116 [22.2%]) vs. 89 [16.5%] on warfarin, p = 0.019) as was the number of heart failure admissions (218 vs. 155, p <0.001). Major bleeding episodes were more frequent with warfarin compared with clopidogrel (p <0.01), but not aspirin (p = 0.22).

Strengths and limitations

This is the largest trial to date investigating antithrombotic agents in heart failure. However, it was terminated prematurely due to problems with enrolment. It raises further concerns about the safety of aspirin in patients with heart failure and the potential for a deleterious interaction with ACEi. The dose of aspirin was higher than in conventional practice in many countries. It is unclear whether lower doses would be more or less effective or any safer than higher doses.

Learning points

- In patients with heart failure, mortality is similar in patients treated with warfarin, clopidogrel, or aspirin.
- Warfarin may be more effective at preventing strokes.

- The rate of bleeding is similar with aspirin 162.5 mg/day and warfarin, but lower with clopidogrel 75 mg/day in this population.
- Patients on aspirin experienced increased hospitalization for heart failure compared to those on warfarin. This may reflect a detrimental effect of aspirin rather than a protective effect of warfarin (refer to the WASH study).

Further reading

- Al-Khadra AS, Salem DN, Rand WM, *et al.* Antiplatelet agents and survival: a cohort analysis from the Studies of Left Ventricular Dysfunction (SOLVD) trial. *J Am Coll Cardiol* 1998; 31: 419–25.
- Lip GY, Gibbs CR. Anticoagulation for heart failure in sinus rhythm: a Cochrane systematic review. *QJM* 2002; 95: 451–9.

Management of diastolic heart failure

A substantial subset of patients diagnosed with 'heart failure' have normal left ventricular systolic function. Many are now classified as having 'diastolic heart failure' or 'heart failure with a preserved ejection fraction' (HF-PEF). Diastolic HF is characterized by delayed relaxation and impaired filling of a stiff, non-compliant left ventricle. However, HF-PEF is probably very heterogeneous and could include patients with RV disease, pulmonary hypertension, valve disease, and long-axis systolic dysfunction. Whilst the majority of patients with LVSD are men aged <75 years, most patients with HF-PEF are women aged >75 years. Hypertension is a common antecedent. There is no robust evidence in favour of any particular therapy for HF-PEF.

I-PRESERVE

Massie BM, Carron PE, McMurray JJ, Komajda M, McKelvie R, Zile MR, Anderson S, Donovan M, Iverson E, Staiger C, Ptaszynska A; I-PRESERVE Investigators. Irbesartan in Patients with Heart Failure and Preserved Ejection Fraction. *N Eng J Med* 2008; 359: 2456–67.

Background

The CHARM-preserved study (see p. 221) suggested that candesartan might improve outcome in patients with HF-PEF. This trial sought to confirm that.

Methods and results

This randomized, double-blind, placebo controlled trial enrolled 4128 patients aged >60 years with symptomatic heart failure and LVEF ≥45%. The patients had to have 'corroborative evidence of heart failure' defined as pulmonary congestion on radiography, echocardiographic findings of left ventricular hypertrophy or left atrial enlargement, or ECG findings of left ventricular hypertrophy or left bundle branch block. Patients were stratified according to background ACEi therapy. A group of 2067 were randomized to receive irbesartan (target dose 300 mg daily) and 2061 to placebo. Mean follow-up was 49.5 months. The primary composite outcome of all-cause mortality and cardiovascular hospitalization occurred in 742 patients (36%) in the irbesartan group and in 763 patients (37%) in the placebo group (OR 0.95, CI 0.86–1.05, p = 0.35). Rates of all-cause mortality were 52.6 and 52.3 per 1000 patient-years in the irbesartan and placebo groups respectively (OR 1.0, CI 0.88–1.14, p = 0.98). There was no difference in the rates of hospitalization (OR 0.95, CI 0.85–1.08, p = 0.44).

Strengths and limitations

The diagnosis of HF-PEF did not apply stringent echocardiographic criteria for diastolic dysfunction, but it is not clear that this would have been useful. A substantial proportion of patients (40%) were taking ACEi. The median NT-proBNP, the best prognostic marker in patients with heart failure whether or not they have LVSD, was <400 ng/L indicating either very stable well-treated patients or an inaccurate diagnosis.

> ### Learning points
>
> ◆ Treatment with irbesartan did not reduce the risk of death or hospitalization for cardiovascular causes in patients with symptomatic heart failure with a preserved LVEF.

Further reading

• Borlaug BA, Paulus WJ. Heart failure with preserved ejection fraction: pathophysiology, diagnosis, and treatment. *Eur Heart J* 2011; 32(6): 670–9.

PEP-CHF

Cleland JGF, Tendera M, Adamus J, Freemantle N, Polonski L, Taylor J; PEP-CHF Investigators. The perindopril in elderly people with chronic heart failure (PEP-CHF) study. *Eur Heart J* 2006; 27(19): 2338–45.

Background

Landmark trials had established that ACE inhibitors were beneficial in patients with heart failure secondary to left ventricular systolic dysfunction, but uncertainty existed about their effects in patients with heart failure and preserved left ventricular ejection/diastolic heart failure.

Methods and results

This randomized, placebo-controlled trial recruited patients aged >70 years, who were on diuretic therapy for heart failure and who had been hospitalized for a cardiac cause within the previous six months. Objective evidence of cardiac dysfunction was required, with at least two out of four echocardiographic features of cardiac dysfunction including left atrial dilatation, mild LVSD, LVH, or diastolic dysfunction (E/A ratio <0.5, mitral inflow deceleration time >280 msec, isovolumic relaxation time >105 msec) except for patients with atrial fibrillation, who required only one echocardiographic criterion. Of 852 patients enrolled, 424 were randomized to perindopril and 426 to placebo. Average follow-up was 26.2 months.

The event rates for the composite primary end point of all-cause mortality or unplanned hospitalization for heart failure were similar for patients assigned to perindopril and placebo (HR 0.919, 95% CI 0.700–1.208, p = 0.54; 107 patients [25.1%] in placebo group vs. 100 [23.6%] in the perindopril group). If analysis was confined to the first year, when compliance with study medication was high; 65 patients (15.3%) assigned to placebo and 46 (10.8%) assigned to perindopril had a primary outcome event (HR 0.69, CI 0.47–1.01, p = 0.055). During the first year of follow-up fewer patients in the perindopril group (8%) had unplanned hospitalization for heart failure than the placebo group (12.4%, HR 0.63, CI 0.41–0.97, p = 0.033). At one year, patients assigned to perindopril had an improved NYHA class (p = 0.03) and exercise capacity.

Strengths and limitations

This study was hampered by insufficient enrolment, a lower than anticipated event rate, and a high rate of cessation of blinded therapy (drug and placebo) after one year. The low event rate suggests that many patients did not have significant cardiac dysfunction, a notion supported by the findings that most patients had only mild symptoms and almost 50% of patients had a plasma concentration of NTproBNP >400 ng/L.

Further reading

● Hogg K, Swedberg K, McMurray J. Heart failure with preserved left ventricular systolic function: epidemiology, clinical characteristics and prognosis. *J Am Coll Cardiol* 2004; 43: 317–27.

● Lenzen MJ, Scholte OP, Reimer WJM, Boersma E, *et al*. Differences between patients with a preserved and a depressed left ventricular function: a report from the Euro-Heart Failure Survey. *Eur Heart J* 2004; 25: 1214–20.

Conclusion

Few other areas of medicine have created such a wealth of evidence and enjoyed so many successes. What is less well appreciated is the large number of interventions that have failed. Many interventions that should have worked in theory failed in practice. Sometimes this will have been due to a failure of the intervention, but on other occasions will have been due to poor study design or inclusion of the wrong population[27, 28, 29, 30]. Most troubling of all is that trial-and-error and serendipity rather than fundamental science has, so far, been responsible for most of the successful treatments for heart failure.

Research on ACE inhibitors for heart failure was peripheral to their development for hypertension; an afterthought that demonstrated that the prognosis of heart failure could be altered and was no longer a death sentence[31, 32]. The success of ACE inhibitors triggered an explosion of interest and subsequently a vast increase in clinical and research resources directed at heart failure. Interestingly, despite a further 25 years of research no new class of pharmacological agent has made a substantial impact on prognosis. Beta blockers, developed in the 1960s, had been condemned as harmful by a small observational study that initiated propranalol in doses of up to 240 mg/day in patients with often quite severe heart failure[33] and it took 30 years for the mistake to be both recognized[34] and then corrected[35]. How many other treatments have been carelessly rejected? Aldosterone antagonists also pre-dated ACE inhibitors by a quarter of a century[36], but were also overlooked for 40 years as a mainstay therapy for heart failure[37].

Clinical scientists have dreamt up various explanations for why these agents work. The data supporting the mechanisms of action are far from convincing. Angiotensin converting enzyme inhibitors probably exert much of their action through bradykinin/prostaglandin pathways rather than interfering with the production of angiotensin II. This explains why the benefits of ACE inhibitors are diminished in the presence of aspirin[38] (an agent for which there is no evidence of benefit beyond six weeks after an acute vascular event and which may be harmful in heart failure[39]) and also why ACE inhibitors appear somewhat superior to angiotensin receptor blockers[40, 41]. Beta blockers were thought to act through blocking the effects of adrenergic receptor stimulation, but studies of centrally acting agents that reduce sympathetic activation demonstrated an adverse effect on outcome[42], whilst an agent, ivabradine, that reduces heart rate without interfering with the sympathetic nervous system appears effective[43]. Perhaps heart rate reduction is the mainstay of beta blocker effect and adrenergic receptor blockade is just a mechanism that generates side effects. Complex explanations for the mechanism of effect of aldosterone antagonists have been proposed, but ultimately diuresis and an increase in potassium may explain all the benefit. So, not only have we discovered good treatments more or less by accident but the mechanism of effect is almost invariably different from what was first expected.

However, the great success in managing heart failure has itself become a problem. More people are surviving longer with the disease and require more care. Inevitably, the incidence of disease and mortality cannot remain out of balance for long. Heart failure progresses, patients deteriorate, and they require more treatment just to 'stand still'. This 'therapeutic treadmill' is likely to be an exhausting exercise for health services and has already triggered new coping strategies such as remote patient care (Telehealth) to maintain or improve the quality of care with finite human resources[44]. Like a dam in a great river, dealing with one aspect of heart failure may stop progression by one route but 'pressures' build up elsewhere and the dam is circumvented or simply overflows. Downstream, the river flows as swiftly as ever. Treatment has been very effective at halting progressive left ventricular remodelling but this has led to a 'morphing' of the disease with pulmonary hypertension, anaemia and renal, vascular, diastolic ventricular, and right ventricular dysfunction becoming more important pathways of progression.

At some point, the clinical science of heart failure will have to go back to basics. First, to identify a robust, objective definition of heart failure so that researchers can be confident that they are studying the same problem. Clinical diagnosis of heart failure is often difficult. Two markers of 'congestion', prescription of loop diuretics and plasma concentrations of natriuretic peptides, are objective and provide much more powerful prognostic information than a clinical diagnosis of heart failure or demonstration of a reduced left ventricular ejection fraction[7,45]. Although diuretics and plasma natriuretic peptide concentration may not be entirely sufficient to confirm a diagnosis of heart failure, the presumption should be that such patients have

heart failure until proven otherwise. Absence of such markers either excludes heart failure as a diagnosis or indicates that therapy has been successful and caused a remission of disease[46]. These markers make identification of heart failure easy in primary or secondary care and create a large, objectively verifiable pool of patients who have unmet needs and require treatment. Whether treatment should be aligned with a particular pathophysiology will depend on the intervention.

That the needs of patients with heart failure are not adequately met by existing therapy is demonstrated not only by their high continuing morbidity and mortality, but by the complex polypharmacy they receive. If an intervention was truly effective, it would abrogate the need for the rest. At some point treatment will need to be rationalized. Are ACE inhibitors needed in patients who are receiving aldosterone antagonists? Do patients receiving ivabradine need a beta blocker? These will be tricky questions to answer.

In conclusion, trying to improve the lot of patients with heart failure is a truly Herculean task. The heart failure 'Hydra' has grown many heads since it was first roused from slumber by the advent of ACE inhibitors. Heart failure is also the 'Proteus' of cardiovascular disease. Never underestimate your opponent.

References

1. Cleland JGF, Cohen-Solal A, Cosin-Aguilar J, *et al*. An International Survey of the Management of Heart Failure in Primary Care. The IMPROVEMENT of Heart Failure Programme. *Lancet* 2002; 360: 1631–9.

2. Cleland J.G.F., Swedberg K, Follath F, *et al*. The EuroHeart Failure Survey Programme: Survey on the Quality of Care Among Patients with Heart Failure in Europe. Part 1: Patient Characteristics and Diagnosis. *Eur Heart J* 2003; 24: 422–63.

3. Lloyd-Jones DM, Larson MG, Leip MS, *et al*. Lifetime Risk for Developing Congestive Heart Failure—The Framingham Heart Study. *Circulation* 2002; 106(24): 3068–72.

4. Khand AU, Shaw M, Gemmel I, Cleland JG. Do discharge codes underestimate hospitalisation due to heart failure? Validation study of hospital discharge coding for heart failure. *Eur J Heart Fail* 2005; 7(5): 792–7.

5. Ingelsson E, Arnlov J, Sundstrom J, Lind L. The validity of a diagnosis of heart failure in a hospital discharge register. *Eur J Heart Fail* 2005; 7(5): 787–91.

6. Torabi A, Cleland JGF, Khan NK, *et al*. The timing of development and subsequent clinical course of heart failure after a myocardial infarction. *Eur Heart J* 2008; 29(7): 859–70.

7. Cleland JGF, Shelton R, Nikitin NP, Ford S, Frison L, Grind M. Prevalence of markers of heart failure in patients with atrial fibrillation and the effects of ximelagatran compared to warfarin on the incidence of morbid and fatal events: A report from the SPORTIF III and V trials. *Eur J Heart Fail* 2007; 9(6–7): 730–9.

8. Cleland JGF, Khand A, Clark AC. The heart failure epidemic: exactly how big is it? *Eur Heart J* 2001; 22(8): 623–6.

9. Torabi A, Rigby AS, Cleland JGF. Declining In-Hospital Mortality and Increasing Heart Failure Incidence in Elderly Patients with First Myocardial Infarction. *J Am Coll Cardiol* 2009; 55(1): 79–81.

10. Khand A, Gemmel I, Clark A, Cleland JGF. Is the prognosis of heart failure improving? *J Am Coll Cardiol* 2000; 36(7): 2284–6.

11. Harjola VP, Follath F, Nieminen MS, *et al*. Characteristics, outcomes, and predictors of mortality at 3 months and 1 year in patients hospitalized for acute heart failure. *Eur J Heart Fail* 2010; 12(3): 239–48.

12. Cleland JGF, McDonagh T, Rigby AS, *et al*. The National Heart Failure Audit for England and Wales 2008–2009. *Heart* 2011; 97(11): 876–86.

13. McDonagh TA, Morrison CE, Lawrence A, *et al.* Symptomatic and asymptomatic left-ventricular systolic dysfunction in an urban population. *Lancet* 1997; 350: 829–33.

14. Davies MK, Hobbs FDR, Davis RC, *et al.* Prevalence of Left-ventricular systolic dysfunction and heart failure in the Echocardiographic Heart of England Screening study: a population based study. *Lancet* 2001; 358(9280): 439–44.

15. Cleland JGF, Clark AL. Delivering the cumulative benefits of triple therapy for heart failure. Too many cooks will spoil the broth. *J Am Coll Cardiol* 2003; 42: 1226–33.

16. Nieminen MS, Brutsaert D, Dickstein K, *et al.* EuroHeart Failure Survey II (EHFS II): a survey on hospitalized acute heart failure patients: description of population. *Eur Heart J* 2006; 27(22): 2725–36.

17. Dickstein K, Cohen-Solal A, Filippatos G, *et al.* ESC Guidelines for the diagnosis and treatment of acute and chronic heart failure 2008: the Task Force for the Diagnosis and Treatment of Acute and Chronic Heart Failure 2008 of the European Society of Cardiology. Developed in collaboration with the Heart Failure Association of the ESC (HFA) and endorsed by the European Society of Intensive Care Medicine (ESICM). *Eur Heart J* 2008; 29(19): 2388–442.

18. Dickstein K, Vardas PE, Auricchio A, *et al.* 2010 focused update of ESC Guidelines on device therapy in heart failure: an update of the 2008 ESC Guidelines for the diagnosis and treatment of acute and chronic heart failure and the 2007 ESC Guidelines for cardiac and resynchronization therapy. Developed with the special contribution of the Heart Failure Association and the European Heart Rhythm Association. *Eur J Heart Fail* 2010; 12(11): 1143–53.

19. Goodlin SJ. Palliative care in congestive heart failure. *J Am Coll Cardiol* 2009; 54(5): 386–96.

20. Johnson MJ, Gadoud A. Palliative care for people with chronic heart failure: when is it time? *J Palliat Care* 2011; 27(1): 37–42.

21. McDonagh TA, Blue L, Clark AL, *et al.* European Society of Cardiology Heart Failure Association Standards for delivering heart failure care. *Eur J Heart Fail* 2011; 13(3): 235–41.

22. Yusuf S, Zucker D, Peduzzi P, *et al.* Effect of coronary artery bypass graft surgery on survival: overview of 10 year results from randomised trials by the Coronary Artery Bypass Graft Surgery Trialists Collaboration. *Lancet* 1994; 344:563–70.

23. Banerjee P, Banerjee T, Khand A, Clark AL, Cleland JGF. Diastolic heart failure—neglected or misdiagnosed? *J Am Coll Cardiol* 2002; 39(1): 138–41.

24. Banerjee P, Clark AL, Nikitin N, Cleland JGF. Diastolic heart failure. Paroxysmal or chronic? *Eur J Heart Failure* 2004; 6: 427–31.

25. Fonarow GC, Adams KFJr, Abraham WT, Yancy CW, Boscardin WJ. Risk stratification for in-hospital mortality in acutely decompensated heart failure: classification and regression tree analysis. *JAMA* 2005; 293(5):572–80.

26. Massie BM, O'Connor CM, Metra M, *et al.* Rolofylline, an Adenosine A1-Receptor Antagonist, in Acute Heart Failure. *N Engl J Med* 2010; 363: 1419–28.

27. Massie BM, Carson PE, McMurray JJ, *et al.* Irbesartan in Patients with Heart Failure and Preserved Ejection Fraction. *N Engl J Med* 2008; 11.

28. Konstam MA, Gheorghiade M, Burnett JC, *et al.* Effects of oral tolvaptan in patients hospitalized for worsening heart failure: the EVEREST Outcome Trial. *JAMA* 2007; 297(12): 1319–31.

29. Mebazaa A, Nieminen MS, Packer M, *et al.* Levosimendan vs. dobutamine for patients with acute decompensated heart failure: the SURVIVE Randomized Trial. *JAMA* 2007; 297: 1883–91.

30. McMurray JJV, Teerlink JR, Cotter G, *et al.* Effects of Tezosentan or Symptoms and Clinical Outcomes in Patients with Acute Heart Failure. The VERITAS Randomized Controlled Trials. *JAMA* 2007; 298(17): 2009–19.

31. Cleland JGF, Dargie HJ, Hodsman GP, *et al.* Captopril in heart failure. A double blind controlled trial. *Br Heart J* 1984; 52(530): 535.

32. Swedberg K, Idanpaan Heikkila U, Remes J; for the CONSENSUS trial study group. Effects of enalapril on mortality in severe congestive heart failure. Results of the Cooperative North Scandinavian Enalapril Survival Study (CONSENSUS). *New Engl J Med* 1987; 316(23): 1429–35.

33. Epstein SE, Braunwald E. The effect of beta-adrenergic blockade on patterns of urinary sodium excretion. *Ann Intern Med* 1966; 65: 20–7.

34. Waagstein F, F.Hjalmarson A, Varnauskas E, Wallentin I. Effect of chronic beta adrenergic receptor blockade in congestive cardiomyopathy. *Br Heart J* 1975; 37: 1022–6.

35. Packer M, Bristow MR, Cohn JN, *et al.* The effect of carvedilol on morbidity and mortality in patients with chronic heart failure. *New Engl J Med* 1996; 334: 1349–55.

36. Settel E. Combined spironolactone-hydrochlorothiazide (Aldactazide) treatment in refractory congestive failure. *Curr Ther Res Clin Exp* 1961; 3: 243–9.

37. Pitt B, Zannad F, Remme WJ, *et al.* The effect of spironolactone on morbidity and mortality in patients with severe heart failure. Randomized Aldactone Evaluation Study Investigators. *N Engl J Med* 1999; 341(10): 709–17.

38. Dagenais GR, pogue J, Fox K, Simoons ML, Yusuf S. Angiotensin-converting-enzyme inhibitors in stable vascular disease without left ventricular systolic dysfunction or heart failure: a combined analysis of three trials. *Lancet* 2006; 368(9535): 581–8.

39. Cleland JGF. Is aspirin 'The Weakest Link' in cardiovascular prophylaxis. The surprising lack of evidence supporting the use of aspirin for cardiovascular disease. *Prog Cardiovasc Dis* 2002; 44: 275–92.

40. Pitt B, Poole Wilson PA, Segal R, *et al.* Effect of losartan compared with captopril on mortality in patients with symptomatic heart failure: randomised trial—the Losartan Heart Failure Survival Study ELITE II. *Lancet* 2000; 355: 1582–7.

41. Dickstein K, Kjekshus J, and the OPTIMAAL steering committee for the OPTIMAAL study group. Effects of losartan and captopril on mortality and morbidity in high-risk patients after acute myocardial infarction: the OPTIMAAL randomised trial. *Lancet* 2002; 360: 752–60.

42. Cohn JN, Pfeffer MA, Rouleau J, *et al.* Adverse mortality effect of central sympathetic inhibition with sustained-release moxonidine in patients with heart failure (MOXCON). *Eur J Heart Fail* 2003; 5(5): 659–67.

43. Swedberg K, Komajda M, Bohm M, *et al.* Ivabradine and outcomes in chronic heart failure (SHIFT): a randomised controlled study. *Lancet* 2010; 376: 875–85.

44. Inglis SC, Clark RA, McAlister FA, *et al.* Structured telephone support or telemonitoring programmes for patients with chronic heart failure. *Cochrane Database Syst Rev* 2010; (8): CD007228.

45. Cleland JG, Yassin A, Arrow Y, *et al.* Outcome of patients discharged on loop diuretic therapy with or without a diagnosis of heart failure. *Eur J of Heart Fail Suppl* 2009. (abstract).

46. Cleland JGF, Coletta A, Freemantle N, Velavan P, Tin L, Clark AL. Clinical Trials Update from the American College of Cardiology Meeting: CARE-HF and the Remission of Heart Failure, Women's Health Study, TNT, COMPASS-HF, VERITAS, CANPAP, PEECH and PREMIER. *Eur J Heart Failure* 2005; 7(5): 931–6.

Chapter 14

Cardiac resynchronization therapy

Dr Ricardo Petraco, Dr Larry Mulligan, and Dr Francisco Leyva

Introduction

The effect of heart failure on survival is comparable to cancer. Despite advances in pharmacological therapy, over half of all patients die within four years of the diagnosis and more than a third die within one year of a first hospitalization. In addition, heart failure has a devastating effect on quality of life, similar to that associated with a stroke, chronic haemodyalisis, and motor neurone disease.

The development of cardiac resynchronization therapy (CRT) over the past decade marks a new era of device therapy for patients with heart failure. Evidence supporting CRT initially emerged from single case studies and small patient series. Subsequently, the findings of large randomized controlled trials have placed CRT firmly within clinical guidelines for the treatment of heart failure. The increasing demand for CRT is testament to the evidence-based practice that characterises modern cardiology.

This is an opportune time to reflect on the history of CRT research. From over 3000 published studies and reviews on the subject, we have selected the ten papers which we feel most adequately represent the evolution of CRT research over the years. Prominent in our approach for this review is the intention to illustrate how research has evolved from exploration of first principles to the emergence of clinically applicable findings from randomized controlled trials.

A pioneering case report

Four-chamber pacing in dilated cardiomyopathy

Cazeau S, Ritter P, Bachdach S, Lazarus A, Limousin M, Henao L, Mundler O, Daubert JC, Mugica J.
Clin Electrophysiol 1994; 17(11 Pt 2): 1974–9.

Background

In the early 1990s, studies failed to show any consistent benefit of atrio-ventricular (AV) delay optimization in patients with heart failure using conventional dual-chamber pacemakers. There was biological plausibility for the principle that an optimal AV delay would optimize ventricular filling, reduce pre-systolic mitral regurgitation, and increase cardiac performance. The role of right ventricular pacing in heart failure, however, was never proven. In 1983, de Teresa and colleagues first described the application of CRT to four patients with a left bundle branch block (see the Further reading list). Delivered epicardially, CRT was shown to lead to a marked improvement in left ventricular function. Despite its significant findings, this study was only published in abstract form and failed to generate widespread interest at the time. It was not until the report of Cazeau *et al.* in 1994, under the auspices of Jacques Mujica, that widespread interest in CRT began to emerge.

Main hypothesis

In a patient with advanced and refractory heart failure, four-chamber pacing (both atria and both ventricles) would lead to haemodynamic and symptomatic benefits.

Methods

A 54-year-old man with advanced heart failure secondary to dilated cardiomyopathy presented to hospital with acute decompensation and pulmonary oedema, which was refractory to medical therapy, including intravenous nitrates and inotropes. His ECG showed sinus rhythm, with a 200 msec PR interval, left bundle branch block (LBBB), and a QRS duration of 200 msec. There was also evidence of intraventricular dyssynchrony on echocardiography (wall motion delay between septal and posterior wall). The patient was submitted to invasive monitoring and four chamber pacing (right atrium, left atrium via coronary sinus, right ventricle, and left ventricle via femoral approach). The atrial leads were connected together using a Y-connector and plugged in the atrial port of a DDD pacemaker generator. The two ventricular leads were connected in a similar fashion to the ventricular port.

Results

Four-chamber pacing (synchronous biatrial and biventricular pacing) led to an acute haemodynamic improvement, with a significant drop in pulmonary capillary wedge pressure (PCWP, from 36 to 25 mmHg) and an increase in cardiac output (from 3.9 to 5.69 L/min). Optimal AV delay was found to be between 95 and 140 msec. The acute results encouraged the investigators to implant a permanent pacemaker with similar settings (using an epicardial LV lead). Within six weeks, the patient experienced a 17 kg weight loss and a dramatic improvement in symptoms (from New York Heart Association—NYHA class IV to II).

Conclusions

This paper reported only a single clinical case with obvious limitations. However, the improvement observed with biventricular pacing was so dramatic that this initial experiment triggered a renewed interest in the application of pacing to the treatment of heart failure. Interestingly, the authors modestly quoted in their conclusions: 'we doubt that this technique will have an impact on long term survival'. Providence would later prove them wrong.

Learning points

◆ This preliminary study clearly demonstrated that the addition of a left heart lead resulted in a major improvement in the patient's function and clinical status.

Further reading

- Auricchio A, Salo RW. Acute hemodynamic improvement by pacing in patients with severe congestive heart failure. *Pacing Clin Electrophysiol* 1997; 20(2 Pt 1): 313–24.
- Cazeau S, Ritter P, Lazarus A, *et al*. Multisite pacing for end-stage heart failure: early experience. *Pacing Clin Electrophysiol* 1996; 19(11 Pt 2): 1748–57.
- Garrigue S, Jaïs P, Espil G, *et al*. Comparison of chronic biventricular pacing between epicardial and endocardial left ventricular stimulation using Doppler tissue imaging in patients with heart failure. *Am J Cardiol* 2001; 88(8): 858–62.
- van Gelder BM, Bracke FA, Meijer A, Lakerveld LJ, Pijls NH. Effect of optimizing the VV interval on left ventricular contractility in cardiac resynchronization therapy. *Am J Cardiol* 2004; 93(12): 1500–3.

- Gras D, Mabo P, Tang T, *et al.* Multisite pacing as a supplemental treatment of congestive heart failure: preliminary results of the Medtronic Inc. In Sync Study. *Pacing Clin Electrophysiol* 1998; 21(11 Pt 2): 2249–55.
- Kerwin WF, Botvinick EH, O'Connell JW, *et al.* Ventricular contraction abnormalities in dilated cardiomyopathy: effect of biventricular pacing to correct interventricular dyssynchrony. *J Am Coll Cardiol* 2000; 35(5): 1221–7.
- Linde C, Rydén L. Pacing in dilated cardiomyopathy. *Pacing Clin Electrophysiol* 1995; 18(7): 1341–5.
- Nelson GS, Berger RD, Fetics BJ, *et al.* Left ventricular or biventricular pacing improves cardiac function at diminished energy cost in patients with dilated cardiomyopathy and left bundle-branch block. *Circulation* 2001; 103(3): 476.
- Nelson GS, Curry CW, Wyman BT, *et al.* Predictors of systolic augmentation from left ventricular preexcitation in patients with dilated cardiomyopathy and intraventricular conduction delay. *Circulation* 2000; 101(23): 2703–9.
- de Teresa E, Chamorro JL, Pulpon A, *et al.* An even more physiological pacing: changing the sequence of ventricular activation. In: Steinbach KG, Laskovics A, eds. Cardiac Pacing. Proceedings of the 7th World Symposium on Cardiac Pacing. Darmstadt, Germany: Steinkopff-Verlag; 1983: 395–401.

The first series of patients

Acute haemodynamic effects of biventricular DDD pacing in end-stage heart failure

Leclercq C, Cazeau S, Le Breton H, Ritter P, Mabo P, Gras D, Pavin D, Lazarus A, Daubert JC. *J Am Coll Cardiol* 1998; 32(7): 1825–31.

Background

Following Cazeau's report of four patients treated with CRT, increasing interest focused on the deleterious effect of electrical dyssynchrony on cardiac function. In addition, the neutral or even deleterious effects of right ventricular pacing in patients with left ventricular systolic dysfunction was being increasingly recognized. At this point, there was a need to further understand the haemodynamic effects of CRT in patients with heart failure.

Main hypothesis

In patients with advanced heart failure and evidence of electrical interventricular dysynchrony (LBBB on ECG), CRT (biventricular pacing) leads to an acute haemodynamic response.

Methods

A total of 18 patients with heart failure (NYHA class III and IV, left ventricular ejection fraction—LVEF of $19 \pm 4.5\%$ and QRS duration of 170 ± 37 msec), on optimal medical therapy, underwent invasive haemodynamic monitoring (pulmonary artery (PA) pressures, PCWP, and cardiac output). Temporary pacing wires were inserted via femoral or subclavian veins and deployed in the right atrial appendage, coronary sinus (to pace the left atrium), right ventricular apex or outflow tract (to pace the right ventricle at different sites), and lateral or posterolateral cardiac veins (to pace the left ventricle). Three different pacing modes were compared at a rate of ten beats per minute (bpm) above spontaneous sinus rate: AAI—biatrial pacing with intrinsic conduction (used as control); DDD RV—pacing the atria followed by RV pacing (apical or septal, whichever provided the highest cardiac output) and DDD BV—pacing the atria followed by biventricular pacing.

Results

Compared with control (AAI pacing), biventricular pacing (DDD BV) was associated with a 35% increase in cardiac index (2.7 ± 7 vs. 2 ± 0.4 L/min/m^2, p <0.001) and a 18.5% reduction in PCWP (22 ± 8 vs. 27 ± 9 mmHg, p <0.001). Compared to right ventricular pacing (DDD RV), biventricular pacing resulted in a smaller (12.5%) but significant improvement in cardiac index (2.7 ± 7 vs. 2.4 ± 0.6 L/min/m^2, p <0.01) and a 9% reduction in PCWP (22 ± 8 vs. 24 ± 8 mmHg, p <0.01). Biventricular pacing was also associated with a non-significant but detectable rise in systolic and diastolic blood pressure compared to control and RV pacing (127 ± 15, 115 ± 10 and 122 ± 6 mmHg, respectively). Interestingly, no haemodynamic response to biventricular pacing was observed in 6/18 patients (33% deemed 'non-responders'). An attempt was made to identify predictors of haemodynamic response to biventricular pacing but the small number of subjects was a clear limitation.

Conclusions

This study enrolled the first series of patients with advanced heart failure and confirmed the acute haemodynamic benefits that could be derived from biventricular pacing suggested by previous case reports. Even a small number of subjects were sufficient to show improvements in cardiac output and a reduction in PCWP.

Learning points

◆ The acute improvement in cardiac function in this small but high impact study provided the initial support for biventricular pacing as a therapeutic option for patients with LBBB, QRS >120 and NYHA class III–IV. With the benefit of hindsight, the issue of 'non-responders' evolved from this work. Patients who did not demonstrate a 10% improvement in cardiac index were labelled as such. Additionally, this observation occurred in 33% of the patients, in agreement with current observations.

Further reading

• Blendea D, Singh JP. Lead positioning strategies to enhance response to cardiac resynchronization therapy. *Heart Fail Rev* 2011; 16(3): 291–303.

• Bordachar P, Ploux S, Ritter P. Three left ventricular leads required for improved haemodynamic and clinical status of a patient with very severe heart failure and a narrow QRS duration. *Europace* 2011;13(3):439. (Epub 20 Dec 2010).

• Delnoy PP, Ottervanger JP, Vos DH, *et al.* Upgrading to biventricular pacing guided by pressure-volume loop analysis during implantation. *J Cardiovasc Electrophysiol* 2011; 22(6): 677–83.

• Duckett SG, Ginks M, Shetty AK, *et al.* Invasive acute hemodynamic response to guide left ventricular lead implantation predicts chronic remodelling in patients undergoing cardiac resynchronization therapy. *J Am Coll Cardiol* 2011 6; 58(11): 1128–36.

• Gold MR, Niazi I, Giudici M, *et al.* A prospective, randomized comparison of the acute hemodynamic effects of biventricular and left ventricular pacing with cardiac resynchronization therapy. *Heart Rhythm* 2011; 8(5): 685–91. (Epub 27 Dec 2010).

• Khan FZ, Virdee MS, Read PA, *et al.* Impact of VV optimization in relation to left ventricular lead position: an acute haemodynamic study. *Europace* 2011; 13(6): 845–52. (Epub 21 Mar 2011).

• Shetty AK, Duckett SG, Bostock J, Rosenthal E, Rinaldi CA. Use of a quadripolar left ventricular lead to achieve successful implantation in patients with previous failed attempts at cardiac resynchronization therapy. *Europace* 2011; 13(7): 992–6. (Epub 22 Feb 2011).

The MUSTIC study

Effects of multisite biventricular pacing in patients with heart failure and interventricular conduction delay

Cazeau S, Leclercq C, Lavergene T, Walker S, Varma C, Linde C, Garrigue S, Kappenberger L, Haywood GA, Santini M, Bailleul C, Daubert JC; Multisite Stimulation in Cardiomyopathies (MUSTIC) Study Investigators. *N Engl J Med* 2001; 344: 873–80.

Background

Case reports and small uncontrolled studies had shown that biventricular pacing was associated with haemodynamic and symptomatic benefit in patients with advanced heart failure and electrocardiographic evidence of dyssynchrony. A controlled trial was needed to assess CRT's efficacy and safety and to start defining its role as a therapeutic modality in heart failure.

Main hypothesis

The study was designed to assess whether multisite pacing would be clinically safe and associated with improvements in symptoms and exercise tolerance in patients with advanced heart failure and evidence of electrical dyssynchrony.

Methods

The study enrolled 67 patients with NYHA class III heart failure due to left ventricular systolic dysfunction, in sinus rhythm and with a QRS duration of more than 150 msec. It was a single-blinded, crossover study in which subjects received a biventricular pacemaker and were randomly assigned to one of two groups: a three-month period of inactive pacing (CRT-off—where the device was set to VVI 40 bpm) or three months of active biventricular pacing (CRT-on). The initial stage was followed by a crossover phase in which the other pacing parameter was used (CRT on vs. off). The primary end point was the distance walked in six minutes. The main secondary end point was the quality of life. Other secondary end points were hospitalization for heart failure, peak oxygen consumption, patient's choice of pacing modality (initial vs. final three-month period), and death from any cause.

Results

Implantation rate was high (92% initial success and 88% with a functional LV lead at the end of study). No significant complications occurred during and immediately after device implantation. Eight patients had the LV lead displaced, of which five were re-positioned successfully. When compared to CRT-off, CRT-on increased the distance walked in six minutes by 23% (399 ± 100 m vs. 326 ±134 m, p <0.001), the quality of life score by 32% (p <0.001), peak oxygen uptake by 8% (p <0.03) and decreased hospitalizations by 66% (3 vs. 9, p <0.05). Cardiac resynchronization therapy-on was the (blinded) choice of pacing modality for 85% of patients (p <0.001).

Limitations

This was a small study not powered to assess hard end points such as mortality. Also, the high number of initial drop-outs may have selected better responders, since the device function was optimized before randomization.

Conclusions

For the first time, in a controlled crossover study, CRT was shown to improve exercise tolerance and quality of life in patients with NYHA class III heart failure and electrocardiographic evidence of dyssynchrony.

Learning points

- This effort was the first step to move from a research study to a study focused on safety and clinical benefit. Although underpowered and not randomized, this study did meet its objective.

Further reading

- Alonso C, Ritter P, Leclercq C, Mabo P, Bailleul C, Daubert JC; MUSTIC Study Group. Effects of cardiac resynchronization therapy on heart rate variability in patients with chronic systolic heart failure and intraventricular conduction delay. *Am J Cardiol*. 2003; 91(9): 1144–7.
- Cazeau S, Leclercq C, Lavergne T, Garrigue S, Bailleul C, Daubert JC; Groupe des investigateurs MUSTIC. (MUSTIC trial). *Arch Mal Coeur Vaiss* 2002; 95 Spec 4(5 Spec 4): 33–6.
- Duncan A, Wait D, Gibson D, Daubert JC; MUSTIC (Multisite Stimulationin Cardiomyopathies) Trial. Left ventricular remodelling and haemodynamic effects of multisite biventricular pacing in patients with left ventricular systolic dysfunction and activation disturbances in sinus rhythm: sub-study of the MUSTIC (Multisite Stimulationin Cardiomyopathies) trial. *Eur Heart J* 2003; 24(5): 430–41.
- Linde C, Braunschweig F, Gadler F, Bailleul C, Daubert JC. Long-term improvements in quality of life by biventricular pacing in patients with chronic heart failure: results from the Multisite Stimulation in Cardiomyopathy study (MUSTIC). *Am J Cardiol* 2003; 91(9): 1090–5.
- Linde C, Leclercq C, Rex S, *et al.* Long-term benefits of biventricular pacing in congestive heart failure: results from the MUltisite STimulation in cardiomyopathy (MUSTIC) study. *J Am Coll Cardiol* 2002; 40(1): 111–8.
- Salukhe TV, Dimopoulos K, Francis D. Cardiac resynchronisation may reduce all-cause mortality: meta-analysis of preliminary COMPANION data with CONTAK-CD, InSync ICD, MIRACLE and MUSTIC. *Int J Cardiol* 2004; 93(2–3): 101–3.
- Varma C, Sharma S, Firoozi S, McKenna WJ, Daubert JC; Multisite Stimulation in Cardiomyopathy (MUSTIC) Study Group. Atriobiventricular pacing improves exercise capacity in patients with heart failure and intraventricular conduction delay. *J Am Coll Cardiol* 2003; 41(4): 582–8.
- Witte K, Thackray S, Clark AL, Cooklin M, Cleland JG. Clinical trials update: IMPROVEMENT-HF, COPERNICUS, MUSTIC, ASPECT-II, APRICOT and HEART. *Eur J Heart Fail* 2000; 2(4): 455–60.

The first randomized, double-blind and controlled CRT trial

Multicenter InSync Randomized Clinical Evaluation (MIRACLE)

Abraham WT, Fisher WG, Smith AL, Delurgio DB, Leon AR, Loh E, Kocovic DZ, Packer M, Clavell AL, Hayes DL, Ellestad M, Trupp RJ, Underwood J, Pickering F, Truex C, McAtee P, Messenger J; MIRACLE Study Group.
N Engl J Med 2002; 346 (24): 1845–53.

Background

Several small, uncontrolled studies had suggested that CRT could be beneficial for patients with heart failure and a broad QRS on the ECG. Improvement in exercise capacity and evidence of left ventricular reverse remodelling had been demonstrated. These hypothesis-generating studies needed to be backed up by a large, blinded, controlled trial which could establish the safety of CRT as a therapeutic tool.

Main hypothesis

Cardiac resynchronization therapy improves symptoms, quality of life, and exercise tolerance in patients with advanced heart failure and optimal medical therapy and would prove to be a safe and clinically applicable therapeutic modality.

Methods

The MIRACLE study was the first randomized, double-blind and controlled trial in CRT. A group of 453 patients with optimally treated NYHA class III/IV heart failure, EF <35% and QRS duration >130 msec were randomly assigned to biventricular pacing or no pacing at all (both groups received the device and were blinded to treatment modality). Primary end points were NYHA functional class, distance walked in six-minute walk test and quality of life (as assessed by the Minnesota Living with Heart Failure score). Secondary end points included peak oxygen consumption, LVEF, and volumes and severity of mitral regurgitation. Other variables analysed included death, worsening of heart failure and days spent in hospital. Intention to treat analyses were used.

Results

Safety of CRT implantation: of the 571 initially enrolled patients, 4 experienced adverse clinical events during implant (2 patients developed complete heart block and 2 died as a complication of the implant). Coronary sinus dissection occurred in 4% and perforation of a cardiac vein in 2%. Left ventricle lead replacement or repositioning was required in 5% of patients. Device related infection requiring explantation occurred in 1.3%.

Primary end points: at six months, CRT was associated with an improvement in all parameters assessed (6-minute walk test: 39 m vs. 10 m; p = 0.005/Quality of life assessment -18 vs. -9 points; p = 0.001/Improvement in NYHA status; p <0.001).

Secondary end points: CRT increased peak oxygen consumption (1.1 ml/kg/min vs. 0.2 ml/kg/min; p = 0.009) and total exercise time on treadmill (time increased by 81 sec vs. 19 sec; p = 0.001). Also, patients with CRT showed a small but consistent evidence of reverse remodelling (LV end-diastolic dimension decreased by 3.5 mm vs. 0.0 mm; p <0.001/LVEF increased by 4.6% vs. -0.2%; p <0.001). Finally, CRT was associated with less hospitalization rates, total hospitalization days, and need for intravenous diuretic therapy (all p <0.05). Death from any cause was not statistically different between CRT and controls (12 vs. 16; p = 0.4)

Limitations

The study had a short follow-up (six months) and was not designed to assess the long-term effects of CRT, a question that would be answered by subsequent larger clinical trials.

Conclusions

The MIRACLE study was the first randomized, controlled, double-blind clinical trial which demonstrated the safety and feasibility of CRT as a treatment modality in heart failure. It also confirmed the findings of previous small studies, showing that CRT was undoubtedly associated with clinical benefits and evidence of improved cardiac function.

Learning points

- The first randomized, double-blind study was successful and led to the development of CRT as a class I treatment.

Further reading

- Adamson PB. Cardiac resynchronization therapy—how big of a miracle? *Curr Heart Fail Rep* 2004; 1(1): 30–5.
- Aranda JM Jr, Conti JB, Johnson JW, Petersen-Stejskal S, Curtis AB. Cardiac resynchronization therapy in patients with heart failure and conduction abnormalities other than left bundle-branch block: analysis of the Multicenter InSync Randomized Clinical Evaluation (MIRACLE). *Clin Cardiol* 2004; 27(12): 678–82.
- Egoavil CA, Ho RT, Greenspon AJ, Pavri BB. Cardiac resynchronization therapy in patients with right bundle branch block: analysis of pooled data from the MIRACLE and Contak CD trials. *Heart Rhythm* 2005; 2(6): 611–5.
- Kron J, Aranda JM Jr, Miles WM, *et al.* Benefit of cardiac resynchronization in elderly patients: results from the Multicenter InSync Randomized Clinical Evaluation (MIRACLE) and Multicenter InSync ICD Randomized Clinical Evaluation (MIRACLE-ICD) trials. *J Interv Card Electrophysiol* 2009; 25(2): 91–6. (Epub 19 Jan 2009).
- León AR, Abraham WT, Curtis AB, *et al.*; MIRACLE Study Program. Safety of transvenous cardiac resynchronization system implantation in patients with chronic heart failure: combined results of over 2000 patients from a multicentre study program. *J Am Coll Cardiol* 2005; 46(12): 2348–56.
- Pires LA, Abraham WT, Young JB, Johnson KM; MIRACLE and MIRACLE-ICD Investigators. Clinical predictors and timing of New York Heart Association class improvement with cardiac resynchronization therapy in patients with advanced chronic heart failure: results from the Multicenter InSync Randomized Clinical Evaluation (MIRACLE) and Multicenter InSync ICD Randomized Clinical Evaluation (MIRACLE-ICD) trials. *Am Heart J* 2006; 151(4): 837–43.
- Reynolds MR, Joventino LP, Josephson ME; Miracle ICD Investigators. Relationship of baseline electrocardiographic characteristics with the response to cardiac resynchronization therapy for heart failure. *Pacing Clin Electrophysiol* 2004; 27(11): 1513–8.
- St John Sutton MG, Plappert T, Abraham WT, *et al.*; Multicenter InSync Randomized Clinical Evaluation (MIRACLE) Study Group. Effect of cardiac resynchronization therapy on left ventricular size and function in chronic heart failure. *Circulation* 2003; 107(15): 1985–90. (Epub 31 Mar 2003).
- Sutton MG, Plappert T, Hilpisch KE, Abraham WT, Hayes DL, Chinchoy E. Sustained reverse left ventricular structural remodeling with cardiac resynchronization at one year is a function of etiology: quantitative Doppler echocardiographic evidence from the Multicenter InSync Randomized Clinical Evaluation (MIRACLE). *Circulation* 2006; 113(2): 266–72.
- Woo GW, Petersen-Stejskal S, Johnson JW, Conti JB, Aranda JA Jr, Curtis AB. Ventricular reverse remodeling and 6-month outcomes in patients receiving cardiac resynchronization therapy: analysis of the MIRACLE study. *J Interv Card Electrophysiol* 2005; 12(2): 107–13.
- Young JB, Abraham WT, Smith AL, *et al.*; Multicenter InSync ICD Randomized Clinical Evaluation (MIRACLE ICD) Trial Investigators. Combined cardiac resynchronization and implantable cardioversion defibrillation in advanced chronic heart failure: the MIRACLE ICD Trial. *JAMA* 2003; 289(20): 2685–94.

Comparison of Medical Therapy, Pacing, and Defibrillation in Heart Failure

Cardiac resynchronization of therapy with or without an implantable defibrillator in advanced heart failure

Bristow MR, Saxon LA, Boehmer J, Krueger S, Kass D, De Marco T, Carson P, DiCarlo L, DeMets D, White BG; for the Comparison of Medical Therapy, Pacing and Defibrillation in Heart Failure (COMPANION) Investigators. *N Eng J Med* 2004; 350: 2140–50.

Background

Cardiac resynchronization therapy was known to improve cardiac function and symptoms in patients with advanced heart failure. However, its mid to long-term impact on major cardiovascular end points, such as death and heart failure events, was not known. Also, the additional benefits of CRT over an implantable defibrillator (ICD) were yet to be investigated. The COMPANION trial was the first randomized, controlled trial which compared CRT (with and without an ICD) against optimal medical therapy in advanced heart failure.

Main hypothesis

In patients with advanced heart failure due to left ventricular systolic dysfunction and evidence of intraventricular conduction delay on the ECG, CRT would reduce the composite end point of death and hospitalization from any cause.

Methods

The COMPANION study was a multi-centre, randomized trial which enrolled 1520 patients with chronic heart failure and the following criteria: NYHA class III or IV; EF <35%; QRS duration >120 msec and PR interval >150 msec; sinus rhythm, and no indication for a pacemaker. Patients were assigned in a 1:2:2 ratio to one of three groups: optimal medical therapy (ACE-i, betablockers, spironolactone, and diuretics), CRT with a defibrillator (CRT-D) and CRT without a defibrillator (CRT-P). Patients and clinicians were not blinded to the assignments. The primary end point was a composite of death from and hospitalization for any cause. The main secondary end point was death from any cause. Other secondary end points analysed were death and hospitalization caused by heart failure. The study was event driven.

Results

Similarly to previous studies, successful implantation rate of the devices was high (90%). Death related to procedure complications occurred in 0.8% and 0.5% of, respectively, CRT-P and CRT-D implants.

Primary end point: when compared to pharmacological therapy alone, CRT-P reduced the risk of death from and hospitalization for any cause (68% vs. 56%; HR 0.81; 95% CI 0.69–0.96; p = 0.014); a similar benefit was found in the CRT-D group (56% HR 0.8; 95% CI 0.68–0.95; p = 0.010). Overall relative risk reduction (RRR) with CRT was 20%; absolute risk reduction (ARR) was approximately 12%.

Secondary end points: there was a significant decrease in the incidence of death from any cause in the CRT-D group (HR 0.64; 95% CI 0.48–0.86; p = 0.004; RRR = 36%), with a marginally significant benefit in the CRT-P group (HR 0.76; 95% CI 0.58–1.01; p = 0.06). Cardiac resynchronization therapy also significantly reduced the incidence of death from or hospitalization for heart failure (CRT-P HR 0.66; 95% CI 0.53–0.87; p = 0.002; RRR = 34% and CRT-D HR 0.60; 95% CI 0.49–0.75; p <0.001; RRR = 40%). Subgroup analysis revealed a greater benefit of CRT-D in patients with non-ischaemic cardiomyopathy, reducing the risk of death from any cause by 50% (HR = 0.50; 95% CI 0.29–0.88; p = 0.015), when compared to pharmacological therapy. The benefit of CRT-D on death from any cause was not statistically significant in patients with ischaemic cardiomyopathy (HR 0.73; 95% CI 0.52–1.04).

Limitations

As with other previous CRT studies, patients and clinicians were not blinded to treatment modality. As a consequence, there was an unexpectedly high withdrawal rate from the pharmacological group (26%), as patients and clinicians opted to have a device implanted.

Conclusions

The COMPANION study was the first large, randomized, controlled clinical trial to demonstrate the effects of CRT in reducing mortality and major cardiovascular events in heart failure. It demonstrated that CRT-D was associated with clinical benefits that go beyond those achieved by CRT-P. The only unanswered question left by the trial was whether CRT-P could reduce death from any cause in this patient population, since the results did not reach statistical significance.

Learning points

◆ The COMPANION study added an important aspect, the impact on death and hospitalization, to the findings from MIRACLE. These two studies provided sufficient proof relating CRT with improved health outcomes.

Further reading

- Anand IS, Carson P, Galle E, *et al*. Cardiac resynchronization therapy reduces the risk of hospitalizations in patients with advanced heart failure: results from the Comparison of Medical Therapy, Pacing and Defibrillation in Heart Failure (COMPANION) trial. *Circulation* 2009; 119(7): 969–77. (Epub 9 Feb 2009).
- Carson P, Anand I, O'Connor C, *et al*. Mode of death in advanced heart failure: the Comparison of Medical, Pacing, and Defibrillation Therapies in Heart Failure (COMPANION) trial. *J Am Coll Cardiol* 2008; 51(22): 2197.
- De Marco T, Wolfel E, Feldman AM, *et al*. Impact of cardiac resynchronization therapy on exercise performance, functional capacity, and quality of life in systolic heart failure with QRS prolongation: COMPANION trial sub-study. *J Card Fail* 2008; 14(1): 9–18.
- Feldman AM, de Lissovoy G, Bristow MR, *et al*. Cost effectiveness of cardiac resynchronization therapy in the Comparison of Medical Therapy, Pacing, and Defibrillation in Heart Failure (COMPANION) trial. *J Am Coll Cardiol* 2005; 46(12): 2311–21.
- Olshansky B, Day JD, Sullivan RM, Yong P, Galle E, Steinberg JS. Does cardiac resynchronization therapy provide unrecognized benefit in patients with prolonged PR intervals? The impact of restoring atrioventricular synchrony: An analysis from the COMPANION Trial. *Heart Rhythm* 2011. (Epub 9 Aug 2011).

- Salukhe TV, Dimopoulos K, Francis D. Cardiac resynchronisation may reduce all-cause mortality: meta-analysis of preliminary COMPANION data with CONTAK-CD, InSync ICD, MIRACLE and MUSTIC. *Int J Cardiol* 2004; 93(2–3): 101–3.
- Salukhe TV, Francis DP, Sutton R. Comparison of medical therapy, pacing and defibrillation in heart failure (COMPANION) trial terminated early; combined biventricular pacemaker-defibrillators reduce all-cause mortality and hospitalization. *Int J Cardiol* 2003; 87(2–3): 119–20.
- Sauer WH, Bristow MR. The Comparison of Medical Therapy, Pacing, and Defibrillation in Heart Failure (COMPANION) trial in perspective. *J Interv Card Electrophysiol* 2008; 21(1): 3–11. (Epub 28 Nov 2007).
- Saxon LA, Bristow MR, Boehmer J, *et al.* Predictors of sudden cardiac death and appropriate shock in the Comparison of Medical Therapy, Pacing, and Defibrillation in Heart Failure (COMPANION) Trial. *Circulation.* 2006; 114(25): 2766–72. (Epub 11 Dec 2006).
- Saxon LA, Olshansky B, Volosin K, *et al.* Influence of left ventricular lead location on outcomes in the COMPANION study. *J Cardiovasc Electrophysiol* 2009; 20(7): 764–8. (Epub 27 Feb 2009).

The effect of CRT alone in reducing total mortality

The effect of cardiac resynchronization on morbidity and mortality in heart failure.

Cleland JGF, Daubert J-C, Erdmann E, Freemantle N, Gras D, Kappenberger L, Tavazzi L; for the Cardiac Resynchronization-Heart Failure (CARE-HF) study investigators. *N Eng J Med* 2005; 352: 1539–49.

Background

It was known that cardiac resynchronization therapy was associated with improvements in left ventricular function and symptoms in patients with advanced heart failure and evidence of electrical dyssynchrony. Also, the COMPANION trial and previous meta-analyses had shown that CRT (with or without a defibrillator) reduced the composite end point of death *and* hospitalization. However, the question as to whether CRT alone could reduce death from any cause was still open. The CARE-HF was a study designed to answer this question.

Main hypothesis

In patients with advanced heart failure due to left ventricular systolic dysfunction and evidence of electromechanical dyssynchrony, CRT would reduce death from any cause without leading to significant complications.

Methods

The CARE-HF study was a multi-centre, international, randomized trial in which 813 patients were enrolled and followed up for a mean of 29.4 months. Inclusion criteria were the following: symptoms of heart failure for at least six weeks, NYHA class III or IV despite optimal pharmacological therapy; left ventricular systolic dysfunction, EF <35% and left ventricular end diastolic diameter—LVEDD >30 mm; QRS interval of at least 150 msec, or 120–150 msec and evidence of two out of three criteria for mechanical dyssynchrony on echocardiography (aortic pre-ejection time >140 msec, interventricular mechanical delay >40 msec or delayed activation of the left ventricular posterolateral wall). Patients with a conventional indication for a pacemaker and those with atrial arrhythmias were excluded. Patients were randomized in a non-blinded fashion to optimal medical therapy with or without CRT (atrial and biventricular pacing without a defibrillator). The primary end point was a composite of death from any cause or hospitalization for a major cardiac event, with only the first event for each patient considered in the analysis. The secondary end points included death from any cause and NYHA and quality of life scores at 90 days.

Results

A group of 409 patients were allocated to the CRT group, with 95% successfully receiving a device; 404 patients were assigned to receive medical therapy only. The groups represented patients with moderate to severe heart failure (only 43% on high dose diuretics) with similar baseline characteristics. The mean duration of follow-up was 29.4 months.

Primary end point: CRT reduced the composite incidence of death from any cause or hospitalization (39% vs. 55%; HR = 0.63; 95% CI 0.51 to 0.77; p <0.001). Cardiac resynchronization therapy also reduced the incidence of death from any cause (20% vs. 30%; HR = 0.64; 95% CI 0.48–0.85; p <0.002).

Secondary end points: CRT increased LVEF, improved indices of electromechanical delay, and reduced end-systolic volumes and amount of mitral regurgitation; it also improved symptoms and the quality of life (p <0.01). In terms of absolute benefit, the number of patients needed to be treated (NNT) with CRT to prevent one death was nine, a benefit similar to pharmacological agents such as beta blockers. Overall benefits were similar among patients with ischaemic and non-ischaemic cardiomyopathy.

Limitations

The study was not blinded to patients or clinicians. Echocardiographic parameters used to define the level of dyssynchrony needed for successful response to CRT are now recognized as inaccurate and may have excluded other patients who could have benefited from device therapy.

Conclusions

The CARE-HF trial was the first randomized-controlled study to show that CRT-pacing (without a defibrillator) reduces mortality from any cause in patients with NYHA class III and IV heart failure and evidence of electrical dyssynchrony. Together with COMPANION, CARE-HF formed the basis of guideline recommendations for the use of CRT.

Learning points

◆ Cardiac resynchronization therapy without a defibrillator can reduce mortality in patients suffering from heart failure and a wide QRS complex.

Further reading

- Berger R, Shankar A, Fruhwald F, *et al.* Relationships between cardiac resynchronization therapy and N-terminal pro-brain natriuretic peptide in patients with heart failure and markers of cardiac dyssynchrony: an analysis from the Cardiac Resynchronization in Heart Failure (CARE-HF) study. *Eur Heart J* 2009; 30(17): 2109–16. (Epub 2 Jun 2009).
- Calvert MJ, Freemantle N, Yao G, *et al.*; CARE-HF investigators. Cost-effectiveness of cardiac resynchronization therapy: results from the CARE-HF trial. *Eur Heart J* 2005; 26(24): 2681–8. (Epub 11 Nov 2005).
- Cleland JG, Freemantle N, Ghio S, *et al.* Predicting the long-term effects of cardiac resynchronization therapy on mortality from baseline variables and the early response a report from the CARE-HF (Cardiac Resynchronization in Heart Failure) Trial. *J Am Coll Cardiol* 2008; 52(6): 438–45.
- Cleland JG, Calvert MJ, Verboven Y, Freemantle N. Effects of cardiac resynchronization therapy on long-term quality of life: an analysis from the CArdiac Resynchronisation-Heart Failure (CARE-HF) study. *Am Heart J* 2009; 157(3): 457–66. (Epub 20 Jan 2009).
- Cleland JG, Daubert JC, Erdmann E, *et al.* Longer-term effects of cardiac resynchronization therapy on mortality in heart failure (the CArdiac REsynchronization-Heart Failure (CARE-HF) trial extension phase). *Eur Heart J* 2006; 27(16): 1928–32. (Epub 16 Jun 2006).
- Cleland JG, Daubert JC, Erdmann E, *et al.*; CARE-HF study Steering Committee and Investigators. Baseline characteristics of patients recruited into the CARE-HF study. *Eur J Heart Fail* 2005; 7(2): 205–14.
- Cleland JG, Freemantle N, Daubert JC, Toff WD, Leisch F, Tavazzi L. Long-term effect of cardiac resynchronisation in patients reporting mild symptoms of heart failure: a report from the CARE-HF study. *Heart* 2008; 94(3): 278–83. (Epub 5 Nov 2007).
- Edner M, Kim Y, Hansen KN, *et al.* Prevalence and inter-relationship of different Doppler measures of dyssynchrony in patients with heart failure and prolonged QRS: a report from CARE-HF. *Cardiovasc Ultrasound* 2009; 7: 1.
- Gervais R, Leclercq C, Shankar A, *et al.*; CARE-HF investigators. Surface electrocardiogram to predict outcome in candidates for cardiac resynchronization therapy: a sub-analysis of the CARE-HF trial. *Eur J Heart Fail* 2009; 11(7): 699–705. (Epub 7 Jun 2009).
- Ghio S, Freemantle N, Scelsi L, *et al.* Long-term left ventricular reverse remodelling with cardiac resynchronization therapy: results from the CARE-HF trial. *Eur J Heart Fail* 2009; 11(5): 480–8. (Epub 14 Mar 2009).
- Richardson M, Freemantle N, Calvert MJ, Cleland JG, Tavazzi L; CARE-HF Study Steering Committee and Investigators. Predictors and treatment response with cardiac resynchronization therapy in patients with heart failure characterized by dyssynchrony: a pre-defined analysis from the CARE-HF trial. *Eur Heart J* 2007; 28(15): 1827–34. (Epub 31 May 2007).
- Uretsky BF, Thygesen K, Daubert JC, *et al.* Predictors of mortality from pump failure and sudden cardiac death in patients with systolic heart failure and left ventricular dyssynchrony: results of the CARE-HF trial. *J Card Fail* 2008; 14(8): 670–5. (Epub 15 Jul 2008).
- Vatankulu MA, Goktekin O, Kaya MG, *et al.* Effect of long-term resynchronization therapy on left ventricular remodeling in pacemaker patients upgraded to biventricular devices. *Am J Cardiol* 2009; 103(9): 1280–4.
- Wikstrom G, Blomström-Lundqvist C, Andren B, *et al.*; CARE-HF study investigators. The effects of aetiology on outcome in patients treated with cardiac resynchronization therapy in the CARE-HF trial. *Eur Heart J* 2009; 30(7): 782–8. (Epub 24 Jan 2009).

A doubtful role for dyssynchrony imaging in patient selection

Results of the Predictors of Response to CRT (PROSPECT) Trial.

Chung E, Leon A, Tavazzi L, Sun J, Nihoyannopoulos P, Merlino J, Abraham W, Guio S, Leclerq C, Bax J, Yu C-M, Gorcsan III J, Sutton M, De Sutter J, Murillo J. *Circulation* 2008; 117(20): 2608–16.

Background

The most widely accepted paradigm underpinning CRT is that the syndrome of heart failure is partly due to dyssynchrony and that correction of dyssynchrony by CRT leads to a clinical benefit. In line with this paradigm, there has been a prevailing hypothesis according to which increasing severity of dyssynchrony pre-implant relates to a better response to CRT. Indeed, numerous single-centre studies in the early part of this century supported this hypothesis.

Main hypothesis

The Predictors of Response to CRT (PROSPECT) study tested the ability of echocardiographic measures of dyssynchrony to predict response to CRT.

Methods

In this prospective multi-centre study, comprising 53 centres in Europe, Hong Kong, and the United States, 498 patients were enrolled with standard CRT indications (NYHA class III or IV heart failure, LVEF ≤35%, QRS ≥130 msec, stable medical regimen). Twelve echocardiographic parameters of dyssynchrony, based on both conventional and tissue Doppler-based methods were utilized in the trial. Quality control of echocardiography was crucial in this study. In this regard, each centre was required to obtain accreditation from the echocardiography core laboratory in its region by providing high-quality images before enrolling any study subjects. Any studies judged to be of insufficient quality by the core laboratory were not included in the analysis. In addition, an independent echocardiographic review committee reviewed the core laboratory data. Response to CRT was evaluated through the use of two separately analysed primary outcomes at six months: heart failure clinical composite score (CCS) and relative change in left ventricular end systolic volume (LVESV). A patient's CCS was classified as one of the following:

◆ Worsened (the patient died or was hospitalized for or associated with worsening heart failure, demonstrated worsening in NYHA class at last observation carried forward, had moderate or marked worsening of patient global assessment score at last observation carried forward, or permanently discontinued CRT because of or associated with worsening heart failure).

◆ Improved (the patient had not worsened as defined above and demonstrated improvement in NYHA class at last observation carried forward or had moderate or marked improvement in patient global assessment score at last observation carried forward).

◆ Unchanged (the patient was neither improved nor worsened). Indicators of positive CRT response were improved clinical composite score and > or = 15% reduction in LVESV at six months.

Results

The CCS was improved in 69% of 426 patients, whereas LVESV decreased ≥15% in 56% of 286 patients with paired data. The ability of the 12 echocardiographic parameters to predict CCS response varied widely, with sensitivity ranging from 6% to 74% and specificity ranging from 35% to 91%; for predicting LVESV response, sensitivity ranged from 9% to 77% and specificity from 31% to 93%. For all the parameters, the area under the receiver-operating characteristics curve for positive clinical or volume response to CRT was ≤0.62.

Conclusions

The authors concluded that no single echocardiographic measure of dyssynchrony could be recommended to improve patient selection for CRT beyond current guidelines. It is the basis of this study that subsequent clinical guidelines for CRT, with the exception of the UK National Institute for Health and Clinical Excellence (NICE) guidance, that mechanical dyssynchrony was excluded as a criterion for patient selection.

Learning points

◆ The PROSPECT trial was unsuccessful in identifying an echocardiographic parameter that would have been used to select patients at risk for being non-responders. However, the trial was designed at a time when novel echocardiographic techniques were being discovered for use in CRT.

Further reading

- Abraham T, Kass D, Tonti G, *et al*. Imaging cardiac resynchronization therapy. *JACC Cardiovasc Imaging* 2009; 2(4): 486–97.
- Aggarwal NR, Martinez MW, Gersh BJ, Chareonthaitawee P. Role of cardiac MRI and nuclear imaging in cardiac resynchronization therapy. *Nat Rev Cardiol* 2009; 6(12): 759–70. (Epub 3 Nov 2009).
- Bilchick KC, Lardo AC. Cardiac resynchronization therapy: application of imaging to optimize patient selection and assess response. *Curr Heart Fail Rep* 2008; 5(3): 119–27.
- Bleeker GB, Mollema SA, Holman ER, *et al*. Left ventricular resynchronization is mandatory for response to cardiac resynchronization therapy: analysis in patients with echocardiographic evidence of left ventricular dyssynchrony at baseline. *Circulation* 2007; 116(13): 1440–8. (Epub 4 Sep 2007).
- Boogers MM, Chen J, Bax JJ. Role of nuclear imaging in cardiac resynchronization therapy. *Expert Rev Cardiovasc Ther* 2009; 7(1): 65–72.
- Breithardt OA. Echocardiographic patient selection for cardiac resynchronization therapy: betting on a dead horse? *JACC Cardiovasc Imaging* 2009; 2(5): 544–7.
- Burri H, Lerch R. Echocardiography and patient selection for cardiac resynchronization therapy: a critical appraisal. *Heart Rhythm* 2006; 3(4): 474–9.
- Chan PS, Khumri T, Chung ES, *et al*. Echocardiographic dyssynchrony and health status outcomes from cardiac resynchronization therapy: insights from the PROSPECT trial. *JACC Cardiovasc Imaging* 2010; 3(5): 451–60.
- Cleland JG, Tageldien A, Buga L, Wong K, Gorcsan J 3rd. Should we be trying to define responders to cardiac resynchronization therapy? *JACC Cardiovasc Imaging* 2010; 3(5): 541–9.
- Da Costa A, Thévenin J, Roche F, *et al*. Prospective validation of stress echocardiography as an identifier of cardiac resynchronization therapy responders. *Heart Rhythm* 2006; 3(4): 406–13.
- Goldenberg I, Moss AJ, Hall WJ, *et al*.; on behalf of the MADIT-CRT Executive Committee. Predictors of Response to Cardiac Resynchronization Therapy in the Multicenter Automatic Defibrillator Implantation Trial With Cardiac Resynchronization Therapy (MADIT-CRT). *Circulation* 2011; 124(14): 1527–36. (Epub 6 Sep 2011).
- Helm RH, Lardo AC. Cardiac magnetic resonance assessment of mechanical dyssynchrony. *Curr Opin Cardiol* 2008; 23(5): 440–6.
- Hsing JM, Selzman KA, Leclercq C, *et al*. Paced Left Ventricular QRS Width and ECG Parameters Predict Outcomes After Cardiac Resynchronization Therapy: PROSPECT-ECG Sub-Study. *Circ Arrhythm Electrophysiol* 28 Sep 2011 (Epub ahead of print).
- Leyva F. Cardiac resynchronization therapy guided by cardiovascular magnetic resonance. *J Cardiovasc Magn Reson* 2010; 12: 64.
- Popovic ZB, Thomas JD. In search of a holy grail: predicting cardiac resynchronization therapy outcomes by echocardiography. *Circ Cardiovasc Imaging* 2008; 1(1): 3–5.

CRT in NYHA classes I and II

Prevention of disease progression by cardiac resynchronization therapy in patients with asymptomatic or mildly symptomatic left ventricular dysfunction: insights from the European cohort of the REVERSE (Resynchronization Reverses Remodeling in Systolic Left Ventricular Dysfunction) trial

Daubert C, Gold MR, Abraham WT, Ghio S, Hassager C, Goode G, Szili-Torok T, Linde C; REVERSE Study Group. *J Am Coll Cardiol* 2009, 54(20): 1837–46.

Background

Cardiac resynchronization therapy was known to be effective in reducing major cardiac events, including total mortality, in patients with optimally treated, NYHA class III and IV heart failure, low EF (35%), and a wide QRS complex (>120 msec). Previous studies had reported that CRT in patients with less advanced disease could lead to improvement in LV function and reverse remodelling. The REVERSE trial aimed to investigate the effects of CRT in patients with NYHA I and II heart failure.

Main hypothesis

Cardiac resynchronization therapy would provide clinical benefits for NYHA class I and II heart failure patients with low ejection fraction (<40%) and a QRS duration of more than 120 msec.

Methods

Six hundred and ten patients with ischaemic and non-ischaemic cardiomyopathy were enrolled. Inclusion criteria were: NYHA class I or II symptoms (asymptomatic or mildly symptomatic patients); EF <40%; QRS duration >120 msec. All patients had a clinical indication for an ICD as per primary prevention guidelines. They were randomized in a 2:1 fashion to CRT-on (n = 419) versus CRT-off (n = 191). The primary end point of the study was a 'HF clinical composite response', which classified patients into three groups: worsened, unchanged, or improved. This composite end point incorporated symptom-based and clinical criteria (hospitalization, etc.) and was used to improve sensitivity of the trial. Secondary end points included LVESV and EF. An intention to treat analysis was used.

Results

At 12 months, CRT-on was not associated with a reduction of HF composite end points when compared to CRT-off (16% of patients with CRT worsened their status compared to 21% without it, p = 0.1). Cardiac resynchronization therapy also showed no benefit on quality of life scores and six-minute walk test. On secondary end points, CRT-on was associated with objective evidence of reverse remodelling. There was a significant reduction in LVESV index (18.4 ± 29.5 ml/m^2 vs. 1.3 ± 23.4 ml/m^2, p <0.001), an effect which was three times greater in patients with non-ischaemic cardiomyopathy compared with those with ischaemic disease. There was also a significant but small improvement in LVEF (from 27% to 31% in the CRT-on group). Cardiac resynchronization therapy was also associated with a delayed time to first hospitalization for heart failure (HR = 0.47, p = 0.03).

Limitations

The 'HF composite response' categorical end point was specifically chosen to improve the sensitivity of the trial to detect relatively small clinical benefits. Despite this unusual end point, CRT was not associated with a significant clinical benefit after 12 months. This suggests REVERSE was a relatively underpowered study to assess major cardiac end points in a population of patients with NYHA class I and II symptoms of heart failure. Also, the relatively small number of subjects widened the confidence interval of LV measurements (volume and ejection fraction).

Conclusions

In a population of patients with mild heart failure symptoms (NYHA I and II) CRT was associated with objective evidence of LV reverse remodelling. These findings suggested that CRT could potentially retard the progression of heart failure in patients with milder symptoms.

Learning points

◆ A review of the literature regarding clinical and echocardiographic assessment of response to CRT shows no clear winner. However, the impact of CRT on reverse remodelling independent of the clinical impact provides similar evidence to that observed in the REVERSE trial.

Further reading

- Linde C, Abraham WT, Gold MR, Daubert C; REVERSE Study Group. Cardiac resynchronization therapy in asymptomatic or mildly symptomatic heart failure patients in relation to etiology: results from the REVERSE (REsynchronization reVErses Remodeling in Systolic left vEntricular dysfunction) study. *J Am Coll Cardiol* 2010; 56(22): 1826–31.
- Linde C, Abraham WT, Gold MR, St John Sutton M, Ghio S, Daubert C; REVERSE (REsynchronization reVErses Remodeling in Systolic left vEntricular dysfunction) Study Group. Randomized trial of cardiac resynchronization in mildly symptomatic heart failure patients and in asymptomatic patients with left ventricular dysfunction and previous heart failure symptoms. *J Am Coll Cardiol* 2008; 52(23): 1834–43. (Epub 7 Nov 2008).
- Linde C, Gold M, Abraham WT, Daubert JC; REVERSE Study Group. Baseline characteristics of patients randomized in The Resynchronization Reverses Remodeling. In Systolic Left Ventricular Dysfunction (REVERSE) study. *Congest Heart Fail* 2008; 14(2): 66–74.
- Linde C, Gold M, Abraham WT, Daubert JC; REVERSE Study Group. Rationale and design of a randomized controlled trial to assess the safety and efficacy of cardiac resynchronization therapy in patients with asymptomatic left ventricular dysfunction with previous symptoms or mild heart failure—the Resynchronization reVErses Remodeling in Systolic left vEntricular dysfunction (REVERSE) study. *Am Heart J* 2006; 151(2): 288–94.
- Linde C, Mealing S, Hawkins N, Eaton J, Brown B, Daubert JC; REVERSE study group. Cost-effectiveness of cardiac resynchronization therapy in patients with asymptomatic to mild heart failure: insights from the European cohort of the REVERSE (Resynchronization Reverses remodeling in Systolic Left Ventricular Dysfunction). *Eur Heart J* 2011; 32(13): 1631–9. (Epub 25 Nov 2010).
- St John Sutton M, Ghio S, Plappert T, *et al*.; REsynchronization reVErses Remodeling in Systolic left vEntricular

dysfunction (REVERSE) Study Group. Cardiac resynchronization induces major structural and functional reverse remodeling in patients with New York Heart Association class I/II heart failure. *Circulation* 2009; 120(19): 1858–65. (Epub 26 Oct 2009).

Multicenter Automatic Defibrillator Implantation Trial With Cardiac Resynchronization Therapy (MADIT-CRT)

Cardiac resynchronization therapy for the prevention of heart failure events

Moss AJ, Hall WJ, Cannom DS, Klein H, Brown MW, Daubert JP, Estes NA, 3rd, Foster E, Greenberg H, Higgins SL. Pfeffer MA, Solomon SD, Wilber D, Zareba W; MADIT-CRT Trial Investigators. *N Engl J Med* 2009, 361(14): 1329–38.

Background

The REVERSE trial demonstrated the effects of CRT on markers of reverse remodelling in patients with mild heart failure, improving LVEF and volumes. However, the impact of CRT on clinical heart failure end points in this population remained unknown.

Main hypothesis

The hypothesis was that CRT (biventricular pacing with ICD) would reduce the risk of death or non-fatal heart failure events in patients with NYHA class I and II heart failure, low EF (<30%), and a QRS duration of more than 130 msec, as compared to patients receiving ICD only.

Methods

This multi-centre trial involved 1820 patients with ischaemic and non-ischaemic cardiomyopathy who fulfilled the following criteria: class I or II NYHA symptoms (asymptomatic or mildly symptomatic patients); LVEF <30%, and a QRS duration >130 msec All patients met the guideline indication for ICD implantation for primary prevention. Therefore, they were randomized in a 3:2 ratio to CRT-D (n = 1089) versus ICD only (n = 731). The primary end point was death from any cause *or* non-fatal heart failure events (defined as the need for intravenous diuretic therapy in an outpatient regimen or an increase in heart-failure regimen during hospitalization), whichever came first. Average follow-up was for 2.4 years. An intention to treat analysis was used.

Results

Cardiac resynchronization therapy reduced the relative incidence of the primary end point (death from any cause *or* non-fatal heart failure events) events by 34% (hazard ratio of 0.66 [0.52–0.84], p = 0.001). The absolute reduction was 8% (185/731 [25.3%] in the ICD-only group vs. 187/1089 [17.2%] in the CRT-ICD group) with an NNT of 12 for 2.4 years. The benefits were mainly driven by a 41% relative reduction of heart failure events, with no difference in total mortality. The effects on heart failure and mortality were present in both ischaemic and non-ischaemic groups (HR of 0.67 and 0.62 respectively). Kaplan-Meier curves started to diverge within two months and continued to separate thereafter. As surrogate end points, CRT also increased EF (by 8% compared to ICD) and reduced LV volumes.

Limitations

This was not a blinded study (patients and doctors knew whether an LV lead was implanted). Physicians responsible for the diagnosis of heart failure events were also not blinded to assignment. Recruitment included 10% of patients with class I and II symptoms who were in class III less than three months before entering the trial (not truly mildly symptomatic patients). Also, the definition of heart failure events was criticized for lack of consistency and objectiveness. Subgroup analysis revealed that benefit occurred only in patients with QRS duration >150ms.

Conclusions

In comparison to ICD therapy, CRT-D reduced heart failure events in patients with milder symptoms (NYHA class I or II), poor ejection fraction, and broad QRS complex, without mortality benefit.

Further reading

- Barsheshet A, Wang PJ, Moss AJ, *et al.* Reverse remodeling and the risk of ventricular tachyarrhythmias in the MADIT-CRT (Multicenter Automatic Defibrillator Implantation Trial-Cardiac Resynchronization Therapy). *J Am Coll Cardiol* 2011; 57(24): 2416–23.

- Goldenberg I, Hall WJ, Beck CA, *et al.* Reduction of the risk of recurring heart failure events with cardiac resynchronization therapy: MADIT-CRT (Multicenter Automatic Defibrillator Implantation Trial With Cardiac Resynchronization Therapy). *J Am Coll Cardiol* 2011; 58(7): 729–37.
- Goldenberg I, Moss AJ, Hall WJ, *et al.*; on behalf of the MADIT-CRT Executive Committee. Predictors of Response to Cardiac Resynchronization Therapy in the Multicenter Automatic Defibrillator Implantation Trial With Cardiac Resynchronization Therapy (MADIT-CRT). *Circulation* 2011; 124(14): 1527–36. (Epub 6 Sep 2011).
- Moss AJ, Brown MW, Cannom DS, *et al.* Multicenter automatic defibrillator implantation trial-cardiac resynchronization therapy (MADIT-CRT): design and clinical protocol. *Ann Noninvasive Electrocardiol* 2005; 10(4 Suppl): 34–43.
- Pouleur AC, Knappe D, Shah AM, *et al.*; MADIT-CRT Investigators. Relationship between improvement in left ventricular dyssynchrony and contractile function and clinical outcome with cardiac resynchronization therapy: the MADIT-CRT trial. *Eur Heart J* 2011; 32(14): 1720–9. (Epub 24 May 2011).
- Singh JP, Klein HU, Huang DT, *et al.* Left ventricular lead position and clinical outcome in the multicenter automatic defibrillator implantation trial-cardiac resynchronization therapy (MADIT-CRT) trial. *Circulation* 2011; 123(11): 1159–66. (Epub 7 Mar 2011).
- Zareba W, Klein H, Cygankiewicz I, *et al.*; MADIT-CRT Investigators. Effectiveness of Cardiac Resynchronization Therapy by QRS Morphology in the Multicenter Automatic Defibrillator Implantation Trial-Cardiac Resynchronization Therapy (MADIT-CRT). *Circulation* 2011; 123(10): 1061–72. (Epub 28 Feb 2011).

CRT and a narrow QRS complex

Cardiac-resynchronization therapy in heart failure with narrow QRS complexes

Beshai J, Grimm R, Nagueh S, Baker J, Beau S, Greenberg S, Pires L, Tchou P; for the RethinQ Study Investigators. *N Eng J Med* 2007; 357: 2461–71.

Background

The benefits of CRT in patients with advanced heart failure and electrocardiographic evidence of dyssynchrony (QRS >120 msec) was already established, with several large-scale clinical trials demonstrating reduction in major cardiovascular events and total mortality. The evidence to use the ECG as a criteria for dyssynchrony was also established, with the most impressive clinical benefit of CRT observed in patients with a broader QRS complex (particularly >150 msec). Small uncontrolled studies suggested that patients with a narrow QRS complex could also potentially benefit from CRT, providing that they had echocardiographic evidence of dyssynchrony. The RethinQ trial was a study which could potentially expand the indications for CRT to patients with heart failure and a narrow QRS complex.

Main hypothesis

Cardiac resynchronization therapy would improve exercise tolerance and oxygen consumption in patients with advanced heart failure, narrow QRS complex, and echocardiographic evidence of dyssynchrony.

Methods

The RethinQ trial was a double-blind, randomized, controlled trial. A group of 172 patients who had an indication for an ICD received a CRT device and were randomly assigned to CRT (CRT and ICD on) or control (CRT-off with ICD-on). The inclusion criteria were: chronic heart failure due to ischaemic or non-ischaemic cardiomyopathy, an LVEF <35%, NYHA class III symptoms, a narrow QRS on a 12-lead ECG (less than 130 msec), and evidence of mechanical dyssynchrony on echocardiography.

Echocardiographic criteria for intraventricular dyssynchrony were: septal-to-posterior wall or septal-to-lateral wall delay of 65 msec or more as assessed by tissue Doppler imaging (TDI); septal-to-posterior wall motion delay of 130 msec or more as assessed by M-mode on paraesternal long axis view. The primary end point was the proportion of patients with an increase in peak oxygen consumption of at least 1 ml/kg/min at six months. Secondary end points included quality of life score, NYHA, six-minute walk test, and echocardiographic markers of reverse LV remodelling (EF and volumes).

Results

At six months, CRT was not associated with improvements in peak oxygen consumption (46% vs. 41%), quality of life score, or six-minute walk test distance. The CRT group had a significant improvement in NYHA class (54% vs. 29%; p = 0.006). Also, there was no difference between the two groups in echocardiographic parameters, such as LV volumes, EF, or degree of mitral regurgitation.

Limitations

The echocardiographic criteria used to established mechanical dyssynchrony were later found to be inaccurate markers of CRT response even in patients with broader QRS complex (PROSPECT study). Moreover, peak oxygen uptake is a doubtful surrogate measure of symptomatic or prognostic benefit in patients with heart failure. For example, the Multicenter InSync ICD Randomized Clinical Evaluation II (MIRACLE ICD II), a randomized, double-blind, parallel-controlled trial, showed that CRT led to an improvement in NYHA class, but not in peak oxygen uptake. It is noteworthy that although the RethinQ study found no benefit in terms of peak oxygen uptake, it did demonstrate an improvement in NYHA class.

Conclusions

Cardiac resynchronization therapy did not improve peak oxygen consumption, exercise tolerance, or quality of life in patients with advanced heart failure, left ventricular systolic dysfunction, narrow QRS complex, and evidence of mechanical dyssynchrony on echocardiography. Despite the negative findings of the RethinQ study, there is still intense interest on the possible application of CRT in the normal QRS duration population. Ongoing randomized controlled studies are addressing this issue.

Learning points

◆ In a focused study on patients with a narrow QRS, the benefit from CRT was not observed in terms of QoL, or six-minute walk test but did improve NYHA class.

Further reading

- Beshai JF, Khunnawat C, Lin AC. Mechanical dyssynchrony from the perspective of a cardiac electrophysiologist. *Curr Opin Cardiol* 2008; 23(5): 447–51.
- Foley PW, Patel K, Irwin N, *et al*. Cardiac resynchronisation therapy in patients with heart failure and a normal QRS duration: the RESPOND study. *Heart* 2011; 97(13): 1041–7. (Epub 21 Feb 2011).
- Holzmeister J, Hürlimann D, Steffel J, Ruschitzka F. Cardiac resynchronization therapy in patients with a narrow QRS. *Curr Heart Fail Rep* 2009; 6(1): 49–56.
- Mehta S, Asirvatham SJ. Rethinking QRS Duration as an Indication for CRT. *J Cardiovasc Electrophysiol* 2011. doi: 10.1111/j.1540-8167.2011.02163.x. (Epub ahead of print) PubMed PMID: 21914019.
- Williams LK, Ellery S, Patel K, *et al*. Short-term hemodynamic effects of cardiac resynchronization therapy in patients with heart failure, a narrow QRS duration, and no dyssynchrony. *Circulation* 2009; 120(17): 1687–94. (Epub 12 Oct 2009).

Conclusions

In this review, we have selected papers which we think most adequately trace the evolution of CRT research. We should not discount the important body of work on electrical and mechanical dyssynchrony that preceded the development of CRT. Equally, we must not discount the ongoing efforts in extending CRT to other patient populations. In our opinion, further work is required on patient selection and refinement of the CRT implantation procedure, as well as the post-procedure optimization of therapy. Ongoing research may confirm our conviction that CRT has a role in patients with less severe symptoms or no symptoms at all, in whom the therapy might halt or retard disease progression. It may also be possible that one day CRT will replace conventional, right-ventricular pacing.

Chapter 15

Non-ischaemic cardiomyopathy

Dr Julian Ormerod and Professor Michael Frenneaux

Introduction

The past four decades have seen an explosion in our understanding of the cardiomyopathies. Increasing understanding of the underlying aetiologies has resulted in reclassification of the disorders and is providing important insights into pathophysiology that may lead to specific therapies, at least in some of these diseases.

Although there had been isolated case reports of what we now know to be this disorder over the previous hundred years, the first systematic description of hypertrophic cardiomyopathy (HCM) was in the late 1950s by the London pathologist Donald Teare. Since then we have learnt that this disease, characterized by left and sometimes right ventricular hypertrophy, is inherited as an autosomal dominant trait, and is usually the result of mutations in genes encoding sarcomere proteins. These mutations cause abnormal sarcomere cross bridge cycling with an 'energy wasting' effect. The resulting cardiac energy impairment results in impaired left ventricular diastolic relaxation during exercise and plays an important role in exercise limitation. Correction of this energy impairment by perhexiline was recently shown to improve diastolic filling during exercise in the non-obstructive form of the disease, increasing exercise capacity and improving symptoms. It has been proposed that cardiac energy impairment, present in genotypically affected individuals before the development of ventricular hypertrophy, may be the stimulus for the development of hypertrophy. Cardiac energetic impairment has also been shown to be present in other forms of cardiomyopathy, including dilated cardiomyopathy, and appears to play an important pathophysiological role in this syndrome also, being associated with a poorer outcome.

Huge advances have been made in the symptomatic treatment of the obstructive form of the disease. Surgical septal myectomy has excellent short and long-term results and in experienced centres can be performed at low risk in those without significant co-morbidities. More recently the less invasive technique of alcohol septal ablation has been developed and is being widely used. It reduces outflow tract gradient by creating a septal infarct, thinning the septum, and reducing the obstruction. There have been no randomized comparisons with surgical myectomy. Long-term results of alcohol ablation are awaited. Concerns have been raised about the potential for increased risk of ventricular arrhythmias due to the associated scar and for the late development of systolic heart failure due to remodelling following the septal infarct.

In the two decades following Teare's description of HCM the disorder was considered to be rare and to be associated with a high risk of sudden cardiac death (SCD). Subsequently it has become clear that it is a relatively common disease—with community echocardiographic studies demonstrating unexplained left ventricular hypertrophy in up to 1 in 500 of the adult population. It became clear that the very high rates of SCD reported in early series were in part the result of tertiary referral bias. Nevertheless, HCM is one of the most common causes of SCD in adolescents and young adults, and especially in athletes. Therefore a major step forward in therapy has come from an understanding of the mechanisms underlying SCD risk and the development of a risk factor algorithm that facilitates targeted deployment of implantable cardio-defibrillators (ICDs) in high-risk patients. A subgroup of patients with HCM develop progressive heart failure due either to restrictive left ventricular systolic physiology or to the development of systolic dysfunction. This progression is associated with a poor outcome and represents a major challenge for future research to understand the pathophysiology and to develop effective therapies. Recent evidence suggests an important role for cardiac fibrosis.

Arrhythmogenic right ventricular cardiomyopathy (ARVC) is another inherited cardiomyopathy that is also a frequent cause of SCD in young adults. It is typically characterized by fibrofatty replacement of the right ventricular free wall following myocyte apoptosis, and this may result in aneurysm formation. The risk of ventricular arrhythmias and SCD is greatest in adolescence and early adult life, but in older patients right ventricular (RV) failure may supervene. Recently it has become clear that left ventricular (LV) involvement is common and indeed some patients may have predominantly left ventricular involvement. Whilst HCM is a disease of the sarcomere it has now become clear that ARVC is a disorder due to mutations of genes encoding one of several proteins crucial for cell-to-cell adhesion. Whilst the majority of cases are autosomal dominant, a small proportion are autosomal recessive, and indeed the first elucidation of the molecular genetics occurred in a recessive form of the disease occurring in the Greek island, Naxos. As well as the cardiac phenotype, affected individuals have woolly hair and palmar-plantar hyperkeratosis due to disturbed cell-to-cell adhesion in the skin. The latter phenotype greatly simplifies clinical diagnosis. A mutation affecting the gene encoding plakoglobin was identified. The disturbed cell-to-cell adhesion causes cellular slippage

and appears to activate proapoptotic pathways. The penetrance of the dominantly inherited forms of the disorder is variable and clinical diagnosis in first degree relatives can be challenging. The recent publication of guidelines for the diagnosis has provided a framework. Cardiac MRI is of particular value in the imaging of these patients.

Athletes are at particularly high risk of SCD. The development of a screening programme for athletes in Italy appears (on the basis of longitudinal data) to have reduced the occurrence of SCD. However, such programmes are fraught with difficulties, including false positives, that can have a huge impact on the wrongly diagnosed athlete, ending their careers. A particular challenge is the distinction between the 'physiological' hypertrophy of some athletes (particularly top level endurance athletes) and HCM. Certain features have now been shown to be very useful. Hypertrophy of more than 13 mm is very rare in Caucasian male athletes but can occasionally be up to 15 mm in black male athletes. In female athletes left ventricular wall thickness is virtually never more than 12 mm. The hypertrophy in athletes' hearts is usually concentric, whereas it is usually (but not necessarily) asymmetric in HCM. The LV and RV diastolic dimensions are usually increased or high normal in athletes' hearts versus reduced or low normal in HCM. The presence of ST-segment depression or T wave inversion in contiguous inferior or lateral ECG leads is highly suggestive that the hypertrophy is due to HCM. Ultimately the final arbiter may be the regression or not of hypertrophy following a period of detraining, but this may be a difficult strategy to institute in a professional athlete.

Dilated cardiomyopathy (DCM) is a disorder associated with enlargement of the left and/or right ventricles associated with reduced ejection fraction (EF). Unlike HCM and ARVC it is not due to a single pathophysiological mechanism but may be the end result of a variety of aetiological factors. Amongst these, it has become clear over the past two decades that if careful family screening is performed, DCM will be found in other first degree family members in up to 40% of cases. The pattern of inheritance is most frequently autosomal dominant. Unlike HCM and ARVC, the molecular genetics does not have a single 'theme'. It appears that mutations of a large variety of genes can result in the phenotype of DCM. These genes include those encoding sarcomere genes, cytoskeletal genes, and nuclear envelope proteins. As noted above, ARVC and DCM phenotypes may present within the same family and in these cases are due to mutations of genes involved in cell-to-cell adhesion. The penetrance is variable and age-related. An interaction with other aetiological factors (e.g. alcohol) may alter the age of onset. Viral infection of the heart can result in acute myocarditis. This may present with acute and severe heart failure and is rare. However, a body of work has been published over the past few years suggesting that subclinical myocarditis followed by viral persistence in the myocardium may be a relatively common cause of DCM. The Berlin group has reported very high rates of enteroviral genome expression (particularly parvovirus) in cardiac biopsies from patients with DCM compared to biopsies from patients with other forms of heart disease. Accordingly, the group are now exploring the role of immunomodulatory therapies, for example with interferon beta-1b, though promising pilot results have yet to translate to clinical effect. Other groups have reported much lower rates of expression of enteroviral genome in DCM patients.

Takotsubo cardiomyopathy was first described by Japanese investigators. It is a syndrome that most commonly occurs in post-menopausal women after an emotional shock or some other form of stress. The clinical presentation is as an acute coronary syndrome (that can be either ST-elevation myocardial infarction or non-ST-elevation myocardial infarction). Echocardiography performed in the first few days classically shows preserved basal systolic function with apical ballooning of the left ventricle, though this classic appearance may resolve quite quickly to a minor wall motion abnormality and subsequently complete normalization. A rarer form has been reported with basal dysfunction and preservation of apical LV function. Plasma troponin is typically mildly or moderately elevated. If serial ECGs are performed, transient QT prolongation will usually be observed. This can result in Torsade de pointes ventricular tachycardia and rarely SCD. The epicardial coronary arteries are normal or near normal. Whilst complete resolution is usual, recurrence occurs in approximately 10% of cases. There has been an explosion of literature regarding this condition in the last few years, and it is now clear that it is far from rare. The pathophysiology is a subject of intense investigation—catecholamine toxicity may be involved.

Hypertrophic cardiomyopathy

Sudden death in hypertrophic cardiomyopathy: identification of high risk patients

Elliott PM, Poloniecki J, Dickie S, Sharma S, Monserrat L, Varnava A, Mahon NG, McKenna WJ. *J Am Coll Cardiol* 2000; 36(7): 2212–8.

Hypertrophic cardiomyopathy is a heritable disease of the myocardium, first described in the nineteenth century by Liouville but elucidated by Teare in his seminal 1958 case series, describing the dominant mode of inheritance for the first time. The penetrance of HCM within a pedigree is generally high but variable, while a minority of cases are currently believed to be sporadic. The condition is probably under-diagnosed, with estimates of prevalence as high as 1:500. Management of HCM involves three main areas: palliation of symptoms, risk assessment, and risk reduction. In those patients with outflow tract obstruction, symptom control is generally achieved with pharmacological reduction of the left ventricular outflow tract gradient using a combination of a beta blocker and disopyramide, but where such a strategy fails, septal reduction using surgery or alcohol ablation may be indicated. Therapy for symptomatic patients with the non-obstructive form is usually with high dose verapamil or diltiazem, or beta blockers, but is generally unsatisfactory. Risk reduction mainly involves targeted implantation of ICDs in patients considered to be at high risk of SCD. Implantation of ICDs carries the standard risks of infection or haemorrhage, but also the specific side effects of inappropriate discharge, which may be particularly troublesome in some people. Accurate stratification of risk is therefore essential.

A 1989 review (McKenna and Camm 1989) summarized evidence from three main sources—a retrospective case series of 254 patients (McKenna *et al.* 1981), a prospective study of ambulatory ECGs in 99 patients (Maron *et al.* 1981), and a prospective study of ambulatory ECGs in 86 patients (McKenna *et al.* 1981)—in an effort to create a systematic framework of risk assessment in patients with HCM. It was already appreciated that family history of sudden death is a risk factor in the patient with HCM. McKenna and Camm brought together evidence from the authors and others regarding non-sustained ventricular tachycardia (NSVT) and abnormal haemodynamic changes during exercise. Syncope was also noted to be an ominous sign. In a subsequent study (Elliott *et al*. 2000) the authors quantified the annual risk for each of the univariate predictors of SCD, and showed the incremental effects of two or more risk factors. This landmark paper forms the basis of the risk stratification used in current clinical practice.

sustained VT will usually undergo implantaion of an ICD irrespective of the presence or absence of other risk factors.

Further reading

- Elliott PM, Gimeno Blanes JR, Mahon NG, Poloniecki JD, McKenna WJ. Relation between severity of left-ventricular hypertrophy and prognosis in patients with hypertrophic cardiomyopathy. *Lancet* 2001; 357(9254): 420–4.
- Geisterfer-Lawrance AA, Kass S, Tanigawa G, *et al*. A molecular basis for familial hypertrophic cardiomyopathy: a beta-cardiac myosin heavy chain gene missense mutation. *Cell* 1990; 62: 999–1006. (First identification of a responsible gene.)
- Liouville H. Retrecessment cardiaque sous aortique. *Gazette Med Paris* 1869; 24: 161–65 (The first description of sub-aortic thickening of the myocardium as a disease entity.)
- Maron BJ, Savage DD, Wolfson JK, Epstein SE. Prognostic significance of 24 hour ambulatory electrocardiographic monitoring in patients with hypertrophic cardiomyopathy: a prospective study. *Am J Cardiol* 1981; 48: 252–7.
- McKenna WJ, Deanfield J, Faruqui A, England D, Oakley CM, Goodwin JF. Prognosis in hypertrophic cardiomyopathy: Role of age, and clinical, electrocardiographic and hemodynamic features. *Am J Cardiol* 1981; 47: 532–38.
- McKenna WJ, England D, Doi YL, Deanfield JE, Oakley CM, Goodwin JF. Arrhythmia in hypertrophic cardiomyopathy: I. Influence on prognosis. *Br Heart J* 1981; 46: 168–72.
- McKenna WJ, Camm AJ. Sudden death in hypertrophic cardiomyopathy. Assessment of patients at high risk. *Circulation* 1989; 80(5): 1489–92. (An early call for an evidence-based method of risk assessment in HCM.)
- Teare RD. Asymmetrical hypertrophy of the heart in young adults. *Br Heart J* 1958; 20: 1–10. (The seminal case series describing heritable hypertrophic cardiomyopathy.)

Learning points

Risk assessment in hypertrophic cardiomyopathy:
- Family history of sudden death in two or more first degree relatives at age <40.
- Abnormal blood pressure response to exercise.
- Recent or recurrent syncope.
- Non-sustained VT.
- Maximum wall thickness >30 mm.
- Left ventricular outflow tract obstruction.

Individual factors have a low positive predictive value for sudden death; stratification is based on consideration of all six. The presence of a single risk factor, or absence of factors imparts an annual risk of sudden death of less than 1%; the presence of two or more factors signifies a high risk and is considered an indication for ICD implantation. Additionally, patients with a prior cardiac arrest should be considered for ICD implant irrespective of other risk factors. Patients who have had a prior cardiac arrest or who have

Alpha-tropomyosin and cardiac troponin T mutations cause familial hypertrophic cardiomyopathy: a disease of the sarcomere

Thierfelder L, Watkins H, MacRae C, Lamas R, McKenna W, Vosberg HP, Seidman JG, Seidman CE. *Cell* 1994; 77(5): 701–12.

As techniques to investigate genetic disease improved, serious heritable diseases such as HCM seemed prime targets for research, with the promise of therapeutic advances stimulating action. Several different mutations were found in the gene encoding the β-Myosin Heavy Chain (β-MHC) in HCM families in the late 1980s and early 1990s. This protein forms part of the force-generating apparatus of the cardiac muscle cell—the functional unit known as the sarcomere. In this paper, the investigators examined the genotypes of five families with inherited HCM. They discovered mutations in two other sarcomeric proteins—α-tropomyosin and troponin T—which can also cause HCM, and this led to the realization that HCM is a disease of the sarcomere itself. This elucidation of the nature of HCM paved the way for a greater understanding of the subtypes of disease seen in different families, and today this work, and the work of others, allows us to give important prognostic information to patients where the genetic lesion has been identified. Though this is still applicable only to a minority of families, it is likely that more subtypes of HCM will be found, with the possibility that therapy will be tailored to specific disease types.

This pioneering early work provided an impetus to the discovery of the genetics of other types of inherited cardiomyopathy and has also shed light upon the pathogenesis of non-heritable disorders of the heart muscle. Unfortunately, the authors' hope that increased understanding would engender therapeutic advances has so far proved unfounded. Finally, this paper reminds us of the technical challenges faced by those at the forefront of genetic research in the era preceding the Human Genome Project, and is a metric of the speed of change in this field.

Learning points

- Myosin heavy chain mutations underlie around 40% of cases of HCM; myosin binding protein c mutations are found in 30–35%.
- Late-onset (fourth decade and beyond) HCM is generally associated with mutations in myosin binding protein c, but other mutations have been reported (e.g. troponin T).
- Different mutations are associated with different phenotypes; the effects of β-MHC mutations are particularly well documented.
- For example, incidence of SCD ranges from high ($Arg^{403}Gln$) to very low indeed ($Leu^{908}Val$).
- The phenotype is also influenced by distant genes, including the angiotensin-converting enzyme (ACE) gene.
- Epigenetic phenomena also contribute to the development and phenotype of an individual's disease.

Further reading

- Geisterfer-Lawrance AA, Kass S, Tanigawa G, *et al*. A molecular basis for familial hypertrophic cardiomyopathy: a beta-cardiac myosin heavy chain gene missense mutation. *Cell* 1990; 62: 999–1006. (The lesion was found to reside in the gene encoding the β-Myosin Heavy Chain.)
- Hejtmancik JF, Brink PA, Towbin J, *et al*. Localization of the gene for familial hypertrophic cardiomyopathy to chromosome 14q1 in a diverse US population. *Circulation* 1991; 83: 1592–7. (Two groups used linkage analysis to localise the genetic lesion to the long arm of chromosome 14.)
- Jarcho JA, McKenna W, Pare JAP, *et al*. Mapping a gene for familial hypertrophic cardiomyopathy to chromosome 14q1. *N Engl J Med* 1989; 321: 1372–8.

Dilated cardiomyopathy genetics

Mutations in sarcomere protein genes as a cause of dilated cardiomyopathy

Kamisago M, Sharma SD, DePalma SR, Solomon S, Sharma P, McDonough B, Smoot L, Mullen MP, Woolf PK, Wigle ED, Seidman JG, Seidman CE. *N Engl J Med* 2000 Dec 7; 343(23): 1688–96.

Dilated cardiomyopathy (DCM) is the commonest primary disease of heart muscle. It is sometimes distinguished from ischaemic cardiomyopathy (which may have a dilated phenotype) by the term idiopathic DCM. Cases may be spontaneous (or perhaps the first of a lineage) or inherited in an autosomal dominant, recessive, X-linked, or mitochondrial manner, though dominant inheritance is the norm. In the late 1990s, several mutations in cytoskeletal proteins (including actin, desmin, δ-sarcoglycan, and dystrophin) were found to cause inherited DCM. These mutations disrupt the structural integrity of the cardiomyocyte and interfere with normal signalling.

In this progressive work, the authors performed a genome-wide linkage study of 21 families with inherited DCM, which implicated a locus on the long arm of chromosome 14; the site of the gene encoding β-MHC. They demonstrated mutations in the sarcomeric proteins troponin T and β-MHC, which had both been previously implicated in HCM. This represents a significant step forward in the understanding of the aetiology of non-ischaemic cardiomyopathy; distinct mutations in the same group of sarcomeric proteins can cause entirely separate inherited conditions. Dilated cardiomyopathy and HCM are distinct at both the macro- and microscopic levels, with disproportionate septal wall thickening, myocyte disarray, and diminished, as opposed to increased, ventricular volumes characterizing the latter. Mutations causing HCM generally increased force generation in the sarcomere, whereas those causing DCM undermined the stability of the same group of proteins, leading to reduced force generation.

Mutations in sarcomeric proteins are now estimated to underlie at least 10% of cases of familial DCM, but, just as importantly, this paper prompted a reassessment of the pathogenesis of cardiomyopathy in general. The search continues: a second major group of causative mutations have been identified in proteins of the nuclear envelope—including lamins A and C—but this avenue is far from exhausted. Future work will also elucidate the frequency of pathogenic mutations in the giant myofibrillar protein, titin, but completing this massive task is at the limit of current genetic techniques.

Learning points

◆ Dilated cardiomyopathy is the commonest cardiomyopathy.
◆ It most commonly presents between the ages of 18–50.
◆ Around 30–40% of cases are inherited.
◆ Up to half of affected individuals, unless transplanted, will die within five years of diagnosis.
◆ Sudden death is at least as common as death from pump failure.
◆ Dilated cardiomyopathy is also a feature of several systemic diseases, including muscular dystrophies, collagen vascular diseases, and glycogen storage disorders.

Further reading

- Li D, Tapscoft T, Gonzalez O, *et al*. Desmin mutations responsible for idiopathic dilated cardiomyopathy. *Circulation* 1999; 100: 461–4.
- Olson TM, Michels VV, Thibodeau SN, Tai YS, Keating MT. Actin mutations in dilated cardiomyopathy, a heritable form of heart failure. *Science* 1998; 280(5364): 750–2. (The first report of a genetic lesion in dilated cardiomyopathy.)

Dilated cardiomyopathy aetiology

Viral persistence in the myocardium is associated with progressive cardiac dysfunction

Kühl U, Pauschinger M, Seeberg B, Lassner D, Noutsias M, Poller W, Schultheiss HP. *Circulation* 2005; 112(13): 1965–70.

Viruses are known to cause myocarditis, a condition that progresses to dilated cardiomyopathy in a variable proportion of cases. However, a school of thought has developed which suggests that viruses may have a causative role in far more cases of cardiomyopathy than previously imagined, with persistence of the virus in heart muscle causing inflammation and eventually heart failure, in the absence of a recognized index illness of myocarditis.

In this observational study, the investigators followed 172 patients to assess the prevalence and clinical significance of persistent virus in the myocardium. These 172 patients were recruited from an initial sample of 841 patients, who had been referred to the centre with likely previous myocarditis or a diagnosis of DCM. The principle recruitment criterion was the presence of viral genomes in the initial myocardial biopsy. Patients with active or recent myocarditis were excluded from this study. In the recruited patients 40% were found to have significant inflammation of the heart at presentation.

Several different persistent viruses were identified and, regardless of its type, clearance of the virus from subsequent myocardial biopsies was associated with a clinical improvement. The most common virus encountered was parvovirus B19 (in 37% of biopsies), and 33% contained enterovirus, with adenovirus and human herpes virus (HHV6) in around 10% each. Different frequencies have been reported in subsequent studies.

This is an influential theory but remains controversial. The causative link between common infections and subsequent disease is very difficult to establish. The majority of adults have been exposed to Coxsackie virus, for example, but most do not develop heart failure. It is often impossible to unpick the influence of several competing aetiologies in a given case of 'idiopathic' DCM—consider as an example a patient with moderate alcohol intake, a temporal association of symptoms with a viral infection, and mild-moderate coronary artery disease—and it may be that the true proportion of cases where viruses are responsible can only be revealed with the advent of specific therapy. At present, this research raises intriguing possibilities for the future, and indeed there have been promising preliminary reports of the use of interferon beta-1b to clear parvovirus in chronic DCM.

Dilated cardiomyopathy energetics

Myocardial phosphocreatine-to-ATP ratio is a predictor of mortality in patients with dilated cardiomyopathy

Neubauer S, Horn M, Cramer M, Harre K, Newell JB, Peters W, Pabst T, Ertl G, Hahn D, Ingwall JS, Kochsiek K. *Circulation* 1997; 96(7): 2190–6.

Magnetic resonance spectroscopy (MRS) provides a non-invasive measure of a variety of compounds in the heart. Since the high-energy phosphate system is in constant flux, the amount of adenosine triphosphate (ATP) alone does not give an accurate indication of the energy status of the myocardium. Consequently, the ratio of phosphocreatine (PCr, the high-energy species in the creatine shuttle unique to muscle) to ATP is used. Patients with severe heart failure have been shown to display reduced PCr:ATP ratio, and this has been interpreted as an impairment of myocardial energetics.

In this cohort study, 39 patients were followed up for 30 months. Myocardial energetic status was measured by P^{31} MRS. Impaired cardiac energetic status, which was prospectively defined as a PCr:ATP ratio less than 1.60, was found in 20 of the group of 39. This group had a significantly increased mortality compared to the 19 heart failure patients with a normal PCr:ATP ratio and unsurprisingly also when compared to a group of 30 healthy volunteers. In a Cox multivariate analysis, myocardial energetics provided significant prognostic information independent of NYHA class.

The study design has certain limitations. Cohort studies can only define associations, and do not provide proof of causation. Despite this, measurable risk factors are useful in real-world medicine, though in this case the measurement technique is by no means widely available. Availability should increase, and technical challenges in patients with a thin myocardium (such as those with DCM) may be less of a problem with future MRI scanners. However, the greatest effect of this work in heart failure management is as a rationale for a new breed of 'metabolic agents' for heart failure. These include perhexiline (an anti-anginal drug originally used in the 1970s) and trimetazidine, which is gaining popularity in continental Europe. Such agents are believed to switch myocardial metabolism from fatty acid to glucose metabolism, with concomitant gains in efficiency. Excitingly, other cardiomyopathies, especially HCM, have been postulated to involve impaired energetics and may well be amenable to therapy with agents such as perhexiline. Recent work performed in our group suggests this may indeed be the case (Abozguia *et al.* 2010).

Learning points

- Impaired myocardial energetic status is an independent risk factor for poor outcome in heart failure.
- Measurement of energetic status can be achieved non-invasively by MR spectroscopy.
- Magnetic resonance spectroscopy, however, remains a research tool at present.

Further reading

- Abozguia K, Elliott P, McKenna W, *et al*. Metabolic modulator perhexiline corrects energy deficiency and improves exercise capacity in symptomatic hypertrophic cardiomyopathy *Circulation* 2010; 122(16): 1562–9. (A randomized controlled trial of perhexiline in HCM.)
- Herrmann G, Decherd GM. The chemical nature of heart failure. *Annals of Internal Medicine* 1939; 12: 1233–44.

(An early recognition that the substrate used by the heart in pathophysiology is important.)

- Lee L, Campbell R, Scheuermann-Freestone M, *et al*. Metabolic modulation with perhexiline in chronic heart failure: a randomized, controlled trial of short-term use of a novel treatment. *Circulation* 2005; 112(21): 3280–8. (A randomized controlled trial of perhexiline in chronic heart failure showed improvement in exercise capacity and quality of life.)

Arrhythmogenic right ventricular cardiomyopathy/dysplasia

Identification of a deletion in plakoglobin in arrhythmogenic right ventricular cardiomyopathy with palmoplantar keratoderma and woolly hair (Naxos disease)

McKoy G, Protonotarios N, Crosby A, Tsatsopoulou A, Anastasakis A, Coonar A, Norman M, Baboonian C, Jeffery S, McKenna WJ. *Lancet* 2000; 355: 2119–24.

Arrhythmogenic right ventricular cardiomyopathy is a dominantly-inherited cardiomyopathy characterized by fatty infiltration and fibrosis of the myocardium, predominantly affecting the right ventricle. This provides the anatomical substrate for electrical disturbance and sudden death. The disease was first described by Marcus and colleagues, in a report of 24 adults with the condition, two of whom were related. A full pedigree was documented in 1988, on the basis of a family with right ventricular cardiomyopathy and effort-induced tachycardia. This form of ARVC is now classed as type 2 (ARVC2) and established the classic autosomal dominant, variable penetrance, inheritance of the disease.

In this paper, McKoy and colleagues reported a deletion mutation in the plakoglobin gene, which was responsible for Naxos disease. This autosomal-recessive condition displays a very similar cardiac phenotype to ARVC, but patients also suffer from palmoplantar keratoderma and woolly hair. Plakoglobin is a cell adhesion molecule and this interesting result raised the possibility of a structural protein basis for ARVC, as in some families with DCM. Further molecular genetic study of this cardiocutaneous disorder laid the path for the current understanding of ARVC as a disease of the desmosome, part of the cell-cell mechanical junctional apparatus in myocytes (and epidermal cells). The dominant forms of classical ARVC tend to affect the heart only, with skin manifestations evident in recessively-inherited diseases.

A variety of mutations in desmosomal proteins have been shown to cause ARVC in the last five years, and genetic testing for relatives of cases is frequent where a genetic mutation is known. Detection of cases by genetic testing is challenging, as not enough is known to definitively distinguish disease-causing mutations from polymorphisms.

Learning points

- Myocytes are gradually lost in ARVC, to be replaced by fibrous and fatty tissue.
- The prevalence is approximately 1:5000.
- It is estimated to be responsible for around 25% of SCD in athletes.
- Ventricular arrhythmias are triggered by episodes of exertion.

Further reading

- Kaplan SR, Gard JJ, Protonotarios N, *et al*. Remodeling of myocyte gap junctions in arrhythmogenic right ventricular cardiomyopathy due to a deletion in plakoglobin (Naxos disease). *Heart Rhythm* 2004; 1(1): 3–11. (Molecular genetic study which established the concept of ARVC as a disease, or group of diseases, of the desmosome.)
- Marcus F, Fontaine G, Guiraudon G, *et al*. Right ventricular dysplasia: a report of 24 adult cases. *Circulation* 1982; 65: 384–98. (The first description of sporadic cases of ARVC.)
- Marcus FI, McKenna WJ, Sherrill D, et al. Diagnosis of Arrhythmogenic Right Ventricular Cardiomyopathy/Dysplasia. Proposed Modification of the Task Force Criteria. Circulation 2010; 121:1533–41. (The most contemporaneous version of the diagnostic criteria for ARVC.)

• Nava A, Canciani B, Daliento L, *et al.* Juvenile sudden death and effort induced tachycardias in a family with right ventricular cardiomyopathy. *Int J Cardiol* 1988; 21(2): 111–26. (First description of the dominant inheritance of ARVC, the specific condition described is now categorized as type 2.)

• Sen-Chowdhry S, Syrris P, McKenna WJ. Genetics of right ventricular cardiomyopathy. *J Cardiovasc Electrophysiol* 2005; 16: 927e35. (An early review of this concept.)

Athletic screening

Screening for Hypertrophic Cardiomyopathy in Young Athletes

Corrado D, Basso C, Schiavon M, Thiene G. *N Engl J Med* 1998; 339: 364–9.

Italy is the only country worldwide to legally mandate a cardiac screening programme for all young adults participating in organized sports. Hypertrophic cardiomyopathy is the commonest cause of sudden death in young athletes, and can be screened for in several ways. History and examination is considered least sensitive, electrocardiography sensitive but not specific, and echocardiography sensitive and specific for HCM but insensitive in diagnosing other serious cardiac conditions. In this prospective observational study of 33,735 young athletes who underwent pre-participation screening in the University of Padua, Corrado and colleagues attempted to show that screening saves lives. This landmark paper prompted soul searching across the globe, and has raised the profile of pre-participation screening, even if other countries still lag behind Italy's example.

In stark contrast to experience from the US, where more than a third of sudden deaths in athletes are caused by HCM, only 1 (2%) of the 49 athletes who died suddenly during the 17-year follow-up had HCM. Twenty-two individuals were diagnosed with HCM during screening. These were all excluded from competition, and none died during the period of follow-up. Sudden death occurred more frequently in athletes than non-athletes less than 35 years in age (relative risk 2.1, 95% CI 1.5–2.9; p <0.001), and in this cohort ARVC was the commonest cause of all sudden death (22%). The rate of HCM diagnosis in this study was rather low compared to some previous community estimates of prevalence (1:1400 compared to 1:500 in Maron, 1997); however, it seems likely that pre-participation screening prevented sudden deaths from HCM, leaving the proportionately more difficult-to-diagnose ARVC as the major killer.

Learning points

♦ Athletes may be at greater risk of sudden death than other young people.
♦ The majority of deaths are cardiac in nature and a proportion can be prevented by screening.
♦ This benefit must be balanced against the harm of preventing young people from taking part in sport and the high cost involved in intensive screening.

Further reading

• Maron BJ. Hypertrophic cardiomyopathy. *Lancet* 1997; 350: 127–33.
• Wheeler MT, Heidenreich PA, Froelicher VF, Hlatky MA and Ashley EA. Cost-Effectiveness of Preparticipation Screening for Prevention of Sudden Cardiac Death in Young Athletes. *Annals of Internal Medicine* 2010; 152(5): 276–286.

Takotsubo cardiomyopathy

Myocardial stunning due to simultaneous multivessel coronary spasms: a review of 5 cases

Dote K, Sato H, Tateishi H, Uchida T, Ishihara M. *J Cardiol* 1991; 21: 203–14.

Takotsubo cardiomyopathy or transient LV apical ballooning syndrome is a non-ischaemic cardiomyopathy that is characterized by acute-onset chest pain and LV dysfunction, with a (classically apical) ballooning of the LV wall, in the absence of significant coronary artery disease. The Japanese name was given in reference to a similarly shaped pot used for catching octopuses. The typical patient is a post-menopausal female and in the majority of cases a history of a stressful event is present within the few days prior to the event. Providing the patient survives the initial episode, LV function recovers within weeks, but may recur. The QT interval is typically prolonged during episodes and episodes of Torsade de pointes VT may occur. The condition can be easily confused with acute myocardial infarction, as electrocardiographic changes are typical, but release of biomarkers of cardiac necrosis is low to moderate at most.

Takotsubo cardiomyopathy is estimated to be the diagnosis in up to 2% of all patients presenting with cardiac chest pain. This work shows that relatively common conditions may still await description and, despite the pace of cardiomyopathy research in recent decades, the future of the field is very exciting.

Conclusion: the future

From the glimpses provided in this chapter it will be clear that there have been huge advances in our understanding of the aetiological basis for the cardiomyopathies—particularly the molecular genetics—and of the pathophysiology of these disorders. However, it must be acknowledged that, thus far, these exciting data have not translated into specific therapies. Our recent paper demonstrating that the metabolic modulator perhexiline partially corrects cardiac energetic impairment in patients with hypertrophic cardiomyopathy, and that this translates into improved symptoms and exercise capacity, may be a forerunner of such therapeutic translation.

Chapter 16

Cardiac failure and transplantation

Dr William Davies and Dr Jayan Parameshwar

Introduction

Cardiac transplantation is arguably the most emotive of operative interventions. The specialty is relatively young, and has undergone considerable evolution since the pioneering days of the 1960s. Many of the major contributors are well recognized for their achievements in both the popular and medical press. The following ten landmark papers are those that have altered the course of the specialty considerably during this time.

Studies on orthotopic homotransplantations of the canine heart

Lower RR, Shumway NE. *Surg Forum* 1960; 11: 18–9.

Norman Edward Shumway was born in Kalamazoo, Michigan, USA on 9 February 1923. Although initially intending to study law, he was drafted into the army and asked to complete an aptitude test with only two outcomes: a career in medicine or dentistry. He passed, chose medicine, and was sent to Vanderbilt University for his medical training. He did his internship in the University of Minnesota where he developed an interest in cardiac surgery. He was made Chief of Cardiothoracic Surgery at Stanford University in 1964, a post he held until his retirement in 1993. In 1967 he announced that Stanford would perform the first human heart transplant when a suitable donor became available. It was not to be, but Christian Barnard acknowledges Shumway's work in the opening paragraphs of his report of the first human cardiac transplant in 1968.

Dr Shumway is considered by many to be the father of cardiothoracic transplantation. He is particularly remembered for his persistence in the face of adversity when initial disappointing outcomes led to many surgeons calling for a suspension of further transplants until the issues surrounding rejection and long-term survival could be overcome. He oversaw a programme that transplanted over 800 hearts. His legacy may be measured also in his ability to teach. Many of the founders of transplant programmes throughout the world can claim to have passed through Shumway's mentorship.

Richard Lower was born in Detroit, and graduated from Amherst College, earning his medical degree from Cornell University in 1955. He was a Surgical Resident at Stanford in 1959, working with Dr Shumway. Initial attempts at transplanting canine hearts had led to a survival record of only seven hours, and Lower undertook much work to refine the surgical techniques. Their report of the refined technique is our first landmark paper.

Published in *Surgical Forum*, the manuscript recounts the technique of canine cardiac transplantation in detail. Experiments were performed on healthy, adult mongrel dogs weighing 17–25 kg. Although the donors and recipients were of comparable size, no other effort was made to attain genetic or phenotypic resemblance.

The donor was first prepared by exposing the heart and great vessels under phenobarbital anaesthesia. Heparin at a dose of 2 mg/kg was given, and the body temperature lowered to 30°C with surface cooling. The recipient was heparinized and prepared for cardio-pulmonary bypass. The oxygenator was to be of the rotating disc type. The recipient heart was exposed through a left thoracotomy and longitudinal pericardiotomy, to allow catheters to be inserted into the vena cavae for delivery of venous blood to the oxygenator. After bypass was initiated, a non-crushing clamp was placed through the transverse sinus for occlusion of the pulmonary artery and aorta. One major technical advance, seen in the early years of animal transplantation, was the fashioning of the atrial anastomosis. Lower and Shumway excised the heart, leaving a common posterior atrial wall containing the ostia of the vena cavae, the pulmonary veins, and a ridge of atrial septum.

Once recipient cardio-pulmonary bypass had been established, the donor heart was excised and immersed in normal saline at 4°C for five minutes. The heart was then transplanted into the recipient animal by joining the atrial walls and atrial septum to the posterior wall of the recipient with a continuous suture. The anastomoses were completed with aortic and pulmonary connections. The aortic anastomosis was not completed until bronchial blood had been allowed to fill the left side of the heart, displacing the air. Unclamping of the aorta allowed re-establishment of coronary blood flow, and the heart was re-warmed and defibrillated as necessary. Bypass was discontinued once the donor heart was able to maintain sufficient cardiac output, and the incisions were closed once haemostasis had been achieved. The total reported duration of cardiac anoxia was approximately one hour.

The recovery from anaesthesia was reportedly uneventful, and during convalescence the dogs ate and exercised normally. Lower and Shumway report a series of eight consecutive transplantations, with five of the recipients living for 6–21 days. Electrocardiograms showed ST-T waves changes compatible with pericarditis and in some instances the P waves were abnormal.

The terminal course was usually very rapid, occurring over 24 hours, during which time the animal became lethargic and tachypnoeic. At post-mortem, the heart was seen to be ecchymotic and oedematous, with generalized dilatation and fibrinoid pericarditis. Microscopic examination showed severe myocarditis, massive round cell infiltration, patchy necrosis, interstitial haemorrhage, and oedema. There was also noted to be widespread lymphadenopathy with a non-specific increase in plasma cells and histiocytes.

Despite these findings, the authors reported normal function of the transplanted, denervated heart during convalescence. They postulate that the difference in survival times may have been due to individual variation in the immunological response of each recipient. Fundamentally, they concluded that if these immunologic mechanisms involved in the host response could be modulated, then the graft may continue to function adequately for the normal life span of the animal.

A Human Cardiac Transplant: an interim report of a successful operation performed at Groote Schuur Hospital, Cape Town

Barnard CN. *S Afr Med J* 1967; 41: 1271–4.

Christian Barnard was born on the 8 November 1922 in Beaufort West, South Africa. He obtained his medical degree from the University of Cape Town in 1945 and completed his early training in Groote Schuur Hospital. In 1956 he travelled to the University of Minnesota to study under Dr Walton Lillehei who, at the time, was one of only two surgeons using the heart-lung bypass machine, the other being John Kirklin at the Mayo Clinic. He returned to South Africa to become the Head of Cardiothoracic Surgery at the University of Cape Town. His younger brother, Marius, also a qualified surgeon, became his assistant.

On 3 December 1967, Barnard became the first surgeon to transplant a human heart into another human. Our second landmark paper is a description of the procedure and early post-operative course, published 27 days later in the *South African Medical Journal*.

The transcript begins: 'On the 3rd December 1967, a heart from a cadaver was successfully transplanted into a 54-year-old man to replace a heart irreparably damaged by repeated myocardial infarction.' Barnard continues to allude to the multi-disciplinary progress over the preceding decades that was necessary to allow this advance, 'the ultimate in cardiac surgery', to happen.

Much of the introduction poses philosophical points: 'The dream of the ancients from time immemorial has been the junction of portions of different individuals, not only to counteract disease but also to combine the potentials of different species.' He continues: 'The modern world has inherited these dreams in the form of the sphinx, the mermaid and the chimera forms of many heraldic beasts.' Barnard acknowledges the contributions of Carrel and Guthrie, at the beginning of the century, and Shumway more recently, describing them as 'brilliant men'.

The description of the operation then begins. The donor recipient matching involved compatible red cell antigens and a similar leucocyte antigen pattern. The donor and recipient were placed on cardiopulmonary bypass in adjacent operating theatres. Once it became obvious that 'death was inevitable' in the donor, the recipient was anaesthetized. Once the donor had been certified dead, confirmed by five minutes of inactivity on the electrocardiogram, heparin was administered and cardiopulmonary bypass rapidly commenced. The body was cooled to 26°C, the aorta cross-clamped and the heart cooled further to 16°C prior to explantation. The excision took two minutes. The heart was placed in a bowl containing Ringer's Lactate solution at 10°C and transferred to the adjacent operating theatre. The heart then underwent extra-corporal perfusion four minutes after explantation.

The recipient was commenced on cardiopulmonary bypass, and cooled to 30°C. The patient's heart was then excised after cross-clamping the aorta proximal to the aortic cannula. The left atrium of the donor heart was first attached to the recipient using double layers of 4-0 continuous silk. The right atrium was anastomosed next, followed by the pulmonary arteries (5-0 silk) and thereafter the aorta (4-0 silk). The left ventricle was vented through the apex and the aortic cross-clamp released. Re-warming was commenced after a bypass time of 165 minutes. At 184 minutes partial bypass was commenced by decreasing venous return to the pump.

Barnard continues: 'With a mid-oesophageal temperature of 36°C and a rectal temperature of 31°C, after a total perfusion duration of 196 minutes, 35 joules of energy were applied to the heart from a DC defibrillator. The first shock was successful in restoring good coordinated ventricular contraction. The heart was beating at a rate of 120/min in nodal rhythm.' The donor heart had been without coronary perfusion for 7 minutes at normothermia, and for 14 minutes at 22°C. It had, thereafter, been perfused by the heart-lung machine for a total period of 117 minutes.

Barnard recounts three areas of particular concentration in the post-operative period: first, the maintenance of a satisfactory cardiac output, second, the suppression of the immunologic reaction to the transplanted organ, and third, the prevention of infection. Cardiac output was assessed by the systolic blood pressure, the venous pressure, the rate and rhythm of the heart, the palpation of the peripheral pulses, measurement of the urine output, the temperature, the acid-base balance, and electrolyte measurements. Isoprenaline was used to treat any decrease in cardiac output, and digoxin used to treat tachycardia.

To detect rejection Barnard used the following parameters; the leucocyte response in the blood, a deterioration in cardiac output, a change in the serum enzyme levels that could indicate myocardial damage, and changes in the voltage of the R wave of the electrocardiograph. Rejection was treated with steroids (both as hydrocortisone and prednisolone), local irradiation of the heart, and azathioprine. Infection was prevented by meticulous asepsis and thorough decontamination of the patient and the surrounding environment.

At this point the manuscript ends with a summary of this 'successful operation'. The only clue contained within the description of the post-operative survival is that the donor heart was irradiated on day 9 post-operatively. In fact, Louis Washkansky (a 54-year-old grocer) survived for a total of 18 days and succumbed to pneumonia. The donor, Denise Darvall, a 24-year-old dressmaker, suffered a serious head injury following a collision with a car on 2 December 1967.

Much has been written about the exact events surrounding this milestone in transplantation. Barnard became an instant celebrity, and in contrast to Shumway, courted and enjoyed the media spotlight. He soon became known as the 'film star surgeon' and is alleged to have had several affairs. He retired in 1983 having operated with rheumatoid arthritis for twenty years. He died in 2001.

Production of severe atheroma in a transplanted human heart

Thomson JG. *Lancet* 1969; 2: 1088–92.

Although several of the early recipients of cardiac transplants did survive for many years, much was to be learnt of the unique pathophysiological processes that followed this daring new intervention in heart disease. JG Thomson was the pathologist on Barnard's team at the Groote Schuur Hospital during those early days. The manuscript recounts the discovery of transplant allograft vasculopathy at post-mortem. A 24-year-old donor heart had been transplanted into a 58-year-old male recipient who survived for 19 months post-transplant. This transplant had taken place on 2 January 1968, two days after the publication of the previous paper. Very severe atheroma with associated luminal narrowing had been seen at post-mortem. Thomson also reported atheroma in the aorta. The recipient was known to be hypercholesterolaemic.

At post-mortem, the pericardium was opened to reveal the coronary arteries of the donor heart. These were broad, bright-yellow, atheromatous structures, clearly visible without sectioning the vessels. Thomson recounts that he had not seen such a high intensity or wide a distribution of coronary atheroma in 40 years of necropsy experience. He also judged the atheromatous process to be remarkably uniform, with no breaks or focal accentuations. The description states that 'in many vessels the yellow atheromatous deposit lay in the deepest portion of the thickened intima and a white lipid-free intimal thickening lay over it'. Thomson noted that many of the cells in the aortic atheromatous plaque were plasma cells, which could only indicate rejection of the donor aorta, a hypothesis supported by the fact that the adjacent recipient aorta was atheroma free. He also describes proliferation in the endothelial lining of the arteries, which subsequently migrate into the thickened intima. Thomson termed the unusual appearance of the coronary disease as 'atheromatous stuffing', with the media becoming stretched and thinned.

The patient had received azathioprine and prednisolone as immunosuppression, and also antilymphocytic globulin in the last year of his life. Despite this, there was severe rejection seen in the myocardium itself, with lymphocytes, histiocytes, and plasma-cells in abundance. In conclusion, Thomson states: 'This case adds another hazard where transplantation is undertaken on account of myocardial insufficiency from atheroma of the coronary arteries. I suggest that such patients with ischaemic heart disease are not suitable for heart transplantation'.

In current practice, chronic allograft vasculopathy is the main manifestation of chronic rejection, and the main cause of late death following transplantation. Improved immunosuppression and the use of statins have, however, delayed the onset and slowed progression of the disease.

Percutaneous Transvenous Endomyocardial Biopsy in Human Heart Recipients. Experience with a New Technique

Caves PK, Stinson EB, Billingham ME, Shumway NE. *Ann Thorac Surg* 1973; 16: 325–36.

In the early days of cardiac transplantation there was much to discover about the optimal peri-operative monitoring and therapy required for success. One of the steepest, and arguably most rewarding, learning curves was in the area of immunosuppression. By the time Philip Caves published our next landmark paper, Shumway's team at Stanford had performed 17 cardiac transplant procedures. Although these initial results had been encouraging, several patients had succumbed to acute rejection, and the group were working hard to perfect the available immunological modification techniques. The diagnosis of acute rejection was often made when the patient had signs and symptoms of severe allograft dysfunction. Very large doses of immunosuppression were then required to reverse the process and overwhelming infection often resulted.

The role of needle biopsy in solid organ transplantation had been well established in the setting of renal transplantation. The previously described techniques for biopsy of the human heart had significant associated mortality, and were not considered suitable in the transplant recipient. However, one technique, pioneered by Sakakibara and Konno in 1963, using a catheter delivered bioptome, held promise. Using this bioptome, the Stanford group was able to successfully perform serial biopsies of their canine orthotopic series without significant morbidity or mortality. Acute graft rejection could, thereafter, be demonstrated histologically, prior to clinical signs of graft dysfunction.

The manuscript describes the initial experience with the Konno-Sakakibara bioptome. The authors report that frequently it was necessary to make several unsuccessful attempts at obtaining endocardial tissue prior to an adequate sample. The Caves-Stanford cardiac biopsy forceps, a modification of the Konno-Sakakibara bioptome, were later developed. These forceps were delivered into the right ventricle (RV) by means of a sheath inserted into the right internal jugular vein using a Seldinger technique. The bioptome was introduced into the right atrium (RA), and then guided using fluoroscopy, across the tricuspid valve and into the RV. The jaws were then opened, and an endocardial biopsy obtained. The forceps was then withdrawn, and the 1–2 mm biopsy specimen removed. In most patients, several such biopsies were taken prior to removal of the internal jugular sheath. Haemostatsis was achieved by sitting the patient upright, and applying pressure manually, preserving the vein for future use. A dressing of antibiotic ointment and gauze was applied once haemostasis had been confirmed. A chest 'roentgenogram' was obtained to rule out an iatrogenic pneumothorax. The procedure was performed on an outpatient basis and invariably took less than five minutes to complete.

The authors, thereafter, outline their indications for biopsy. First, it was put forward as a useful tool in the pre-operative assessment of a potential transplant candidate. In the first two months post-transplant, a baseline biopsy was taken at the time of transplant, one in the first 14 days, and again if any functional change in the graft was seen. Biopsies were also taken following treatment of an acute rejection episode, and routinely every ten days for the first two months. In suspected episodes of rejection, a biopsy was taken immediately, and then after a seven-day course of heightened immunosuppression. Thereafter biopsies were taken periodically in the long-term survivors. Excellent correlation was seen between the endocardial biopsy histological pattern and post-mortem biopsies in those unfortunate patients that died soon after diagnosis of an episode of acute rejection.

In conclusion, the authors reaffirm their belief that the principal determinant of long-term survival following cardiac transplantation is the successful management of these acute episodes of rejection. The novel technique of safe endocardial biopsy allowed, for the first time, the diagnosis of acute rejection before functional changes in the graft. It is indeed remarkable, that this endomyocardial biopsy technique has altered so little in the subsequent 40 years, and still remains the gold standard investigation for the diagnosis of transplant rejection.

Cyclosporin A initially as the only immunosuppressant in 34 recipients of cadaveric organs: 32 kidneys, 2 pancreas and 2 livers

Calne RY, Rolles K, Thiru S, McMaster P, Craddock GN, Aziz S, White DJG, Evans DB, Dunn DC, Henderson RG, Lewis P. *Lancet* 1979; 2: 1033–6.

Our last two landmark papers have concentrated on the early and reliable diagnosis of the biggest threat to graft survival in the post-transplant period, namely acute rejection. However, in the early days of cardiac transplantation, the therapeutic armamentarium to combat this immunological threat was limited. Indeed the initial survival benefit from cardiac transplantation was so poor, that many surgeons demanded a moratorium on further procedures until the immunological issues had been more thoroughly assessed and addressed.

Perhaps the single greatest advance in the transplant field, and a manuscript responsible for the renaissance of cardiac transplantation in the last two decades of the twentieth century, was the work performed in Cambridge, UK, by Sir Roy Calne on cyclosporin A (now termed ciclosporin). Sir Roy performed the first liver transplantation in Europe in 1968, the world's first combined liver, heart and lung transplant in 1986, and the first intestinal transplant in the UK in 1992.

In 1978, Calne and his team began a pilot study of cyclosporin A in 34 recipients of cadaveric organs: 32 kidneys, 2 pancreas, and 2 livers. The starting dose of cyclosporin was between 10 and 25 mg/kg/day. Twenty of the recipients were off their steroid prescription at one year, and 16 received no additional immunosuppressive agents at any time. In this period, no kidney had been lost through rejection, and only one acute rejection crisis had been reported.

These impressive short-term benefits did not come without complications. Cyclosporin had previously been shown to be nephrotoxic, a side effect that could be largely overcome by the judicious use of pre-hydration and mannitol. Of the 16 who received only cyclosporin, two developed self-limiting viral infections, one developed cytomegalovirus, and one patient's allograft had become infected with bacteria and had to be removed. One patient presented with a gastroduodenallymphoma which was resected.

Many cyclosporin treated recipients had mild derangement of their liver function tests, and all tended to resolve with reduction in dose. Most patients had an increase in growth of hair on their face and body, and several developed gum hypertrophy. Tremor, which was common in the early post-operative period, tended to resolve with time.

In their discussion, the authors are realistic about the limitations restricting the more widespread use of cyclosporin in solid organ transplantation. At the time, little was known about the pharmacodynamics of cyclosporin in man, and no suitable animal model had been developed. Since cyclosporin was fat soluble, they hypothesized that it was most likely to be excreted in bile, an explanation underlying the effects of deranged liver function on its potency. The exact mode of action of cyclosporin was also elusive, although it was hypothesized that it was the first partially selective immunosuppressive drug, acting at an early stage of differentiation of the T-cells. The authors quickly realized that cyclosporin was particularly attractive as it could be used as a steroid sparing agent, avoiding the inherent steroidal side effects. Ciclosporin has remained as a cornerstone of all immunosuppressive regimens for twenty years.

Heart-Lung transplantation: successful treatment for patients with pulmonary vascular disease

Reitz BA, Wallwork JL, Hunt SA, Pennock JL, Billingham ME, Oyer PE, Stinson EB, Shumway NE. *N Eng J Med* 1982; 306: 557–64.

By 1982, significant strides had been made in the optimal management of patients after cardiac transplantation. The ciclosporin era was beginning and early mortality post surgery improving. Although both heart and lung transplants were becoming more frequent, there had been no human recipient of a combined heart and lung transplant. As both congenital and acquired lung conditions often result in myocardial compromise, the attraction of a combined heart-lung block from a healthy donor was obvious. This report summarizes the clinical course of three patients who underwent this novel procedure between March and July 1981.

Patient 1 was a 45-year-old woman with primary pulmonary hypertension. Her mean pulmonary artery pressure by cardiac catheterization was 50, with a cardiac index of 1.9 litres. Despite aggressive vasodilatation, the patient's functional status deteriorated relentlessly and she consented to the procedure. The donor was a 15-year-old boy who was declared brain dead after a severe head injury. The operation report mentions the preservation of both phrenic nerves on pericardial pedicles, and explantation of the native block through incision in the aorta, right atrium, and trachea. Both the recurrent laryngeal and vagal nerves were preserved. The trachea was anastomosed first (4-0 prolene) followed by the aorta (also 4-0 prolene). The right atrial cuff was anastomosed to the recipient's right atrium with 3-0 prolene. Weaning from bypass occurred without incident and the patient was extubated 36 hours later. The patient was discharged 85 days post-operatively, a delay caused by two significant episodes of cardiac rejection. At ten months' follow-up she was enjoying an excellent functional status.

Patient 2 was a 30-year-old man suffering with Holt-Oram syndrome. He was diagnosed with large atrial and ventricular septal defects at the age of 12, by which time he had developed a significant increase in his pulmonary vascular resistance. The donor was to be a 25-year-old man who had met the brain stem death criteria following a motor vehicle accident. Despite initial pulmonary oedema, no episodes of acute cardiac rejection were found, and he was discharged on day 45 post-operatively. At early follow-up, right heart catheterization revealed normal pressures, pulmonary function tests were satisfactory, and the side-effects of the ciclosporin immuno-suppression minimal.

Patient 3 was a 29-year-old woman who had been diagnosed with transposition of the great arteries, with both atrial and ventricular septal defects in infancy. She had undergone a Baffes procedure (a palliative procedure using a homograft to connect the inferior vena cava to the left atrium) aged two, but had recently become severely limited by breathlessness. A palliative Mustard procedure (the construction of a baffle to transport the oxygenated blood in the pulmonary veins into the systemic right ventricle) brought only temporary functional improvement. The operation was complicated by the previous cardiac surgeries, and haemostasis proved very difficult to achieve. The patient died of multi-organ failure on day 4 post-operatively.

Shumway's team attributed their success to prior experience with heart-lung transplantation in the primate, to the use of cyclosporin A, and to the perceived anatomic and physiologic advantages of combined heart-lung transplantation. Their hope that this procedure would prove of benefit to those with end-stage pulmonary vascular disease and congenital heart defects has since been recognized. Indeed there is initial evidence that patients receiving a heart-lung transplant are less likely to develop cardiac allograft vasculopathy when compared to a matched group of heart-only recipients. However, most patients die of obliterative bronchiolitis, a form of chronic rejection of the lungs.

Value of peak oxygen uptake for optimal timing of cardiac transplantation in ambulatory patients with heart failure

Mancini D, Eisen H, Kussmaul W, Mull R, Edmonds HL, Wilson JR. *Circulation* 1991; 83: 778–86.

It has been said that patients who undergo cardiac transplantation trade one fatal disease process for a different set of iatrogenic disease processes that are also inevitably fatal. Even with the advances over the last 40 years, the average life expectancy of a cardiac transplant recipient is still a little over ten years. The crux of the listing process is to identify those with the poorest prognosis without transplant, and defer those patients with a slightly better prognosis until necessary.

Listing criteria for prospective transplant recipients prior to the work described in our next landmark paper had been subjective. Many physicians relied upon New York Heart Association (NYHA) functional status, resting ejection fraction, and haemodynamic data. Mancini *et al.* from the Hospital of the University of Pennsylvania were the first to risk stratify patients with cardiac failure according to their peak VO_2. Peak VO_2 is defined as the peak oxygen consumption measured during maximal exercise testing. It provides an objective assessment of the functional capacity of the subject if anaerobic threshold is reached during exercise. It is proportional to the cardiac output with exercise. The authors also showed that it was a good predictor of mortality in ambulatory patients with cardiac failure.

The study design was to use peak VO_2 to separate all ambulatory referrals into three categories. Group one were patients accepted for transplantation (VO_2 max <14 ml/kg/min); group two were patients rejected due to preserved exercise capacity (VO_2 max >14 ml/kg/min); and group three were candidates with a poor exercise capacity (VO_2 max <14 ml/kg/min) but who were not suitable for transplant for non-cardiac reasons. Patients could cross from group one to two and vice versa depending on changes in their VO_2 max.

Patients with preserved exercise capacity had survival rates of 94% and 84% at one and two-year follow-up, respectively. Patients in group one and three had similar survival rates; 70% at one year, although this is likely to be an overestimate as patients were removed from this survival curve following transplantation. These transplanted patients from group one had survival rates of 83% and 76% at one and two years, respectively.

These results suggested, for the first time, that peak exercise VO_2 could provide valuable prognostic data, and allow objective allocation to transplant waiting lists. The authors, therefore, advocated routine determination of exercise capacity in all ambulatory patients with heart failure considered for cardiac transplantation. This has since become standard practice in transplant centres around the world.

Effect of Pravastatin on outcomes after cardiac transplantation

Kobashigawa JA, Katznelson S, Laks H, Johnson JA, Yeatman L, Wang XM, Chia D, Terasaki PI, Sabad A, Cogert GA, Trosian K, Hamilton MA, Moriguchi JD, Kawata N, Hage A, Drinkwater DC, Stevenson LW.
N Eng J Med 1995; 333: 621–7.

Allograft coronary artery disease remained a significant problem, even when acute rejection was well controlled with the advent of ciclosporin based immunosuppression. Most immunosppressive regimes have an adverse effect on the lipid profile of recipients. Bile acid binding agents used to lower cholesterol were not suitable in transplant recipients because of their potential to affect the absorption of immunosuppressive drugs. The introduction of HMG-CoA reductase inhibitors in the late 1980s led to a resurgence in interest in this field but there were early reports of a higher incidence of rhabdomyolysis with lovastatin when combined with ciclosporin. Unlike lipophillic HMG-CoA reductase inhibitors, pravastatin is hydrophilic, and, therefore, less likely to cause these side effects.

This study reports a prospective, randomized, open-label trial in patients with cardiac transplants to assess the effect of pravastatin on cholesterol lowering, rejection, survival, and the development of coronary vasculopathy. Ninety-seven patients were enrolled between July 1992

and February 1994, 47 being randomly assigned to pravastatin and 50 to no pravastatin. Immuosuppression was accomplished using cyclosporine, azathrioprine, and prednisolone. All patients who showed signs of cardiac failure underwent myocardial biopsy. The primary end points for the study included the effects of pravastatin on cholesterol levels, cardiac rejection, survival, and the development of cardiac vasculopathy.

The beneficial effects on survival were seen at one year, far too early for effects on allograft vasculopathy to be the mechanism. One putative mechanism for this effect may be that pravastatin has an effect on the function of natural killer cells, another example of the pleiotropic effects of statins.

The final answer as to the direct mechanisms of action of the statins post-transplantation has yet to be fully explained. Current interest has been focused on the role of statins on the circulating progenitor cell population for both vascular scaffold and the cardiomyocyte. Statins are now commenced routinely in all heart transplant recipients in the immediate post-operative period.

An Implantable Permanent Left Ventricular Assist System for Man

Portner PM, Oyer PE, Jassawalla JS, Miller PJ, Chen H, LaForge DH, Skyte KW. *Trans Am Soc Artif Intern Organs* 1978; 24: 98–101.

Dr Peer Portner (1940 to 2009) was a pioneer in the field of mechanical circulatory assist devices. He attended McGill University in Montreal and graduated with a Doctor of Philosophy degree in Experimental Nuclear Physics in 1968. He founded Novocor Medical Corporation in 1979 to develop on a commercial scale the Novocor LVSA, the device used in the world's first successful bridge to transplant in Stanford in 1984. Our landmark paper is the first published description of the Dual Pusher Plate Blood Pump Left Ventricular Assist Device.

The body of the manuscript concentrates on the engineering physics behind the solenoid energy converter and the seamless elastomeric sac which is symmetrically deformed by the pump pusher plates. All surfaces and machine-body interfaces were designed to cause minimal red cell trauma, and to provide maintenance free implantability. The LVAS was designed for long-term use in man, and, as such, was a landmark in the therapeutic armamentarium available to the physicians and surgeons treating patients with end-stage cardiac failure.

Advanced Heart Failure Treated with Continuous-Flow Left Ventricular Assist Device

Slaughter MS for the HeartMate II Investigators. *N Engl J Med* 2009; 361: 2241–51.

The first generation of ventricular assist devices (like the HeartMate XVE) provided pulsatile flow. This made them relatively large and harder to implant. The HeartMate XVE was also dogged by mechanical failure after a year of support. Continuous flow devices are smaller, easier to implant, and appear to be reliable for several years of use. They do, however, need anticoagulation with warfarin and anti-platelet agents. The HeartMate II is one such continuous flow device that has been compared to the HeartMate XVE in patients who were deemed not to be suitable for heart transplantation.

The study was a multi-centre study conducted in the United States enrolling patients with advanced heart failure that were ineligible for cardiac transplantation, and whose heart failure was refractory to optimal medical management. Exclusion criteria included irreversible severe renal, pulmonary, or hepatic dysfunction or the presence of active infection. Patients were thereafter randomly assigned, in a 2:1 ratio, to either a continuous-flow LVAD or a pulsatile-flow LVAD. Extensive demographic data was collated prior to implantation, as well as device performance data, laboratory results, and medication use at regular intervals post-operatively.

The primary composite end point was survival at two years free of disabling stroke or re-operation to replace the device.

Those receiving the continuous-flow device were statistically more likely to survive free of disabling stroke and re-operation at two years (p <0.001). Of these criteria, re-operation and death were the two elements of the composite that were more significant in the pulsatile-flow group. The continuous-flow device group also had a lower rate of repeat hospitalization, with an improved quality of life and functional capacity.

This study showed improvements in the rate of survival, quality of life, functional capacity and device durability with a continuous-flow design of LVAD. Indeed, the survival rate amongst the continuous-flow group was twice that reported in the study. The authors conclude that permanent left ventricular assist device therapy, in selected patients, provides long-term haemodynamic support that is linked both to longevity and quality of life. The HeartMate II is now approved by the Food and Drug Administration for long-term support in patients with advanced heart failure and the number of implants is likely to increase rapidly in the next few years.

Conclusions

The major hurdle to the more widespread therapeutic use of organ transplantation is donor availability. Although work is underway to use non-heart beating donors to expand this pool, it is unlikely that demand will be met. Left ventricular assist devices will continue to improve due to technological advances, leading to a concomitant improvement in the quality of life for recipients. There are no major clinical trials underway at present in the field of cardiac transplantation. The hope for transplant recipient longevity rests with the translation from bench-to-bedside of the phenomenon of immunological tolerance.

Part IV

Hypertension

Chapter 17

Systemic arterial hypertension

Dr Kaleab Asrress and Professor Bryan Williams

Introduction

Cardiovascular disease is the leading cause of death in the world[1]. Individually, ischaemic heart disease (IHD) is the leading, and cerebrovascular disease the second leading, cause of mortality in all regions of the world apart from sub-Saharan Africa[2,3]. The impact of hypertension is significant, with an estimated 47% of all IHD and 54% of all stroke being attributable to high blood pressure (BP)[4]. It should be noted, however, that there has been a major decline in cardiovascular disease mortality in Western Europe, the USA, and Japan over the past 40 years[5,6]. There are multiple factors underlying these favourable trends but more widespread and improved control of hypertension has certainly played a major role[7,8,9]. Several landmark studies over the past 50 years have been instrumental in this process, particularly in exploring the underlying epidemiology, defining individual risk factors, and assessing treatment strategies. Selecting a short list from this immense body of work has not been an easy task, with many important papers not making the final selection. What we can say is that those presented here are truly landmark in every sense of the word, and we hope to convince the reader of the reasons for this.

Epidemiology

Epidemiologic assessment of the role of blood pressure in stroke: The Framingham study

Kannel WB, Wolf PA, Verter J, McNamara PM. *JAMA* 1970; 214: 301–10.

Background

Much of our current understanding about the role of BP in cardiovascular disease can be attributed to decades of high quality research conducted upon the much-studied town of Framingham. This was established in 1949 with the aim of securing epidemiological data on atherosclerotic and hypertensive cardiovascular disease[10]. Their first major report, after 14 years of follow-up, provided a critical insight into the relationship between BP and coronary artery disease (CAD)[11]. Though the relationship between hypertension and CAD was already well established, this was a ground-breaking study in many ways, none more so than in establishing the link with BP to the risk of stroke.

Methods

Since 1949, the National Heart Institute has been conducting a long-term prospective study in Framingham, Massachusetts, of factors related to the development of cardiovascular disease and stroke. A group of 5208 subjects between the ages of 30 and 62 had their BP recorded biennially, at three separate times during a single consultation. Hypertension was arbitrarily designated present at 160/95 mmHg or greater, normotension at 140/90 mmHg or below, with the rest recorded as borderline. Minimum criteria for diagnosing a stroke were established. Surveillance of the population during their biennial visit included a neurological examination; those suspected of having suffered a stroke being examined by a second observer as well as a neurologist. Patients hospitalized with a suspected stroke were examined by a neurologist during the acute phase. Surviving stroke victims had their condition re-evaluated during each visit to the research clinic. Follow-up was reasonably complete, with less than 2% completely lost to follow-up over 14 years.

Results

In 14 years of follow-up, 65 men and 70 women developed a focal neurological deficit of abrupt onset meeting the minimum criteria for diagnosis of stroke. The incidence of all the major cardiovascular sequelae, including stroke, increased in direct proportion to the BP, even in the normotensive range, without any identifiable critical or safe value. Analysis showed that systolic and diastolic BPs were of equal importance, and significant whether the pressure was labile or not. Risk of stroke was of equal significance across different sex and age groups.

Conclusions and clinical implications

This study showed clearly that control of hypertension whether labile or fixed, systolic or diastolic, at any age, in either sex appeared central in preventing stroke.

It dispelled many a misconception held at the time and ushered in a paradigm shift in the management of this disease process. These findings were also central in instructing the design of future epidemiological and interventional studies that would later improve and refine the management of hypertension in the prevention of cardiovascular disease.

Learning points

- Systolic and diastolic hypertension are equally important in the aetiology of stroke.
- Both labile and fixed hypertension should be treated.
- Mean arterial pressure was no better at predicting stroke than systolic pressure alone.
- Elevated BP was equally important across different age groups.
- Both sexes were equally susceptible to stroke from elevated BP.

Further reading

- Kannel WB, Wolf PA, Verter J, McNamara PM. Epidemiologic assessment of the role of blood pressure in stroke: the Framingham Study. 1970. *JAMA* 1996; 276(15): 1269–78.
- Turnbull F, Kengne AP, MacMahon S. Blood pressure and cardiovascular disease: tracing the steps from Framingham. *Prog Cardiovasc Dis* 2010; 53(1): 39–44.

Age-specific relevance of usual blood pressure to vascular mortality: a meta-analysis of individual data for one million adults in 61 prospective studies

Lewington S, Clarke R, Qizilbash N, Peto R, Collins R. Prospective Studies Collaboration. *Lancet* 2002; 360(9349): 1903–13.

Background

Several epidemiological studies have been published examining the relationship between BP and vascular disease mortality. These have produced valuable information; however, there is likely to be an appreciable random error resulting in different studies producing apparently different results. This is particularly an issue at the lower BP levels, where the mortality levels are relatively low. This can, to some extent, be overcome by performing meta-analyses[12,13,14]. The selected landmark study by Lewington *et al.* is a meta-analysis examining the relationship between BP and vascular mortality. It has several advantages over earlier meta-analyses. First, it is large, including over one million patients from 61 cohorts involving 120,000 deaths. Second, individual patient records were available for each of these participants, allowing detailed analysis. Third, individuals with pre-existing vascular disease were excluded to avoid reverse-causality, that is, preventing the effects of pre-existing vascular diseases on BP. Appropriate time-dependent adjustments were also made for 286,000 repeat measurements, to correct for what they term 'regression dilution'.

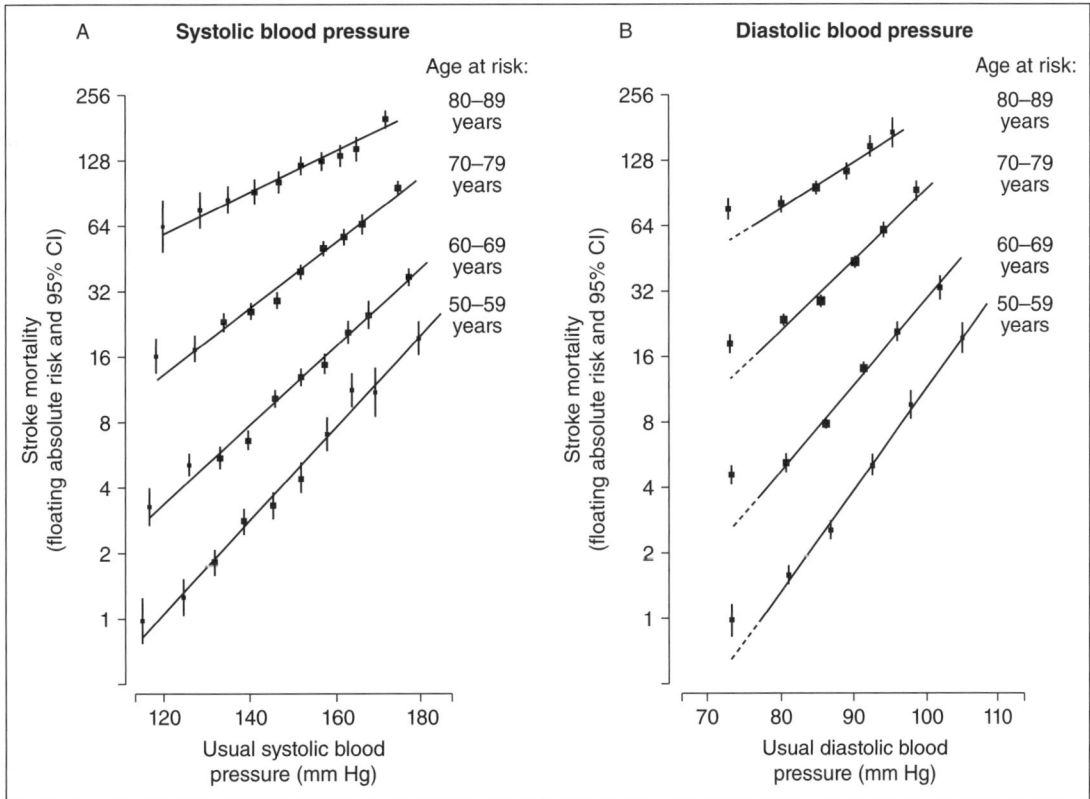

Figure 17.1 Stroke mortality rate in each decade of age versus usual blood pressure at start of that decade.

Reproduced from Lewington S, *et al.* Prospective Studies Collaboration 2002: Age-specific relevance of usual blood pressure to vascular mortality: a meta-analysis of individual data for one million adults in 61 prospective studies. *Lancet* 2002; 360(9349): 1903–13, with permission from Elsevier.

Methods

A key aspect leading to the success of this project is the fact that collaboration was sought and achieved from the investigators of all prospective observational studies in which data on BP, blood cholesterol, date of birth, and sex had been recorded at a baseline screening visit, and in which cause and date of death had been routinely sought[15]. The analysis amounted to 5000 person-years of follow-up. The primary risk factors for the meta-analysis were age, and the systolic and diastolic BPs. Five age ranges and ten systolic BP categories yielded a total of 50 different groups, one of which was taken as the reference group, with a hazard ratio of 1.0.

Results

During 12.7 million person-years at risk (mean of 12 years to death), there were 11,960 deaths attributed to stroke, 34,283 to IHD, 10,092 to other vascular causes, 60,797 to non-vascular causes, with a further 5584 deaths of unknown cause. This meta-analysis showed that with increasing years throughout middle and old age, BP is strongly and directly related to vascular, and overall mortality, without any evidence of a threshold down to at least 115/75 mmHg. For example, at the ages of 60–69, each difference in systolic BP of 20 mmHg (roughly 10 mmHg diastolic BP) was associated with slightly more than a two-fold difference in the risk of stroke death and with almost two-fold difference in death from IHD and from other vascular causes. Figure 17.1 demonstrates the stroke mortality rate in each decade of age versus usual BP at the start of that decade. Similar striking relationships with BP are seen with IHD mortality, as well as other vascular mortality (non-stroke, non-IHD).

Conclusions and clinical implications

This major meta-analysis on the subject demonstrated that throughout middle and old age, BP is strongly and directly related to stroke, IHD, and overall mortality. It also confirmed that risk extends to lower levels of BP than currently treated for. Furthermore, at around the time of publication, there was debate on whether there might be a threshold level of systolic BP, at about 140–160 mmHg, below which lowering BP further would not be associated with lower disease risks[16]. This meta-analysis was therefore important in highlighting this large, previously undefined, group as being at risk, and potentially benefiting from intervention. Although patients with pre-existing vascular disease at baseline were excluded from the present study, the results suggest that those who are at high risk because of pre-existing disease would gain particular benefit from lowering BP, even if they would currently be classified as normotensive.

Learning points

- Blood pressure throughout middle and old age is directly related to stroke, IHD, and other vascular mortality.
- There does not appear to be a lower limit for normal BP. Risk is continuous down to at least a BP of 115/75 mmHg.

Blood pressure treatment

Effects of treatment on morbidity in hypertension. Results in patients with diastolic blood pressures averaging 115 through to 129 mmHg

VA Cooperative Study Group. *JAMA* 1967; 202: 1028–34.

Background

The association between hypertension and adverse outcomes, including stroke and myocardial infarction (MI), was being established around the time of this publication. However, data on the benefits of treating high BP was limited. Though there was data to support the treatment of malignant hypertension, effectiveness of treating less severe forms was disputed[17,18]. This study was the first randomized, controlled trial in hypertension, and set out to answer this question.

Methods

The investigation was centred on male patients without signs of accelerated hypertension at study enrolment, whose diastolic BPs prior to treatment averaged 115–129 mmHg. All potential subjects were hospitalized for one week for pre-randomization assessment. Severity of hypertension was assessed in five categories, one for average diastolic BP, and the other four for markers of hypertensive end organ damage to optic fundi, brain, heart, and kidney. This was the basis on which subjects were stratified into those suffering with mild, moderate, or severe hypertension. The latter were excluded from the trial. The trialists then went to extraordinary lengths to ensure a compliant cohort of patients. After the initial in-patient assessment, eligible subjects went into a second pre-randomization phase, following discharge. They were given two placebos, one of which contained riboflavin, which produces a yellow fluorescence of urine under ultraviolet light. They were then followed up at monthly intervals, by a physician, for up to four months. The assessment of reliability was based on their attendance at clinic, urine testing, and strict pill counts. These subjects then underwent double-blind randomization to either active treatment (hydrochlorothiazide plus reserpine plus hydralazine hydrochloride), or placebo.

Follow-up was monthly for the first two months and bimonthly thereafter. Annual examinations included a physical examination, chest X-ray, electrocardiogram, and blood tests. End points were death; class A events, defined as hypertensive complications listed in the protocol which required treatment with known active agents and permanent removal from the protocol; class B events were defined as events that did not require permanent discontinuation of protocol treatments.

Results

In the study, 143 hypertensive males, average age 51 years (range 30–73), with average diastolic BPs of 115–129 mmHg were randomized to either active treatment (hydrochlorothiazide plus reserpine plus hydralazine hydrochloride) or placebo. Average follow-up was approximately 18 months across the two groups. There was a significant drop in the diastolic BP in the active treatment group (from four-month follow-up to study completion) with no significant change in the placebo group.

There were four deaths and ten class A events in the placebo group compared to zero in the treatment group. The deaths were related to cardiovascular disease (dissecting aortic aneurysm in two, ruptured aortic aneurysm in one, and sudden death in one). Class A events included grade 3–4 hypertensive retinopathy, cerebrovascular haemorrhage, dissecting aortic aneurysm, subarachnoid haemorrhage, and congestive cardiac failure.

Treatment failures were not predefined in the protocol, but were those events not meeting the specific criteria for any one class A event but were considered to be life threatening enough for protocol drugs to be removed and treatment instituted with known antihypertensive agents. There were seven such events in the placebo group compared to one in the active group. There were six class B events in the placebo group compared to one in the active group.

The authors analysed the results in many ways. What remains clear is that there is a large significant reduction in adverse events with active anti-hypertensive treatment over a very short period of treatment.

Conclusions and clinical implications

There are two important messages to come from this seminal work in the field of hypertension. First, whilst essential hypertension was generally regarded as a slowly progressive disease, it can be shown that there is an extremely high incidence of severe complications. Second, over a relatively short period of treatment with antihypertensives, patients with diastolic BPs of 115 mmHg or more can have a significant reduction in event rates. Observed was a particularly high incidence of fundoscopic manifestations of accelerated hypertension which has important implications in the age-group studied, who are on the whole of working age. The results established the practice of fundoscopy in patients with what might be considered as mild levels of hypertension.

Learning points

◆ Diastolic BPs in the region of 115–129 mmHg are associated with a high incidence of severe complications over a short period of time.
◆ Treatment in this group with a combination of thiazides, reserpine, and hydralazine is associated with a significant reduction in cardiovascular events.
◆ Clinical assessment and surveillance in this cohort should include markers of end organ damage to the eyes, kidneys, brain, and heart.

Design of specific inhibitors of angiotensin converting enzyme: a new class of orally active antihypertensive agents

Ondetti MA, Rubin B, Cusgman DW. *Science* 1977; 196: 441–4.

Background

The design of specific inhibitors of the renin-angiotensin-aldosterone system (RAS) has heralded a new class of orally active therapies important in not only treating hypertension but also several facets of the cardiovascular disease spectrum. Before embarking on a description of this important work, it is instructive to appraise the discovery and evolution of earlier anti-hypertensive therapies.

The first group of medications to control hypertension were associated with significant side effects, limiting their use, including methyldopa, reserpine, pentaquine, hydralazine, and guanethidine. Diuretics were the first group of drugs to effectively reduce hypertension without causing undue adverse effects. They were discovered by chance in the 1930s when patients taking sulphonamides to treat bacterial infections reported large diuresis on taking the medication. This was tested in patients with heart failure, who improved dramatically, but investigators concluded that sulphonamides were too toxic for prolonged or routine use[19]. Through a process of trial and error, the formula for sulphonamide was modified, resulting in the discovery of chlorothiazide, a relatively safe but effective diuretic which when administered to ten hypertensive patients, reduced their BP to almost normal levels within a few days[20]. The discovery of the prototype beta blocker, propranolol, by James Black[21], who was subsequently awarded the Nobel Prize, provided another class of anti-hypertensives (as well as anti-anginals, which was their original design). A number of beta blockers with different characteristics soon became available. A quest for similar drugs led to the development of verapamil. Later studies showed that verapamil was not actually a beta blocker at all, but worked by blocking the entry of calcium into cells, which led to the development of other calcium channel antagonists, as well as an understanding of the importance of intracellular calcium metabolism in muscle contraction. Clinical research revealed that as well as lowering BP, beta blockers and calcium channel antagonists reduced the risk of stroke and MI by one-third. Problems still arose from the non-specific nature of their action that often led to frequent side effects. There were also hypertensive patients who were inadequately controlled on a combination of diuretic, calcium channel antagonists, and beta blockers. The discovery of the RAS, a powerful highly specific control system for BP, led to the development of an important class of drugs in this field.

Discovery of ACE-inhibitors

The importance of the kidney as a major guardian of BP control began to be suspected in the mid-nineteenth century. In 1872 Frederick Akbar Mohamed, an Indian doctor working at Guy's hospital, was able to make crude measurements of BP and showed that patients with kidney disease also had enlarged hearts and high BP. Many years of laboratory work from different groups followed to better understand the mechanisms by which the kidneys controlled BP. The importance of renin and later angiotensin converting enzyme (ACE) in the control of BP became established. The concept of ACE-inhibitors took several more years to develop.

Workers in the banana plantations of south-western Brazil were known to collapse suddenly after being bittern by a pit viper. Work began identifying, purifying, and testing the blood-pressure lowering substance in snake venom. David Cushman and Miguel Ondetti, working for Squibb pharmaceuticals in New Jersey, were able to make a synthetic version of the substance which when injected into volunteers as well as hypertensive patients resulted in significant drops in BP. The major problem was that this substance was too big to be absorbed by the gut and could therefore not be given in oral form. After many years of effort, and over 2000 diverse compounds tested, it was not possible to modify this substance into a compound that had the desired chemical properties and could be taken orally. Help came from an unexpected source in the form of a pancreatic digestive enzyme called carboxypeptidase A.

To gain further insight into its action in the body, Byers and Wolfenden, developed a simple but highly potent inhibitor of carboxypeptidase A, benzylsuccinic acid[22]. Cushman and Ondetti had noticed that the structure of carboxypeptidate A was similar to ACE so the discovery of a potent inhibitor to the former provided a new approach to creating an inhibitor to the latter. What followed was an elegant series of experiments logically modifying the chemical structure of this pancreatic enzyme inhibitor, eventually culminating in the synthesis of captopril, described in this landmark paper published in *Science*. This approach, of specifically designing compounds for a precise chemical fit, resulted in the development of the next generation of ACE inhibitors including enalapril and lisinopril, and subsequently angiotensin receptor blockers and direct renin inhibitors.

Conclusions and clinical implications

The development of captopril and related ACE inhibitors was the best example of drug design whereby molecules are constructed for a precise fit with a molecular receptor. Apart from resulting in a hugely important class of drugs for the treatment of hypertension and other cardiovascular disorders, it promoted this approach of structure-based drug design that has subsequently been applied successfully to many other disorders, including HIV and cancer.

Learning points

◆ The renin-angiotensin-aldosterone system is a powerful mechanism for the control of BP.
◆ The design of captopril highlighted the importance of drug design based on a chemical understanding to modify molecular structures, an approach used in the design of many other drugs.

Further reading

● Dustan HP, Roccella EJ, Garrison HH. Controlling hypertension. A research success story. *Arch Intern Med* 1996; 156(17): 1926–35.
● Ferreira SH. A Bradykinin-potentiating factor (BPF) present in the venom of Bothrops Jararca. *Br J Pharmacol Chemother* 1965; 24: 163–9.

Effects of an angiotensin converting enzyme inhibitor, ramipril, on cardiovascular events in high-risk patients

Yusuf, S, Sleight, P, Pogue, J, Bosch, J, Davies, R, Dagenais, G. The Heart Outcomes Prevention Evaluation Study Investigators. *N Engl J Med* 2000; 342: 145–53.

Background

At the time of designing this study it was known that activation of the RAS has an important role in increasing the risk of cardiovascular events. Angiotensin converting enzyme inhibitors had been shown in several trials to reduce the risk of MI in patients with low ejection fraction (EF). Subsequent analyses of these trials showed that this effect was independent of EF, heart disease, concomitant use of medications, diabetes status, and BP. This suggested that ACE inhibitors might have a role in preventing MI in a broad range of patients, which instructed this trial design.

Methods

A total of 9297 patients with high cardiovascular risk, ≥55 years of age, who had evidence of vascular disease in the form of CAD, stroke, peripheral vascular disease, or diabetes plus one other cardiovascular risk factor (hypertension, elevated total cholesterol levels, low high-density lipoprotein cholesterol levels, cigarette smoking, or documented microalbuminuria) were randomized to receive ramipril 10 mg once per day or placebo. Patients with low EF were excluded. The primary outcome was a composite of MI, stroke, or death from cardiovascular causes.

There was a range of pre-specified secondary and other outcomes. There was a run-in phase where all eligible subjects received 2.5 mg ramipril once per day for 7–10 days, followed by placebo for 10–14 days. A total of 1035 patients were subsequently excluded because of non-compliance, abnormal serum creatinine, or potassium levels, or withdrawal of consent. After subsequent randomization, patients in the treatment group received ramipril 2.5 mg once per day for one week, 5 mg for the next three weeks, and then 10 mg. The trial was a two-by-two factorial study evaluating both ramipril and vitamin E. The effects of vitamin E reported separately showed no effect on cardiovascular outcomes[23].

Results

After five years of follow-up, 651 patients assigned to the ramipril group (14.0%) reached the primary end point, compared to 826 patients assigned to placebo (17.8%). This equated to a 22% reduction in the primary outcome of MI, stroke, or death from a cardiovascular cause. There were also significant reductions in each of these outcomes taken individually in the treatment group. In terms of secondary outcomes, there was a significant reduction in death from any cause, revascularization procedures, cardiac arrest, heart failure, worsening angina, a new diagnosis of diabetes, and complications related to diabetes.

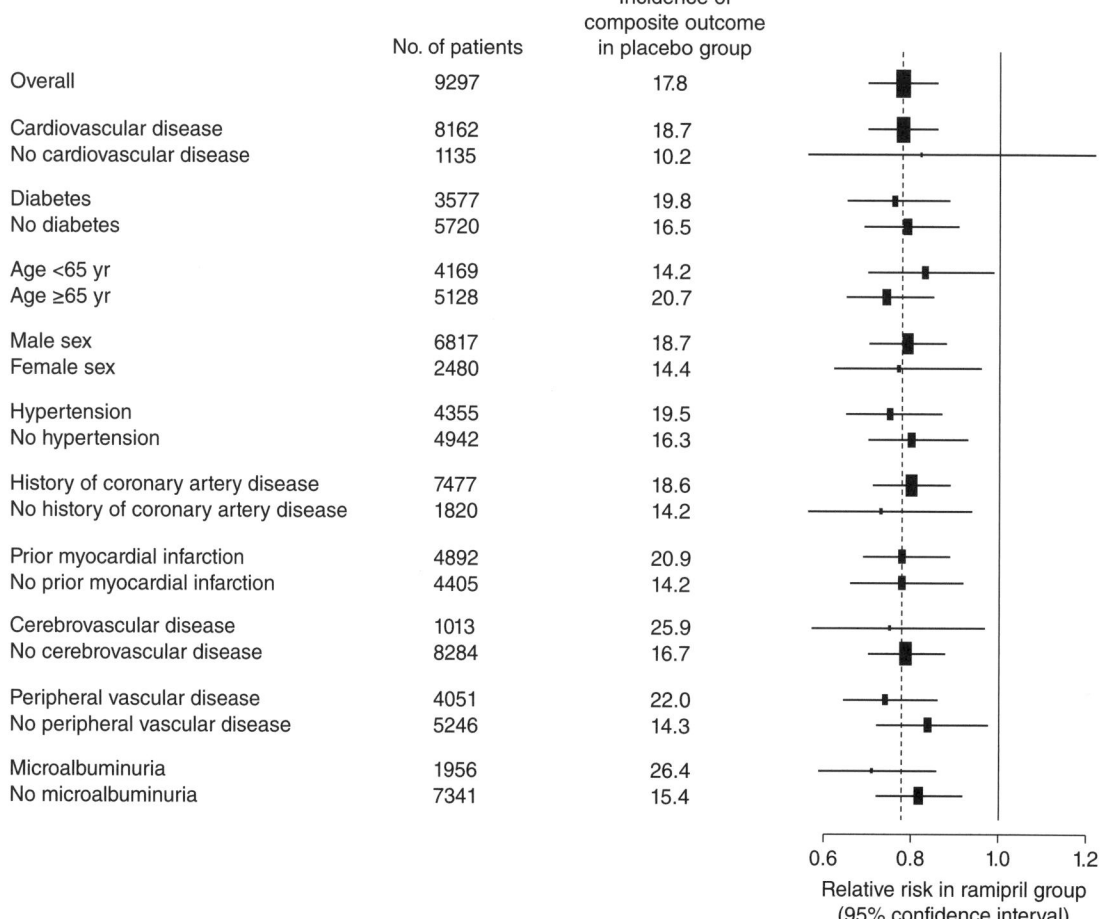

Figure 17.2 The beneficial effects of treatment with ramipril on the composite outcome of myocardial infarction, stroke, or death from cardiovascular causes overall and in various pre-defined subgroups.

Reproduced from Yusuf S, *et al*. Effects of an Angiotensin-Converting–Enzyme Inhibitor, Ramipril, on Cardiovascular Events in High-Risk Patients: The Heart Outcomes Prevention Evaluation Study Investigators. *NEJM* 2000; 342: 145–53, with permission. Copyright © (2000) Massachusetts Medical Society. All rights reserved.

Figure 17.2 shows the overall results, as well as the range of pre-defined subgroups that derived a benefit in the primary outcome from receiving ramipril. A broad range of patients were included in the study, including those with manifestations of CAD, cerebrovascular disease, or peripheral vascular disease, or diabetes and one other cardiovascular risk factor. Ramipril was beneficial in all these groups.

Conclusions and clinical implications

The Heart Outcomes Prevention Evaluation (HOPE) study demonstrated the benefit of ramipril in significantly reducing rates of death, MI, and stroke in a broad range of patients at high cardiovascular risk. Treatment with ramipril appeared to have protective effects on both the vasculature and the myocardium. There was only a small reduction in BP (3/2 mmHg), suggesting that ramipril has beneficial effects independent of reduction in BP— although this has remained controversial and almost all of the benefit of ramipril was seen in the subgroup with a BP >140/90 at baseline. Benefits were observed among patients that were already taking a number of effective treatments to reduce cardiovascular risk, such as aspirin, beta blockers, and lipid-lowering agents, indicating that the inhibition of ACE offers an additional approach to the prevention of atherothrombotic complications. Although not technically a study of 'hypertension', many of the subjects were treated hypertensive patients. Consequently, this study had a major impact on the use of RAS blockade as a mainstay of modern antihypertensive treatment strategies.

Learning points

- Ramipril given to a broad range of patients at high cardiovascular risk, reduced major cardiovascular and cerebrovascular events.
- This benefit is derived despite a seemingly modest reduction in BP, implicating RAS in exerting additional direct mechanisms on the heart and vasculature.

- Ramipril reduced the incidence of and complications from diabetes, highlighting its importance in this group of patients.
- The question as to whether this was a class effect of ACE inhibitors or indeed whether similar effects could be expected from angiotensin receptor blockade remained unanswered.

Telmisartan, ramipril, or both in patients at high risk for vascular events

The ONTARGET Investigators, Yusuf S, Teo KK, Pogue J, Dyal L, Copland I, Schumacher H, Dagenais G, Sleight P, Anderson C. *N Engl J Med* 2008; 358: 1547–59.

Background

At the time of study design, trials of ACE inhibitors had convincingly demonstrated their benefit in reducing rates of death, MI, and stroke among patients at high cardiovascular risk. Data on the use of angiotensin receptor blockers (ARBs) was less robust, but benefit had been shown in those with impaired left ventricular function unable to take ACE inhibitors[24]. The same group showed that the addition of an ARB to ACE inhibitor in patients with chronic heart failure resulted in an additional reduction in cardiovascular events[25]. This trial set out to test the ARB temisartan against ramipril in patients at high cardiovascular risk, and whether the combination of the two drugs was superior to ramipril alone. The population tested was similar to the HOPE study (see previous paper) where ramipril had been shown to have benefit.

Methods

Patients with coronary, peripheral, or cerebrovascular disease or diabetes with end-organ damage were enrolled in the study. After a three-week run-in period patients underwent double-blind randomization, with 8,576 assigned to receive 10 mg of ramipril per day, 8,542 assigned to receive 80 mg of telmisartan per day, and 8,502 assigned to receive both drugs. The primary composite outcome was death from cardiovascular causes, MI, stroke, or hospitalization for heart failure.

Results

At a median follow-up of 56 months, mean BP was lower in both the telmisartan (0.9/0.6 mmHg lower) and the combination therapy group (2.1/1.4 mmHg) compared to the ramipril group. The primary outcome had occurred in 16.5% of the ramipril group as compared to 16.7% in the telmisartan group, which was not a significant difference. The telmisartan group had a lower rate of cough and angio-oedema, but had a higher rate of hypotensive symptoms. In the combination therapy group there was no significant reduction in the primary outcome, but treatment was associated with a significantly higher rate of hypotensive symptoms, syncope, and renal dysfunction compared to the ramipril group.

Conclusions and clinical implications

The Ongoing Telmisartan Alone and in Combination with Ramipril Global Endpoint (ONTARGET) trial was the fourth and largest comparative hypertension trial, and confirmed that ARBs were non-inferior to ACE inhibitors at reducing hard cardiovascular end points in high-risk patients. Similarly, combination therapy, which despite lowering BP further, conferred no additional benefit in reducing cardiovascular events and was associated with more side effects. The results have been extremely important in instructing clinical practice.

Learning points

- Ramipril and telmisartan appear to provide similar benefit in reducing cardiovascular events in patients at high cardiovascular risk.
- The combination of ramipril and telmisartan is associated with more side effects without conferring additional benefit, and combination therapies of ACE-inhibition + ARBs have no place in the routine management of hypertension.
- This data has been generally interpreted as showing that ACE-inhibition and ARBs are broadly equivalent with regard to CVD prevention, but with ARBs less likely to induce side effects.

Major outcomes in high-risk hypertensive patients randomized to angiotensin-converting enzyme inhibitor or calcium channel blocker vs diuretic

The Antihypertensive and Lipid-Lowering Treatment to Prevent Heart Attack Trial (ALLHAT). The ALLHAT Officers and Coordinators for the ALLHAT Collaborative Research Group. *JAMA* 2002; 288: 2981–97.

Background

The first two classes of anti-hypertensives, thiazide diuretics and beta blockers were used in early clinical trials to demonstrate the benefit of lowering BP. Since then, other classes of anti-hypertensives, namely ACE inhibitors, alpha blockers, and calcium channel antagonists have become available, and shown in placebo-controlled trials to reduce cardiovascular events in patients with hypertension. Their relative value compared with older, less expensive, therapies was unclear, particularly which therapy to use first. This clearly has major clinical, public health, and economic implications. The ALLHAT study was an ambitious study that set out to answer this question.

Methods

Participants aged ≥55 years with hypertension and at least one other cardiovascular risk factor were enrolled from 623 North American centres. Patients with impaired left ventricular function were excluded. Individuals already on anti-hypertensives continued their medications until the point of randomization, at which point they stopped taking all previous medications. Double-blind randomization was to chlorthalidone, amlodipine, lisinopril, or doxazosin. Target BP in each group was less than 140/90 mmHg, achieved by titrating the assigned drug and where necessary adding open-label agents at the physician's discretion (atenolol, clonidine, or reserpine) and if a further agent was required, hydralazine. The primary outcome was combined fatal CAD or non-fatal MI. Secondary outcomes were all-cause mortality, stroke, combined CHD (primary outcome, coronary revascularization, or angina with hospitalization), and combined cardiovascular disease (combined CHD, stroke, treated angina without hospitalization, heart failure, and peripheral arterial disease).

Results

A total of 42,418 patients were enrolled. After one year of follow-up chlorthalidone was found to be superior to doxazosin, resulting in termination of this arm, and results reported early[26]. A group of 33,357 patients continued in the other arms, and at a mean follow-up of 4.9 years the primary outcome occurred in 2956 participants with no difference between treatments groups. For amlodipine versus chlorthalidone, secondary outcomes were similar, except for a higher six-year rate of heart failure with amlodipine. There has been concern about the validity of the heart failure diagnosis and subsequent studies have shown that CCBs are effective at preventing heart failure in hypertensive patients. For lisinopril versus chlorthalidone, lisinopril had higher six-year rates of combined cardiovascular disease, stroke, and heart failure.

The authors reported no differences in subgroups for the comparison of amlodipine and chlorthalidone. The only notable subgroup differences were an increased risk of stroke and combined cardiovascular disease in the ACE inhibitor group in black but not in non-black patients. Amongst black patients, follow-up BP was substantially higher in the ACE inhibitor group than in the chlorthalidone group. Otherwise, among pre-specified subgroups of interest defined by age, sex, race, and diabetes, results were remarkably consistent.

In terms of safety end points, six-year rates of hospitalization for gastrointestinal bleeding were not significant across the different treatment arms. Angio-oedema occurred in 0.1, 0.1, and 0.4% in the chlorthalidone, amlodipine, and lisinopril groups respectively and was notably more common in people of African/Caribbean descent. Prior observational data had previously pointed to an increased the risk of cancer, gastrointestinal bleeding, and all-cause mortality with calcium channel antagonists, particularly the dihydropyridines. The results from ALLHAT did not support this finding.

Conclusions and clinical implications

The ALLHAT study is the largest and one of the most important trials in hypertension, profoundly affecting the way it is treated. It compared simultaneously four classes of anti-hypertensives and showed that the thiazide-like diuretic chlorthalidone was equivalent to ACE-inhibition or CCB at preventing the primary end-point of the trial, i.e. cornonary heart disease. This led the Joint National Committee 7 guidelines published in 2003 to recommend that because the diuretic was cheaper and non-inferior to the alternative treatments, then this should be the preferred first line therapy for hypertension. ALLHAT also confirmed long-held views that ACE inhibitors were less effective at lowering blood pressure and thus less effective at preventing stroke in people of Black African/Caribean descent in whom angiooedema was also more common with this treatment. Finally, ALLHAT refuted prior saftey concerns from observational and case controlled studies which had suggested CCBs might be associated with less effective protection against CHD and an increased risk of cancer and gastrointestinal bleeding.

Each of the medications substantially reduced BP, although the extent of BP reduction was not equivalent. The BP differences between amlodipine and chlorthalidone were small and balanced (lower systolic BP for chlorthalidone and lower diastolic for amlodipine). Lisinopril was less effective at lowering BP than chlorthalidone, especially in people of Black African/Caribbean descent.

What is clear from ALLHAT is that the results provide definitive data on one important aspect of hypertension management—the best initial therapy. The findings have resulted in a positive return to prescribing thiazide diuretics and away from more expensive alternatives.

Further Reading

- Stafford RS, Bartholomew LK, Cushman WC, Cutler JA, Davis BR, Dawson G, Einhorn PT, Furberg CD, Piller LB,

> ### Learning points
>
> - Chlorthalidone is superior to lisinopril and amlodipine in preventing the adverse sequelae of cardiovascular disease.
> - All three drug classes show good safety and tolerability profiles.
> - The ACE inhibitors should not be used as first-line therapy in the black population.
> - The demographic heterogeneity and consistency of subgroup findings suggest that ALLHAT results can be generalized to the hypertensive population at large.

Pressel SL, Whelton PK; ALLHAT Collaborative Research Group. Impact of the ALLHAT/JNC7 Dissemination Project on thiazide-type diuretic use. *Arch Intern Med.* 2010; 170(10): 851–8.
- Kostis JB, Cabrera J, Cheng JQ, Cosgrove NM, Deng Y, Pressel SL, Davis BR et al. Association between chlorthalidone treatment of systolic hypertension and long-term survival. *JAMA.* 2011; 306: 2588–93.

Dilemmas in the management of hypertension

Treatment of Hypertension in Patients 80 Years of Age or Older

Beckett NS, Peters R, Fletcher AE, Staessen JA, Liu L, Dumitrascu D. *N Engl J Med* 2008; 358: 1887–98.

Background

Leading up to the publication of this study, debate remained as to whether treating hypertension in patients 80 years or older was beneficial. Although the risk of stroke increases continuously with increasing BP, it has been shown that the risk of stroke attenuates with increasing age. Furthermore, epidemiological studies have suggested that BP and risk of death are inversely related in people ≥80 years. Whether this was due to increased risks of therapy for BP reduction or reverse causation due to conditions that may be associated with blood-pressure reduction (such as cancer, dementia, MI, and heart failure) was not clear. Furthermore, there was the real potential for BP lowering to lead to increased adverse effects in the very elderly (especially postural hypotension and falls) as a consequence of their less

flexible cardiovascular haemodyanics. What added to this uncertainty was that randomized controlled trials published to date have either excluded those ≥80 years or have recruited too few to show a difference between treatments. The meta-analyses available at the time were not robust enough to give meaningful results. The Hypertension in the Very Elderly Trial (HYVET) aimed to resolve this issue.

Methods

The HYVET study was a randomized, double-blind, placebo-controlled trial performed in 195 centres in 13 countries in Europe, China, Australasia, and North Africa. Patients enrolled were ≥80 years and had a sustained systolic BP of 160 mmHg or more. Patients were instructed to stop all anti-hypertensive treatment and to take a single placebo daily for at least two months and to undergo two BP measurements two months apart. Subsequently, if the mean BP was between 160 and 199 mmHg, patients underwent randomization to either the diuretic indapamide (sustained release, 1.5 mg) or a matching placebo. The ACE inhibitor perindopril (2 or 4 mg) or a matching placebo was added if necessary to achieve the target BP of 150/80 mmHg. The primary end point of the trial was any stroke (fatal or non-fatal, not including transient ischaemic attacks). Secondary end points included all-cause death, death from cardiovascular causes, death from cardiac causes, and death from stroke.

Exclusion criteria included a contraindication to use of the trial medications, accelerated hypertension, secondary hypertension, haemorrhagic stroke in the previous six months, heart failure requiring treatment with antihypertensives, defined biochemical abnormalities, gout, a diagnosis of clinical dementia, and a requirement of nursing care.

Results

A total of 4,761 patients entered the placebo run-in phase. Of these, 3,845 were randomized to the two arms of the study. Age range at entry was 80–105 years, with 73% in the 80–84 age range. At two years, the mean BP was 15.0/6.1 mmHg lower in the active-treatment group compared to the placebo group. After a median follow-up of 1.8 years active treatment was associated with a 30% reduction in the rate of fatal or non-fatal stroke, a 39% reduction in the rate of death from stroke, a 21% reduction

in the rate of death from any cause, a 23% reduction in the rate of death from cardiovascular causes, and a 64% reduction in the rate of heart failure. Fewer serious adverse events were reported in the active-treatment group.

Conclusions and clinical implications

Hypertension in individuals ≥80 years is common. The HYVET trial unequivocally shows that treatment of hypertension with indapamide, and the addition of perindopril where necessary, aiming to achieve a target BP of 150/80 mmHg is beneficial and is associated with reduced risks of death from stroke, death from any cause, and heart failure. The results show that it is never too late to start anti-hypertensives in the elderly population, expanding the spectrum for which there is evidence of a treatment benefit, and providing a mandate to recommend treatment in this age group, the fastest growing segment of the population.

Learning points

- Systolic BP >160 mmHg, in people of ≥80 years should be treated to a target of 150 mmHg, which results in reductions in cardiovascular events.
- The combination of a thiazide diuretic and ACE inhibitor, where necessary, should be the treatments recommended in this age group.

Prognostic Significance of Left Ventricular Mass Change During Treatment of Hypertension

Devereux RB, Wachtell K, Gerdts E, Boman K, Nieminen MS, Papademetriou V, Rokkedal J, Harris K, Aurup P, Dahlöf B *JAMA* 2004; 292: 2350–56.

Background

An increase in left ventricular mass is associated with many chronic diseases, including aortic stenosis, regurgitant valvular heart disease, obesity, diabetes, and MI. The most common cause, however, is hypertension. The increase in left ventricular mass is thought to represent a reaction to pressure or volume overload. In the short term, this may be of benefit in allowing the heart to compensate for increased wall stress and prevent potential haemodynamic compromise. In the long term, the ventricular remodelling leading to hypertrophy independently predicts adverse outcomes in diverse populations, including hypertension. This was first noted in

the Framingham Heart Study (see previous Landmark Paper). These findings suggest that the level of left ventricular mass and mass reduction during treatment of hypertension may provide independent information about disease progression or control, though the data available at the time were conflicting. A further contentious issue was whether some specific types of drugs, such as ACE inhibitors or calcium channel blockers, may be more effective than others in reducing increased left ventricular mass associated with hypertension. This pre-specified substudy of the Losartan Intervention For Endpoint Reduction in Hypertension (LIFE) study[27] set out to resolve these issues.

Methods

A prospective cohort substudy of the LIFE randomized clinical trial was conducted from 1995 to 2001. A total of

941 prospectively identified patients aged 55–80 years with essential hypertension and electrocardiographic left ventricular hypertrophy had left ventricular mass measured by echocardiography at enrolment in the LIFE trial and thereafter followed up annually. Participants were aged 55–80 years; had BPs of 160–200 mmHg systolic, 95–115 mmHg diastolic, or both, during placebo treatment; and had not experienced an MI or stroke within six months; and did not require treatment with a beta blocker, ACE inhibitor, or ARB. Following randomization, blinded treatment was begun with losartan 50 mg, or atenolol 50 mg, and matching double placebo and up-titrated by adding hydrochlorothiazide, 12.5 mg, followed by increasing study medication to 100 mg with a target BP of <140/90 mmHg. The main outcomes were a composite of cardiovascular death, fatal or non-fatal MI, and fatal or non-fatal stroke.

Results

Baseline characteristics of this substudy were similar to the entire LIFE population. There were no significant differences between the two treatment groups. Median follow-up was 4.8 years. Blood pressure, heart rate, and left ventricular mass all decreased substantially during the first year; thereafter, BP and heart rate decreased only slightly. In contrast, left ventricular mass continued to decrease markedly from 12 to 24 months, with further small reductions throughout follow-up.

The composite end point occurred in 104 patients (11%). The multivariate Cox regression model showed a strong association between lower in-treatment left ventricular mass index (LVMI-LV mass divided by body surface area) and the reduced rate of the composite end point over and above that predicted by reduction in BP. In-treatment LVMI was also associated with lower cardiovascular mortality, stroke, MI, and all-cause mortality independent of treatment arm and systolic BP. These lower rates of the composite end point with in-treatment reduction in LVMI were seen in women and men, older patients versus younger than 65 years, patients with and without diabetes, and in black and non-black patients.

Conclusions and clinical implications

In-treatment reductions in echocardiograpic left ventricular mass are associated with greater reductions in cardiovascular events. This was independent of the degree of BP reduction, or treatment modality. This suggests that a strategy in which an active effort is made to reduce left ventricular mass may have important clinical benefits. In an accompanying study, by the same group, analysis of another pre-specified subgroup of the LIFE study was presented—those with electrocardiographic evidence of left ventricular hypertrophy[28]. They showed that less severe, in-treatment, electrocardiographic, left ventricular hypertrophy was associated with lower likelihood of cardiovascular events, independent of BP lowering and treatment modality. These studies, taken together, suggest that left ventricular hypertrophy in the context of hypertension is an independent cardiovascular risk factor that requires attention. They support a role for evaluating left ventricular hypertrophy at the time of hypertension diagnosis and, at the very least, for considering changes in left ventricular mass when tailoring long-term antihypertensive therapy.

Learning points

- Left ventricular mass is an independent predictor of cardiovascular events in patients with hypertension.
- Reduction of left ventricular mass on anti-hypertensive therapy is associated with reduced cardiovascular events, independent of BP treatment and drugs used.
- An assessment of left ventricular mass, either echocardiographic or electrocardiographic, should be made at the time of hypertension diagnosis and used to tailor long-term therapy.

New mechanisms

Differential impact of blood pressure-lowering drugs on central aortic pressure and clinical outcomes

Williams B, Lacy PS, Thom SM, Cruickshank K, Stanton A, Collier D, Hughes AD, Thurston H, O'Rourke M CAFÉ Investigators, Anglo-Scandinavian Cardiac Outcomes Trial Investigators, CAFÉ Steering Committee and Writing Committee. *Circulation* 2006; 113: 1213–25.

Background

Since the invention of the sphygmomanometer and the early observations in the late nineteenth century of the link between elevated BP and diseases of the heart and kidneys, almost everything that we have learnt about hypertension is based on the simple non-invasive measurements of brachial artery BP. There is an overwhelming body of evidence showing that elevated brachial BP is a powerful predictor of major cardiovascular events, and reducing it with medications is associated with reduced risk of death, stroke, and MI, as well as many other important clinical end points. With the development of multiple classes of anti-hypertensives, several studies have been designed to test their efficacy. In head-to-head studies, beta blockers have fallen short of other classes in preventing hypertensive complications. The beta blocker, atenolol, was tested against the ARB, losartan, in the Losartan Intervention For Endpoint reduction (LIFE)[27], and against amlodipine in the Anglo-Scandinavian Cardiovascular Outcomes Trial (ASCOT)[29]; both studies favouring the non-beta blocker treatment arms. Various authors tried to explain these findings based on the improved brachial cuff control in the non-beta blocker arms, or perhaps wider effects beyond BP reduction.

An alternative explanation was that various classes of anti-hypertensives have profoundly different effects on pulse wave morphology, arterial wave reflection, and thus central haemodynamic parameters, despite similar brachial artery pressures. The Conduit Artery Function Evaluation (CAFE) study, a substudy of ASCOT, examined the impact of two different BP lowering regimes on central aortic pressures and hemodynamics derived from radial artery applanation tonometry and pulse wave analysis.

Methods

Participants already recruited into ASCOT were eligible for recruitment into the CAFE study. In the ASCOT study participants were randomized into two BP lowering arms (atenolol ± bendoflumethiazide or amlodipine

± perindopril). Recruitment to CAFE began one year after commencement of ASCOT, and a total of 2,199 participants were recruited from five ASCOT study centres.

The study used radial artery applanation tonometry and pulse wave analysis[30] to calculate derived central BPs and other parameters using a commercially available system. Applanation tonometry measurements were obtained at scheduled ASCOT follow-up visits and by the end of the study an average of 3.4 measurements per patient had been recorded. The mean follow-up time after the initial tonometry measurement was approximately

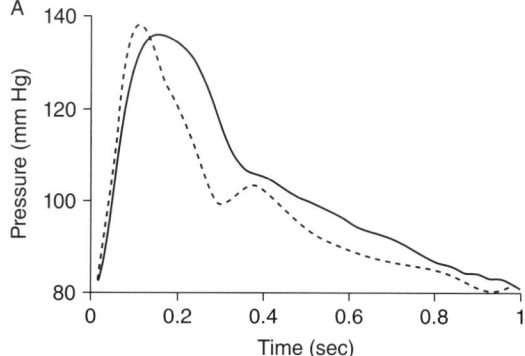

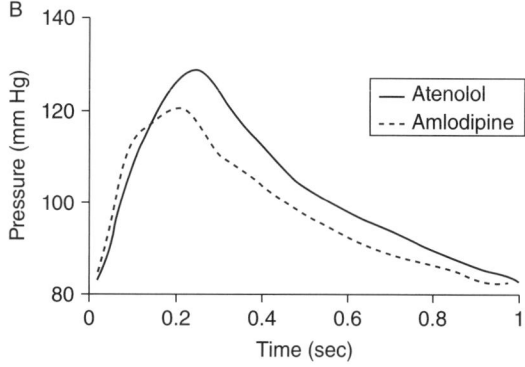

Figure 17.3 Examples of peripheral (A) and corresponding radial artery applanation tonometry and pulse wave analysis derived central aortic (B) waveforms from patients of equal age treated with atenolol (solid line) or amlodipine (broken line) achieving equivalent brachial BPs.

Reproduced from Williams B. *et al.* CAFE Investigators, Anglo-Scandinavian Cardiac Outcomes Trial Investigators, CAFE Steering Committee and Writing Committee. Differential impact of blood pressure-lowering drugs on central aortic pressure and clinical outcomes. *Circulation* 2006; 113: 1213–25, with permission from Wolters Kluwer Health.

three years for each treatment group. Brachial BP was measured according to the ASCOT protocol using a validated, semi-automated oscillometric device.

Results

The CAFE participants were well matched between treatment arms and well matched against all participants in ASCOT. Despite similar brachial systolic pressures between treatment groups (0.7 mmHg; 95% CI, ~0.4–1.7; p = 0.2), there were substantial reductions in central aortic pressures with the amlodipine regimen (central aortic systolic BP, 4.3 mmHg; 95% CI, 3.3–5.4; p~0.0001; central aortic pulse pressure, 3.0 mmHg; 95% CI, 2.1–3.9; p = 0.0001). Figure 17.3 shows representative averaged radial artery waveforms and the resulting derived central aortic waveforms from individual patients with similar brachial BPs treated with either atenolol or amlodipine monotherapy.

To evaluate whether BP and tonometry-derived hemodynamic indexes were related to clinical outcomes in the CAFE cohort, a Cox proportional-hazards model showed that central pulse pressure was significantly associated with a post-hoc defined composite outcome of total cardiovascular and renal outcomes, which was consistent after adjustment in three separate Cox regression models.

Conclusions and clinical implications

The CAFE trial is the first study to investigate prospectively the hypothesis that alternative BP lowering medications might affect central aortic pressures differently despite similar effects on brachial BPs in a large cohort of patients. The results showed significant differences in central aortic pressure and haemodynamics in favour of calcium channel blocker versus beta blocker therapy. This finding is based on the relative inability of beta blockers to reduce the magnitude of the reflected augmentation wave, an observation made from earlier smaller studies, and provides a potential mechanism to explain differences in clinical outcomes between the two treatment arms in ASCOT. This has resulted in a move away from beta blockers as a first-line treatment for hypertension. The CAFE trial has also served to highlight a method of better understanding the central pharmacodynamics of anti-hypertensive drugs. Simple-to-use devices now exist that can measure central aortic systolic pressure[31], with the potential to have a major impact on cardiovascular trials and clinical practice.

Learning points

- Different classes of anti-hypertensives affect central aortic pressure differently, despite similar brachial cuff pressures.
- Calcium channel antagonists reduce central aortic pressure to a greater extent compared to beta blockers.
- Central aortic pressure differences impact on major cardiovascular and renal events.

Further reading

- Cecelja M, Jiang B, McNeill K, *et al.* Increased wave reflection rather than central arterial stiffness is the main determinant of raised pulse pressure in women and relates to mismatch in arterial dimensions: a twin study. *J Am Coll Cardiol* 2009; 54(8): 695–703.
- Safar ME, Levy BI, Struijker-Boudier H. Current Perspectives on Arterial Stiffness and Pulse Pressure in Hypertension and Cardiovascular Diseases. *Circulation* 2003; 107(22): 2864–9.

Diabetes and blood pressure

Prevention of diabetic nephropathy by pharmacological amelioration of glomerular capillary hypertension

Zatz R, Dunn BR, Meyer TW, Anderson S, Rennke HG, Brenner BM. *J Clin Invest* 1986; 77: 1935–30.

Background

Diabetic nephropathy develops in a large proportion of patients with type 1 diabetes, significantly increasing the risk of end-stage renal failure, transplantation, and death. It has been shown that patients with newly diagnosed type 1 diabetes exhibit a state of glomerular hyperfiltration, as well as in experimental diabetes in animals. In similar models, glomerular structural injury can be effectively prevented despite significant hyperglycaemia as long as glomerular pressures and flows are artificially maintained within normal limits. These findings therefore suggest that haemodynamic, rather than metabolic factors are important in the initiation and progression of diabetic glomerulopathy. While data existed showing that hypertension worsened diabetic nephropathy, and treatment of hypertension in established nephropathy ameliorated the condition, the basic science studies suggested that anti-hypertensive therapy in normotensive diabetic subjects may protect against glomerular disease by reducing glomerular hydraulic pressure. This study was the first to test this hypothesis.

Methods

Three groups of age and weight-matched adult male rats were studied. Two groups underwent induction of streptozotocin diabetes (an established model for type 1 diabetes)[32], with the third undergoing a sham procedure. Diabetic rats received enough insulin to maintain stable moderate hyperglycaemia, in addition one group of diabetic rats were treated with the ACE inhibitor enalapril. Measurements included whole kidney and single-nephron glomerular filtration rate, glomerular plasma flow, glomerular hydraulic pressure, transcapillary hydraulic pressure gradient, and urinary protein. Histological examination of the kidneys was performed at 14 months.

Results

Average kidney weight, whole kidney and single-nephron glomerular filtration rate, and glomerular plasma flow rate were elevated to similar levels in both groups of diabetic rats, compared to the control rats. Non-enalapril treated diabetic rats exhibited significant increases in mean glomerular capillary hydraulic pressure and transcapillary hydraulic pressure gradient, compared with the enalapril-treated diabetic rats and normal controls. This group also developed marked and progressive albuminuria, with subsequent histological examination of the kidneys showing a high incidence of glomerular structural abnormalities.

Conclusions and clinical implications

These findings suggest that preventing glomerular capillary hypertension in diabetics effectively protects against the subsequent development of glomerular nephropathy and proteinuria. This protection was despite moderate hyperglycaemia, supporting the view that haemodynamic rather than metabolic factors predominate. This study was seminal in instructing large-scale human studies that established the importance of BP in the pathophysiology of diabetic nephropathy. At a time when clinicians were puzzled as to the best way of preventing or reducing the incidence of diabetic nephropathy, basic science research provided some timely answers. This was instrumental in changing clinical practice, increasing the use of ACE inhibitors for nephroprotection long before trials in humans confirmed this.

Learning points

- Diabetic nephropathy results largely from increased glomerular capillary pressure.
- Blood pressure is likely to be a major factor in the pathophysiology of diabetic nephropathy.
- Angiotensin converting enzyme inhibitors can protect against the development of diabetic nephropathy despite hyperglycaemia in an animal model of type 1 diabetes.

The effect of angiotensin converting enzyme inhibition on diabetic nephropathy

Lewis EJ, Hunsicker LG, Bain RP, Tohde RD. The Collaborative Study Group. *N Engl J Med* 1993; 329: 1456–62.

Background

Diabetic nephrophathy, characterized by proteinuria and a gradual decline in glomerular filtration rate develops in approximately one-third of insulin-dependent patients. Most patients reach end-stage renal failure within ten years after the onset of proteinuria. Studies have shown that treatment of hypertension slows the rate of decline in renal function. However, animal studies (see Landmark Paper above) have shown that ACE inhibitors could reduce glomerular damage in this setting by mechanisms independent of their hypertensive effects. This trial was designed to test this hypothesis.

Methods

Eligible patients between 18–49 years of age were enrolled if they had insulin-dependent diabetes for at least seven years, with onset before the age of 30, had diabetic retinopathy, urinary protein excretion of ≥500 mg/24 hrs, and a serum creatinine concentration of ≤2.5 mg/dl (221 micromol/l). Patients already on ACE inhibitor or calcium channel antagonists were eligible provided that their blood pressure could be kept within the requirements of the trial without these medications. Double-blind randomization was to either captopril 25 mg three times per day or an identical looking placebo three times daily. The BP goal was a systolic below 140 mmHg and diastolic below 90 mmHg. The primary end point was a doubling of the baseline serum creatinine to at least 2.0 mg/dl (177 micromol/l). Secondary outcomes included length of time to the combined end points of death, dialysis, and transplantation, and changes in renal function.

Results

A group of 207 patients were randomized to captopril and 202 to placebo, and followed up to a median of three years. Baseline characteristics of the two groups were well matched, apart from a higher urinary protein excretion in the placebo arm. Twenty-five patients in the captopril group reached the primary end point of a doubling of serum creatinine concentration compared to 43 in the placebo group (p = 0.0007). This equated to a 48% relative risk reduction of the primary end point with captopril, which was greatest (76%) in the subgroup with the worst creatinine concentrations (<2 mg/dl). Captopril treatment was also associated with a 50% reduction in the risk of the combined end points of death, dialysis, and transplantation. This was independent of the small difference in BP between the two groups.

Conclusions and clinical implications

This study provided the first definitive evidence in humans of the beneficial effects of ACE inhibitors in preserving renal function in patients with insulin-dependent diabetic nephropathy, as well as reducing death and both the need for dialysis and transplantation, compared to placebo. This effect was independent of its anti-hypertensive properties, and supported the view that ACE inhibitors are superior to other anti-hypertensives in this setting, and should be the recommended therapy. It also fostered other trials that have established ACE inhibition as the standard of care in diabetics with hypertension.

Learning points

- Diabetics with nephropathy have a high risk of developing end-stage renal failure.
- The use of ACE inhibitors can significantly retard the progression of nephropathy as well as reducing death.
- These effects are independent of its anti-hypertensive action.
- Angiotensin converting enzyme inhibitors should be recommended for all diabetic patients with nephropathy.

Tight blood pressure control and risk of macrovascular and microvascular complications in type 2 diabetes: UKPDS 38

UK Prospective Diabetes Study Group. *BMJ* 1998; 317: 703–13.

Background

The United Kingdom Prospective Diabetes Study (UKPDS) was the largest clinical research study into type 2 diabetes ever conducted. The study was conceived in 1976. A group of 5,102 patients with newly diagnosed type 2 diabetes was recruited across 23 centres within the UK between 1977 and 1991. Patients were followed up for an average of ten years to answer important questions about the management of the disorder, including whether intensive use of pharmacological therapy to lower blood glucose levels would result in clinical benefits; whether the use of various sulfonylurea drugs, the biguanide drug metformin, or insulin have specific therapeutic advantages or disadvantages[33]; and the optimal target BP control in hypertensive diabetics.

The latter question centres around the observation that in the general population, treating hypertension reduces the incidence of stroke and MI, together with the fact that in patients with type 1 diabetes that have microalbuminuria or overt nephropathy, tight BP control reduces microalbuminuria, deterioration in renal function, and the development of end-stage renal disease. Whether the same was true in type 2 diabetes was not clear.

Methods

Hypertensive patients with type 2 diabetes who had been recruited to the UKPDS were studied. Of the 4,054 patients recruited in the 20 centres participating in the hypertension in diabetes study, 1544 (38%) had hypertension, defined in 727 patients as a systolic BP >160 mmHg and/or a diastolic BP >90 mmHg, or in 421 patients receiving antihypertensive treatment as a systolic pressure of >150 mmHg and/or a diastolic pressure >85 mmHg. A group of 1,148 patients fulfilled the inclusion criteria and 758 were randomized to tight BP control, aiming for <150/85 mmHg, with 400 patients given captopril and 358 atenolol as the main treatment; 390 patients were allocated to less tight control of BP, aiming for <180/105 mmHg, but avoiding treatment with ACE inhibitors or beta blockers.

Twenty-one clinical end points were predefined in the study protocol and could be defined as fatal and non-fatal, related to diabetes, deaths related to diabetes, and all-cause mortality. Surrogate measures of microvascular disease included urinary albumin excretion and retinal photography.

Results

Median follow-up was 8.4 years. There were no significant differences in glycaemic control based on glycated-haemoglobin measurements. Mean BP during follow-up was significantly reduced in the tight BP control group (144/82 mm Hg) compared with the group assigned to less tight control (154/87 mmHg) (p <0.0001). There were significant reductions in several end points in the group assigned to tight BP control, including a 24% reduction in diabetes related end points, 32% in deaths related to diabetes, and 37% reduction in microvascular end points. After nine years of follow-up, 29% of patients in the tight BP control group required three or more anti-hypertensives to achieve the target BP.

Conclusions and clinical implications

The UKPDS trial is the largest study ever undertaken in the management of type 2 diabetes, at a time when the incidence of the disease is increasing at an alarming rate. The hypertension study clearly showed the benefit of tight BP control in newly diagnosed patients in reducing the risk of any non-fatal or fatal diabetic complications and of deaths related to diabetes; which was independent of glycaemic control. It promoted the control of BP in these patients to the forefront of their management, having a major impact on clinical practice and public health policy.

Learning points

♦ Hypertension in patients with type 2 diabetes is associated with major microvascular and macrovascular complications, independent of glycaemic control.
♦ Tight BP control to a target of at least <150/85 mmHg should be achieved with the use of ACE inhibitors and beta blockers. (Note, current guidelines advocate much tighter control.)
♦ Multiple classes of anti-hypertensives may be required to achieve target BP.

Chapter conclusions

The aforementioned landmark studies in hypertension presented here have had a fundamental impact on the way we practice medicine, from the early epidemiological studies identifying hypertension as a major risk factor, through to developing pharmacological treatment strategies and identifying specific treatment targets in diverse populations. In many ways the identification of hypertension as a risk factor and the development of subsequent strategies for treatment has been a classic paradigm for translational medicine, encompassing all aspects of the translational pathway from epidemiology, novel drug discovery, the development of clinical trial technology through to their impact on treatment guidelines and ultimately public health. However, there is no room for complacency and many challenges remain. More than one billion people in the world have high blood pressure, much of the increased incidence occurring in the developing world. Although, not emphasized in the landmark papers, lifestyle plays a major role in the aetiology of hypertension, usually on a background of genetic susceptibility. For many years, the pharmaceutical industry has had spectacular success in identifying new drug targets for hypertension but they have now become a victim of their own success. These treatments have become progressively more effective and are associated with minimal side effects. The majority of these proven and effective treatments are fast becoming generic and low cost. This may now divert the focus of discovery away from hypertension to new areas on the assumption that hypertension is 'sorted'. This would be unfortunate because this is still one of the largest and most important disease areas and treated patients still experience residual risk which is potentially amenable to better therapies in selected patient groups.

So where will this field go in the next ten years? There is now renewed focus on the vascular ageing process which is accelerated by high blood pressure. This has led to the recognition that perhaps we treat too late, when much of the structural damage, the harbinger of risk, is already done and irreversible. Thus, future research will focus on better phenotyping of early hypertension to better stratify people at increased risk at an earlier stage, facilitating earlier interventions. This, in turn, will most likely identify new mechanisms for early disease and new targets for early intervention, thereby preventing the evolution of the life course of the condition rather than simply focusing on preventing events at the end of the process. The biotechnology revolution yielding improved non-invasive diagnostics will assist with better phenotyping and disease stratification. Technology is also making its way into treatment with the recent emergence of radiofrequency ablation of renal nerves, providing interesting therapeutic options and improved understanding of the role of renal sympathetic afferent nerves in the regulation of blood pressure and perhaps also the metabolic syndrome commonly associated with high blood pressure; other strategies to try and provide a more permanent resolution of high blood pressure are likely to evolve.[34,35,36]

A noticeable absence from the landmark papers is genetic studies. Whilst there has been considerable investment in such large-scale studies, perhaps not surprisingly single culprit genes have not been identified and are unlikely to be for the vast majority with this condition. That said, improved phenotyping, whole genome sequencing, epigenetics and better understanding of the environmental influences on blood pressure (which are demonstrably strong) may yield new insights.

Finally, aside from the above, a rather simple but fundamental question remains to be answered. How should we diagnose and monitor hypertension: clinic blood pressure, home blood pressure or ambulatory blood pressure? At what threshold should we treat, or should we abandon the concept of thresholds and treat on the basis of risk alone, potentially lowering what would have been otherwise classed as a normal blood pressure in high-risk people? How low should we go in lowering blood pressure? Is there a J curve; if so, who does it apply to and at what blood pressure level? The answers to such questions will inform future clinical practice. In so doing, we must not lose sight of the scale of the problem in its simplest form. High blood pressure remains one of the world's biggest killers, a silent killer that needs robust public health policies worldwide for detection and to facilitate access to this most cost effective of interventions. Meanwhile, it is interesting to reflect on how far we have come from the 1930s when a British Professor of Medicine said: 'The greatest danger to a man with high blood pressure lies in its discovery, because then some fool is certain to try and reduce it'[37]. Today, the evidence suggests that the greatest danger to a man with hypertension is complacency with regard to its detection and treatment.

References

1. Mathers C, Fat DM, Boerma JT, World Health Organization. *The Global Burden of Disease: 2004 Update*. Geneva, Switzerland, World Health Organization. 2008.

2. Murray CJ, Lopez AD. Mortality by cause for eight regions of the world: Global burden of disease study. *Lancet* 1997; 349(9061): 1269–76.

3. Lopez AD, Mathers CD, Ezzati M, Jamison DT, Murray CJ. Global and regional burden of disease and risk factors, 2001: Systematic analysis of population health data. *Lancet* 2006; 367(9524): 1747–57.

4. Lawes CM, Vander Hoorn S, Rodgers A, International Society of Hypertension. Global burden of blood-pressure-related disease, 2001. *Lancet* 2008; 371(9623): 1513–8.

5. From the centers for disease control and prevention. Decline in deaths from heart disease and stroke - United States, 1900–1999. *JAMA* 1999; 282(8): 724–6.

6. Levi F, Lucchini F, Negri E, La Vecchia C. Trends in mortality from cardiovascular and cerebrovascular diseases in Europe and other areas of the world. *Heart* 2002; 88(2): 119–24.

7. Antikainen RL, Moltchanov VA, Chukwuma C, *et al.* Trends in the prevalence, awareness, treatment and control of hypertension: The WHO MONICA project. *Eur J Cardiovasc Prev Rehabil* 2006; 13(1): 13–29.

8. Du X, Cruickshank K, McNamee R, *et al.* Case-control study of stroke and the quality of hypertension control in north-west England. *BMJ* 1997; 314(7076): 272–6.

9. Vartiainen E, Sarti C, Tuomilehto J, Kuulasmaa K. Do changes in cardiovascular risk factors explain changes in mortality from stroke in Finland? *BMJ* 1995; 310(6984): 901–4.

10. Dawber TR, Meadors GF, Moore FE. Epidemiological approaches to heart disease: The Framingham Study. *Am J Public Health Nations Health* 1951; 41(3): 279–81.

11. Kannel WB, Schwartz MJ, McNamara PM. Blood pressure and risk of coronary heart disease: The Framingham Study. *Dis Chest* 1969; 56(1): 43–52.

12. MacMahon S, Peto R, Cutler J, *et al.* Blood pressure, stroke, and coronary heart disease. Part 1, prolonged differences in blood pressure: Prospective observational studies corrected for the regression dilution bias. *Lancet* 1990; 335(8692): 765–74.

13. Cholesterol, diastolic blood pressure, and stroke: 13,000 strokes in 450,000 people in 45 prospective cohorts. Prospective studies collaboration. *Lancet* 1995; 346 (8991–8992): 1647–53.

14. Blood pressure, cholesterol, and stroke in Eastern Asia. Eastern stroke and coronary heart disease collaborative research group. *Lancet* 1998; 352(9143): 1801–7.

15. Collaborative overview ('meta-analysis') of prospective observational studies of the associations of usual blood pressure and usual cholesterol levels with common causes of death: Protocol for the second cycle of the prospective studies collaboration. *J Cardiovasc Risk* 1999; 6(5): 315–20.

16. Port S, Demer L, Jennrich R, Walter D, Garfinkel A. Systolic blood pressure and mortality. *Lancet* 2000; 355(9199): 175–80.

17. Perera GA. Antihypertensive drug versus symptomatic treatment in primary hypertension. Effect on survival. *J Am Med Assoc* 1960; 173: 11–3.

18. Goldring W, Chasis H. Antihypertensive drug therapy; an appraisal. *Arch Intern Med* 1965; 115: 523–5.

19. Schwartz WB. The effect of sulfanilamide on salt and water excretion in congestive heart failure. *N Engl J Med* 1949; 240(5): 173–7.

20. Freis ED, Wanko A, Wilson IM, Parrish AE. Treatment of essential hypertension with chlorothiazide (diuril); its use alone and combined with other antihypertensive agents. *J Am Med Assoc* 1958; 166(2): 137–40.

21. Black JW, Stephenson JS. Pharmacology of a new adrenergic beta-receptor-blocking compound (nethalide). *Lancet* 1962; 2(7251): 311–4.

22. Byers LD, Wolfenden R. Binding of the by-product analog benzylsuccinic acid by carboxypeptidase A. *Biochemistry* 1973; 12(11): 2070–8.

23. Yusuf S, Dagenais G, Pogue J, Bosch J, Sleight P. Vitamin E supplementation and cardiovascular events in high-risk patients. The heart outcomes prevention evaluation study investigators. *N Engl J Med* 2000; 342(3): 154–60.

24. Granger CB, McMurray JJ, Yusuf S, *et al.* Effects of candesartan in patients with chronic heart failure and reduced left-ventricular systolic function intolerant to angiotensin-converting-enzyme inhibitors: The charm-alternative trial. *Lancet* 2003; 362(9386): 772–6.

25. McMurray JJ, Ostergren J, Swedberg K, *et al.* Effects of candesartan in patients with chronic heart failure and reduced left-ventricular systolic function taking angiotensin-converting-enzyme inhibitors: The charm-added trial. *Lancet* 2003; 362(9386): 767–71.

26. Major cardiovascular events in hypertensive patients randomized to doxazosin vs chlorthalidone: the antihypertensive and lipid-lowering treatment to prevent heart attack trial (ALLHAT). ALLHAT Collaborative Research Group. *JAMA* 2000; 283(15): 1967–75.

27. Dahlöf B, Devereux RB, Kjeldsen SE, *et al.* Cardiovascular morbidity and mortality in the losartan intervention for endpoint reduction in hypertension study (LIFE): A randomised trial against atenolol. *Lancet* 2002; 359(9311): 995–1003.

28. Okin PM, Devereux RB, Jern S, *et al.* Regression of electrocardiographic left ventricular hypertrophy during antihypertensive treatment and the prediction of major cardiovascular events. *JAMA* 2004; 292(19): 2343–9.

29. Dahlöf B, Sever PS, Poulter NR, *et al.* Prevention of cardiovascular events with an antihypertensive regimen of amlodipine adding perindopril as required versus atenolol adding bendroflumethiazide as required, in the Anglo-Scandinavian cardiac outcomes trial-blood pressure lowering arm (ASCOT-BPLA): A multicentre randomised controlled trial. *Lancet* 2005; 366(9489): 895–906.

30. O'Rourke MF, Pauca A, Jiang XJ. Pulse wave analysis. *Br J Clin Pharmacol* 2001; 51(6): 507–22.

31. Williams B, Lacy PS, Yan P, Hwee CN, Liang C, Ting CM. Development and validation of a novel method to derive

central aortic systolic pressure from the radial pressure waveform using an n-point moving average method. *J Am Coll Cardiol* 2011; 57(8): 951–61.

32. Mansford KR, Opie L. Comparison of metabolic abnormalities in diabetes mellitus induced by streptozotocin or by alloxan. *Lancet* 1968; 1(7544): 670–1.

33. Intensive blood-glucose control with sulphonylureas or insulin compared with conventional treatment and risk of complications in patients with type 2 diabetes (UKPDS 33). UK prospective diabetes study (UKPDS) group. *Lancet* 1998; 352(9131): 837–53.

34. Krum H, Schlaich M, Whitbourn R, Sobotke PA, Sadowski J, Bartus K, *et al.* Catheter-based renal sympathetic denervation for resistant hypertension: a multicentre safety and proof-of-principle cohort study. *Lancet* 2009; 373: 1275–81.

35. Symplicity HTN-2 Investigators. Renal sympathetic denervation in patients with treatment-resistant hypertension (The Symplicity HTN-2 Trial): a randomised controlled trial. *Lancet* 2010; 376: 1903–09.

36. Symplicity HTN-1 Investigators. Catheter-based renal sympathetic denervation for resistant hypertension. Durability of blood pressure reduction out to 24 months. *Hypertension* 2011; 57: 911–917.

37. Hay J. The significance of a raised blood pressure. *Br Med J* 1931; 2: 43–7.

Chapter 18

Pulmonary arterial hypertension

Dr Christopher Valerio and Dr Gerry Coghlan

A note on terminology

The term 'pulmonary hypertension' will be used to refer to an elevation of pulmonary artery pressure due to any cause; the terms primary pulmonary hypertension (PPH, in use to 2003) and pulmonary arterial hypertension (PAH, term introduced in 1998) will be used according to the terms used in the work under discussion (see Table 18.1).

Introduction

In many respects the field of PAH remains in its adolescence. The work of Ernst von Romberg in the nineteenth century established the existence of a disease affecting the pulmonary arteries[1], and then in the middle of the twentieth century Paul Wood detailed the haemodynamic consequences[2]. In the 1970s there was a recognition that PPH was a condition that needed to be understood. The first international meeting dedicated to PPH was held in 1973. Particular interest existed at that time because of an outbreak of pulmonary hypertension associated with use of the anorexigen, aminorex fumarate. It would be 25 years before the next meeting in Evian.

Table 18.1 Classification of pulmonary hypertension from Evian (1998) and Dana Point (2008)

Evian classification of pulmonary hypertension

1 Pulmonary arterial hypertension
   1.1 Primary pulmonary hypertension
     (a) Sporadic
     (b) Familial
   1.2 Related to:
     (a) Collagen vascular disease
     (b) Congenital systemic to pulmonary shunts
     (c) Portal hypertension
     (d) HIV infection
     (e) Drugs/toxins (anorexigens/other)
     (f) Persistent pulmonary hypertension of the newborn
     (g) Other

2 Pulmonary venous hypertension
   2.1 Left-sided atrial or ventricular heart disease
   2.2 Left-sided valvular heart disease
   2.3 Extrinsic compression of central pulmonary veins
     (a) Fibrosing mediastinitis
     (b) Adenopathy/tumours
   2.4 Pulmonary veno-occlusive disease
   2.5 Other

3 Respiratory system and/or hypoxemia
   3.1 Chronic obstructive pulmonary disease
   3.2 Interstitial lung disease
   3.3 Sleep disordered breathing
   3.4 Alveolar hypoventilation disorders
   3.5 Chronic exposure to high altitude
   3.6 Neonatal lung disease
   3.7 Alveolar-capillary dysplasia
   3.8 Other

4 Pulmonary hypertension due to chronic thrombotic and/or embolic disease
   4.1 Thromboembolic obstruction of proximal pulmonary arteries
   4.2 Obstruction of distal pulmonary arteries
     (a) Pulmonary embolism (thrombus, tumour, OVA and/or parasites, foreign material)
     (b) In-situ thrombosis
     (c) Sickle cell disease

5 Pulmonary hypertension due to disorders directly affecting the pulmonary vasculature
   5.1 Inflammatory
     (a) Schistosomiasis
     (b) Sarcoidosis
     (c) Other
   5.2 Pulmonary capillary hemangiomatosis

Dana point classification

1 Pulmonary arterial hypertension
   1.1 Idiopathic PAH
   1.2 Heritable PAH
     1.2.1 BMPR2
     1.2.2 ALK 1, endoglin (with or without hereditary haemorrhagic telangiectasia)
     1.2.3 Unknown
   1.3 Drug and toxin-induced PAH
   1.4 Associated with:
     1.4.1 Connective tissue disease
     1.4.2 HIV infection
     1.4.3 Porto-pulmonary hypertension
     1.4.4 Congenital heart disease
     1.4.5 Schistosomiasis
     1.4.6 Chronic haemolytic anaemia
   1.5 Persistent pulmonary hypertension of the newborn
   1.6 Pulmonary veno-occlusive disease

2 Pulmonary hypertension owing to left heart disease
   2.1 Systolic dysfunction
   2.2 Diastolic dysfunction
   2.3 Valvular heart disease

3 Pulmonary hypertension owing to lung diseases and/or hypoxia
   3.1 Chronic obstructive pulmonary disease
   3.2 Interstitial lung disease
   3.3 Other pulmonary diseases with mixed restrictive and obstructive pattern
   3.4 Sleep-disordered breathing
   3.5 Alveolar hypoventilation disorders
   3.6 Chronic exposure to high altitude
   3.7 Developmental abnormalities

4 Chronic thromboembolic pulmonary hypertension (CTEPH)

5 Pulmonary hypertension with unclear or multifactorial mechanisms
   5.1 Haematologic disorders: myeloproliferative disorders, splenectomy
   5.2 Systemic disorders: sarcoidosis, pulmonary Langerhans cell histiocytosis, lymphangioleiomyomatosis, neurofibromatosis, vasculitis
   5.3 Metabolic disorders: glycogen storage disease, Gaucher disease, thyroid disorders
   5.4 Others: tumoural obstruction, fibrosing medlastinitis, chronic renal failure on haemodialysis

Reprinted from Rich S. Executive summary from the World Symposium on Primary Pulmonary Hypertension 1998. Evian, France. World Health Organization 1998, with permission, and from Simonneau *et al.* Update Clinical Classification of Pulmonary Hypertension. *Journal of the American College of Cardiology* 54(Supplement S), S43–S54, 2009, with permission from Elsevier.

Subsequent world symposia in Venice (2003) and Dana Point (2008) each provide a progress summary of the developments in the field of pulmonary hypertension[4,5]. The classification and diagnostic criteria have also been reviewed at each world symposium (see Tables 18.1 and Table 18.2).

By 1980 associations had been demonstrated with recurrent thrombo-embolism, portal hypertension, scleroderma, and systemic lupus erythematosis. Since then new diseases have been described with an increased incidence of PAH, for example HIV[6], and revisiting well-known diseases has uncovered hallmark pathological changes of PAH, for example schistosomiasis[7]. Recently, our understanding of the genetic basis of PAH has led to the term 'heritable' PAH being preferred over familial[8]. Culprits for drug-induced PAH now include fenfluramine, dexfenfluramine, and toxic rapeseed oil, with substances such as amphetamines and L-tryptophan likely candidates. We expect that left heart disease is still the likeliest explanation for pulmonary hypertension, detected by echocardiography. Hypoxia driven pulmonary hypertension is also far more common than PAH and attention has returned to these two more common clinical phenomena. However, attempts to apply lessons learned from PAH have met with limited success, whereas our management of PAH has perhaps benefitted from

Table 18.2 Functional classification of pulmonary hypertension modified after the NYHA functional classification according to the World Health Organization 1998

Class I—Patients with pulmonary hypertension but without resulting limitation of physical activity. Ordinary physical activity does not cause undue dyspnoea or fatigue, chest pain, or near syncope.

Class II—Patients with pulmonary hypertension resulting in slight limitation of physical activity. They are comfortable at rest. Ordinary physical activity causes undue dyspnoea or fatigue, chest pain or near syncope.

Class III—Patients with pulmonary hypertension resulting in marked limitation of physical activity. They are comfortable at rest. Less than ordinary physical activity causes undue dyspnoea or fatigue, chest pain, or near syncope.

Class IV—Patients with pulmonary hypertension with inability to carry out any physical activity without symptoms. These patients manifest signs of right heart failure. Dyspnoea and/or fatigue may even be present at rest. Discomfort is increased by any physical activity.

avoiding mistakes made in these fields. Chronic thrombo-embolic pulmonary hypertension (CTEPH) has become an increasingly important diagnosis to make, as outcomes following thrombo-endarterectomy are unmatched by medical therapy.

Our understanding of PAH has moved on from histopathological and physiological changes to a more detailed analysis of molecular mechanisms. The categorization of different associations of PAH with similar pathological features has promoted concerted research efforts. Occasionally, it has been the differences rather than the similarities, which have driven things forward. Many developments have been derived from work in general vascular biology, for example the discovery of endothelin-1[9]. Subsequent analysis of the pathways in the lungs has led to this molecule being regarded as a key player in PAH. Arguably, the clearest evidence for the role of endothelin-1 in PAH is the efficacy of the endothelin receptor antagonists.

By far the most dramatic change in the field of PAH has been the development of specific therapies in the last twenty years. Only a small minority of patients with a vasodilator response can expect any benefit from calcium channel blockade and for other patients treatment was, in effect, palliative up to 1990. Heart failure management with diuretics and digoxin has been augmented with anticoagulation to prevent intravascular thrombosis and oxygen for patients with hypoxaemia. First, intravenous prostacyclin analogues (epoprostenol), then endothelin receptor antagonists (bosentan) and phosphodiesterase-5 inhibitors (sildenafil) have demonstrated efficacy. Demonstrating improvements in survival has proved more challenging due to the short duration of trials, but a meta-analysis of randomized, controlled trials has confirmed the benefit exists[10]. A secondary effect of trials in PAH is the importance of the six-minute walk distance as the principal measure of disease progression.

Within this chapter we have tried to include those papers which have, by themselves, provoked a shift in our understanding of PAH (and one relating to CTEPH) and have moved the field forward. Many of the developments in our understanding have come from work in cardiovascular biology and risen to prominence in piecemeal fashion. As is always the case with research, the uncertainty of experimentation means that many studies in PAH do not stand alone. They are reliant on previous trials or lacked power to show a conclusive result. This has been a continuing problem in PAH trials as ethical considerations restrict the use of mortality end points and the number of cases remain relatively small. However, we have been able to select the most worthy papers in pulmonary hypertension; they demonstrate the ingenuity and originality of the researchers, feature coherent scientific arguments firmly supported by appropriate data, and still stand up as examples of how to conduct research in a rare, but important disease.

Primary pulmonary hypertension: a histopathologic study of 80 cases

Bjornsson J, Edwards WD. *Mayo Clin Proc* 1985; 60(1): 16–25.

The diagnosis of PPH does not require histological examination of lung tissue, but different pathological variants had been observed. In this paper the authors set out to determine the relative frequency of the histopathological features seen in PPH. Their tissue source was predominantly autopsy specimens from the Mayo clinic, which included samples from 80 patients obtained between 1930 and 1983. Whilst none of their exclusion criteria (notably this included clinical evidence of pulmonary embolism) were unreasonable, as a retrospective study they had no way to assess for bias in specimen retention. Only basic clinical information was gleaned from patient records. A standardized systematic review of the available lung tissue with grading and description of important features was undertaken. They applied specific criteria to distinguish between organized thrombi and plexiform lesions. They classified their findings as follows:

- Thrombo-embolic pulmonary hypertension: thrombi of various ages with eccentric intimal proliferation and fibrosis.
- Primary plexogenic pulmonary arteriopathy: plexiform lesions (even in the presence of thrombi) or concentric intimal proliferation and fibroelastosis.
- Pulmonary venous hypertension: chronic pulmonary congestion without pulmonary venous thrombosis.
- Pulmonary veno-occlusive disease: eccentric fibrosis and organized thrombi in small pulmonary veins with chronic pulmonary congestion.
- Primary medial hypertrophy: only arterial medial thickening.
- Arteritis: partial destruction of vascular walls with obstructive intimal or luminal thrombosis.

By this classification most of the cases were in fact thrombo-embolic pulmonary hypertension (56%), with a significant number of primary plexogenic pulmonary arteriopathy (28%). The common findings were medial hypertrophy, intimal proliferation and fibrosis, fibrinoid degeneration and necrosis, and thrombosis. The medial hypertrophy seen in primary plexogenic pulmonary arteriopathy was graded as more severe. Scattered thrombi were seen in several forms of PPH, with platelet-fibrin thrombi seen lining the vascular channels in plexogenic arteriopathy. The clinical diagnoses might be called in to question in some of these cases but this was not the purpose of the study. Although many images are shown within the paper to illustrate their findings, there was no blinding or even independent observation. But again, the clearly laid out rationale and large sample size means that the few significant findings are hard to ignore. The finding of pathological lesions that explain the haemodynamic changes in pulmonary hypertension has helped to determine PPH conditions and develop therapies.

Learning points

- There is a high prevalence of thrombo-embolic changes in clinical PPH cases.
- *In situ* thrombosis occurs in histological PPH providing a rationale for anticoagulation.

Further reading

- Fuster V, Steele PM, Edwards WD, Gersh BJ, McGoon MD. Primary pulmonary hypertension: natural history and the importance of a thrombotic etiology. *Circulation* 1984; 70: 580–7.
- Wagenvoort CA, Wagenvoort N. Primary pulmonary hypertension: a pathologic study of the lung vessels in 156 clinically diagnosed cases. *Circulation* 1970; 42: 1163–84.

High-dose calcium channel-blocking therapy for primary pulmonary hypertension: evidence for long-term reduction in pulmonary arterial pressure and regression of right ventricular hypertrophy

Rich S, Brundage BH. *Circulation* 1987; 76(1): 135–41.

Vasodilator agents used in systemic hypertension had been tried in PPH with mixed results. To resolve the question this study examined the effects of high dose calcium channel blockers (CCB) on haemodynamic measures in PPH. Thirteen patients who met USA national registry criteria for PPH were enrolled. This small sample had a mean age of 36 years; very much lower than that reported by current registries. In retrospect, the high proportion of patients who responded to therapy seems remarkable. Pulmonary and femoral artery catheters were left *in situ* following baseline haemodynamic studies. Initial challenge with nifedipine (20 mg) or diltiazem (60 mg) was followed by further oral doses of CCB every hour with full haemodynamic recordings until either a positive response or adverse event occurred, for example systolic BP falling below 90 mmHg. A positive response was defined as a 50% reduction in pulmonary vascular resistance (PVR) and a 33% fall in mean pulmonary artery pressure (mPAP). The cumulative dose of drug deemed effective was then re-administered every 6–8 hours. If side effects were pronounced patients were started on lower doses, which were then up-titrated to the effective dose before discharge. Digoxin was initiated to counteract any negative inotropic effects of CCBs. Patients also returned for a repeat right heart catheter a year later.

The point of interest was how many patients responded to CCBs and what haemodynamic improvements were achieved. Comparisons were made between the responder and non-responder group. Obviously the responder group had, by definition, better haemodynamics following treatment. The results show that the five patients who did not respond without side effects had a larger fall in systemic arterial pressure. Follow-up data showed that one of the eight responders died after six months (after dose reduction). Six responders were symptom free, World Health Organization functional class (WHO FC) I with another in class II (see Table 18.2). Four of the five patients with data from one year showed sustained improvement with respect to haemodynamic measures. The fact that the titration schedule was so regimented and the data for each patient is presented at logical points of interest during the titration is key. It was absolutely necessary at that time to show that CCBs could work in PPH. Less cumbersome systems have subsequently been developed to determine whether someone is a responder. However, the tenet of pulmonary hypertension: that CCBs should be used in those who respond to vasodilator challenge has remained and current treatment guidelines recognize this. The immediate beneficial outcome was to illustrate that in a select group of patients there was an effective treatment for this progressive condition.

Learning points

- A small minority of patients with PPH may respond to high dose CCB therapy.

Further reading

- Montani D, Savale L, Natali D, *et al.* Long-term response to calcium-channel blockers in non-idiopathic pulmonary arterial hypertension. *Eur Heart J* 2010; 31(15): 1898–907.
- Rich S, Kaufmann E, Levy PS. The effect of high doses of calcium-channel blockers on survival in primary pulmonary hypertension. *N Engl J Med* 1992; 327(2): 76–81.

Survival in patients with primary pulmonary hypertension. Results from a national prospective registry

D'Alonzo GE, Barst RJ, Ayres SM, Bergofsky EH, Brundage BH, Detre KM, Fishman AP, Goldring RM, Groves BM, Kernis JT, Levy PS, Pietra GG, Reid LM, Reeves JT, Rich S, Vreim CE, Williams GW, Wu M.
Ann Intern Med 1991; 115: 343–9.

The first world symposium on pulmonary hypertension had collected and reviewed the available data, but concluded that much more work needed to be done. It was recognized that a multi-centre collaboration would be needed to obtain a clearer understanding of the disease. In 1981, a prospective registry of 32 centres in the USA began to enrol patients. The intention was to describe the natural history of PPH. It was also intended to allow for analysis of factors associated with survival. Pulmonary hypertension was defined as mPAP greater than 25 mmHg at rest or 30 mmHg with exercise. A diagnosis of PPH was only accepted after post-capillary pulmonary hypertension, significant lung disease, thrombo-embolic disease, sickle cell anaemia, intravenous drug use and collagen vascular disease had been excluded. The date of the diagnostic right heart study was used as the index date for survival analysis. A group of 194 patients were enrolled in just over four years. The only end point of interest was death; this was subcategorized into sudden death, death due to right ventricular failure or other. Patients were seen at least every six months at the clinical centres and survival status recorded. Data collected at baseline was used for univariate analysis and then multiple variable Cox regression analysis for association with survival.

By the time of conclusion there had been 106 deaths, with 60 patients remaining under active follow-up. Thirteen patients were censored for heart-lung transplantation and fifteen were lost to follow-up. A group of 124 patients were followed up for at least a year, with an estimated survival of 68% (95% confidence intervals [CI] 61–75%). Estimated three-year survival was 48% and five-year survival only 34%. In the group, 47% of patients were recorded to have died from right ventricular failure, with a further 26% listed as sudden deaths. Linear regression identified several variables associated with survival, that is, 95% CI for the odds ratio (OR) did not overlap unity: WHO FC IV compared with I–III (OR 2.38) and WHO FC III or IV compared with I and II (OR 1.93). The presence of Raynaud's phenomenon carried an OR of 2.11, diffusion capacity for carbon monoxide (DLco) OR 0.97, mean right atrial pressure (RAP, OR 1.99), mPAP (OR 1.16), cardiac index (OR 0.62), PVR index (OR 1.04), and pulmonary arterial oxygen content (OR 0.91). Multiple variable regression analysis of survival time showed a high degree of inter-correlation between mean RAP, mPAP, and cardiac index. However, when these parameters were inserted separately in regression analyses with the presence of Raynaud's, WHO FC IV status, and DLco they remained the only significant factors. A formula was derived from these results to predict survival outcome in future patients.

At the time of publication this represented the largest cohort of PPH cases. Although larger registries have since been reported this will remain the definitive study of the natural history of PPH as now all patients will receive targeted therapies. Differences in management between centres cannot be discounted and the inclusion criteria are outdated; HIV was unknown when the registry was started. The formula has been used in multiple subsequent studies, where no control group is available, to derive a predicted survival for populations. The use of measures of right ventricular function, RAP, and cardiac index, as prognostic markers has stood firm.

Learning points

- Survival in untreated PPH is poor: 68%, 48%, and 34% at one, three, and five years, respectively.
- Mortality in PPH is associated with poor right ventricular function.

Further reading

- Rich S, Dantzker DR, Ayres SM, *et al.* Primary pulmonary hypertension. A national prospective study. *Ann Intern Med* 1987; 107(2): 216–23.

Experience and results with 150 pulmonary thrombo-endarterectomy operations over a 29-month period

Jamieson SW, Auger WR, Fedullo PF, Channick RN, Kriett JM, Tarazi RY, Moser KM. *J Thorac Cardiovasc Surg* 1993; 106(1): 116–26.

The treatment of CTEPH by thrombo-endarterectomy was performed infrequently. With little evidence or experience in this matter a potentially curative treatment was being overlooked. It is important to be clear that thrombo-endarterectomy is distinct from pulmonary embolectomy, sometimes employed in the setting of acute pulmonary embolism. Thrombo-endarterectomy is performed via a median sternotomy incision with two periods of circulatory arrest required, one for each side. Following dissection of the main vessels a proximal incision is made in the pulmonary artery and then the dissection plane is established. The dissection is extended distally to lobar segmental or subsegmental levels and the endarterectomy specimen may include intima and media as well as organized thrombus. A period of reperfusion is conventional before tackling the contralateral side. The post-operative course can be difficult, with persistent pulmonary hypertension and secondary reperfusion oedema.

This paper, presented to the American Association for Thoracic Surgery annual meeting, reviews the development of thrombo-endarterectomy and outcomes over 150 consecutive cases by one surgeon. As the paper reports many patients referred for surgery (>150) were awaiting a decision or had deferred. The reasons are not explained beyond this. Three criteria were applied to determine suitability: accessible chronic thrombi, no life-threatening comorbidities, and PVR >300 dyne/s/cm^5. None of these were absolute and more distal thrombi were accepted as experience increased. Of the patients who underwent surgery, over 90% were in WHO FC III or IV. Inferior vena cava filters were placed before surgery in all cases.

Within the series there is consideration of the learning curve of the operator and changes to the procedure and

patients is acknowledged. There is no comparison with results of other centres or patients in whom surgery was not performed. The main concerns of this series were in-hospital mortality (8.7%) and changes in pulmonary haemodynamics post-operatively. Cardiac output increased by 1.8 L/min, mPAP and PVR fell by 19.6 mmHg and 637.5 dyne/s/cm^5, respectively. The duration of circulatory arrest is also discussed and its effect on complications. Unfortunately, no long-term follow-up data is provided to demonstrate the overall effect on survival or possible recurrence. The lack of any control group precludes the authors from making any firm statements beyond quoting mortality and complication rates. The detailed description and discussion of technical aspects of the surgery is the reason why this paper changed practice. It has taken many years for data to come out from other centres and reproduce these findings. Uncovering CTEPH is an absolute must in the assessment of pulmonary hypertension because of the possibility of restoring normal haemodynamics through surgical intervention. By demonstrating the ability of their surgical centre to improve they showed the way forward for others to follow.

Learning points

- Surgical thrombo-endarterectomy improves haemodynamics in chronic thromboembolic pulmonary hypertension.

Further reading

- Archibald CJ, Auger WR, Fedullo PF, *et al*. Long-term outcome after pulmonary thrombo-endarterectomy. *Am J Respir Crit Care Med* 1999; 160(2): 523–8.

A comparison of continuous intravenous epoprostenol (prostacyclin) with conventional therapy for primary pulmonary hypertension

Barst RJ, Rubin LJ, Long WA, McGoon MD, Rich S, Badesch DB, Groves BM, Tapson VF, Bourge RC, Brundage BH, Koerner SK, Langleben D, Keller CA, Murali S, Uretsky BF, Clayton LM, Jobsis MM, Blackburn SD, Shortino D, Crow JW. The Primary Pulmonary Hypertension Study Group. *N Engl J Med* 1996; 334: 296–302.

Although treatment was in use for PPH this consisted of heart failure therapy plus warfarin, with CCBs reserved for patients who responded to vasodilator therapy. None of these options had been established in prospective randomized trials to improve survival. Having conducted an eight-week trial which showed haemodynamic improvement with epoprostenol, a randomized but open trial, as mandated by the delivery system, was conducted over 12 weeks in multiple centres across the USA. Patients with PPH who met criteria for entry into the national registry and were in functional class III or IV despite optimal medical therapy were studied. The baseline data presented are typical for PPH: female preponderance, mPAP ~60 mmHg with a PVR of 1280 dyncs/s/cm⁵ and average six-minute walk distance (6MWD) of 300 metres. All 81 patients had a baseline right heart catheter study with a short infusion of epoprostenol. After randomization, either a continuous infusion of intravenous epoprostenol was added to conventional therapy or conventional therapy was given alone. The 41 patients given epoprostenol

received tunnelled central venous access and training before discharge from hospital. Follow-up study visits took place at one, six, and twelve weeks. The specified end points were exercise capacity, quality of life, haemodynamics, and survival.

In the epoprostenol group, 6MWD improved from 316 m to 348 m, with a decline from 272 to 257 m in the conventional therapy group. There were reported improvements in quality of life scores with epoprostenol and 40% of patients improved their functional class. Haemodynamic assessments at 12 weeks showed a clear advantage with epoprostenol, an adjusted fall in mPAP of 6.7 mmHg and PVR of 392 dynes/s/cm⁵. The major finding was improved survival with epoprostenol; during the study period eight patients died, all in the control group (see Figure 18.1). The short duration of the study did not allow for proper assessment of side effects (jaw pain), adverse events (catheter-related sepsis and paradoxical embolism), and infusion problems. Demonstrating the haemodynamic effects of epoprostenol in all patients from baseline studies removes the potential bias of having a non-responder group. It is as a result of this study that epoprostenol is considered the gold-standard treatment for PAH and is still the recommended first-line therapy for patients in WHO FC IV. Drug trials that have followed have arguably been more constrained by ethical considerations and it is only after meta-analysis that survival benefit with other PAH therapies has been demonstrated.

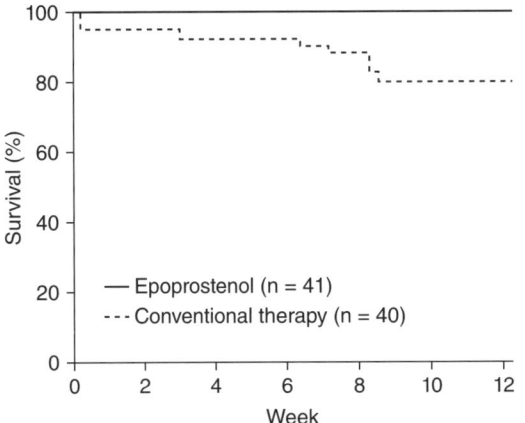

Figure 18.1 Survival among the 41 patients treated with epoprostenol and the 40 patients receiving conventional therapy.

Learning points

◆ Continuous intravenous infusion of epoprostenol improves survival in PPH.

Further reading

● Badesch DB, Tapson VF, McGoon MD, *et al.* Continuous intravenous epoprostenol for pulmonary hypertension due to the scleroderma spectrum of disease. A randomized, controlled trial. *Ann Intern Med* 2000; 132: 425–34.

Executive Summary from the World Symposium on Primary Pulmonary Hypertension 1998

Rich S (ed.). World Health Organization http://web.archive.org/web/20020408173726/http://www.who.int/ncd/cvd/pph.html (accessed 12/07/2010).

This is not a research paper as such, but a combined effort from the leading clinical scientists in the field. They met at the second world symposium on PPH in Evian and this document is a summary of the discussions and opinions from the meeting. The different sections cover pulmonary hypertension in a systematic fashion, but a few areas of note follow.

In the pathology section the vascular abnormalities are discussed layer by layer. The proliferation of endothelium and molecular changes were associated with increased Factor VIII antigen, VEGF receptor, Kdr, eNOS, and endothelin-1. Smooth muscle cell and fibroblast interconversion and medial hypertrophy are mentioned, with a request for better application of the understanding of normal vascular development to pulmonary hypertension. The plexiform lesion is remarked as a mystery, being a mass of disorganized vessels. There follows a new protocol for the pathological assessment of lungs, a standard which all were capable of following and one of the reasons why the document was so influential in driving forward research. Moving onto pathobiology, new work on potassium channels, vasoconstrictor/vasodilators, prostacyclin synthase, nitric oxide, inflammation, serotonin, angiogenesis, thrombosis, haemodynamics and shear stress, and the extracellular matrix are all covered.

The next section dealt with risk factors for developing pulmonary hypertension, including drugs (aminorex, fenfluramine, dexfenfluramine, and toxic rapeseed oil) and demographic factors (female gender). The genetics of 94 families with heritable PAH are considered, as are the clinical implications of screening (likelihood of only 0.6–1.2% of having PPH if one first degree relative is affected). The use of echocardiography for screening of first degree relatives with PPH is mentioned, as is the value of screening in scleroderma irrespective of symptoms, but in systemic lupus erythematosis, other connective tissue diseases, and HIV, only in the presence of symptoms. Patients being assessed for liver transplant are also recommended to have screening echocardiograms.

Although quite prescriptive, again there is helpful guidance on what to assess when using echocardiography, MRI, CT, and right heart catheterization with vasodilator testing.

Therapeutic options are covered, including the appropriate use of CCB (only in those with a vasodilator response), inotropes (including digoxin), anticoagulation, prostaglandins (which had recently been evaluated), and nitric oxide. A positive response to a vasodilator challenge is defined: 10 mmHg reduction in mPAP without a fall in cardiac output. Detailed guidance and discussion of the value of atrial septostomy is provided. The benefit of transplantation and timing of referrals is discussed.

The final section is perhaps the most banal but important: nomenclature and diagnostic classification. For the first time several conditions associated with pulmonary hypertension are grouped together with PPH in what we would now refer to as group 1 or PAH (see Table 18.1). This had tremendous significance in widening the possible beneficiaries of targeted therapy and making the condition attractive for business development. This success can be illustrated by the number of drugs now on the market for PAH.

Learning points

- A standardized protocol was provided for assessing histological specimens to aid the clinician.
- New nomenclature and classification of pulmonary hypertension had been formulated.

Further reading

- Humbert M, McLaughlin VV (eds). Proceedings of the 4th World Symposium on Pulmonary Hypertension. *J Am Coll Cardiol* 2009; 54(S): S1–S117.

BMPR2 haploinsufficiency as the inherited molecular mechanism for primary pulmonary hypertension

Machado RD, Pauciulo MW, Thomson JR, Lane KB, Morgan NV, Wheeler L, Phillips JA, Newman J, Williams D, Galiè N, Manes A, McNeil K, Yacoub M, Mikhail G, Rogers P, Corris P, Humbert M, Donnai D, Martensson G, Tranebjaerg L, Loyd JE, Trembath RC, Nichols WC. *Am J Hum Genet* 2001; 68(1): 92–102.

Familial PAH refers to the autosomally dominant inherited form of PAH that is similar to idiopathic PAH. Within a rare disease the existence of several affected families enabled mapping of the gene locus to chromosome 2q33. This international collaboration briefly reported that the responsible gene on this locus coded for the bone morphogenetic protein receptor 2 (BMPR2) a member of the transforming growth factor-β superfamily. This paper sets out the spectrum of mutations and the functional impact thereof, as the beginning of the road to elucidating the mechanism causing PAH. DNA samples were taken from members of 47 separate affected families and three sporadic cases of PAH. Following polymerase chain reaction (PCR) amplification and gene sequencing the mutations were tested against a panel of 150 chromosomes from normal individuals. Plasmids were constructed by digesting BMPR2 cDNA. Bone morphogenetic protein receptor 2 mutations were identified in 23 families and the three sporadic cases of PAH. Fifteen of the mutations lead to a truncated BMPR2 molecule, with PCR quantification techniques showing reduced values, consistent with heterozygosity, for several of the cases studied. The mutations found were dispersed throughout the gene and included frameshift, nonsense, and deletions. Analysis of messenger RNA obtained from lung tissue of one patient yielded both normal BMPR2 product and code missing several exons. Cell transfection using code for two of the BMPR2 mutations resulted in

reduced functional activity in response to the BMP4 ligand compared with wild type. The age of disease onset showed wide variability in these cases. The type of BMPR2 mutation did not correlate with the number of family members affected or age of onset.

Although many individuals were identified, the variable mutations and consequent heterogeneity mean there is no clear single line of thought. The paper is a conglomeration of several experiments, which can make it difficult to follow. The discovery of the genetic mechanism of PAH, from demonstrating BMPR2 mutations in sporadic cases, has led to a whole new direction of research in the hope of exploiting this pathway.

Learning points

- Heterozgous BMPR2 mutations of many kinds occur with the phenotypic result of PAH.
- Familial PAH probably occurs as a result of a 'two hit' process.

Further reading

- International PPH Consortium, Lane KB, Machado RD, Pauciulo MW, *et al.* Heterozygous germline mutations in BMPR2, encoding a TGF-beta receptor, cause familial primary pulmonary hypertension. *Nat Genet* 2000; 26(1): 81–4.

Bosentan therapy for pulmonary arterial hypertension

Rubin LJ, Badesch DB, Barst RJ, Galie N, Black CM, Keogh A, Pulido T, Frost A, Roux S, Leconte I, Landzberg M, Simonneau G. *New Eng J Med* 2002; 346(12): 896–903.

Endothelin-1 produces potent vasoconstriction in experimental studies and elevated levels are seen in lungs of PAH patients. An endothelin receptor antagonist had shown haemodynamic benefit in phase II studies. The Bosentan Randomized Trial of Endothelin Receptor Antagonist Therapy was the first of many studies with

bosentan in PAH. The two objectives were to demonstrate efficacy of bosentan in PAH and also assess the higher strength dose: 250 mg twice daily. This double-blind, placebo-controlled, randomized study was limited to a duration of 16 weeks. A follow-on open label study was available for most patients. In the group, 213 patients who met the contemporary diagnostic criteria for PAH at rest (mPAP >25mmHg, wedge <15 mmHg, PVR >240 dyne/s/cm⁵) in WHO FC III or clinically stable in class IV with a 6MWD of 150–450 m were eligible. Only patients with primary PAH or scleroderma or systemic lupus erythematosis-related PAH were recruited. The change in 6MWD from baseline to week 16 was the primary end point, with change in Borg dyspnoea index and WHO FC and time to clinical worsening events as secondary measures.

At 16 weeks 6MWD in the placebo group had fallen by 8 m, in contrast the bosentan-treated group 6MWD had improved by 44 m (35 m in the 125 mg twice daily group, see Figure 18.2). Subgroup analysis demonstrated that although treatment effect was similar in primary PAH and scleroderma-associated PAH the effect was to prevent deterioration in the latter group, that is, bosentan only increased 6MWD by 3 m from baseline but a decline of 40 m was seen in patients with scleroderma on placebo. Patients with an mPAP <50 mmHg or a cardiac index >2.3 L/min/m² were also less likely to see a beneficial change in exercise capacity. The overall effect on Borg dyspnoea index and WHO FC did not reach significance. The effect of bosentan in delaying time to clinical worsening was significant at 16 weeks with no difference between doses. Although greater improvement in 6MWD was seen with high dose bosentan the apparent lack of dose effect in the prevention of clinical worsening and the high rate of liver enzyme abnormalities (14%) meant the authors did not endorse the 250 mg twice daily regimen. The success of this study in proving benefit by means of six-minute walk testing after a brief double-blind period is perhaps the beginning of a problem afflicting all

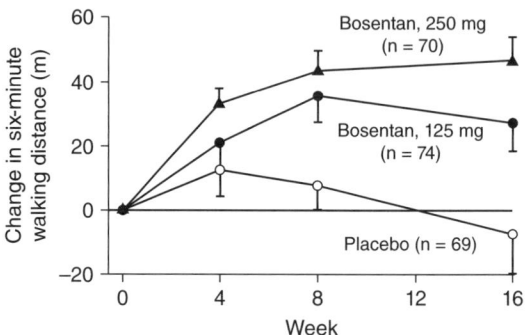

Figure 18.2 Mean (± SE) change in six-minute walking distance from baseline to week 16 in the placebo and bosentan groups.

subsequent PAH trials. Criticism frequently rests on two things: short duration of blinded treatment and failure to demonstrate survival benefit.

Learning points

♦ Bosentan improves exercise capacity in PAH.

Further reading

● Channick RN, Simonneau G, Sitbon O, et al. Effects of the dual endothelin-receptor antagonist Bosentan in patients with pulmonary hypertension: a randomised placebo-controlled study. Lancet 2001; 358: 1119–23.

Pulmonary arterial hypertension in France: results from a national registry

Humbert M, Sitbon O, Chaouat A, Bertocchi M, Habib G, Gressin V, Yaici A, Weitzenblum E, Cordier JF, Chabot F, Dromer C, Pison C, Reynaud-Gaubert M, Haloun A, Laurent M, Hachulla E, Simonneau G.
Am J Respir Crit Care Med 2006; 173(9): 1023–30.

The American registry had been a success and produced very helpful data, but the classification of PAH had changed. The relatively narrow definition used for PPH in the 1980s and 1990s had been broadened to include HIV and collagen vascular disease. With this new arrangement 17 university hospitals in France joined together to create a registry of all their PAH patients from 2002. They aimed to provide estimates of prevalence and incidence and describe the clinical and haemodynamic

parameters of this current cohort. Their definition of PAH required an mPAP >25 mmHg with a wedge pressure <15 mmHg. Patients with respiratory disease (FEV₁, FVC, or TLC <60% predicted) were excluded since they were deemed prone to develop pulmonary hypertension secondary to chronic respiratory diseases. Incidental cases (n = 121) were diagnosed between October 2002 and 2003, with prevalent cases (n = 553) being those diagnosed prior to October 2002. The date of diagnosis was taken as the date of right heart catheter study.

The calculated annual incidence of PAH in France from this study was 2.4 cases per million. The prevalence of idiopathic PAH was 5.9 cases per million, with 15 cases per million for all cause PAH. The mPAP was lower in incident cases, as was the ratio of females to males. Despite this, 81% of incident cases were in WHO FC III or IV at diagnosis, with an estimated mean of 27 months elapsing between the onset of symptoms and diagnosis. A comparison of haemodynamic data between the incident and prevalent cases showed that mPAP was lower in incident cases; however, other parameters were nearly identical (right atrial pressure (RAP), wedge, cardiac index, SvO_2, PVR index).

The breakdown of PAH subtypes was: idiopathic 39.2%, connective tissue disease 15.3%, congenital heart disease 11.3%, portal hypertension 10.4%, anorexigen 9.5%, HIV 6.2%, and familial 3.9%, with 4.3% having evidence of two co-existent causes (typically HIV and portal hypertension). Vasodilator response was only demonstrated in a small minority of patients (5.8%). Estimated one-year survival was 88.4% in the incident population; this compared favourably with the calculated estimate of 71.8% using the above D'Alonso formula.

This was the first descriptive study of a national population since the Evian re-classification. Whilst replicating earlier work, but in a different population (geographically and chronologically), the importance of descriptive studies should not be underestimated when dealing with rare diseases such as PAH. The key point, that is still relevant today, was the high proportion of patients with marked symptoms at diagnosis.

> **Learning points**
>
> ◆ Patients with PAH present late after disease onset with marked symptoms and haemoydnamic disturbance.
> ◆ One-year survival in PAH has possibly improved to 88% for contemporary diagnoses.

Addition of sildenafil to long-term intravenous epoprostenol therapy in patients with pulmonary arterial hypertension

Simonneau G, Rubin L, Galiè N, Barst RJ, Fleming TR, Frost AE, Engel PJ, Kramer MR, Burgess G, Collings L, Cossons N, Sitbon O, Badesch DB; for the Pulmonary Arterial Hypertension combination Study of Epoprostenol Sildenafil (PACES) Study Group. *Ann Intern Med* 2008; 149: 521–30.

Although many specialists were already treating patients with two therapies for PAH, there were no randomized, controlled trials to back up this practice. The Bosentan Randomized trial of Endothelin Antagonist Therapy for PAH (BREATHE-2) study assessed the combination of bosentan and epoprostenol as initial therapy with equivocal results. The goal of the 16-week multi-centre, double-blind, placebo-controlled patient-centred episode system (PACES) study was to show that combining sildenafil with epoprostenol improved 6MWD (primary end point). Idiopathic, familial, anorexigen, connective tissue disease related PAH patients were eligible, plus patients with congenital defects repaired more than five years earlier. Patients were over 18 years of age with a 6MWD in the range 100–450 m and were not allowed to be taking bosentan. Entry required long-term intravenous epoprostenol therapy (defined as more than three months) with a stable dose for four weeks. Randomization was on a 1:1 basis but stratified by cause (idiopathic vs. other) and six 6MWD (above or below 325 m). Follow-up was every four weeks to sixteen weeks and included up-titration to 40 then 80 mg sildenafil three times a day. Of the 267 patients randomized, nine patients (eight in the placebo group) were lost to follow-up.

There were no significant differences between the two groups at baseline. The sildenafil group achieved an improvement in 6MWD of 29.8 m compared with 1 m in the placebo group (p <0.001). Due to missing observations and lost patients several statistical tests were run to cover the permutations of the protocol deviations, all confirming significance. Patients with baseline walk distances greater than 325 m or idiopathic PAH appeared to derive more benefit. Haemodynamic measures improved with sildenafil therapy (placebo adjusted differences): mPAP -3.8 mmHg, RAP -2.1 mmHg, cardiac output + 0.9 L/min, heart rate -3.6 bpm, mixed venous

O_2 + 6.9%, PVR -173 dyne/s/cm^5. Time to clinical worsening criteria in this study included adjustment of epoprostenol dose by >10% due to clinical deterioration. This event occurred first in nine patients on placebo, but none on sildenafil and probably accounts for much of the difference in time to clinical worsening (p = 0.002 at 112 days by stratified log-rank). Although there were seven deaths in the placebo group and none with sildenafil therapy this was not formally tested for significance. A large number of adverse events and side effects were reported in both groups, but fewer than 10% discontinued treatment. The study does not provide evidence for the efficacy of up-front combination therapy (i.e. at diagnosis) and, as with most PAH trials, survival benefit is not proven. However, it does show that combination therapy can improve exercise capacity in PAH and has given impetus to combination treatment.

> ### Learning points
>
> - Combination therapy by means of the addition of sildenafil to intravenous epoprostenol improves exercise capacity and haemodynamic measures in PAH.

Further reading

- Hoeper MM, Faulenbach C, Golpon H, Winkler J, Welte T, Niedermeyer J. Combination therapy with bosentan and sildenafil in idiopathic pulmonary arterial hypertension. *Eur Respir J* 2004; 24: 1007–10.
- Humbert M, Barst RJ, Robbins IM, *et al.* Combination of bosentan with epoprostenol in pulmonary arterial hypertension: BREATHE-2. *Eur Respir J* 2004; 24: 353–59.

Connective tissue disease-associated pulmonary arterial hypertension in the modern treatment era

Condliffe R, Kiely DG, Peacock AJ, Corris PA, Gibbs JS, Vrapi F, Das C, Elliot CA, Johnson M, DeSoyza J, Torpy C, Goldsmith K, Hodgkins D, Hughes RJ, Pepke-Zaba J, Coghlan JG. *Am J Respir Crit Care Med* 2009; 179(2): 151–7.

Connective tissue disease associated pulmonary arterial hypertension (CTD-PAH) comprises the second largest group of patients in most PAH registries and clinical trials. Studies had mostly focused on scleroderma (SSc-PAH) and reported poor survival, despite more favourable haemodynamics when compared with idiopathic PAH. This study utilized data from the UK registry of patients with CTD-PAH. All incident cases were entered into local databases at diagnosis. The 2003 Venice diagnostic criteria were used and therefore exercise-induced PAH was included. Patients with an FVC <60% or with fibrosis covering more than one-third of the lung field on high resolution CT scan were labelled as respiratory associated pulmonary hypertension. Patients were followed up as clinically required to censor date. Data for FVC, DLco, and walk distance were available for 79%, 71%, and 82% of patients respectively.

One, two, and three-year survival in SSc-PAH without significant respiratory disease was 78%, 58%, and 47%, respectively. Nearly two-thirds of these patients received targeted PAH therapies. Risk factor analysis showed that young age, female gender, high mixed venous oxygen content, and WHO FC I/II were predictors of better outcomes.

Amongst the 42 patients with exercise-induced PAH the mean time to PAH at rest was 838 days. The calculated incidence of CTD-PAH rose to 1.27 cases per million population per year in 2005. The prevalence of CTD-PAH at the end of the study was 3.57 cases per million. Although other diseases were studied only enough cases of systemic lupus erythematosis were included to give an estimate of one year survival at 78%.

This is the largest study of CTD-PAH with haemodynamic data looking at CTD-PAH. It covers a broad range of CTD-PAH rather than just scleroderma. However, the data is entirely observational and no comment can be made about the impact of new therapies. The definition of respiratory associated pulmonary hypertension is also unvalidated.

> ### Learning points
>
> - Scleroderma is the predominant pathology in CTD-PAH and better screening strategies are needed to identify patients.

◆ Connective tissue disease associated pulmonary arterial hypertension confers a poor prognosis but this may be better in diagnoses other than scleroderma.

Further reading

- Chung L, Liu J, Parsons L, *et al.* Characterization of connective tissue disease-associated pulmonary arterial hypertension from REVEAL: identifying systemic sclerosis as a unique phenotype. *Chest* 2010; 138(6): 1383–94

Accuracy of Doppler Echocardiography in the Hemodynamic Assessment of Pulmonary Hypertension

Fisher MR, Forfia PR, Chamera E, Housten-Harris T, Champion HC, Girgis RE, Corretti MC, Hassoun PM. *Am J Respir Crit Care Med* 2009; 179: 615–21.

Although Doppler estimates the Right Ventricular Systolic Pressure (RVSP) or Pulmonary Artery Systolic Pressure (PASP) rather than mPAP, echocardiography is the recommended screening tool for pulmonary hypertension. It offers a non-invasive assessment of right heart pressures. However, echo derived parameters have (so far) failed to provide useful end points in clinical trials. Difficulty obtaining Doppler waveforms in patients with lung disease led to this group challenging the belief that echocardiographic estimates of right heart pressures provide an accurate guide. Hence, they conducted a prospective study in PAH patients who underwent right heart catheter studies. Demographic data suggest a representative sample, although some were patients with non-PAH pulmonary hypertension. The design was simple; within an hour of patients having a right heart catheter study, blinded transthoracic echocardiography was performed to a standardized protocol. They then compared values derived from echo for: RAP, PASP, and cardiac output with those derived from the invasive studies conducted less than an hour earlier. Analysis was made using correlation accuracy assessments and Bland-Altman analysis. Accuracy was pre-defined as 95% limits of agreement within +/- 10 mmHg for PA pressure estimates and +/- 1 L/min for cardiac output measurements. Although the correlation coefficient between Doppler derived PASP and invasive assessment was 0.66 (p <0.001) only 48% were within 10 mmHg of invasively measured pressure. This is illustrated by the Bland-Altman plot, which derives a bias of 0.6 mmHg, but the 95% limits of agreement were at + 38.8 and -40.0 mmHg. Overestimation of RAP was responsible for half of the Doppler overestimates of PASP. Removing these and looking at the trans-tricuspid gradient did improve matters but limits were still outwith 30 mmHg in either direction.

Echocardiography derived cardiac output estimates were also judged to be inaccurate from the study data.

The strength of the study lies in not assuming a commonly held belief and identifying the correct methods with which to assess the question. Whilst good correlation was replicated the correct determinant of accuracy was applied to this problem with unequivocal, if surprising results. There are many questions it does not resolve about echocardiography, such as those of reproducibility and inter-observer variation. What it doesn't do is prove that there is something better, which should replace echocardiography, it is a negative study in many senses. It has provoked a re-evaluation of how we, as clinicians, should interpret this Doppler derived data. In fact, it has helped improve echocardiographic screening by demonstrating that trans-tricuspid gradient by itself is more helpful than with the addition of best guess RAP. No one should be falsely reassured by a normal Doppler derived PASP in the face of clear symptomatic and clinical evidence of pulmonary hypertension.

Learning points

- Good correlation does not mean accurate prediction.
- Doppler echocardiography derived values for PASP are likely to be inaccurate.

Further reading

- Bland JM, Altman DG. Statistical methods for assessing agreement between two methods of clinical measurement. *Lancet* 1986; 1: 307–10.

Conclusion: the future

So what does the future hold for PAH? We can expect the number of available treatments to rise and expand beyond the three pathways targeted currently. There are 136 studies in PAH listed on clinicaltrials.gov using: soluble guanylate cyclase activators, platelet derived growth factor receptor inhibitors, vasoactive intestinal peptide, prostaglandin receptor agonists, protein kinase C inhibitors, tetrahydrobiopterin analogues, noradrenaline and serotonin reuptake inhibitors, multiple kinase inhibitors, and antioxidants. Other therapeutic avenues, such as transplantation of autologous endothelial progenitor cells or the use of right ventricular assist devices may prove helpful. Our understanding of the pathobiology of PAH is far from complete, even the downstream effects of BMPR2 mutations have not been fully elucidated. It is possible this will yield more disease associations or lead to refinement of the classification of pulmonary hypertension. Many clinicians have already started to look outside PAH for possible situations where therapies may be of benefit. Our knowledge of the interactions between the left heart and the lungs with the pulmonary circulation will be challenged by this.

Beyond treatment, the greatest hope for improving outcomes lies with detecting PAH at an earlier stage. An ongoing study: Early, simple and reliable DETECTion of pulmonary arterial hypertension (PAH) in Systemic Sclerosis (SSc) (DETECT), anticipates improvements in the screening strategy for scleroderma patients. Screening of relatives may be enhanced as more genes implicated in heritable PAH are discovered. There are a plethora of possible biomarkers in PAH and future experience should lead us to a rational use of widely available assays. Imaging in PAH has been a difficult problem due to the conformation of the right ventricle, but there is much promise in MRI. A large study demonstrating which measures predict survival is required. Further developments in echocardiography techniques such as 3D modelling and speckle tracking are being applied to PAH. Despite previous attempts to diminish the role of invasive right heart studies they have remained integral and will do so for the foreseeable future. It is possible that application of intravascular imaging technologies may make right heart studies even more informative.

Whilst the hope is that we may be able to find a way to arrest the underlying disease process and prevent the right ventricle failing, it may be that this is dependent on catching this progressive disease early enough.

References

1. Romberg E. Über Sklerose der Lungenarterie. *Deutsches Archiv für klinische Medicin*, Leipzig, 1891–1892, 48: 197–206.
2. Wood P. Pulmonary hypertension. *Modern Concepts of Cardiovascular Disease* 1959; 28: 513–8.
3. Rich S (ed.). *Executive Summary from the World Symposium on Primary Pulmonary Hypertension* 1998. World Health Organization. http://web.archive.org/web/20020408173726/http://www.who.int/ncd/cvd/pph.html (accessed 12/07/2010)
4. Galié N, Rubin LJ (eds). Pulmonary Arterial Hypertension Epidemiology, Pathobiology, Assessment, and Therapy. *J Am Coll Cardiol* 2004; 43(S): S1–S90.
5. Humbert M, McLaughlin VV (eds). Proceedings of the 4th World Symposium on Pulmonary Hypertension. *J Am Coll Cardiol* 2009; 54(S): S1–S117.
6. Mehta NJ, Khan IA, Mehta RN, Sepkowitz DA. HIV-related pulmonary hypertension: analytic review of 131 cases. *Chest* 2000; 118: 1133–41
7. Lapa M, Dias B, Jardim C, *et al*. Cardiopulmonary manifestations of hepatosplenic schistosomiasis. *Circulation* 2009; 119(11): 1518–23.
8. Simonneau G, Robbins IM, Beghetti M, *et al*. Updated Clinical Classification of Pulmonary Hypertension. *J Am Coll Cardiol* 2009; 54(S): S43–54
9. Yanagisawa M, Kurihara H, Kimura S, *et al*. A novel potent vasoconstrictor peptide produced by vascular endothelial cells. *Nature* 1988; 332(6163): 411–5.
10. Galiè N, Manes A, Negro L, Palazzini M, Bacchi-Reggiani ML, Branzi A. A meta-analysis of randomized controlled trials in pulmonary arterial hypertension. *Eur Heart J* 2009; 30: 394–403.8.

Part V

Valvular heart disease

Chapter 19

Epidemiology and intervention

Dr Hasan Jilaihawi, Dr Natalia Briceno, Dr Joerg Seeburger,
and Professor Friedrich Mohr

Introduction

The last 50 years have witnessed significant advances and rapid innovations in cardiothoracic surgery; none more so than valvular surgery, which has now become a routine procedure in the modern era with excellent perioperative results. One of the predominant catalysts to this evolution in cardiac surgery has been the invention of the heart-lung machine in the early 1950s. In the case of valvular disease, where the initial focus lay in treating mitral valve stenosis by valvotomy, this new tool afforded a direct view of the pathology and therefore advanced the complexity of surgical treatment that was possible. Dwight Harken, a pioneering US Army cardiac surgeon, was one of the first to replace the aortic valve with a so-called 'cage-ball' valve in 1960, intriguing the wider surgical audience. Engineers and surgeons worked together looking for the Holy Grail in the management of valve disease.

Starr and Edwards were able to successfully replace the mitral valve with their prosthesis in 1960, but due to concerns with regard to haemodynamics and haemolysis, future mechanical valves consisted of a single or divided-disc instead of the early ball-cage constructions.

First attempts at using autologous homografts in 1962, or the Ross-procedure, showed promising results, with much of the emphasis now being placed on implanting biological or artificial valvular prostheses. In 1964, Duran and Gunning implanted a xenograft based on porcine material in the aortic position of a dog, but the early results were disappointing due to rapid valve deterioration. Multi-staged chemical treatment and washout procedures improved the long-term durability of these artificial prostheses and by the 1970's, studies provided adequate follow-up results for more than 15 years.

Although valve replacement became the primary therapy in the 1960s and 1970s, the mortality rates were still high. Therefore, pioneers like McGoon, Kay, David, Yacoub, and Carpentier worked on the idea of preserving the valve and its structure, especially for the mitral valve. Subsequent work by Carpentier and Duran strengthened the concept of valvular repair, and soon the results of the mitral repair technique, depending on the pathology, exceeded those that had been replaced. Further developments with modified cardiopulmonary bypass techniques and myocardial protection opened up the concept for less invasive procedures. Again, Carpentier was one of the first that operated on a mitral valve using video assistance through a small right-sided port access. Inspired by that, various approaches with partial sternotomies or intercostal entries dominated the development of minimally invasive valve surgery in the 1990s. Additionally, specialized surgical techniques, for example the annuloplasty and artificial chordae replacement for mitral valve repair, emerged to become the gold-standard technique and generated excellent operative and long-term results.

A new concept for treating valvular diseases is the percutaneous transcatheter valve implantation. Currently, it is mainly used for patients with high logistic EuroScores and excessive perioperative risk. The idea is to avoid the potential risk of using an extracorporeal circulation by performing a beating heart procedure. The transapical or transfemoral aortic valve replacement and the percutaneous mitral valve repair (MitraClip - Abbott Vascular, Illinois, USA) have demonstrated acceptable results thus far, but much more needs to be known about long-term durability of these prostheses. What is promising has been the increasingly prevalent collaboration between the cardiac surgeon and the interventional cardiologist to the point where self-styled Heart Teams will become mandatory, rather than desirable, in all high-volume specialist cardiac centres.

In this chapter we aim to highlight several critical steps in the development of the modern treatment of valvular heart disease.

Pulmonary valve

Percutaneous replacement of pulmonary valve in a right-ventricle to pulmonary-artery prosthetic conduit with valve dysfunction

Bonhoeffer P, Boudjemline Y, Saliba Z, Merckx J, Aggoun Y, Bonnet D, Acar P, Le Bidois J, Sidi D, Kachaner J. *Lancet* 2000; 356(9239):1403–5.

Purpose

Conduits with valves or without valves have been used surgically to repair congenital defects, by providing continuity between the right ventricle and pulmonary artery. However, these conduits frequently become stenosed and insufficiency of the conduit can occur, leading to reoperations. Stenting of the conduit percutaneously can delay the need for surgery. This can, however, lead to worsening of the insufficiency as the valve often has to be sacrificed. The authors of this paper developed a new system for percutaneous stent implantation combined with valve replacement. This was initially trialled in animal models with good results and they present the first human application in this paper.

Patient

The patient was a 12-year-old boy with pulmonary atresia and a ventricular septal defect (VSD) who had previously had a central aortopulmonary shunt at age 11 days and a right modified Blalock-Taussig shunt at ten months of age. At the age of four he had a total repair with closure of the VSD and insertion of an 18 mm Carpentier-Edwards conduit from the right ventricle (RV) to the pulmonary artery.

Study

The patient was symptomatic with New York Heart Association (NYHA) class II symptoms and significant stenosis and insufficiency of the conduit, leading to moderate dilatation of the RV. Both ethics approval and written consent from the patient's parents were obtained. A bovine jugular valve was used in this procedure, which was fixed to a platinum stent and inserted percutaneously.

Trial end points measured

Study end points included haemodynamic measurements post-procedure via angiography, including systolic pressure ratio between the RV and the aorta, function of the valve also via angiography and echocardiography with Doppler and with diastolic pulmonary-arterial pressures. Other study end points included the occurrence of any clinical events post-procedure. Size and systolic function of the RV were also measured as an end point.

Results

Angiography was performed pre- and post-procedure. Pre-procedure angiography revealed a calciferous narrowing of the Carpentier-Edwards conduit. Pressure measurements revealed a systolic right ventricular pressure of 80 mmHg, and a systolic systemic pressure of 95 mmHg. Pulmonary arterial pressures distal to the stenosis were 30/8, with a mean gradient of 16 mmHg.

The bovine valve was inserted successfully into the degenerated valve of the conduit. Haemodynamic measurements post-procedure showed a small reduction of the systolic pressure ratio between the RV and aorta from 85% to 66%. After one month the pressure ratio had decreased further to almost 50%. There was also an increase in the diastolic pulmonary-arterial pressures (30/16, mean 20 mmHg) showing good valve function.

Echocardiography was performed and did confirm residual obstruction in the conduit, with a competent pulmonary valve examined with Doppler. Five days after the procedure the systolic function and the size of the RV were normal.

After one month of follow-up the patient was in NYHA class I and repeat Doppler confirmed no insufficiency of the valve. There was only partial relief of the obstruction, however, due to the calcific nature of the obstruction being resistant to dilatations.

Study limitations

This study only investigated the use of this procedure in one patient. Follow-up was reported for a short period of time.

Study strengths

This study demonstrates a successful pioneering technique that represents a huge advance in the management of valvular heart disease in general.

Why is this a landmark paper?

This paper was the first of its kind to show a successful percutaneous valve implantation in humans. This represents an important paradigm shift in the management of valvular heart disease traditionally managed by open heart surgery.

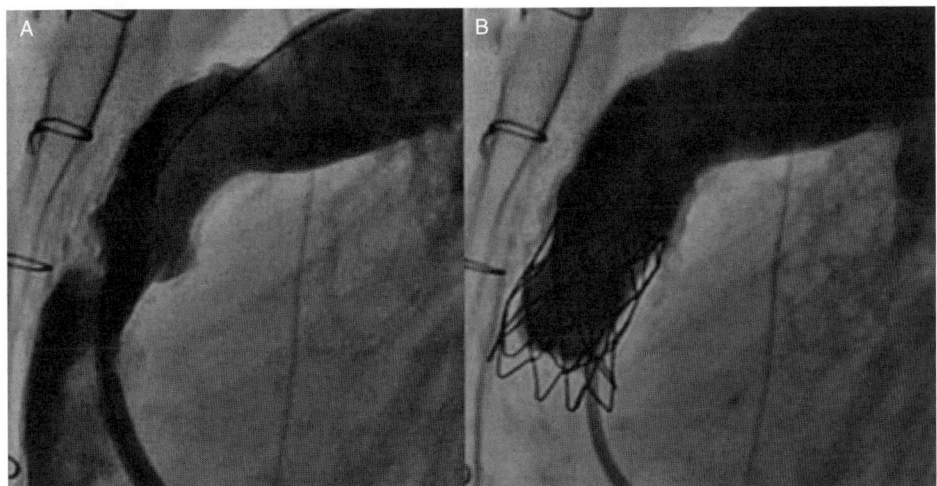

Figure 19.1 This patient presented with tetralogy of Fallot and pulmonary atresia with severe pulmonary regurgitation. Angiograms are shown demonstrating (A) preimplantation conduit obstruction and pulmonic regurgitation and (B) relief of obstruction and a competent valve after transcatheter pulmonary valve replacement with the Melody valve.

Reproduced from McElhinney DB, *et al*. Short and medium-term outcomes after transcatheter pulmonary valve placement in the expanded multicenter US melody valve trial. *Circulation* 2010; 122(5): 507–16, with permission from Wolters Kluwer Health.

Impact on clinical practice and management of specific disease process

The device in this reported case was the precursor to the Melody percutaneous pulmonary valve implant (PPVI), which is now used worldwide for the treatment of degenerated right ventricular outflow tract (RVOT) conduits. This may extend the lifetime of surgical conduits and reduce the threshold for re-intervention in chronic conduit failure and, in turn, prevent RV failure earlier.

Conclusion

Percutaneous valve implantation became a reality after this case and has revolutionized the surgical management of valvular heart disease. It represents an important advance in the management of congenital heart disease, with PPVI offering a less invasive alternative to surgery for degenerated RVOT conduits.

Learning points

- ◆ Percutaneous implantation of a biologic heart valve was first shown in this case performed in France in 2000.

- ◆ Percutaneous pulmonary valve implant is a safe and effective treatment for degenerated RVOT conduits.
- ◆ The calcific nature of these conduits made residual stenosis a problem in the early experience.

Further reading

- McElhinney DB, Hellenbrand WE, Zahn EM, *et al*. Short and medium-term outcomes after transcatheter pulmonary valve placement in the expanded multicenter US melody valve trial. *Circulation* 2010; 122(5): 507–16. (Epub 19 Jul 2010). An updated analysis of the multi-centre US Melody valve trial supports the safety and efficacy of PPVI with the Melody valve in over 120 patients. Stent fracture and residual gradients were identified as important shortcomings to be resolved (see Figure 19.1).
- Nordmeyer J, Lurz P, Khambadkone S, *et al*. Pre-stenting with a bare metal stent before percutaneous pulmonary valve implantation: acute and 1-year outcomes. *Heart* 2011; 97(2): 118–23. (Epub 21 Oct 2010). This study describes the important technical refinement of pre-stenting of the RVOT with a bare metal stent prior to PPVI, a strategy which appears to reduce the incidence of both stent fracture and residual obstruction.

Aortic valve

A comparison of outcomes in men 11 years after heart-valve replacement with a mechanical valve or bioprosthesis

Hammermeister KE, Sethi GK, Henderson WG, Oprian C, Kim T, Rahimtoola S. Veterans Affairs Cooperative Study on Valvular Heart Disease. *N Engl J Med* 1993; 328(18): 1289–96.

Purpose

Mechanical prosthetic valves are very durable. However, they come with the added risk of bleeding because they necessitate long-term anticoagulation with warfarin. Bioprosthetic valves function more like human valves, but are not as durable long term. This study sought to compare mechanical prosthetic heart valves with bioprostheic heart valves through the vehicle of a randomized controlled trial (RCT).

Patients

Between 1977 and 1982, 575 men, who were scheduled to undergo either MV replacement or aortic valve

replacement (AVR), were randomly assigned to receive either a mechanical prosthetic valve (Bjork-Shiley spherical disc mechanical heart valve) or a bioprosthetic valve (Hancock porcine-heterograft bioprosthetic valve). Inclusion criteria included those patients who had not previously undergone valve replacement, no active endocarditis, no contraindication to anticoagulation, a diameter of >21 mm for an aortic prosthesis or >27 mm for a mitral prosthesis, a life expectancy of three or more years excluding heart disease, and that the patient was able to give written informed consent.

Study design

This was a RCT seeking to compare outcomes in patients who were recruited and randomly assigned to receive either a prosthetic or bioprosthetic valve. Statistical analyses were performed using the Kaplan-Meier estimator of survival. The log rank statistic was used to compare outcomes between the two groups.

Treatment

Treatment was valve replacement with either a mechanical prosthetic or bioprosthetic heart valve.

Trial end points measured

Primary end points included the length of time to death from any cause, including operative mortality, and the length of time to the first occurrence of a valve-related complication. This included systemic embolism, bleeding, prosthetic valve endocarditis, valve thrombosis, non-thrombotic valve obstruction, prosthetic valvular regurgitation, and reoperation on the randomly assigned valve for any other reason.

Follow-up

Follow-up was performed up to 11 years after valve replacement. These patients were followed up at bi-annual clinic visits from 1977 to 1985, where data was collected on death, valve-related complications, functional status, and adequacy of anticoagulation. Subsequent follow-up was performed through a mailed questionnaire and telephone consultations where data was collected solely on death and valve-related complications. These were reviewed by a committee blinded to the type of valve inserted. Two patients were lost to follow-up but were thought to still be alive.

Results

The mean age of entry was 59 ± 8 years, 76% of patients were in NYHA functional class III or IV. Angiographically demonstrable coronary artery disease (CAD) was present in 44% of patients. The baseline characteristics of both groups were the same, including post cardiac catheterization data showing no significant differences between the groups in valve gradient, orifice area, or left ventricular function.

There was no difference in operative mortality between the study groups according to valve type or location. Operative mortality overall was 8%, and 11% for the subgroup of patients with coronary artery disease. Coronary artery bypass graft (CABG) surgery was performed in 79% of patients with CAD. There was no significant difference in operative mortality between the groups in this particular population.

There was no significant difference in the probability of death between patients who underwent aortic or MV replacement, with or without CABG and whether or not

the patient received a prosthetic or bioprosthetic valve. There was also no significant difference between the two study groups with regards to death from all causes (p = 0.57), deaths from cardiac causes alone (p = 0.22), and valve related deaths only (p = 0.07). There was also no significant difference in the second primary end point (the length of time to the first valve-related complication) between the two cohorts. There was no significant difference in the occurrence of systemic embolism between the two study groups in either the aortic (p = 0.49) or MV position (p = 0.61).

A total of 155 patients had one or more clinically important bleeding episodes and there were higher rates of these bleeding episodes in those who received a mechanical prosthetic valve. There was no difference between those receiving an aortic or MV. The 11-year probability of bleeding complications combined for both positions was 0.42 for mechanical valves and 0.26 for bioprosthetic valves (p <0.001). Anticoagulation was recorded as being used in one or more of the six-month follow-up visits in 32% of the patients with aortic bioprosthesis and 63% of those with a mitral bioprosthesis. Some 108 patients had one or more serious bleeding episodes (including bleeding from the GI tract, brain, and urinary tract). More serious bleeding episodes occurred in the study group receiving bioprosthetic valves (p <0.001).

Both prosthetic valve endocarditis and prosthetic valve thrombosis, which both resulted in catastrophic outcomes, had similar rates in both study groups. Paravalvular regurgitation occurred significantly more among patients having a mechanical MV replacement than those receiving a bioprosthesis. This also extended to those undergoing AVR. Thirty-one patients had structural valve failure (all of these had bioprosthetic heart valves implanted). Mitral bioprosthetic valves were more likely to fail compared to aortic bioprosthetic valves. For the aortic position, patients with a bioprosthetic valve implanted had a trend towards a shorter time to reoperation (p = 0.07) compared to those with mechanical AVs. The difference observed was due to reoperation for structural valve failure and to the necessity of changing valves at the initial operation. This difference was not observed in those patients undergoing MV replacements (MVRs).

The difference in the distribution of death between those receiving an aortic bioprosthetic valve and those receiving a mechanical valve was of borderline statistical significance. Only 6% of deaths among patients with a bioprosthetic heart valve were due to structural valve failure. There was no significant difference in the distribution of deaths between those patients with mitral bioprosthetic or mechanical valves.

Study limitations

Based on the US Veterans Affairs (VA) healthcare system, this trial only studied one particular population (middle-aged and older men) so the study results cannot be extrapolated to other populations, including women and younger patients in general. They also studied the use of older prostheses, not in widespread use today. This trial also used high intensity anticoagulation therapies, which may in part explain the high risk of bleeding in those patients with a mechanical heart valve. Only 12% of those with bleeding episodes had a prothrombin ratio greater than what was recommended in the protocol. There is also a limitation in the duration of the patients followed up as some latent valve complications may have been missed and reoperation rates may also have been different.

Study/trial strengths

This was a large multi-centre RCT. Randomization occurred in the operating room, allowing there to be no significant difference in the baseline characteristics between the two study populations. Follow-up was excellent, with only two out of the 575 patients randomly assigned lost to follow-up.

Why is this a landmark paper?

This paper's results have influenced current surgical management of valve disease, forming the basis of evidence to guide choice of prosthesis.

Impact on clinical practice and management of specific disease process

This trial, combined with the Edinburgh Heart Valve Trial, forms the basis of recommendations for choice of prosthesis still implemented today. For the aortic position, American College of Cardiology/American Heart Association (ACC/AHA) guidelines suggest the following as a Class IIa indication:

'A mechanical prosthesis is reasonable for AVR in patients under 65 years of age who do not have a contraindication to anticoagulation. A bioprosthesis is reasonable for AVR in patients under 65 years of age who elect to receive this valve for lifestyle considerations after detailed discussions of the risks of anticoagulation versus the likelihood that a second AVR may be necessary in the future.' Similar guidelines are stated for the mitral position later in the document.

Conclusion

No significant differences were found in the primary end points between bioprosthetic valves and mechanical valves. This was due to the higher risk of bleeding in the mechanical valve group balanced by the higher rates of structural valve failure in the bioprosthetic group. There were no differences found in overall death, valve complications, and reoperation rates between the two study groups.

Learning points

- There is no significant difference in outcome with regards to overall mortality and valve-related complications between bioprosthetic and mechanical prosthetic valves.
- There are more serious bleeding rates in those patients receiving a mechanical valve. However, there are higher rates of structural failure in those receiving a bioprosthetic valve.
- The investigators recommended the use of prosthetic valves in patients who are younger (age <60) and those requiring a MV replacement.
- Due to higher risks of bleeding in the elderly, older patients should receive a bioprosthetic valve.

Further reading

- Hammermeister K, Sethi GK, Henderson WG, Grover FL, Oprian C, Rahimtoola SH. Outcomes 15 years after valve replacement with a mechanical versus a bioprosthetic valve: final report of the Veterans Affairs randomized trial. *J Am Coll Cardiol* 2000; 36: 1152– 8. Fifteen-year follow-up of the same study, essentially revealing the same findings, but better survival with mechanical than bioprosthetic AVR, predominantly in the <65 age group, driven by structural valve failure.
- Oxenham H, Bloomfield P, Wheatley DJ, *et al.* Twenty year comparison of a Bjork-Shiley mechanical heart valve with porcine bioprostheses. *Heart* 2003; 89(7): 715–21. Twenty-year follow-up of the Edinburgh Heart Valve Study. No difference in long-term mortality was found but with bioprostheses, structural valve deterioration was observed at 8–10 years in the mitral position and 12–14 years in the aortic position.
- Rahimtoola SH. Choice of prosthetic heart valve in adults an update. *J Am Coll Cardiol* 2010; 55(22): 2413–26. Review. An authoritative contemporary review to guide choice of prosthesis based on available evidence.

A randomized trial of intensive lipid-lowering therapy in calcific aortic stenosis

Cowell SJ, Newby DE, Prescott RJ, Bloomfield P, Reid J, Northridge DB, Boon NA; Scottish Aortic Stenosis and Lipid Lowering Trial, Impact on Regression (SALTIRE) Investigators. *N Engl J Med* 2005; 352(23): 2389–97.

Purpose/hypothesis

Calcific aortic stenosis (AS) is a disease that affects primarily the elderly. It is mediated by a chronic inflammatory process that is felt to be similar to atherosclerosis. It has been found that progression of AS is affected by the degree of stenosis, valvular calcification, and hypercholesterolaemia. Aortic stenosis is a known feature in some patients with severe homozygous familial hypercholesterolaemia. Prior observational studies in AS have shown that the use of statins are associated with delay in disease progression. The aim of this study was to investigate whether high dose statins halt the progression or induce regression of calcific AS.

Patients

Eligibility criteria included patients >18 years with calcific AS, an aortic-jet velocity of at least 2.5 m/s, and AV calcification on echocardiography.

Exclusion criteria were childbearing potential without contraception, active or chronic liver disease, a history of alcohol or drug abuse, severe MV stenosis (valve area <1 cm^2), severe mitral or aortic regurgitation, left ventricular dysfunction (ejection fraction – EF <35%), a planned AVR, intolerance of statins, statin therapy or a potential benefit from statin therapy, a baseline serum total cholesterol concentration <150 mg/dL (4 mmol/L), and a presence of a permanent pacemaker or implantable cardiac debrillator.

Of the patients screened, 445 were eligible for inclusion, 173 agreed to participate, and 155 underwent randomization.

Study/trial design

This was a randomized, double-blind, placebo controlled trial comparing 80 mg of atorvastatin with placebo. Patients were randomized between March 2001 and April 2002 by the minimization technique. This incorporated the following eight variables: age, sex, smoking, hypertension, diabetes mellitus, serum cholesterol concentration, aortic jet velocity, and AV calcium score.

Assessment of valvular stenosis was performed through echocardiography using M-mode and pulsed and continuous wave Doppler. The measurements were averaged from three cardiac cycles. Both peak and mean AV pressure gradients and AV area (AVA) were calculated.

Spiral CT was performed to view the AV and assess the amount of calcification. The trial was to be terminated early in the event of a negative effect of treatment or a strong benefit of treatment. Intention to treat analyses were used for all clinical outcome variables. Two tailed tests were used throughout and two sided p values of <0.05 were considered to be statistically significant.

Trial end points measured

There were two primary end points: progression of stenosis (assessed with echo) and progression of valvular calcification (measured by CT). Secondary end points were a composite of clinical end points such as death from cardiovascular causes, AVR, or hospitalization attributable to severe AS. Other secondary end points included AVR, death from any cause, hospitalization for any cause, and hospitalization for cardiovascular causes.

Follow-up

Patients were assessed at baseline, two months, and six months thereafter for a minimum of two years. Patients were evaluated with echocardiography and CT. They also had details about their functional status and adverse events documented.

Treatment

Atorvastatin 80 mg was compared with placebo.

Results

A total of 77 patients were assigned to receive atorvastatin and 78 received placebo. They were followed for a mean of 25 months. As a result of the randomization technique all baseline characteristics were similar between the two groups. Low-density lipoprotein cholesterol concentration (LDL-C) remained static in the placebo group; however, it decreased by 53% in the statin group (p <0.001).

Intensive lipid therapy had no effect on the rate of change in the aortic-jet velocity or valvular calcification.

Serum LDL-C concentrations did not correlate with disease progression demonstrated on echo or CT. There were slightly less patients reaching secondary end points in the atorvastatin group but this was not found to be statistically significant.

Subgroup analyses comparing the mild to moderate and severe AS patients revealed a trend to faster progression in the severe AS group. However, the overall study findings were consistent regardless of the severity of the stenosis at baseline.

There were similar rates of adverse events in both study groups. Four patients in the placebo group and seven patients in the statin group discontinued the drug due to gastrointestinal side effects. There were no cases of rhabdomyolysis and no serious adverse events.

Study/trial limitations

There were patients recruited for the study with severe AS and the authors suggest this may have attenuated the possible benefit of statin use as they were unlikely to have an affect on the disease at such an advanced stage. The subgroup analysis, however, showed similar results. Follow-up may have been shorter than necessary to see a benefit in the treatment group. However, there was no trend to benefit later on in patients followed up for a longer period of time. The study was also not powered sufficiently to assess effects on secondary outcomes.

Study/trial strengths

This was a well-designed RCT performed in a single coordinating centre. As a result, a consistent and reproducible method to assess severity of AS was used. A minimization technique was also used to ensure that there were no differences in baseline between the two study groups, despite the relatively small number of patients studied.

Why is this a landmark paper?

Although the outcomes were negative in this study, it provided an important step forward in understanding the mechanisms of aortic disease progression. Despite prior studies showing that both AS and atherosclerosis have similar putative aetiologies, this study did not show a benefit of using high dose statin therapy in patients with calcific AS, separating the processes mechanistically. The authors postulate that this difference could be due to, in contrast to coronary disease, a virtual absence of smooth muscle cell proliferation and lipid-laden macrophages, with earlier and more aggressive calcification.

Impact on clinical practice and management of specific disease process

As a result of this work it is not recommended to start statin therapy in patients with calcific AS unless there is co-existing vascular disease. The paper has provided the basis of several studies to further understand the progression of this increasingly prevalent disease.

Conclusion

High dose statins in this trial did not halt the progression of AS. There was also no evidence found to suggest there was a relationship between serum LDL levels and progression of AS.

Learning points

- Prior studies have suggested that the processes that cause calcific AS are similar to vascular atherogenesis.
- In contrast to studies for coronary atherosclerotic disease progression, this trial did not show benefit in the use of high dose statins for AS progression.
- Although atherogenesis is central to coronary disease progression, mineralization may be more important in the deterioration of AS.

Further reading

- Chan KL, Teo K, Dumesnil JG, Ni A, Tam J; ASTRONOMER Investigators. Effect of lipid lowering with rosuvastatin on progression of aortic stenosis: results of the aortic stenosis progression observation: measuring effects of rosuvastatin (ASTRONOMER) trial. *Circulation* 2010; 121(2): 306–14. (Epub 4 Jan 2010). Similarly negative study with rosuvastatin.
- Miller JD, Weiss RM, Heistad DD. Calcific aortic valve stenosis: methods, models, and mechanisms. *Circ Res* 2011; 108(11): 1392–412. Review. Valuable contemporary overview of potential mechanisms of AS progression and the future of basic and clinical research in this field.
- Rossebø AB, Pedersen TR, Boman K, *et al.* Intensive lipid lowering with simvastatin and ezetimibe in aortic stenosis.; SEAS Investigators. *N Engl J Med* 2008; 359(13): 1343–56. (Epub 2 Sep 2008). With 1873 patients studied, the SEAS study remains the largest randomized trial to investigate the effects of lipid-lowering (with simvastatin and ezetimibe) on disease progression in patients with mild to moderate AS. It helped to affirm the negative findings of the SALTIRE study.

Aortic stenosis with severe left ventricular dysfunction and low transvalvular pressure gradients: risk stratification by low-dose dobutamine echocardiography

Monin JL, Monchi M, Gest V, Duval-Moulin AM, Dubois-Rande JL, Gueret P. *J Am Coll Cardiol* 2001; 37(8): 2101–7.

Purpose/hypothesis

At the time of this paper, there was little data on risk statification for patients with severe AS, LV dysfunction, and low transcatheter gradients. The investigators sought to apply dobutamine stress echocardiography (DSE) for this purpose.

Patients/trial participants

This was a prospective observational study. Patients were enrolled with severe native AS (valve area ≤1 cm²) with severe LV systolic dysfunction (LVEF ≤ 30%) or a mean pressure gradient ≤40 mmHg. Patients with AR more than mild, atrial fibrillation (AF), and severe comorbidities were excluded. A total of 45 patients were recruited to the study.

Study/trial design

Patients underwent DSE prior to decisions being made by the referring physician, who had knowledge of the results. Patients were classified into two groups on the basis of presence or absence of contractile reserve (defined as an increase in SV of ≥20% on DSE).

Dobutamine was titrated initially at 5 μg/kg/min and then upwards in 2.5 μg/kg/min increments to a maximum of 20 μg/kg/min. An increase in heart rate ≥10 beats/min was defined as an end point for test termination. Transaortic gradient, AVA, and stroke volume were calculated at each dose titration, by standard echocardiographic methods.

Treatment

Surgery or medical therapy was decided at the discretion of the referring physicians. Although the referring physicians had knowledge of the DSE results, there were no criteria for this decision imposed by the study.

Trial end points measured

Perioperative (30 day) and long-term survival were compared according to surgery or medical therapy and presence or absence of contractile reserve.

Follow-up

Follow-up was to a median of 24 months from the time of DSE (range 8–39).

Results

Thirty-day (peri-operative) mortality after surgery was 8% (n = 24) in those with contractile reserve and 50% (n = 6) without. Absence of contractile reserve conferred a relative risk of peri-operative mortality of 6.0 (95% CI 1.3–28, p = 0.014).

There was no significant difference in long-term outcomes in those who did not undergo surgery, regardless of presence or absence of contractile reserve. Of those who underwent surgery, survival at five years was 88% in those with contractile reserve and only 25% at 12 months in those without it.

In the Cox proportional hazards model, patients undergoing surgery had a significant advantage compared to medical therapy if contractile reserve was present (HR—hazard ratio for death 0.13, 95% CI 0.002–0.49, p = 0.003), but a significant disadvantage compared to medical therapy if contractile reserve was absent (HR for death 19.6, 95% CI 2.7–142, p = 0.003). This remained the case after adjustment for baseline age, diabetes, hypertension, and chronic obstructive pulmonary disease.

Study/trial limitations

This was a small study that represented only 5% of referrals evaluated by the authors over the enrolment period. The group undergoing surgery without contractile reserve was very small (n = 6), limiting how definitive this study could be. Although there was some attempt to adjust for baseline characteristics, this was a non-randomized study, and as such is subject to confounding factors, some of which may not have been known or corrected for.

Why is this a landmark paper?

At the time of the study, there was no known baseline predictor of surgical outcome in low gradient AS with LV dysfunction. This was the first study to demonstrate the value of DSE to risk stratify such patients prior to surgical AVR.

Impact on clinical practice and management of specific disease process

This study has formed the basis of the assessment of low gradient AS in the setting of significant LV dysfunction. Dobutamine stress echocardiography has become central to the risk stratification of such patients.

Conclusion

Dobutamine stress echocardiography provides important prognostic information on the outcome of low-gradient AS in the setting of significant LV dysfunction.

Learning points

- Dobutamine stress echocardiography can be used safely as a diagnostic tool in severe AS.
- It is of value in the risk stratification of low gradient, low EF AS.
- The prognosis of such patients in the presence of contractile reserve is excellent after AVR.
- Absence of contractile reserve confers a poor prognosis if managed with surgical AVR, and such patients appear best managed medically.

Further reading

- Monin JL, Quéré JP, Monchi M, et al. Low-gradient aortic stenosis: operative risk stratification and predictors for long-term outcome: a multicenter study using dobutamine stress hemodynamics. *Circulation* 2003; 108(3): 319–24. (Epub 30 Jun 2003). The authors confirmed their findings in a subsequent larger multi-centre DSE study of 136 patients.
- Tribouilloy C, Lévy F, Rusinaru D, et al. Outcome after aortic valve replacement for low-flow/low-gradient aortic stenosis without contractile reserve on dobutamine stress echocardiography. *J Am Coll Cardiol* 2009; 53(20): 1865–73. This propensity-matched study compared five-year outcomes of AVR to medical therapy if contractile reserve was absent with DSE in low-flow, low-gradient AS. It found that, despite a higher operative mortality than AVR with contractile reserve, there was a significant long-term survival benefit compared to medical therapy.

Percutaneous transcatheter implantation of an aortic valve prosthesis for calcific aortic stenosis: first human case description

Cribier A, Eltchaninoff H, Bash A, Borenstein N, Tron C, Bauer F, Derumeaux G, Anselme F, Laborde F, Leon MB. *Circulation* 2002; 106(24): 3006–8.

Purpose/hypothesis

The investigators sought to deploy a bioprosthetic valve mounted on a balloon expandable stent frame within a calcified severely stenotic AV. The concept was based on the observation by the authors that such a stent could effectively open the calcified leaflets of a cadaveric AV without coronary occlusion or disruption to the mitral apparatus.

Patient

The patient was a compassionate case with no other therapeutic option. He was a 57-year-old man who had been turned down for conventional AVR by several surgeons on the basis of multiple comorbidities and haemodynamic instability. His comorbidities included severe peripheral vascular disease, silicosis, and chronic pancreatitis.

He presented with cardiogenic shock and subacute ischaemia of the right leg. He had a severely calcified bicuspid AV with mean gradient 30 mmHg, AVA 0.6 cm², and poor LV function (EF 14%). There was no contractile reserve on DSE.

The patient initially underwent balloon aortic valvuloplasty (BAV) via trans-septal route (given the severe peripheral vascular disease) with a 20 mm balloon with initial improvement but deteriorated a week later with cardiogenic shock refractory to inotropes.

Study/trial design

This was a first-in-man compassionate use case performed after *in vitro* and animal model testing.

Treatment

The procedure was performed under local anaesthesia with light sedation. With 24Fr venous access, a standard trans-septal puncture was performed and a straight wire passed antegradely across the AV through a balloon flotation catheter and exchanged for a 260 cm stiff wire. This wire was then snared through a 5Fr arterial contralateral sheath and exteriorized. The percutaneous valve was then crimped onto a 3 cm long balloon (diameter 23 mm). It was placed at the level of the AV calcification and the balloon rapidly inflated and deflated. There was mild paravalvular regurgitation noted with a mean transcatheter transaortic gradient of 6 mmHg. Both coronary ostia were patent (see Figure 19.2).

Trial end points measured

Trans-oesophageal echocardiography (TOE) was used to assess valve area by planimetry, mean transvalvular gradient, and LV function.

Follow-up

Valve function was assessed by TOE immediately post-procedure and at seven days and two-weekly intervals thereafter.

Results

The patient had a dramatic early improvement with a significant amelioration of heart failure symptoms, and was able to mobilize, having been previously bed-bound. Aortic valve area by planimetry remained 1.5–1.6 cm² with mean transvalvular gradient a maximum of 15 mmHg. **Left ventricular** systolic function remained poor.

However, several complications occurred, including a pulmonary embolus on day three, septicemia day ten, and progressive right leg ischemia leading to amputation at ten weeks. The patient died 17 weeks after valve implantation from failure of wound healing and sepsis.

Study/trial limitations

This was a single-patient case report that led to a number of subsequent studies and developments in the technology culminating in a RCT.

Why is this a landmark paper?

This was the first demonstration that a bioprosthetic valve could be successfully inserted by transcatheter route to the aortic position and function well.

Impact on clinical practice and management of specific disease process

This study paved the way for a revolutionary technology that has changed clinical practice in valvular heart disease, permitting AV implantation by a minimally invasive transcatheter method that enables patients previously regarded as inoperable to be effectively treated.

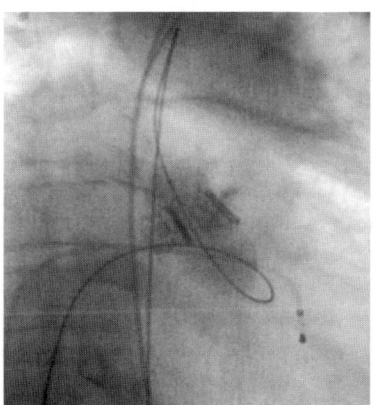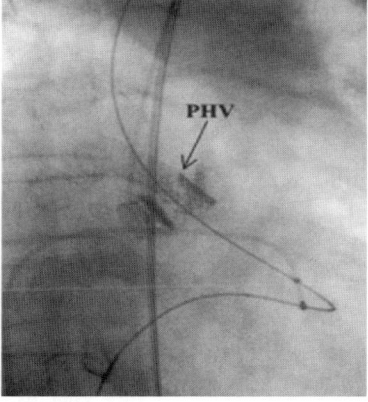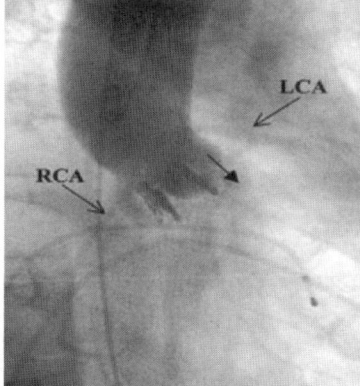

Figure 19.2 Percutaneous heart valve (PHV) delivery within the native calcific valve. Left: maximal balloon inflation (23 mm) for valve delivery. Middle: the PHV in position at mid-part of the native aortic valve, pushing aside the calcific leaflets. Right: supraaortic angiogram after PHV implantation showing no aortic regurgitation across the PHV and a mild paravalvular regurgitation (arrow). Both coronary ostia are patent and removed from the valve prosthesis. LCA = left coronary artery; RCA = right coronary artery.

Reproduced from Cribier A, *et al*. Percutaneous transcatheter implantation of an aortic valve prosthesis for calcific aortic stenosis: first human case description. *Circulation* 2002; 106(24): 3006–8, with permission from Wolters Kluwer Health.

Multiple transcatheter AV devices have been and are in development, and this therapy has dramatically transformed how severe calcific AS is managed worldwide.

Conclusion

This was the first transcatheter AV implantation (TAVI) in man, performed successfully in a patient with overwhelming comorbidities that made conventional surgery prohibitive.

Learning points

- A transcatheter valve mounted on a stent was inserted in the aortic position antegrade via transseptal approach.
- Several other approaches have developed, including the retrograde transfemoral approach, transapical, transaxillary/trans-subclavian, and trans-thoracic aortic.
- This proof of concept has led to the successful development of many other transcatheter AV devices.

Further reading

- Andersen HR, Knudsen LL, Hasenkam JM. Transluminal implantation of artificial heart valves. Description of a new expandable aortic valve and initial results with implantation by catheter technique in closed chest pigs. *Eur Heart J* 1992; 13(5): 704–8. First reported animal study of a TAVI device.
- Lichtenstein SV, Cheung A, Ye J, *et al.* Transapical transcatheter aortic valve implantation in humans: initial clinical experience. *Circulation* 2006; 114(6): 591–6. (Epub 31 Jul 2006). First reported experience of a transapical approach to TAVI. Other approaches have also been developed, including trans-axillary and transaortic (thoracic aorta).
- Webb JG, Chandavimol M, Thompson CR, *et al.* Percutaneous aortic valve implantation retrograde from the femoral artery. *Circulation* 2006; 113(6): 842–50. (Epub 6 Feb 2006). First experience of a retrograde transfemoral TAVI technique that has now become the most popular approach.

Transcatheter aortic-valve implantation for aortic stenosis in patients who cannot undergo surgery

Leon MB, Smith CR, Mack M, Miller DC, Moses JW, Svensson LG, Tuzcu EM, Webb JG, Fontana GP, Makkar RR, Brown DL, Block PC, Guyton RA, Pichard AD, Bavaria JE, Herrmann HC, Douglas PS, Petersen JL, Akin JJ, Anderson WN, Wang D, Pocock S; PARTNER Trial Investigators. N Engl J Med 2010; 363(17): 1597–607. (Epub 22 Sep 2010).

Purpose/hypothesis

At the time of this publication, TAVI had shown considerable promise as a less invasive option to surgery for severe AS, and its use had grown significantly since the first-in-man case in 2002. There was, however, a lack of robust evidence for this treatment. Therefore, the investigators sought to compare outcomes of TAVI to medical therapy in a randomized study.

Patients/trial participants

Patients were enrolled to this part of the trial (cohort B) if they had severe symptomatic AS and were considered inoperable by at least two surgeon investigators. Inclusion criteria were AVA <0.8 cm^2 and mean AV gradient ≥40 mmHg, or peak aortic velocity ≥4 m/s. Inoperability was defined on the basis of 'coexisting conditions that would be associated with a predicted probability of 50% or more of either death by 30 days after surgery or a serious irreversible condition'. Cohort A was reported at a later date and randomized high risk but operable patients to TAVI or surgical AVR. Exclusion criteria included the following: 'bicuspid or noncalcified AV, acute myocardial infarction, substantial coronary artery disease requiring revascularization, LVEF <20%, a diameter of the aortic annulus of less than 18 mm or more than 25 mm, severe (>3+) mitral or aortic regurgitation, a transient ischemic attack or stroke within the previous six months, and severe renal insufficiency'.

Study/trial design

It was a multi-centre trial involving 21 sites (17 in the USA). This part of the trial (cohort B) randomized patients to standard therapy or TAVI in a 1:1 fashion.

Treatment

Under general anaesthesia with TOE and fluoroscopy guidance, patients underwent TAVI by a retrograde transfemoral venous route, using the Edwards Sapien valve. The crimped valve was inflated at the aortic annulus at the time of rapid transvenous RV pacing.

Trial end points measured

Intention to treat analyses were performed. The primary end point was death from any cause. The co-primary end point was a composite of time to death or repeat hospitalization related to the valve or procedure. There were a number of pre-specified secondary end points, including cardiovascular death, rate of stroke and MI, valve performance by echocardiography, NYHA status, and six-minute walk test (6MWT).

Follow-up

There was an independent core laboratory for analysis of echocardiograms and electrocardiograms. All patients were followed up for at least a year.

Results

A total of 358 patients were randomized to TAVI (n = 179) or standard therapy (n = 179). All were followed for at least one year (median 1.6). After randomization, the median time to TAVI was six days. Of 179 randomized to TAVI, six did not receive TAVI due to various factors, including death prior to the procedure, annular sizing or unsuccessful femoral access. Of the 173 who underwent TAVI, 6.4% died within 30 days. Over the course of the study, 83.8% of the standard therapy group underwent BAV.

Regarding intention-to-treat analysis, 30 day mortality was 5% in the TAVI group and 2.8% in the standard therapy group, and one-year mortality 30.7% in the TAVI group and 50.7% in the standard therapy group (p <0.001). In the first year, only five patients needed to be treated with TAVI to prevent one death and only three to prevent death/repeat hospitalization. This benefit was offset by an excess of stroke or TIA (at 30 days: 6.7% in the TAVI group vs. 1.7% in the standard therapy group, p = 0.03; at one year: 10.6% in the TAVI group vs. 4.5% in the standard therapy group, p = 0.04). However, the rate of death or major stroke remained considerably lower in the TAVI arm (at one year: 33% vs. 51.3%, p <0.001). There was a significant symptomatic amelioration, with an improvement in 6MWT with TAVI, but not with standard therapy. There were accompanying improvements in AVA and gradients by echocardiography in the TAVI group.

Study/trial limitations

The trial had strict exclusion criteria, including significant peripheral vascular disease and end-stage renal failure. It included only patients unsuitable for surgery. Thus, its findings cannot be extrapolated to all patients with AS and further studies for intermediate and low risk patients are planned. The excess of stroke with TAVI has generated an important focus for future technologies to reduce neuroembolic phenomena.

Why is this a landmark paper?

This study demonstrated a significant and dramatic survival benefit in patients who would otherwise be left untreated. For this reason, TAVI is regarded as the greatest technological advance in interventional cardiology since the advent of coronary stenting. It was a well-designed study that has initiated a revolution in how patients with AS are managed in the USA. It has been the basis of forthcoming trials in intermediate and low-risk patients suffering from AS worldwide.

Impact on clinical practice and management of specific disease process

This was a pivotal US study for TAVI and has resulted in FDA approval of this technology. In Europe, it has given further justification for the widespread use of TAVI for AS in high-risk patients and has made TAVI a commonly used alternative to conventional surgery.

Conclusion

In this randomized study of patients with severe AS who could not undergo surgery, TAVI reduced one-year mortality from any cause by 20% when compared to standard therapy. The authors of this study put this forward as a strong argument for TAVI to be the new standard of care for patients with severe AS, who are ineligible for surgical AVR.

Learning points

◆ Transcatheter aortic valve implantation is a minimally invasive interventional approach to AS.

◆ It confers a significant survival benefit in patients that cannot undergo surgery.

◆ When compared to standard therapy, TAVI offers significant improvements in survival, rates of hospitalization, and functional status.

◆ Its benefit is partially offset by an excess of stroke that appears principally peri-procedural, but the rate of death/stroke is still considerably lower in the TAVI group. See Figure 19.3.

Further reading

● Reynolds MR, Magnuson EA, Lei Y, *et al.*; for the Placement of Aortic Transcatheter Valves (PARTNER) Investigators. Health-Related Quality of Life After Transcatheter Aortic Valve Replacement in Inoperable Patients With Severe Aortic. *Circulation* 2011; 124(18): 1964–72. (Epub 3 Oct 2011). Sub-study of cohort B demonstrating significant improvements in quality of life achieved by TAVI over standard therapy.

● Smith CR, Leon MB, Mack MJ, *et al.*; PARTNER Trial Investigators. Transcatheter versus surgical aortic-valve replacement in high-risk patients. *N Engl J Med* 2011; 364(23): 2187–98. (Epub 5 Jun 2011). Report of cohort A of the PARTNER trial, which randomized high-risk surgical candidates to TAVI or standard surgical AVR and demonstrated non-inferiority between both management strategies for the primary end point of all-cause mortality.

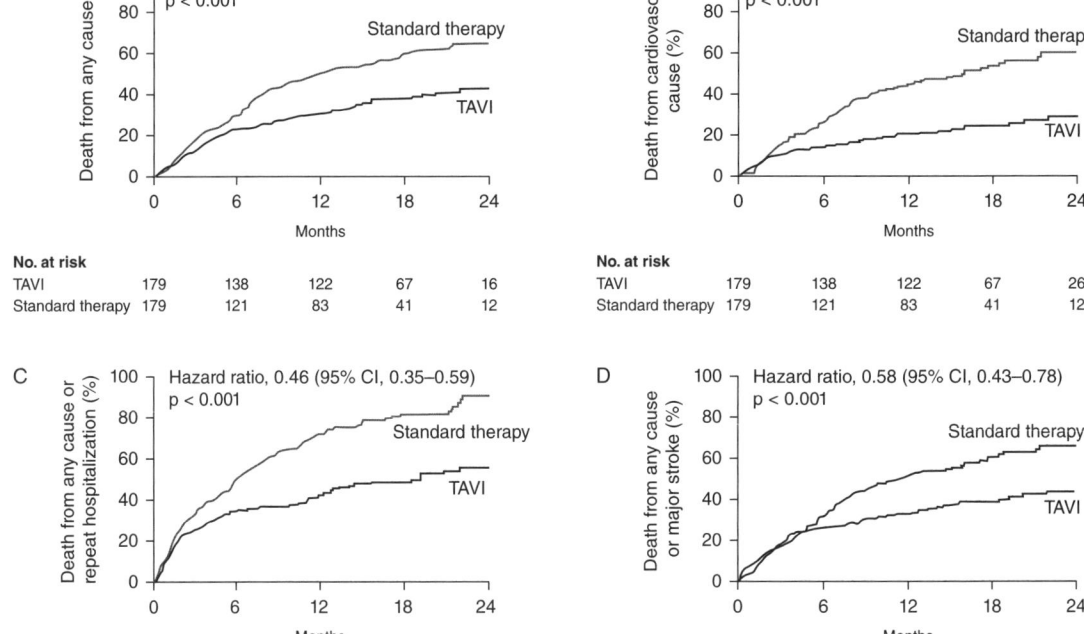

Figure 19.3 Time-to-event curves for the primary end point and other selected end points. Event rates were calculated with the use of Kaplan-Meier methods and compared with the use of the log-rank test. Deaths from unknown causes were assumed to be deaths from cardiovascular causes.

Mitral valve

Clinical application of transvenous mitral commissurotomy by a new balloon catheter

Inoue K, Owaki T, Nakamura T, Kitamura F, Miyamoto M. *J Thorac Cardiovasc Surg* 1984; 87: 394–402.

Purpose/hypothesis

Commissurotomy of MV leaflets in patients with mitral stenosis (MS) was solely performed via thoracotomy up until the advent of transcatheter commissurotomy. The investigators developed a new catheter that used the expansile force of a balloon to open up a stenotic valve. This is the first study that investigated this procedure allowing mitral commissurotomy without open surgery in human subjects.

Patients/trial participants

The procedure was performed in six patients. Echocardiography and cardiac catheterization revealed that each patient had MS of a moderate to severe degree with pliable leaflets, with no significant calcification at the MV, and no thrombus in the left atrium.

Study/trial design

Six patients were initially recruited to this observational study.

Treatment

The balloon used was made of double layers of rubber tubing and a nylon meshwork provided reinforcement. The unique design allowed the balloon to change shape at different stages of the procedure. The distal half inflated first, then the proximal part, and finally the middle section inflated. Two different shaped balloons were trialled, the first had a pillow shape at full inflation and the second had a barrel shape. The balloon was inflated by manually inserting carbon dioxide gas from a syringe attached to the other end of the catheter. The tip of the balloon was protected by a hard shell for easy passage across the atrial septum.

The catheter size was 9Fr. It had a double lumen to allow for guidewire use and measurement of pressures. A guidewire was initially inserted into the left atrium through the saphenous vein and trans-septal puncture under local anaesthesia. The balloon catheter was then advanced over the guidewire and pushed into the left atrium. The patient was then given heparin. A 7Fr pigtail catheter was then inserted into the LV via the left femoral artery to aid in measuring the mitral gradient. The balloon was then placed across the mitral orifice and fully inflated to separate the fused commissures by its expansile force.

Trial end points measured

End points from cardiac catheterization included mean left atrial pressure, a mean diastolic pressure gradient across the MV and a mean systolic gradient across the AV. Orifice size on 2D echocardiography was also measured, as was the presence of regurgitation during LV angiogram.

Follow-up

Reported follow-up was at 2–16 months post procedure.

Results

Six patients underwent the procedure: the first two with the pillow shaped balloon and the last four with the barrel shaped balloon. The procedure was unsuccessful in the second patient as the catheter was not able to pass through the stenotic MV. In all other patients the procedure was successful, with substantial reductions in gradient without significant regurgitation post procedure.

The first two successful cases were described in more detail. The first was that of a 33-year-old man who presented with exertional dyspnoea. He was found to be in AF and 2D echocardiography revealed a stenotic mitral orifice with good dome formation by the anterior leaflets of the MV during diastole. The mean diastolic pressure across the valve fell from 13 mmHg to 6 mmHg. Echocardiography confirmed an increase in the size of the orifice post procedure, and LV angiogram revealed no significant MR The procedure was uncomplicated and he made a good recovery, and one week post procedure was cardioverted into sinus rhythm. Cardiac catheterization was repeated one month after the procedure, which revealed a left atrial pressure of 11 mmHg and a mean gradient of 7 mmHg.

The second successful case was a 45-year-old woman who also presented with exertional dyspnoea. A 2D echocardiography confirmed a stenotic MV with pliable leaflets. The mitral orifice was dilated twice. Immediately after each dilatation, its efficacy was evaluated by measuring the MV gradient, by 2D echocardiography and by auscultating the heart for any murmurs. After dilatation, mean left atrial pressure dropped from 16 mmHg to 5 mmHg. A 2D echocardiography confirmed significant dilatation of the MV orifice. She was well and asymptomatic seven months post procedure.

Study/trial limitations

A small case series of only six patients was presented. Follow-up was limited to only 2–16 months post procedure. With the exception of the two case reports presented, there is a paucity of presented data for the remainder of patients in the study.

Study/trial strengths

This report incorporates the first clinical case of percutaneous mitral commissurotomy performed by Japanese surgeon Kanji Inoue in 1982. It is an elegant technique that was successfully performed under local anesthesia in five of the first six patients attempted.

Why is this a landmark paper?

This was the first description of a procedure that has revolutionized the approach to MS worldwide. An almost identical technique is still practised today, predominantly using the Inoue balloon.

Impact on clinical practice and management of specific disease process

Mitral stenosis has declined precipitously due to the reduction of the burden of infectious disease and rheumatic fever globally. However, percutaneous balloon mitral valvotomy remains the treatment of choice for MS. It is one of the few interventional procedures that carries a class I indication for the treatment of symptomatic moderate or severe MS, with level of evidence 'A' by ACC/AHA guidelines.

Conclusion

Percutaneous balloon mitral valvotomy (PBMV) is a straightforward procedure when managed by an experienced operator working in a high volume centre, performed under local anaesthesia. It is still practised today in a very similar manner to how it was first reported over 20 years ago.

Learning points

- ◆ Percutaneous balloon mitral valvotomy is a less invasive alternative to surgical commissurotomy for MS.
- ◆ In this early report, it was associated with procedural success in 5 of 6 patients, with dramatic reductions in mitral gradients but no significant increase in MR.
- ◆ Its mechanism of action is commissural separation and it is ideally suited to the soft, pliable leaflets seen in rheumatic MS.

Further reading

- Chandrashekhar Y, Westaby S, Narula J. Mitral stenosis. *Lancet* 2009; 374(9697): 1271–83. (Epub 9 Sep 2009). Review. Excellent comprehensive overview of MS, from epidemiology to evidence-based contemporary management.
- Reyes VP, Raju BS, Wynne J, *et al.* Percutaneous balloon valvuloplasty compared with open surgical commissurotomy for mitral stenosis. *N Engl J Med* 1994; 331(15): 961–7. Randomized trial (60 patients) of PBMV to open mitral valvotomy, demonstrating better hemodynamic outcomes at three years with PBMV.
- Turi ZG, Reyes VP, Raju BS, *et al.* Percutaneous balloon versus surgical closed commissurotomy for mitral stenosis. A prospective, randomized trial. *Circulation* 1991; 83(4): 1179–85. Small randomized trial (40 patients) of PBMV to closed commisurotomy, demonstrating similar hemodynamic outcomes.

Valve repair improves the outcome of surgery for mitral regurgitation: a multivariate analysis

Enriquez-Sarano M, Schaff HV, Orszulak TA, Tajik AJ, Bailey KR, Frye RL. *Circulation* 1995; 91(4): 1022–8.

Purpose/hypothesis

In several univariate analyses, MV repair has been found to be associated with better clinical outcomes as it maintains normal valve architecture and has been shown to have lower peri- and post-operative complications. However, previous studies did not adjust for differences in baseline characteristics. This study was performed to compare outcomes in patients post-MV repair versus those having replacement surgery using a multivariate analysis.

Patients

Patients had acquired mitral regurgitation (MR) and had had a pre-operative echo within six months before surgery to allow for assessment of LV function. Exclusion criteria included patients with prior MV surgery, previous or associated aortic or tricuspid valve replacement (patients with tricuspid valve repair were not excluded), and those with MR of an ischaemic or functional aetiology. Patients with concomitant CABG surgery were not excluded.

Study design

During the period examined a total of 2183 patients had MV surgery; 654 of these had isolated MR, and 409 of that group had organic MR and a pre-operative echocardiogram. Of the 409, 195 had valve repair and 214 had valve replacement.

Echocardiography was performed at a mean of 24 +/- 31 days before surgery. Ejection fraction was estimated by two independent observers in all patients, and was also calculated through angiography in 219 patients. Group comparisons were performed using a standard t-test or chi-squared test. Year of surgery was included in the multivariate analysis to allow for the possibility of confounding treatment strategies. The operative variables were also added to the models.

Treatment

Treatment was either valve repair or replacement, with or without CABG.

Trial end points measured

Trial end points included overall survival, late survival, operative mortality, post-operative LV function, rate of reoperation, rate of thromboembolism, and rate of bacterial endocarditis. Other end points included use of coumadin treatment and of significant haemorrhage.

Follow-up

Clinical follow-up continued until just over two years after the first patient treated or death. It was 98% complete.

Results

Parameters studied in the multivariate analysis included age, sex, year of surgery, NYHA class, recent onset of MR, AF, creatinine, presence of coronary artery disease, and hypertension. Echocardiographic parameters included left atrial diameter, LV systolic and diastolic diameters, wall thickening, and EF. Surgical parameters included method of correction and associated CABG surgery. Baseline characteristics were compared. The patients who underwent repair were more likely to be in NYHA class I or II (p = 0.0013). They were also most likely to have a history of CCF, AF, a worse creatinine, and coronary stenoses of >70%.

The overall survival rate after valve repair was significantly higher than that after valve replacement (p = 0.0004) and similar to the survival of an age/sex-matched population without disease (see Figure 19.4). After multivariate analysis, valve repair was found to be an independent favourable predictor of overall survival (p = 0.0001). This was observed irrespective of concomitant CABG surgery.

There was a lower rate of operative mortality (defined as a death within one month of surgery or during same hospitalization) in patients who underwent valve repair (p = 0.002). Late survival was also investigated. This was performed in 375 patients. There were higher rates of coronary disease, LV dysfunction, valvular complications, non-cardiac events, and unknown events in the patients who underwent valve replacement. In terms of reoperation rate there was no significant difference between both groups. This was similarly found with rates of thromboembolism and bacterial endocarditis. Patients with valve repair were less likely to be on warfarin and were free of significant haemorrhage.

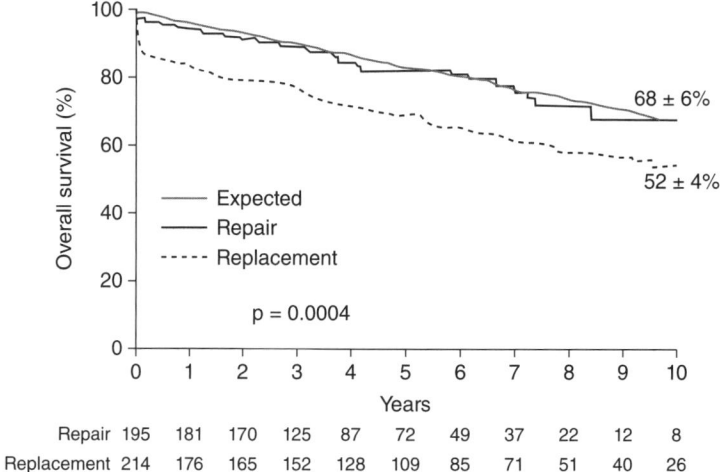

Figure 19.4 Plot of overall survival compared for valve repair and valve replacement groups (p = 0.0004). The expected survival rate for the total of 409 patients is also represented. The numbers at the bottom indicate, for each interval, the number of patients at risk.

Reproduced from Enriquez-Sarano M, *et al*. Valve repair improves the outcome of surgery for mitral regurgitation. A multivariate analysis. *Circulation* 1995; 91: 1022–8, with permission from Wolters Kluwer Health.

Study/trial limitations

One of the end points investigated was post-operative EF and the authors suggested that this may not be reliable since echocardiography was utilized. There was also a suggestion that EF may not have been measured post-operatively at the same time in each patient and that not all patients underwent a post-operative echocardiogram. The other limitation is the difference in baseline characteristics in each group. This was a non-randomized study, making it difficult to compare the two groups. There was also no mention as to how the clinicians decided on which operative procedure to use.

Study strengths

This was a large single-centre study with a large population pool. Sufficient follow-up was performed and a large amount of data was obtained for each patient enrolled. Multivariate analysis was performed to account for differences in baseline characteristics.

Why is this a landmark paper?

This study was one of the first to compare MVR with repair and has now influenced guidelines on the surgical

management of MR. When feasible, with its low operative risk and lower post-operative morbidity, valve repair is now considered a first-line surgical therapy.

Impact on clinical practice and management of specific disease process

Current ESC and ACC/AHA guidelines concur that, when technically possible, valve repair is the preferred surgical management of patients with severe MR. This is due to the findings of this and other studies which have indicated that MV repair carries a lower perioperative mortality, improved survival, better preservation of post-operative LV function, and lower long-term morbidity. In cases where the anatomy is favourable for repair, this is the advised treatment strategy in patients that have an indication for surgery in organic MV disease.

Conclusion

This study of 195 valve repairs and 214 valve replacements demonstrated that valve repair was an independent predictor of improved survival.

Learning points

♦ Mitral valve repair confers a lower post-operative mortality and morbidity compared to valve replacement after adjusting for differences in baseline characteristics.

♦ In surgery for MR, repair is preferred if technically feasible.

Further reading

Although the landmark paper described showed excellent outcomes from MV repair, important exclusions were ischaemic/functional non-ischaemic MR. The outcomes in these pathologies are less clear and discussed in the papers below:

● Alfieri O, De Bonis M. Mitral valve repair for functional mitral regurgitation: is annuloplasty alone enough? *Curr Opin Cardiol* 2010; 25(2): 114–8.

● DiBardino DJ, ElBardissi AW, McClure RS, Razo-Vasquez OA, Kelly NE, Cohn LH. Four decades of experience with mitral valve repair: analysis of differential indications, technical evolution, and long-term outcome. *J Thorac Cardiovasc Surg* 2010; 139(1): 76–83; discussion 83–4.

● LaPar DJ, Kron IL. Should all ischemic mitral regurgitation be repaired? When should we replace? *Curr Opin Cardiol* 2011; 26(2): 113–7. Review.

● Rao C, Murphy MO, Saso S, *et al.* Mitral valve repair or replacement for ischaemic mitral regurgitation: a systematic review. *Heart Lung Circ* 2011; 20(9): 555–65.

Also of interest:

● Cohn LH, Kowalker W, Bhatia S, *et al.* Comparative morbidity of mitral valve repair versus replacement for mitral regurgitation with and without coronary artery disease. *Ann Thorac Surg* 1988; 45(3): 284–90. This earlier paper demonstrated *lower* mortality and late emboli in patients undergoing MV repair when compared to replacement.

Quantitative determinants of the outcome of asymptomatic mitral regurgitation

Enriquez-Sarano M, Avierinos JF, Messika-Zeitoun D, Detaint D, Capps M, Nkomo V, Scott C, Schaff HV, Tajik AJ. *N Engl J Med* 2005; 352(9): 875–83.

Purpose/hypothesis

With improvements in surgical techniques, it was suggested that surgery might be beneficial in some asymptomatic patients with MR that were traditionally managed medically. Although guidelines advised quantitative methods of assessing MR, at the time of this publication, both these methods and outcomes in the absence of symptoms were not clearly delineated. This prospective study therefore sought to investigate whether a quantitative assessment of MR in asymptomatic patients correlated independently with outcome and could help in stratifying risk.

Patients

Patients were enrolled over a nine-year period with at least mild MR. Inclusion criteria comprised isolated (single valve) and pure (without stenosis) MR and the absence of symptoms. Exclusion criteria included MR secondary to ischaemic heart disease or cardiomyopathy, early or late systolic regurgitation, structurally normal valves, associated MS or AV disease, a history of previous valve repair or replacement, congenital or pericardial heart disease, or an EF <50%.

Study design

This was a prospective study where patients were examined at baseline and their past medical history and examination findings were documented. Mitral regurgitation was quantified with Doppler and 2D echocardiography using at least two of three validated methods and the average was taken to obtain the regurgitant volume per beat and the area of the effective regurgitant orifice (ERO). At echocardiography, LV diameters, volumes, and EFs were also measured. Standard statistical methods including student's t-test and Kaplan-Meier methods were used to compare outcomes between groups.

Trial end points measured

Trial end points were death from any cause, death from cardiac causes, and cardiac events. Cardiac events included death from cardiac causes, new AF, or congestive cardiac failure.

Follow-up

Overall follow-up was up to a maximum of 11.7 years. However, mean duration of follow up after diagnosis was 2.7 years under medical management and 5.1 years under medical and surgical management.

Results

The majority of patients were male and in their 60s, with MV prolapse being the most common aetiology of MR. A group of 224 patients (49%) were treated medically, with 232 patients being treated medically first then moving on to surgery. Among the patients with MR managed medically 56 patients died, and in a univariate analysis the degree of MR correlated strongly with survival. The five-year survival rate was highest in those with an ERO of less than 20 mm^2 (91%), and lowest in patients with an ERO of at least 40 mm^2 (58%, p <0.01) in those treated medically (see Figure 19.5).

In multivariate analysis, survival was independently predicted by increasing age, diabetes, and a larger regurgitant orifice (all p values <0.01). After adjustment for various factors and co-morbidities including age, sex, EF, diabetes, the ERO independently predicted survival. The adjusted risk ratio for death from any cause was 1.20 for each 10 mm^2 increment. These findings were not found for regurgitant volume, which was found to be less predictive of survival.

Both regurgitant volume and orifice size predicted the risk of death from cardiac causes, although orifice size had a greater predictive power. Seventy-four patients died during the follow-up period. The five-year mortality rate did not differ from the general population in the different orifice size groups (this is after accounting for post-operative survival rates).

During follow-up, 91 patients had a cardiac event. The five-year rates of cardiac events differed according to regurgitant orifice size, with up to 62% of patients having a cardiac event in those with an orifice of >40 mm^2 (p <0.01). There was also a significant difference in event rate when correlated with regurgitant volume. And these were both found to be independently predictive. Surgery was found through Cox proportional-hazards analysis to be associated with a reduced risk of death. There appeared to be a larger survival benefit in those patients undergoing surgery for larger regurgitant orifices.

Study/trial limitations

This was a single-centre study and therefore this investigation's population dynamics may differ from the general population. The use of echocardiography, albeit with a standardized methodology, may still have had inter- and intra-observer variability, which is not described in the paper. Importantly, it was an observational study and, although it stratified risk in an asymptomatic population with severe MR, the investigators' conclusion that a high ERO should prompt early surgery is not entirely proven due to the absence of randomized data to surgery.

Study strengths

This trial was a large prospective study which was reasonably powered to address its important clinical question. No patients were lost to follow-up. Full baseline characteristics were documented and data on several outcomes were obtained. Multivariate analyses were performed to adjust for confounding factors.

Why is this a landmark paper?

This was the first study of its kind to investigate whether quantitative assessment of MR predicted outcome in the absence of symptoms. Up until this study, the general consensus was to manage patients with MR medically until they developed symptoms, or develop LV systolic dysfunction on echocardiography. However, this study showed that asymptomatic patients with severe MR classified by a regurgitant orifice have a significantly worse outcome. This includes both a higher overall mortality and cardiac death, and a six times higher risk of developing cardiac events. Therefore, given improved surgical techniques, there is a now growing trend to intervene earlier in these patients.

Impact on clinical practice and management of specific disease process

This study increased the awareness that asymptomatic MR is not a benign phenomenon and requires aggressive echocardiographic follow-up to ensure no deterioration in LV function or progressive ventricular dilatation. It has only partially impacted current ESC guidelines, which dictate that patients should have surgical intervention even if they are asymptomatic if their LV systolic function is impaired, if there is evidence of pulmonary hypertension or if they have AF. In contrast, more in line with this study, the ACC/AHA guidelines advocate surgery for asymptomatic patients with severe MR and normal LV function if there is >90% likelihood of successful valve repair in a high volume centre. Both committees' guidelines concur that non-operated asymptomatic severe MR requires close serial echocardiographic

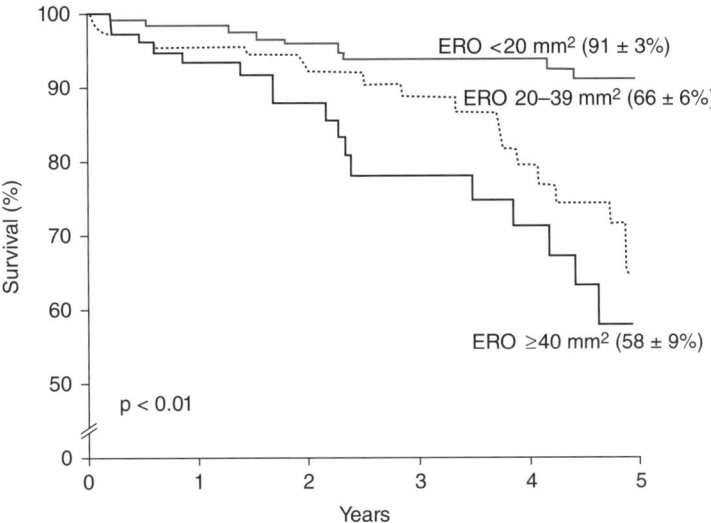

Figure 19.5 Kaplan-Meier estimates of the mean (± SE) rates of overall survival among patients with asymptomatic mitral regurgitation under medical management, according to the effective regurgitant orifice (ERO). Values in parentheses are survival rates at five years.

monitoring for changes in function and cavity dimensions every six months.

Conclusion

This study found that the quantitative grading of organic isolated MR is a strong independent predictor of clinical outcome. It provides a strong rationale for intervening early surgically, before symptoms develop, especially since the advent of MV repair surgery.

Learning points

- Patients with asymptomatic organic MR with an ERO >40 mm^2 or a regurgitant volume of at least 60 ml are at a higher risk of mortality and have a higher rate of cardiac events.
- Quantitative methods (regurgitant orifice size and volume) are strong predictors of clinical outcome.
- These patients should therefore be considered for early surgical intervention or be closely monitored echocardiographically.

Further reading

- Bonow RO, Carabello BA, Chatterjee K, *et al.*; 2006 Writing Committee Members; American College of Cardiology/American Heart Association Task Force. Focused update incorporated into the ACC/AHA 2006 guidelines for the management of patients with valvular heart disease: a report of the American College of Cardiology/American Heart Association Task Force on Practice Guidelines (Writing Committee to Revise the 1998 Guidelines for the Management of Patients With Valvular Heart Disease): endorsed by the Society of Cardiovascular Anesthesiologists, Society for Cardiovascular Angiography and Interventions, and Society of Thoracic Surgeons. *Circulation* 2008; 118(15): e582.
- Vahanian A, Baumgartner H, Bax J, *et al.*; Task Force on the Management of Valvular Heart Disease of the European Society of Cardiology; ESC Committee for Practice Guidelines. Guidelines on the management of valvular heart disease: The Task Force on the Management of Valvular Heart Disease of the European Society of Cardiology. *Eur Heart J* 2007; 28(2): 245.

Minimal invasive mitral valve repair for mitral regurgitation: results of 1339 consecutive patients

Seeburger J, Borger MA, Falk V, Kuntze T, Czesla M, Walther T, Doll N, Mohr FW. *Eur J Cardiothorac Surg* 2008; 34(4): 760–5. (Epub 30 Jun 2008).

Purpose/hypothesis

At the time of this paper, minimally invasive MV repair had been increasingly used, but concerns had been expressed regarding the quality of results, particularly given the limited exposure of the MV and the specialist tools and experience required. The authors sought to evaluate the safety and efficacy of minimally invasive mitral repair for MR, in a large series of patients.

Patients

Patients studied were those in a single institution undergoing minimally invasive MV repair for significant MR over an eight-year period.

Study/trial design

Retrospective observational cohort study.

Treatment

Patients underwent cardiopulmonary bypass and underwent three chest wall incisions. First, a right lateral mini-thoracotomy 5–6 cm in length was performed in the fourth intercostal space. This was lateral to and under the nipple in men and just below the breast (in the submammary crease) in women. The procedure was video assisted using a small 1 cm port in the second intercostal space on the right. There was also a small 0.5 cm incision in the third intercostal space to insert an aortic cross clamp.

Trial end points measured

Operative outcomes studied included mean incision length of the right lateral mini-thoracotomy, total operating time, duration of bypass, and aortic cross-clamp time. Clinical outcomes studied included need for reoperation, neurological complications, post-procedural hospital stay, and mortality, both as a 30-day outcome and as the Kaplan-Meier estimate for survival at five years. Freedom from MV-related reoperation at five years was also studied.

Follow-up

Follow-up was performed by mailed questionnaire or telephone conversation with the patient or family members with additional medical information from the physicians involved in the patients' care. Follow-up was 99% complete and was for a mean of 28.1 ± 23.9 months after surgery.

Results

Between 1999 and 2007, 1339 patients had minimally invasive MV repair. Many patients had concomitant AF ablation in 26.2%, tricuspid surgery in 6%, and PFO/ASD closure in 6.6%. The mean age was 60.3 ± 12.7 years, with 61.2% male and 6.1% having had prior cardiac operations. The mean preoperative MR grade was 3.3 ± 0.6, with the primary cause being myxomatous disease in the majority of patients, and the mean EF 59.2 ± 15.1%.

Mean total operation time was 165 ± 47 min, mean bypass duration was 121 ± 38 min, and mean lateral thoracotomy incision length was 5.3 ± 1.1 cm. Reoperation for bleeding occurred in 5.1% of patients. Overall, 11.7% of patients did not require intermediate or intensive care and went directly to a post-anaesthetic care unit. Neurological impairment post-surgery was seen in 3.1% (1% major). Total hospital stay was 12.4 ± 9.8 days. Thirty-day mortality was 2.4%. Mild or less MR was achieved in 96.9% of patients. Survival at five years (Kaplan-Meier estimate) was 82.6%, with freedom from valve-related reoperation in survivors 96.3% at five years.

Study/trial limitations

There was no comparator group, either randomized or non-randomized, to place the favourable results in context. Comparisons to conventional techniques are therefore made in the discussion in relation to historical published data of best surgical practice.

Criteria for decision making for MV repair were poorly specified. Although pre-operative NYHA status is reported as 2.7 ± 1.2, the proportion of asymptomatic patients is not explicitly stated. Nevertheless, this constitutes real-world experience in a single, world-renowned, high-volume centre and is representative of usual clinical practice.

Why is this a landmark paper?

This was an important first proof of concept that minimally invasive techniques could be applied to MV repair with results that are indirectly comparable to conventional surgery.

Impact on clinical practice and management of specific disease process

This paper laid the foundation for the present era of minimally invasive mitral surgery, with or without robotic assistance.

Conclusion

Minimally invasive MV repair appears to be a safe and effective therapy for MR in a high-volume centre under experienced hands.

Learning points

◆ Mitral valve repair is the gold-standard therapy for the treatment of MR.

◆ Large series have documented excellent results for MV repair with a standard sternotomy.

◆ Minimally invasive MV repair is safe, effective, and feasible in the vast majority of patients with MR.

Further reading

● Chitwood WR Jr, Rodriguez E, Chu MW, *et al*. Robotic mitral valve repairs in 300 patients: a single-center experience. *J Thorac Cardiovasc Surg* 2008; 136(2): 436–41.
This study shows similarly effective results and short hospital stays with robotic MV repair.

● Lee TC, Desai B, Glower DD. Results of 141 consecutive minimally invasive tricuspid valve operations: an 11-year experience. *Ann Thorac Surg* 2009; 88(6): 1845–50.
This study shows that a similar approach is feasible for tricuspid valve repair.

● McClure RS, Cohn LH, Wiegerinck E, *et al*. Early and late outcomes in minimally invasive mitral valve repair: an eleven-year experience in 707 patients. *J Thorac Cardiovasc Surg* 2009; 137(1): 70–5.
Similarly excellent outcomes achieved by an American centre using a minimally invasive approach.

● Seeburger J, Borger MA, Doll N, Walther T, Passage J, Falk V, Mohr FW. Comparison of outcomes of minimally invasive mitral valve surgery for posterior, anterior and bileaflet prolapsed. *Eur J Cardiothorac Surg* 2009; 36(3): 532–8. (Epub 22 May 2009). This paper shows similar results where prolapse is the underlying aetiology of MR, regardless of which leaflet is involved.

Percutaneous repair or surgery for mitral regurgitation

Feldman T, Foster E, Glower DG, Kar S, Rinaldi MJ, Fail PS, Smalling RW, Siegel R, Rose GA, Engeron E, Loghin C, Trento A, Skipper ER, Fudge T, Letsou GV, Massaro JM, Mauri L; EVEREST II Investigators. *N Engl J Med* 2011 364(15): 1395–406.

Purpose/hypothesis

A surgical approach for MV repair involves approximation of anterior and posterior mitral leaflets and the creation of a double orifice, described for treatment of degenerative MR, usually with an annuloplasty ring. It was hypothesized that similar results could be achieved using a transcatheter device (MitraClip, Abbott Vascular) that also approximates the two leaflets of the MV. This device is delivered via trans-septal puncture from right to left atrium from an initial transfemoral venous access route.

Patients

Patients were treated in 37 centres in the United States or Canada. They had to have symptomatic, chronic grade 3+ or grade 4+ MR, and an LVEF ≥25% with an LV end-systolic diameter (LVESD) ≤55 mm. Alternatively, if they were asymptomatic, they had to have one of the following:

1. LVEF 25–60%
2. LVESD 40–55 mm
3. New AF
4. Pulmonary hypertension

There were also anatomical inclusion criteria, which, broadly speaking, were of the principal regurgitant jet originating from malcoaptation of the middle scallops of the anterior and posterior leaflets.

Study design

This was a RCT of transcatheter MV repair using the MitraClip versus MV surgery (2:1 ratio). There was an echocardiographic core lab that assessed the MR at baseline and at various time-points post-procedure. The Harvard Clinical Research Institute was contracted by Abbott Vascular to perform data management, analysis, and clinical-event adjudication.

Treatment

The MitraClip procedure was performed under general anaesthesia with fluoroscopic and transoesophageal echocardiographic guidance. The device was steered in the left atrium after trans-septal puncture, and moved to the left ventricle with opening and grasping of the leaflets with the clip. Failure to reduce the MR grade to 2+ or less was addressed either with removal of the clip and regrasping or insertion of a second clip. Patients with residual MR of ≥3+ despite these manoeuvres underwent elective MV surgery.

Trial end points measured

There were separate safety and efficacy end points pre-specified. The primary safety end point was the rate of major adverse events at 30 days (composite of death, MI, reoperation for failed MV surgery, non-elective cardiovascular surgery for adverse events, stroke, renal failure, deep wound infection, mechanical ventilation for more than 48 hours, gastrointestinal complication requiring surgery, new onset permanent AF, septicaemia and transfusion of ≥2 units of blood).

The primary end point for efficacy was a composite of freedom from death, surgery for MV dysfunction and from grade 3+ or 4+ MR at 12 months. There were additional pre-specified secondary end points, including change in LV dimension and volumes, NYHA class, and quality of life scores.

Follow-up

Outcomes were followed to 12 months for the purposes of the study and this manuscript. Yearly clinical and echocardiographic evaluations are planned in future for a total of five years of follow-up.

Results

A total of 279 patients were randomly assigned (Mitra-Clip 184, MV surgery 95). Some patients withdrew consent before treatment (3% of MitraClip, 16% surgery group). Of those receiving MitraClip, 23% had grade 3+ or 4+ MR before discharge and were referred for surgery. In the surgery group, all 80 patients treated had MR ≤grade 2+.

The rates of the primary efficacy end point were 55% in the MitraClip group and 73% in the surgery group (intention to treat analysis). Of those with successful in-hospital results, the primary efficacy end point was 72% in the MitraClip group and 88% in the surgery group (p = 0.02).

At two years, there was an equal 11% mortality in both groups. There was 22% surgery for valve dysfunction in the MitraClip group and 4% in the surgery group.

The proportion of those with 3+ /4+ MR at two years was 20% and 22%, respectively.

Regarding the primary safety end point, there was a rate of major adverse events at 30 days of 15% in the MitraClip group and 48% in the surgery group; this was predominantly driven by need for blood transfusion, with the respective rates 5% and 10% when blood transfusion events were excluded.

With respect to secondary end points, there was a reduction in end-diastolic and end-systolic volumes in both groups. At 12 months NYHA status of grade III/IV was 2% in the MitraClip group and 13% in the surgery group. Although not a prespecified analysis, MitraClip efficacy was non-inferior to surgery in those with depressed LV function or those over 70 years of age.

Study/trial limitations

The study was randomized, but non-blinded; more patients discontinued participation in the study than in the surgery group. The composite primary safety end point did not distinguish between the severity of specific adverse outcomes. The separation of safety and efficacy end points has created considerable confusion. The safety advantage of the MitraClip was predominantly driven by a lower rate of transfusion compared to the surgical arm, and criteria for transfusion were not standardized. Lastly, the device can only be performed in anatomically suitable patients.

Why is this a landmark paper?

This study is the first to demonstrate favourable outcomes for a percutaneous therapy for MR. Increased safety and similar results at two years were attained with the MitraClip when compared to a surgical benchmark.

Impact on clinical practice and management of specific disease process

The Mitraclip device is now an integral part of treatment for patients with anatomically suitable MR in Europe, mainly applied to treat high-risk patients with functional MR.

Conclusion

The MitraClip device is an important advance in the evolution of MV surgery, with a truly percutaneous approach that is safe and effective in selected patients.

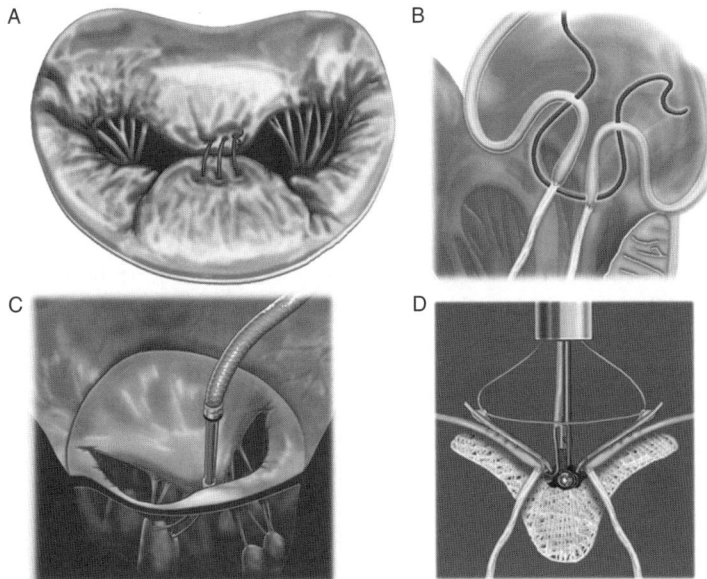

Figure 19.6 (A) The surgical technique involves a continuous suture of the free edge of the leaflets at the site of the regurgitation, here in the A2-P2 area. A double orifice valve is created. (B) The sutures engage the free edge of the facing leaflets. (C) The MitraClip is also implanted in the A2-P2 region. Once proper leaflet grasping is confirmed, the clip is closed to enhance coaptation. (D) The free edges of the leaflets are engaged between the clip arms and the grippers, and the clip is closed.

Reproduced from Maisano F, *et al.* The evolution from surgery to percutaneous mitral valve interventions: the role of the edge-to-edge technique. *J Am Coll Cardiol* 2011; 58(21): 2174–82, with permission from Elsevier.

Learning points

- The edge-to-edge technique is a technically simple approach to MR developed by Italian surgeon Ottavio Alfieri in the 1990s (see Figure 19.6).
- A percutaneous adaptation of this employs the MitraClip device, inserted via a transvenous route with trans-septal puncture.
- Favourable safety data was achieved when compared to conventional surgery.
- The efficacy remains inferior, at least acutely, to surgery, which currently restricts its widespread commercial use to patients at high surgical risk.

Further reading

- Auricchio A, Schillinger W, Meyer S, *et al.*; PERMIT-CARE Investigators. Correction of Mitral Regurgitation in Nonresponders to Cardiac Resynchronization Therapy by MitraClip Improves Symptoms and Promotes Reverse Remodeling. *J Am Coll Cardiol* 2011; 58(21): 2183–9. Multi-centric European observational study showing an improvement in MR using the MitraClip in patients that have not responded to cardiac resynchronization therapy.
- Maisano F, La Canna G, Colombo A, Alfieri O. The Evolution from Surgery to Percutaneous Mitral Valve Interventions: the Role of the Edge-to-Edge Technique. *J Am Coll Cardiol* 2011; 58(21): 2174–82. A valuable overview of the rationale and application of edge-to-edge repair from first conception as a surgical approach to the contemporary percutaneous technique. See Figure 19.6.
- Rudolph V, Knap M, Franzen O, et al. Echocardiographic and Clinical Outcomes of MitraClip Therapy in Patients not Amenable to Surgery. *J Am Coll Cardiol* 2011; 58(21): 2190–5. Large single-centre European non-randomized experience demonstrating an improvement in patients not amenable to surgery.
- St Goar FG, Fann JI, Komtebedde J, Endovascular edge-to-edge mitral valve repair: short-term results in a porcine model. *Circulation* 2003; 108(16): 1990–3. (Epub 6 Oct 2003). First animal report of the MitraClip in 14 pigs.

Conclusion

Aiming for the future necessitates looking back in history. The development of modern interventional techniques to manage valvular heart disease has been fascinating from the beginning in the early decades of the last century to landmark studies for catheter-based treatment. Many different steps, interactions, ideas, methods, and concepts have been followed by cardiac specialists to improve patient care. Complete anatomical replacement with a bulky and non-physiologic prosthesis of the mitral valve, for instance, has been replaced in many centres by delicate and sophisticated repair procedures. It is not even necessary anymore to completely open the chest since minimally invasive techniques have proven to be highly applicable and safe. Mini-sternotomy to endoscopic and robotic surgery and further to transcatheter repair strategies, all mark the development of modern mitral valve treatment. This also holds true for aortic valve replacement, which has recently developed to a rather simple and straightforward procedure. Thus, treatment of valvular heart disease remains a changing and continually evolving environment with many new ideas in the pipeline and a huge potential for many approaches to be considered as landmarks of the future. However, all of these new techniques and devices must be compared against the excellent results of the current standard of care for valvular heart disease.

Chapter 20

Endocarditis

Dr James Harrison and Dr Bernard Prendergast

Introduction

Since the original description of endocarditis by William Osler in 1885 and its association with bacteraemia by Emanuel Libman in 1906, the epidemiology of this elusive condition has changed significantly. Despite significant advances in diagnosis and treatment, infective endocarditis remains a dangerous disease, particularly for people at risk because of a prosthetic valve, congenital heart disease, or a history of infective endocarditis, in whom morbidity and mortality approach 50%.

Recent decades have seen *Staphylococcus aureus*, often acquired as a result of nosocomial infection or intravenous drug abuse, overtake oral streptococci as the most common pathogen in infective endocarditis in developed nations. Infective endocarditis is also increasingly frequent in the elderly and in those with no previous documentation of valvular heart disease.

With these changes in mind, over the past few years international bodies of authority have significantly revised guidelines for the prevention, diagnosis, and treatment of infective endocarditis. Perhaps the most dramatic change is the reduction in antibiotic prophylaxis before dental and other invasive procedures. These guidelines also emphasize the important role of echocardiography in making an early diagnosis of infective endocarditis and that surgery should be performed earlier than previously recommended.

Unlike some other areas of cardiovascular medicine, the literature on endocarditis is not awash with large multi-centre, randomized, controlled trials, which reflects the challenging nature and heterogeneity of the condition. This chapter includes some of the most important clinical publications concerning the epidemiology, diagnosis, complications, and treatment of infective endocarditis and its possible prevention using antibiotic prophylaxis.

Bacteremia associated with toothbrushing and dental extraction

Lockart PB, Brennan MT, Sasser HC, Fox PC, Paster BJ, Bahrani-Mougeot FK. *Circulation* 2008; 117: 3117–25.

Background

Guidelines for the prevention of infective endocarditis have historically focused on bacteraemia following dental procedures. However, daily oral activities (including chewing and toothbrushing) cause a transient bacteraemia, resulting in annual cumulative exposure thousands to millions times greater than that caused by tooth extraction.

Several previous studies have produced conflicting incidence figures for bacteraemia following single tooth extractions (0–100%) and toothbrushing (0–57%). This double-blind, placebo-controlled study compared the incidence, duration, nature, and magnitude of bacteraemia (focusing on organisms which have been both isolated from blood after dental procedures and reported to cause infective endocarditis) following single tooth extractions and toothbrushing. The impact of amoxicillin prophylaxis before single tooth extraction was also studied.

Methods

A group of 290 patients presenting to a single US centre over a three-year period for extraction of at least one tooth was randomized to one of three interventions: (1) toothbrushing (each quadrant for 30 seconds), (2) single tooth extraction with amoxicillin prophylaxis, (3) single tooth extraction with an identical placebo. In groups (2) and (3), amoxicillin/placebo was given one hour before extraction. Baseline aerobic and anaerobic blood cultures were taken before toothbrushing/extraction and subsequently at 1.5, 5, 20, 40, and 60 minutes after the intervention. Patients randomized to the toothbrushing group underwent their extraction after completion of the study or at a subsequent visit. Blood samples were cultured for a maximum of two weeks and polymerase chain reaction (PCR) was used for bacterial identification and quantification.

Results

The overall incidence of bacteraemia at any of the six time points was 32%, 56%, and 80% for the toothbrushing, amoxicillin prophylaxis, and placebo groups respectively (p <0.0001). Of the 98 bacterial species identified, only 32 had previously been associated with infective endocarditis. When considering these 32 species alone, the incidence of bacteraemia was 23%, 33%, and 60% respectively (p <0.0001). The highest incidence of bacteraemia

occurred in the first five minutes following the procedure.

At 20 minutes, the placebo group had a significantly higher number of positive cultures (10%) than the amoxicillin (1%) and toothbrushing groups (1%) (p = 0.001). This persisted to 40 minutes.

Conclusions

This study demonstrated that amoxicillin prophylaxis one hour before a single tooth extraction does reduce the incidence of bacteraemia compared with a placebo. Perhaps more importantly, it showed that there is a substantial bacteraemia involving infective endocarditis-causing species following two minutes of toothbrushing. Antibiotic prophylaxis before invasive dental procedures may, therefore, be a token gesture, and general dental hygiene is probably more important for prevention of infective endocarditis.

Learning points

- The evidence for the role of antibiotic prophylaxis before dental procedures in preventing infective endocarditis is limited.
- Toothbrushing results in a significant bacteraemia, which cumulatively may be more important than a single tooth extraction/dental procedure.
- The importance of general dental hygiene must be stressed to those patients at risk of infective endocarditis.

Further reading

- Oliver R, Roberts GJ, Hooper L. Penicillins for the prophylaxis of bacterial endocarditis in dentistry. *Cochrane Database Syst Rev* 2004; 2: CD003813.
- Roberts GJ. Dentists are innocent! 'Everyday' bacteremia is the real culprit: a review and assessment of the evidence that dental surgical procedures are a principal cause of bacterial endocarditis in children. *Pediatr Cardiol* 1999; 20: 317–25.
- Roberts GJ, Jaffray EC, Spratt DA, *et al.* Duration, prevalence and intensity of bacteraemia after dental extractions in children. *Heart* 2006; 92: 1274–7.

International guidelines on antibiotic prophylaxis for infective endocarditis

Habib G, Hoen B, Tornos P, Thuny F, Prendergast B, Vilacosta I, Moreillon P, de Jesus Antunes M, Thilen U, Lekakis J, Lengyel M, Müller L, Naber CK, Nihoyannopoulos P, Moritz A, Zamorano JL; ESC Committee for Practice Guidelines. Guidelines on the prevention, diagnosis, and treatment of infective endocarditis (new version 2009): Task Force on the prevention, diagnosis, and treatment of infective endocarditis of the European Society of Cardiology; European Society of Clinical Microbiology and Infectious Diseases; International Society of Chemotherapy for Infection and Cancer. *Eur Heart J* 2009; 30: 2369–413.

Wilson W, Taubert K.A, Gewitz M, Lockhart PB, Baddour LM, Levison M, Bolger A, Cabell CH, Takahashi M, Baltimore RS, Newburger JW, Strom BL, Tani LY, Gerber M, Bonow RO, Pallasch T, Shulman ST, Rowley AH, Burns JC, Ferrieri P, Gardner T, Goff D, Durack DT; American Heart Association Rheumatic Fever, Endocarditis, and Kawasaki Disease Committee; American Heart Association Council on Cardiovascular Disease in the Young; American Heart Association Council on Clinical Cardiology; American Heart Association Council on Cardiovascular Surgery and Anesthesia; Quality of Care and Outcomes Research Interdisciplinary Working Group. Prevention of infective endocarditis: guidelines from the American Heart Association: a guideline from the American Heart Association Rheumatic Fever, Endocarditis, and Kawasaki Disease Committee, Council on Cardiovascular Disease in the Young, and the Council on Clinical Cardiology, Council on Cardiovascular Surgery and Anesthesia, and the Quality of Care and Outcomes Research Interdisciplinary Working Group. *Circulation* 2007; 116: 1736–54.

NICE Short Clinical Guidelines Technical Team: Prophylaxis against infective endocarditis: antimicrobial prophylaxis against infective endocarditis in adults and children undergoing interventional procedures. London, National Institute for Health and Clinical Excellence, 2008.

Table 20.1 Summary of current international guidelines for antibiotic prophylaxis in infective endocarditis

	American Heart Association, 2007	National Institute for Health and Clinical Excellence, 2008	European Society of Cardiology, 2009
High-risk patients	Previous IE	Previous IE	Previous IE
	Prosthetic valve	Prosthetic valve	Prosthetic valve or prosthetic material used for valve repair
	Unrepaired or incompletely repaired cyanotic congenital heart disease	Acquired valvular heart disease with stenosis or regurgitation	Cyanotic congenital heart disease (without surgical repair or with residual defects, palliative shunts or conduits)
	Congenital heart disease repaired with prosthetic material (for 6 months after the procedure)	Structural congenital heart disease, including surgically corrected or palliated structural conditions; excluding isolated ASD, fully repaired VSD/PDA, endothelialized closure devices	
	Valve disease in cardiac transplant recipients		Congenital heart disease repaired with prosthetic material (for 6 months if complete repair, indefinite if residual defect)
		Hypertrophic cardiomyopathy	
Procedures requiring prophylaxis	Dental procedures involving manipulation of gingival tissue, the periapical region of teeth, or perforation of the oral mucosa	Gastrointestinal and genitourinary procedures where there is suspected pre-existing infection	Dental procedures requiring manipulation of the gingival or periapical region of the teeth or perforation of the oral mucosa
	Invasive procedures of the respiratory tract needing incision or biopsy of the mucosa		

Antibiotic prophylaxis to prevent infective endocarditis in patients with high-risk cardiac lesions has been traditional cardiac and dental practice for over half a century, despite limited evidence of benefit. The efficacy of antibiotic prophylaxis for infective endocarditis has never been demonstrated in a randomized, controlled trial.

The American Heart Association (AHA), the United Kingdom National Institute for Health and Clinical Excellence (NICE), and the European Society of Cardiology (ESC) have all suggested a dramatic reduction in the emphasis on antibiotic prophylaxis before dental and other invasive procedures. Importantly, they suggest that prophylaxis is no longer indicated for native valve disease, nor for invasive respiratory, gastrointestinal, or genitourinary procedures. This means that for the majority of patients, antibiotic prophylaxis is no longer recommended.

Innovative French guidelines in 2002 were the first to suggest a reduction in the practice of antibiotic prophylaxis, by restricting prophylaxis to those with the highest risk of the disease and its consequences. These also stressed the importance of general oral hygiene in the prevention of infective endocarditis.

Subsequent guidelines from the AHA in 2007 are very similar to those from the ESC in 2009, but include cardiac transplant recipients with valvular heart disease in the high-risk category and also recommend prophylaxis for invasive procedures of the respiratory tract needing mucosal incision or biopsy.

These changes are not, however, as far-reaching as controversial guidelines published by the NICE in 2008.

These suggested an end to the practice of antibiotic prophylaxis for dental procedures altogether, restricting prophylaxis very specifically to those with high-risk cardiac lesions, undergoing gastrointestinal or genitourinary procedures where there is suspected pre-existing infection (when antibiotics would be used anyway).

Learning points

- The efficacy of antibiotic prophylaxis for infective endocarditis has never been demonstrated in a randomized controlled trial. However, this does not mean that it is ineffective.
- Recent guidelines from the AHA, NICE, and ESC have suggested a dramatic reduction in the use of antibiotic prophylaxis.
- A careful approach by cardiologists, dentists, and general practitioners is required to explain these changes to patients, many of whom have taken antibiotic prophylaxis before dental work for many years and have previously been warned about the significant dangers of infective endocarditis.

Further reading

- Danchin N, Duval X, Leport C. Prophylaxis of infective endocarditis: French recommendations 2002. *Heart* 2005; 91: 715–8.

New criteria for diagnosis of infective endocarditis: utilization of specific echocardiographic findings

Durack DT, Lukes AS, Bright DK. Duke Endocarditis Service. *Am J Med* 1994; 96: 200–9.

Background

Infective endocarditis is often a challenging condition to diagnose, in part because of the very variable and often non-specific clinical presentation. In 1981, von Reyn *et al.* published *Infective Endocarditis: an Analysis Based Upon Strict Case Definitions*. They proposed four diagnostic categories: 'definite', 'probable', 'possible', and 'rejected', with specific criteria for each category.

These were initially widely adopted, but as the use of echocardiography became more widespread, the failure of the von Reyn criteria to include echocardiographic findings became increasingly apparent. Additional criticisms were the emphasis on predisposing heart disease and an artificially high number of 'rejected' cases.

Methods

In 1994, the Duke Endocarditis Service proposed the following new criteria (see Table 20.2). These new criteria were compared with the von Reyn criteria in 405 episodes in 353 patients between 1985 and 1992.

Table 20.2 The Duke criteria

Definite infective endocarditis

Pathologic criteria:

◆ Microorganisms: demonstrated by culture or histology in a vegetation, or in a vegetation that has embolized, or in an intracardiac abscess, or

◆ Pathologic lesions: Vegetation or intracardiac abscess present, confirmed by histology showing active endocarditis

Clinical criteria:

◆ 2 major criteria, or

◆ 1 major and 3 minor criteria, or

◆ 5 minor criteria

Possible infective endocarditis

Findings consistent with infective endocarditis that fall short of 'definite,' but not 'rejected.'

Rejected

Firm alternate diagnosis for manifestations of endocarditis, or
Resolution of manifestations of endocarditis, with antibiotic therapy for 4 days or less, or
No pathologic evidence of infective endocarditis at surgery or autopsy, after antibiotic therapy for 4 days or less

Major criteria

◆ Positive blood culture for infective endocarditis

◆ Typical microorganism for infective endocarditis from 2 separate blood cultures

◆ Viridans streptococci, Streptococcus bovis, HACEK group, or

◆ Community-acquired Staphylococcus aureus or enterococci, in the absence of a primary focus, or

◆ Persistently positive blood culture, defined as recovery of a microorganism consistent with infective endocarditis from:

  • Blood cultures drawn more than 12 hours apart, or
  • All of 3 or a majority of 4 or more separate blood cultures, with first and last drawn at least 1 hour apart

◆ Evidence of endocardial involvement

◆ Positive echocardiogram for infective endocarditis

  • Oscillating intracardiac mass, on valve or supporting structures, or in the path of regurgitant jets, or on implanted material, In the absence of an alternative anatomic explanation, or
  • Abscess, or
  • New partial dehiscence of prosthetic valve, or new valvular regurgitation (increase or change in pre-existing murmur not sufficient)

Minor criteria

◆ Predisposition: predisposing heart condition or intravenous drug use

◆ Fever: ≥38.0°C (100.4°F)

◆ Vascular phenomena: major arterial emboli, septic pulmonary infarcts, mycotic aneurysm, intracranial haemorrhage, conjunctival haemorrhages, Janeway lesions

◆ Immunologic phenomena: glomerulonephritis, Osler's nodes, Roth spots, rheumatoid factor

◆ Microbiologic evidence: positive blood culture but not meeting major criterion or serologic evidence of active infection with organism consistent with infective endocarditis

◆ Echocardiogram: consistent with infective endocarditis but not meeting major criterion

Reproduced from Durack DT, *et al*. New criteria for diagnosis of infective endocarditis: utilization of specific echocardiographic findings. *The American Journal of Medicine* 1994; 3: 200–9. Duke Endocarditis Service, with permission of Elsevier.

Results

Some 204 (50%) of the cases in 185 patients were classi-fied as 'definite' endocarditis, with 69 (34%) being patho-logically proven at surgery or autopsy. There were 149 (37%) 'possible' and 52 (13%) 'rejected' cases among the remaining 168 patients.

Of the pathologically proven cases 55 (80%) were clas-sified as 'definite' by the new Duke criteria, whereas only 35 (51%) were classified into the analogous 'probable' category by the von Reyn criteria (p <0.0001). Twelve (17%) pathologically confirmed cases were rejected by the von Reyn criteria, but none were rejected by the Duke criteria. Of the remaining 336 cases not proven patho-logically, 71 (21%) were 'probable' by von Reyn criteria compared with 135 (40%, p <0.01) by Duke criteria.

Conclusions

Introduction of the Duke criteria, with the inclusion of echocardiographic findings, increases the number of definite diagnoses that can be made on clinical grounds. The diagnosis of infective endocarditis is often difficult and uncertain and carefully defined criteria are therefore helpful. This study showed the Duke criteria to be supe-rior to the older von Reyn criteria.

The modified Duke criteria

The Duke criteria have a sensitivity of >80%, high specificity, and negative predictive value. Nevertheless, they have shortcomings, particularly the broad nature of the 'possible' category. The modified Duke criteria pro-posed the following amendments:

- ◆ 'Possible' defined as one major criterion and one minor criterion or three minor criteria.
- ◆ Removal of the minor criterion 'Echocardiogram: consistent with infective endocarditis but not meeting major criterion', given the widespread use of transoesophageal echocardiography.
- ◆ Bacteraemia due to *Staphylococcus aureus* or positive Q-fever serology should both be adopted as major criteria.

Further reading

- Li JS, Sexton DJ, Mick N, *et al.* Proposed modifications to the Duke criteria for the diagnosis of infective endocarditis. *Clin Infect Dis* 2000; 30: 633–8. (Epub 3 Apr 2000).

Impact of cerebrovascular complications on mortality and neurologic outcome during infective endocarditis: a prospective multicentre study

Thuny F, Avierinos J-F, Tribouilloy C, Giorgi R, Casalta J-P, Milandre L, Brahim A, Nadji G, Riberi A, Collart F, Renard S, Raoult D, Habib G. *Eur Heart J* 2007; 28: 1155–61.

Background

Embolic events complicate 20–50% of cases of infective endocarditis (although this risk falls rapidly following the initiation of appropriate antibiotic therapy) and are responsible for some of its most devastating consequences. Brain injury, due to vegetation, embolization, or mycotic aneurysm rupture during the active phase of infective endocarditis, is most commonly symptomatic, but may be silent and detected on imaging alone. This prospective study at two French hospitals analysed the risk of death according to the type of cerebrovascular injury in patients with a definite diagnosis of infective endocarditis.

Methods

Between 1990 and 2005, 496 patients with definite infective endocarditis (according to Duke criteria) were entered into the study. They underwent blood cultures, transthoracic and transoesophageal echocardiography within 48 hours of admission and a cerebral CT was per-formed on admission on all patients recruited after 1993 (n = 453). Antibiotic therapy was initiated upon diagno-sis. Cerebrovascular injury was diagnosed based on clini-cal and CT findings and categorized as silent cerebral embolism, transient ischaemic attack (TIA), ischaemic stroke, or intracerebral haemorrhage. Follow-up data were collected from medical notes at the end of the study, with end points of overall mortality, neurological mortality, and post-operative neurological exacerbation (either post-operative neurological death or worsening of cerebral damage).

Results

Cerebrovascular complications occurred in 109 (22%) patients, being more common in those with mitral valve endocarditis. Silent cerebral embolism was seen in 17 patients, ischaemic stroke in 50 patients, TIA in

30 patients, and primary intracerebral haemorrhage in 12 patients. During a median follow-up period of 2.9 years, 139 (28%) patients died, of whom 33 had had cerebrovascular complications. There was no statistically significant difference in mortality in those with cerebrovascular complications compared with those without. However, when patients were stratified according to the type of cerebrovascular complication, those with stroke (ischaemic or haemorrhagic) had a significant excess mortality (hazard ratio 1.7, p = 0.02), whereas those with silent embolism or TIA did not (hazard ratio 0.9, p = 0.64). In multivariate analysis, mortality was predicted by a low GCS and mechanical prosthetic valve endocarditis. When surgery was performed in patients after a cerebrovascular complication, neurological exacerbation was rare and only observed in those with symptomatic stroke.

Conclusions

This study showed that mortality in infective endocarditis depends on the type of cerebrovascular complication and that only symptomatic stroke (not silent embolism or TIA) is associated with excess mortality, particularly in the context of reduced GCS or prosthetic valve endocarditis.

Learning points

- Cerebral embolism in infective endocarditis can have devastating consequences.
- There is no excess mortality in those with silent cerebral embolism or TIA.
- There is excess mortality in those with symptomatic stroke (ischaemic or haemorrhagic).
- Current ESC guidelines suggest that for patients with aortic or mitral vegetations exceeding 10 mm in size and with one or more embolic events (which may be silent and detected radiologically), urgent surgery is indicated.

Further reading

- Hart RG, Foster JW, Luther MF, Kanter MC. Stroke in infective endocarditis. *Stroke* 1990; 21: 695–700.
- Piper C, Wiemer M, Schulte HD, Horstkotte D. Stroke is not a contraindication for urgent valve replacement in acute infective endocarditis. *J Heart Valve Dis* 2001; 10: 703–11.

Risk of embolism in infective endocarditis: prognostic value of echocardiography: a prospective multicentre study

Thuny F, Disalvo G, Belliard O, Avierinos J-F, Pergola V, Rosenberg V, Casalta J-P, Gouvernet J, Derumeaux G, Larussi D, Ambrosi P, Calabro R, Riberi A, Collart F, Metras D, Lepidi H, Raoult D, Harle J-R, Weiller P-J, Cohen A, Habib G. *Circulation* 2005; 112: 69–75.

Background

Despite advances in diagnosis and treatment, infective endocarditis remains a dangerous disease, with a high incidence of serious complications. Previous studies attempting to identify predictors of embolism and mortality had produced conflicting results, largely due to the heterogeneity of the cases studied and small sample sizes. In particular, the prognostic role of echocardiography in assessing vegetation size and mobility (and thereby predicting complications) was unclear. As a result, international guidelines on the indications for surgery have varied significantly.

This prospective study at four European centres assessed the predictive role of transoesophageal echocardiography (TOE) in definite cases of infective endocarditis.

Methods

From 1993 to 2003, 384 patients with infective endocarditis according to Duke criteria were enrolled into the study. They underwent blood cultures, serology, transthoracic echocardiography (TTE), TOE, and cerebral and abdominal CT within 48 hours of admission, with antibiotic therapy starting upon diagnosis.

Echocardiographic findings were reviewed by two experienced echocardiographers blinded to the clinical status. The presence, maximal length, and mobility of vegetations were recorded and mobility was recorded using a four-point scale:

- Absent—fixed vegetation with no independent motion.
- Low—vegetation with fixed base, but mobile free edge.
- Moderate—pedunculated vegetation remaining within same chamber throughout cardiac cycle.
- Severe—prolapsing vegetation crossing leaflet coaptation plane during cardiac cycle.

The end points recorded were total embolic events, embolic events after initiation of antibiotics, and one-year mortality.

Results

On admission, 103 (27%) patients had already had an embolic event, including 46 (12%) with stroke. A further 28 (7%) patients had embolic events after starting antibiotic therapy, giving a total of 131 (34%) embolic events. TTE and TOE identified vegetations in 94 (24%) and 320 (83%) patients, respectively. Vegetation length was predictive of an embolic event after starting antibiotics and was larger in those with new embolic events than in those without (median length 15.5 vs. 9 mm, p <0.001). A threshold of 10 mm was identified as having the greatest predictive value by receiver operating characteristic (ROC) curve analysis. New embolic events occurred in 14% of patients with a vegetation length >10 mm, but in only 1% of patients with a vegetation length ≤10 mm (p <0.001). Severe vegetation mobility was also strongly predictive of new embolic events. Total one-year mortality was 21%. ROC curve analysis showed a vegetation length >15 mm to be independently predictive of one-year mortality (relative risk 1.7, p = 0.03).

Conclusions

This study showed that vegetation length is strongly predictive of new embolic events after starting antibiotic therapy (>10 mm) and one-year mortality (>15 mm). TTE and TOE are therefore recommended early in the course of the disease and frequently throughout its course, and allow early identification of those patients at high risk of embolism or death.

Learning points

- Vegetation length is predictive of embolic events and one-year mortality.
- Transthoracic echocardiography and TOE should be performed early in the course of infective endocarditis to identify those patients at high risk.
- Current (2009) ESC guidelines suggest that, in the absence of embolism, urgent surgery is indicated for patients with aortic or mitral vegetations exceeding 10 mm in size and with other factors suggesting a poor prognosis (heart failure, persistent infection, or abscess). Following one or more embolic events (which may be silent and/or detected radiologically), urgent surgery is indicated even if these poor prognostic features are absent.

Further reading

- Di Salvo G, Habib G, Pergola V, *et al*. Echocardiography predicts embolic events in infective endocarditis. *J Am Coll Cardiol* 2001; 37: 1069–76.
- Steckelberg JM, Murphy JG, Ballard D, *et al*. Emboli in infective endocarditis: the prognostic value of echocardiography. *Ann Intern Med* 1991; 114: 635–40.

A randomized trial of aspirin on the risk of embolic events in patients with infective endocarditis

Chan K-L, Dumesnil J, Cujec B, Sanfilippo A, Jue J, Turek M, Robinson T, Moher D. *J Am Coll Cardiol* 2003; 42: 775–80.

Background

Embolism is one of the leading causes of morbidity and mortality in infective endocarditis. In patients receiving antibiotic therapy, there is no additional medical therapy known to reduce the risk of embolism. Platelets form a significant component of vegetations seen in infective endocarditis and animal models had suggested that aspirin treatment was associated with their more rapid resolution. This double-blind, placebo-controlled, randomized, multi-centre study investigated the effect of aspirin on the frequency of embolic events in native or prosthetic valve endocarditis.

Methods

A group of 115 patients aged 16–80 with definite infective endocarditis was entered into the study between 1994 and 1998. Patients were excluded if they had right-sided endocarditis, perivalvular abscess, probable surgery within seven days, current aspirin use, previous gastrointestinal bleeding/active peptic ulcer disease, bleeding problems, or an allergy/intolerance to aspirin. Patients were randomized to either 325 mg aspirin (n = 60) or placebo (n = 55) once daily for four weeks. In patients with mechanical prosthetic valves, anticoagulation was continued. There was no difference in antibiotic therapy between the two groups.

The primary outcome measure was symptomatic embolism affecting the brain or other organs. Secondary outcomes were subclinical stroke, death, major or minor bleeding, valve surgery, and echocardiographic progression of valvular involvement.

Results

There was no significant difference in the number of clinical embolic events in patients on aspirin (17 [28%]) or placebo (11 [20%]) (odds ratio 1.62, p = 0.29). Overall bleeding (major or minor) was higher in the aspirin group, but did not reach statistical significance (p = 0.075). There was no suggestion that aspirin increased the risk of cerebral haemorrhage (p = 0.182).

In 46 patients (23 in each group), serial echocardiography was used to monitor vegetation size at baseline and at four weeks. There was no significant difference between the aspirin and placebo groups, with both showing a reduction in vegetation size.

Conclusions

In patients already receiving antibiotic therapy for infective endocarditis, the addition of aspirin does not reduce the frequency of embolic events, nor does it affect the reduction in size of vegetations over time. Aspirin is likely to be associated with an increased risk of major and minor bleeding complications and does not have a direct role in the management of infective endocarditis.

> ### Learning points
>
> ◆ Aspirin does not have a direct role in the management of infective endocarditis and does not reduce the frequency of embolic events.

Further reading

- Chan KL, Tam J, Dumesnil JG, et al. Effect of long-term aspirin use on embolic events in infective endocarditis. *Clin Infect Dis* 2008; 46: 37–41.
- Tornos P, Almirante B, Mirabet S, Permanyer G, Pahissa A, Soler-Soler J. Infective endocarditis due to *Staphylococcus aureus*: deleterious effect of anticoagulant therapy. *Arch Intern Med* 1999; 159: 473–5.

Current features of infective endocarditis in elderly patients

Durante-Mangoni E, Bradley S, Selton-Suty C, Tripodi M-F, Barsic B, Bouza E, Cabell C, Ramos A, Fowler Jr V, Hoen B, Konecny P, Moren A, Murdoch D, Pappas P, Sexton D, Spelman D, Tattevin P, Miro J, van der Meer J, Utili R. *Arch Int Med* 2008; 168: 2095–103.

Background

The epidemiology of infective endocarditis has changed significantly in recent decades and the elderly population has seen the largest relative rise in incidence. This is thought to be due to the increasing prevalence of undiagnosed valve disease (in a recent French series, 47% of patients presenting with infective endocarditis did not have previously documented cardiac disease) and the increasing use of invasive medical procedures and prosthetic medical devices. Previous studies had attempted to characterize infective endocarditis in the elderly population, but with conflicting results.

This multinational, prospective observational cohort study evaluated clinical features, and outcome of infective endocarditis in relation to age.

Methods

A group of 2759 consecutive patients with infective endocarditis (according to modified Duke criteria) were enrolled between 2000 and 2005 and were stratified into two groups: 18–64 years old (n = 1703) and 65 years old or older (n = 1056, defined as 'elderly' in this study). The groups were further subdivided into non-drug use, native valve infective endocarditis (n = 1553) and community-acquired infective endocarditis (n = 1843).

Risk factors, predisposing conditions, source of infection, clinical features, course, and outcome were all analysed.

Results

In the elderly group, the proportion of females was higher (p = 0.001), with more cases of prosthetic valve endocarditis (p <0.001) and healthcare related endocarditis (p <0.001). Elderly patients were more likely to have mitral regurgitation or non-rheumatic aortic stenosis as a predisposing cardiac condition. Almost half of the 2759 patients had at least one chronic illness before the onset of infective endocarditis: diabetes mellitus, gastrointestinal, and genitourinary malignancy were most commonly noted.

Elderly patients were significantly more likely to have undergone an invasive procedure in the six months before presentation (p <0.001 compared with younger patients) and more likely to have a pacemaker or ICD (p <0.001).

In both patient groups, *Staphylococcus aureus* was the most common causative pathogen, with viridans group Streptococci responsible for only half as many cases.

Clinical evidence of infective endocarditis was found less often in elderly patients: rates of embolism, immune-mediated phenomena, and septic complications were all less frequent. Fewer vegetations and more abscesses were seen in the elderly group. Elderly patients had a higher rate of in-hospital mortality (25 vs. 13%, p <0.001) and age ≥65 years was an independent predictor of mortality.

Conclusions

Infective endocarditis is an increasing problem in the elderly population due to prolonged life expectancy, the increasing prevalence of valvular heart disease in this group, and greater use of invasive procedures and prosthetic material. Fewer cases of infective endocarditis are now secondary to oral streptococci, and *Staphylococcus aureus* (frequently acquired as a result of nosocomial infection) is now the most common pathogen, with attendant higher mortality. In this study age ≥65 years was an independent risk factor for mortality.

Learning points

- The incidence of infective endocarditis is increasing in the elderly population.
- Oral streptococci are no longer the most common causative pathogen in infective endocarditis, and more cases are now due to *Staphylococcus aureus*.
- Mortality from infective endocarditis is higher in the elderly population and its presentation often more insidious.

Further reading

- Dhawan VK. Infective endocarditis in elderly patients. *Clin Infect Dis* 2002; 34: 806–12.
- Hoen B, Alla F, Selton-Suty C, *et al*. Changing profile of infective endocarditis: results of a 1-year survey in France. *JAMA*. 2002; 288: 75–81.
- Nkomo VT, Gardin JM, Skelton TN, Gottdiener JS, Scott CG, Enriquez-Sarano M. Burden of valvular heart diseases: a population-based study. *Lancet* 2006; 368: 1005–11.

Conclusion

Infective endocarditis is an evolving disease with a persistently high mortality and morbidity, even in the modern era of advanced diagnostic imaging, improved antimicrobial chemotherapy, and potentially curative surgery. Despite these advancements, the incidence of the disease has remained unchanged over the past few decades and may even be increasing. Chronic rheumatic heart disease is now an uncommon antecedent, whereas degenerative valve disease of the elderly, intravenous drug abuse, valve replacement, and vascular instrumentation have become increasingly common, coinciding with an increase in staphylococcal infections and those caused by fastidious organisms. Furthermore, previously undetected pathogens are now being identified with the disease and multidrug resistant bacteria challenge conventional treatment regimens.

The future is likely to see the development of new antibacterial agents, particularly those targeted at drug-resistant Gram positive cocci, and modified biomaterials may reduce the risk of infective endocarditis in patients with artificial heart valves or other intracardiac prosthetic material. The reduction in antibiotic prophylaxis before dental and other invasive procedures, suggested by recently revised international guidelines, may (if these recommendations prove misguided) result in a rise in the incidence of infective endocarditis. A randomized controlled trial of antibiotic prophylaxis, which would up to now have been deemed unethical, may now be a realistic proposition.

The changing face of infective endocarditis seems set to challenge the endeavours of cardiologists, microbiologists, and cardiac surgeons for many years to come.

Part VI

Cardiac imaging

Chapter 21

Echocardiography

Dr Christopher Steadman and Professor Mark Monaghan

Introduction

It is difficult to imagine how much echocardiography has evolved since the first recordings of movement of the mitral valve were made by Edler and Hertz in Sweden in the 1950s. Since that time ultrasound technology has grown so much that it's difficult to appreciate that the detailed, real-time 3D cardiac images we can obtain today are based upon the same basic principle that those pioneers used 50 years ago. As the technology has improved, the range of clinical applications of echo has also increased and now it is one of the most widely used diagnostic techniques for the assessment of cardiac pathology in both adults and children.

The technological advances in echocardiography have included progression from basic, single-dimensional recordings of individual cardiac structures to real-time 3D dimensional imaging of the entire heart. Improvements in transducer technology, computer processing power, and digital image processing/storage have made these advances possible. Image quality and resolution have also improved with the advent of the transoesophageal approach (in selected patients), harmonic imaging and the use of contrast agents. Thanks to these advances, echo has now become the first-line technique for the assessment of left ventricular function, the evaluation of valvular heart disease and the diagnosis of congenital heart disease.

In addition, it has evolved as a pivotal diagnostic technique in the assessment of patients with suspected endocarditis, cardio-embolic stroke, and in the functional assessment of coronary artery disease. More recently, the technique has been increasingly used to guide interventional procedures for structural heart disease.

Most of the landmark papers chosen for this section have been included because they represent either the first or the most widely quoted publications that marked a significant step forward in the development of echocardiography. Every single paper demonstrates an important and, in the authors' opinions, pivotal advance in technology and/or clinical application of this most pervasive of all cardiac diagnostic techniques.

Oesophageal echocardiography

Frazin L, Talano JV, Stephanides L, Loeb HS, Kopel L, Gunnar RM. *Circulation* 1976; 54: 102–8.

Background

Cardiac ultrasound was first introduced in 1954 and subsequently became an important diagnostic tool. It was widely recognized that external ultrasound was limited when the transducer is a significant distance from the heart, such as in obesity or chronic obstructive pulmonary disease (COPD). To obviate these problems a group from Illinois, USA, developed and clinically tested an oesophageal transducer in this study.

Methods and results

Thirty-eight patients were studied; the exact breakdown was not detailed but 20 were selected because of poor quality anterior echoes and included a mix of normal subjects, patients with cardiac disease, and patients with obesity or COPD. First, standard transthoracic echocardiography (TTE) of that era was performed with an external transducer. In the same sitting transoesophageal echocardiography (TOE) was performed. The oesophageal transducer was a 9 mm non-focused 3.5 MHz device in a rounded casing for easy swallowing. It was attached to a 3 mm coaxial cable. Patients usually fed the transducer themselves after gargling xylocaine. M-mode echocardiography was obtained of the aortic root, aortic valve, left atrium (LA), and mitral valve. The procedure lasted approximately ten minutes.

In the 18 patients in whom TTE was successful, measurements correlated well with TOE; particularly aortic valve opening (r = 0.86), LA dimensions (r = 0.96), and anterior mitral valve leaflet excursion (r = 0.97). However, the correlation was weaker for aortic root dimensions (r = 0.67) and the posterior mitral valve leaflet was rarely visualized. Of the 20 patients with unobtainable TTE the success of TOE was demonstrated with examples although the total number of successful TOE studies in this group was not reported.

Strengths and limitations

This was a pioneering study introducing a novel technique. The rigorous scientific evaluation of the results is perhaps slightly lacking; correlation coefficients do not measure agreement between the two methods, only the relationship between the results, and the success rate of TOE was not reported. However, this is more acceptable given this was a proof of concept study.

Conclusions

This study introduced the novel concept of TOE. The swallowing of the probe enabling it to get close to cardiac structures was clearly markedly different from TTE, but also new manipulations were required to obtain the images with advancing and withdrawal of the probe and medial and lateral rotation more important than the tilting used in TTE. This study demonstrated a proof of concept that images could be obtained using TOE when TTE was unsuccessful. However, it was also noted that improved detail could be obtained with TOE, and this improved resolution remains an important indication for contemporary TOE. The authors recognized the limitations at that stage; they were unable to obtain left ventricular (LV) dimensions mainly due to lack of transducer control. The authors were already working on an external cable to control transducer position, which has continued to the current day where fine control of modern probes is possible.

This was the first step in developing a technique which modern cardiology relies upon in many situations, including the assessment of valve disease (particularly the mitral valve), diagnosis of infective endocarditis, guidance of interventions (including valvuloplasty, closure of septal defects and transcatheter aortic valve implantation (TAVI)), and intra-operative use in cardiac surgery.

Learning points

- ◆ Established proof of concept: TOE was possible.
- ◆ Utility of TOE when TTE images unobtainable.
- ◆ Potential for higher resolution images with TOE.
- ◆ Provided platform for development of contemporary TOE vital for:
  - ● Diagnostics (valve disease, endocarditis).
  - ● Guiding intervention (mitral valvuloplasty, TAVI, defect closure).
  - ● Peri- and intra-operative guidance of cardiac surgery.

Further reading

- ● Fisher EA, Stahl JA, Budd JH, Goldman ME. Transesophageal echocardiography: procedures and clinical application. *J Am Coll Cardiol* 1991; 18: 1333–48.
- ● Pedersen WR, Walker M, Olson JD, *et al.* Value of transesophageal echocardiography as an adjunct to transthoracic echocardiography in evaluation of native and prosthetic valve endocarditis. *Chest* 1991; 100: 351–6.
- ● Rittoo D, Sutherland GR, Currie P, Starkey IR, Shaw TR. The comparative value of transesophageal and transthoracic echocardiography before and after percutaneous mitral balloon valvotomy: a prospective study. *Am Heart J* 1993; 125: 1094–105.

Continuous-wave Doppler echocardiographic assessment of severity of calcific aortic stenosis: a simultaneous Doppler-catheter correlative study in 100 adult patients

Currie PJ, Seward JB, Reeder GS, Vlietstra RE, Bresnahan DR, Bresnahan JF, Smith HC, Hagler DJ, Tajik AJ. *Circulation* 1985; 71: 1162–9.

Background

Prior to the advent of continuous-wave (CW) Doppler, assessment of aortic stenosis (AS) by echocardiography consisted of looking at valve opening with M-mode echocardiography and 2D images to assess calcification and mobility. To determine the pressure drop across the valve cardiac catheterization was required with either simultaneous readings taken in the aorta and LV or by measurement of the pull-back gradient from LV to aorta. The development of CW Doppler enabled pressure gradients to be estimated across stenotic valves and had been reported in small numbers of patients with comparisons to non-simultaneous invasive measures. This study sought to validate this emerging technique in a large number of adult patients with simultaneous invasive pressure readings.

Method and results

One hundred consecutive adults (age ≥50 years, mean age 69) were studied. Males and females were well represented (55 males) and 90% of patients were in sinus rhythm. The presence or absence of coexisting valve disease is not reported, although 97% of patients had coronary angiography (with 61% of these having ≥50% stenosis). All patients had CW Doppler echocardiographic examination at the time of cardiac catheterization, with a 2 MHz non-imaging transducer in multiple sites and positions to find the maximum velocity. In addition, 46 patients also underwent a further non-simultaneous Doppler study within seven days. The Doppler maximum pressure gradient was estimated using the modified Bernoulli equation (gradient = 4 x velocity^2). On cardiac catheterization the valve gradient was assessed by pull-back from LV to aorta in 37 patients, and from simultaneous LV and aortic measurements in 63 (the LV pressure was recorded by trans-septal catheterization in 33 and retrograde catheterization through the aortic valve in 30). The peak-to-peak gradient was determined from the pull-back and the maximum pressure gradient from the simultaneous recordings. Doppler traces and simultaneous LV and aortic pressure waveforms were digitized at 10 msec intervals with gradients calculated at each interval allowing the mean gradient to be derived (see Figure 21.1).

The maximum Doppler-determined gradient correlated strongly with both the simultaneous maximum catheter gradient (r = 0.92, standard error of the estimate (SEE) 15 mmHg) and the peak-to-peak gradient (r = 0.91, SEE 15 mmHg). The peak-to-peak gradient was significantly lower than both Doppler and catheter derived maximum gradients. The mean Doppler and catheter gradients correlated closely (r = 0.92, SEE 10 mmHg). Left ventricular dysfunction and coronary artery disease (CAD) did not affect the accuracy of

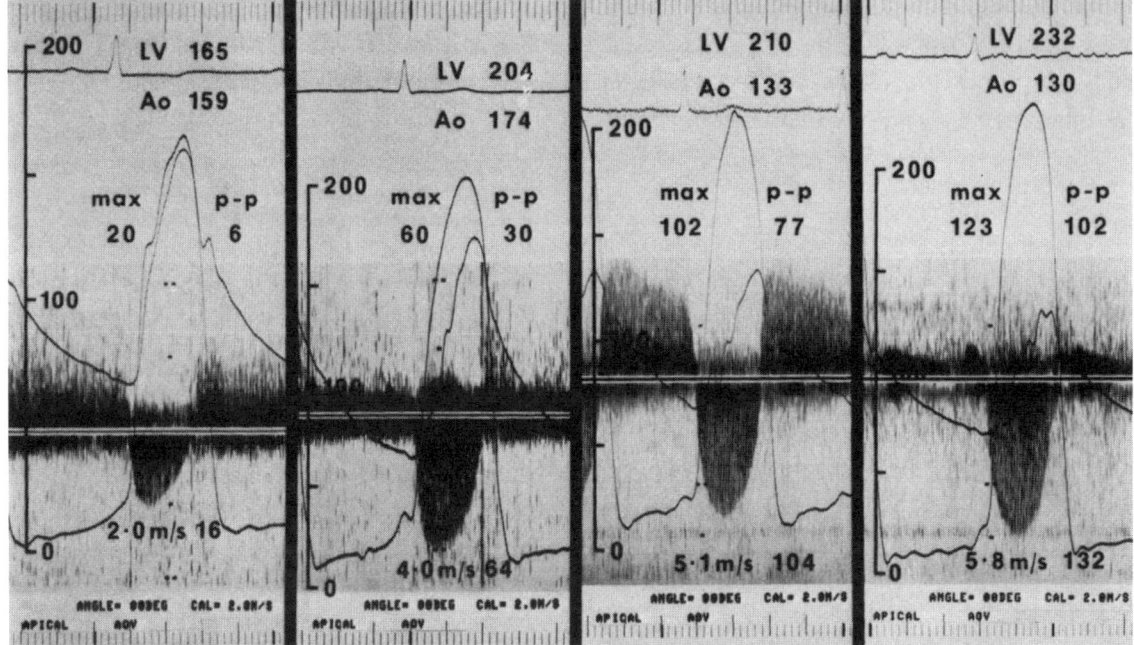

Figure 21.1 A composite of simultaneous Doppler-catheter pressure measurements in four patients with variable severity of aortic stenosis in whom dual-catheter left ventricular (LV) and ascending aortic (Ao) pressure measurements were obtained. The maximum catheter (max) gradient is greater than the peak-to-peak (p-p) catheter gradient at each level of stenosis. The maximum Doppler-derived gradients accurately measure the simultaneously recorded maximum catheter gradient, but overestimate the peak-to-peak catheter gradient. The Doppler calibration markers are 2 m/sec apart.

Reproduced from Currie PJ. Continuous-wave Doppler echocardiographic assessment of severity of calcific aortic stenosis: a simultaneous Doppler-catheter correlative study in 100 adult patients. *Circulation* 1985; 71: 1162–9, with permission from Wolters Kluwer Health.

Doppler measurements. The maximum Doppler gradient from the second echocardiogram completed in 46 patients correlated less well with the maximum catheter gradient than the simultaneous echocardiogram (r = 0.79, SEE 24 mmHg vs. r = 0.95, SEE 12 mmHg, p <0.001).

Strengths and limitations

The strength of this study is that a large number of patients were studied of the age range typically affected by AS and so this is representative of clinical practice. The correlation coefficients (r) need to be interpreted with caution; r measures the strength of relation between the two measurements not the agreement between them. The SEE should be focused on when making comparisons between the two methods in this study, and this shows typical values between 10 and 15 mmHg. This is very supportive of the validity of the use of CW gradients and as the authors

have demonstrated this is strengthened by performing catheterization and echocardiography simultaneously. A particular strength of this study is that the presence of CAD has been shown not to affect the results; CAD is prevalent in patients with AS but often not well described in clinical studies. The limited information regarding coexisting valve disease is perhaps a concern and additionally the validity of the measurements in rhythms other than sinus rhythm is not fully answered.

Conclusions

This landmark study confirmed that CW Doppler was a reliable tool for accurately determining pressure gradients across the valve, and this is now established clinical practice. It should be noted, however, that correct alignment of the ultrasound beam to the aortic velocity jet is vital for accurate assessment. Continuous-wave

Doppler needs to be used in conjunction with other imaging data, including assessment of aortic valve area, and confounding clinical situations such as severe LV dysfunction also need to be considered when making assessments of valve severity.

♦ Continuous-wave Doppler needs to be used in association with other assessments of stenosis severity.
♦ Catheter derived pull-back measurements underestimate true peak aortic valve gradients.

Learning points

♦ Continuous wave Doppler is a reliable way of assessing aortic valve gradients.
♦ Doppler measurements are valid with coexisting coronary artery disease.
♦ Use with caution in some clinical scenarios; arrhythmia, severe LV dysfunction, coexisting valve disease.

Further reading

● Lange RA, Hillis LD. Dobutamine stress echocardiography in patients with low-gradient aortic stenosis. *Circulation* 2006; 113: 1718–20.
● Otto CM. Valvular aortic stenosis: disease severity and timing of intervention. *J Am Coll Cardiol* 2006; 47: 2141–51.
● Taylor R. Evolution of the continuity equation in the Doppler echocardiographic assessment of the severity of valvular aortic stenosis. *J Am Soc Echocardiogr* 1990; 3: 326–30.

Complementary value of two-dimensional exercise echocardiography to routine treadmill exercise testing

Armstrong WF, O'Donnell J, Dillon JC, McHenry PL, Morris SN, Feigenbaum H. *Ann Intern Med* 1986; 105: 829–35.

Background

Treadmill exercise testing with ECG monitoring is the commonest test performed for diagnosis of CAD, determined by symptoms and ECG changes. Whilst this is simple and inexpensive there are problems, particularly with false positives in certain patient groups, notably females. This study sought to examine the role of exercise echocardiography in determining the presence or absence of CAD.

Methods and results

Ninety-five patients (79% male) referred to a chest pain clinic were evaluated. Patients with previous coronary artery bypass grafts (CABG) or percutaneous coronary intervention (PCI) were excluded, but known CAD or previous myocardial infarction (MI) were not exclusions. Only five patients were not taking any medication at the time of assessment. Testing was performed in a tertiary centre and patients had often had non-diagnostic studies elsewhere prior to referral. Treadmill tests were performed according to a modified Balke protocol (a protocol with three-minute increments with an increase in speed and gradient from stage I to II then only increasing gradient). Heart rate, blood pressure, and three bipolar

ECG leads were monitored. The ECG response was graded as normal, ischaemic (≥1 mm of horizontal or downsloping ST depression or a negative U wave with associated chest pain), or non-diagnostic (chest pain without ECG changes, atypical chest pain with ECG changes or LBBB). Coronary angiography was performed within four weeks and CAD was considered present if there was ≥50% luminal stenosis. Resting echocardiography was conducted in the left lateral position with standard parasternal short and long-axis views and apical four and two-chamber views, optimal transducer positions were marked. Immediately after exercise the patient stepped off the treadmill and underwent a repeat echocardiogram at the marked positions. Images were recorded on video tape and the best rest and exercise loops prepared offline. This was then assessed for all patients by a single experienced echocardiographer blinded to other data. Wall motion was judged as normal, hypokinetic, akinetic, dyskinetic, or hyperkinetic at rest and exercise. An ischaemic study was defined as development of a new regional wall motion abnormality (RWMA). The RWMA were ascribed a coronary territory; right coronary—right ventricle, inferior wall and inferior septum of LV, left anterior descending—anterior wall, anterior septum, and apex of LV, circumflex—posterolateral wall of LV.

Thirty-four patients had normal resting ECGs, 25 had non-specific changes or LBBB, and 36 had evidence of previous MI. Eighty patients had CAD; 35 single-vessel, 21 double-vessel, and 24 triple-vessel. A RWMA was seen (at rest, exercise or both) in 70 of the 80 patients with CAD (sensitivity 88%). Of the 15 patients without CAD on routine treadmill testing seven had a normal response; one had an abnormal response and six were non-diagnostic. After exercise echocardiography 13 were classified as normal whereas two were falsely classified with CAD.

The most interesting group were the 59 patients without prior infarction and normal or non-specific changes on ECG; 44 had CAD, 15 did not. Twenty-one had a normal routine treadmill test, of which 13 had CAD, exercise echo did detect a further 11 patients with CAD, but still missed 10. Twenty had an ischaemic routine test, of which 19 had CAD; exercise echo did correctly identify the single false-positive. However, it also incorrectly assessed one of the patients with CAD as the exercise echo was negative. Of the 16 ambiguous routine tests; six did not have CAD; exercise echo correctly indentified all of these six, but exercise echo was positive in only 8 of the 12 with CAD. Overall sensitivity of exercise echo was 80%, specificity 87%, positive predictive value 95%, and negative predictive value 59%.

In the 36 patients with prior infarction, 35 had rest or exercise induced RWMA. Obviously the existence of CAD is not in doubt in this group but the incidence of exercise induced RWMA and co-existence of current stenoses ≥50% was not reported.

Strength and limitations

The fact that the echo was performed immediately after exercise but not at peak exercise may limit the detection of some transient RWMA and lead to underdetection of CAD. Only three-lead ECG was used for routine testing, potentially limiting detection of ischaemic changes. The analysis of the echo by an observer blinded to the other information reinforces the validity of the results. Most patients were male, reflecting standard referrals to chest pain clinic, but the usefulness of exercise echo in females

therefore may have been undervalued. Analysis by sex was not presented, which may have been interesting.

Conclusions

In those without previous MI exercise echo did improve the detection of CAD from 43% (19 of 44) with an ischaemic routine treadmill test to 80% (35 of 44). In those with an ambiguous routine test exercise echo gave the correct diagnosis in 78% (14 of 18). A strength of exercise echo is the positive predictive value of 95%; patients with a positive test are likely to have CAD. However, a negative test is limited by the weak negative predictive value of 59%; 9 of 21 with a negative test did in fact have CAD, the majority (6 patients) having single-vessel disease. Exercise echo improves the diagnostic yield from routine treadmill exercise, equivalent to radionuclide techniques, and therefore is preferable given the lack of exposure to ionizing radiation. If routine use is not locally feasible it should be considered where previous routine testing has been ambiguous. A negative test, however, should be interpreted in the clinical context and patients at high risk for CAD should still be considered for further investigation.

> ## Learning points
>
> - Routine treadmill testing with 3-lead ECG monitoring is limited for detection of CAD.
> - Exercise echo improves the positive predictive value (95%) in those without known CAD.
> - The negative predictive value of exercise echo is limited (59%) and therefore negative tests should be interpreted with caution in those at high clinical risk.

Further reading

- Holland DJ, Prasad SB, Marwick TH. Contribution of exercise echocardiography to the diagnosis of heart failure with preserved ejection fraction (HFpEF). *Heart* 2010; 96: 1024–8.
- Metz LD, Beattie M, Hom R, Redberg RF, Grady D, Fleischmann KE. The prognostic value of normal exercise myocardial perfusion imaging and exercise echocardiography: a meta-analysis. *J Am Coll Cardiol* 2007; 49: 227–37.

A new concept in echocardiography: harmonic imaging of tissue without use of contrast agent

Caidahl K, Kazzam E, Lidberg J, Neumann AG, Nordanstig J, Rantapaa DS, Waldenstrom A, Wikh R.
Lancet 1998; 352: 1264–70.

Background

With improving 2D image quality it became possible to assess LV function more accurately. However, endocardial border definition was frequently suboptimal, hindering analysis. Trans-pulmonary contrast agents were developed so that the endocardial border could be more easily determined. Harmonic imaging utilizing the second harmonic frequency improved the visualization of the microbubbles in the contrast. The authors of this study had noted that use of harmonic imaging appeared to improve border definition even before contrast was given, if the gain was appropriately increased. The hypothesis of this study was therefore that harmonic imaging would improve border detection despite the absence of contrast agents.

Methods and results

Seventy-one participants were studied. Greyscale measurements were performed in five patients with ischaemic heart disease and 22 with systemic sclerosis, along with 22 corresponding age and sex-matched controls. Left ventricular ejection fraction (EF) was determined in a further 22 patients with ischaemic heart disease.

Patients were investigated in the left lateral position. For grey-scale evaluation an HDI-3000 scanner (ATL, USA) was used with a 2.5 MHz broadband transducer operating in fundamental mode (transmitting and receiving at 2.75 MHz) and harmonic mode (transmitting at 1.67 MHz and receiving at 3.33 MHz). No changes in output energy were made. For LVEF evaluation a Sequoia scanner (Acuson, USA) was used, equipped with a 3.5MHz transducer operating in fundamental mode and harmonic mode (transmitting at 1.75 MHz and receiving at 3.5 MHz). Fundamental and harmonic images were recorded on Super-VHS in midventricular, parasternal, and short-axis views for grey-scale assessment and apical four and two-chamber views for LVEF. Author-developed computer software was used to measure grey values on either side of the endocardium and within the myocardium segmentally, and normalized for the range of grey values within the segment. Simpson's biplane method was used to calculate LVEF, with the endocardial border traced on two separate occasions. The endocardial border was also assessed subjectively on a scale from 1 = not

visualized to 8 = good. An image was deemed unacceptable if more than one segment had a score of ≤2.

Harmonic imaging gave significantly increased computer-measured endocardial brightness and improved subjective score with mean improvement of brightness by 87% and qualitative score by 2.19 (both p <0.001). This was true in both systole and diastole. Myocardial brightness was also improved. Harmonic imaging provided significantly less basis for visibility drop-out, with minimum endocardial grey values (relative to the image mean) significantly higher for harmonic imaging compared with fundamental imaging (57% vs. 23% in diastole and 83% vs. 33% in systole, both p <0.001). Reproducibility of LVEF measurements was assessed using Bland-Altman methods. Harmonic imaging provided narrower 95% limits of agreement; this was only displayed graphically, but examining the figures the range of differences was approximately -16% to +16% for harmonic imaging and -22% to +24% for fundamental imaging. Harmonic imaging improved the number of acceptable views, with the most marked effect in the two-chamber view, followed by short axis and lastly four-chamber.

Strengths and limitations

Patients with systemic sclerosis are not common echo subjects and were chosen due to possible changes in endocardial and myocardial properties. However, the study included normal controls and patients with ischaemic heart disease, which are representative of general clinical practice. The predominant strength of the study was including both qualitative and quantitative assessment and relating this to a real world measurement—LVEF.

Conclusions

Harmonic imaging improves endocardial border definition and improves reproducibility of LVEF measurement. At this time it had been reported that only two-thirds of patients had images suitable for LVEF measurement, the dissemination of this technique likely improved this. There have been vast leaps in technology and image quality in modern ultrasound scanners, but despite these advances harmonic imaging is still used to further improve image quality, highlighting the importance of this paper.

Further reading

• Franke A, Hoffmann R, Kuhl HP, *et al.* Non-contrast second harmonic imaging improves interobserver agreement and accuracy of dobutamine stress echocardiography in patients with impaired image quality. *Heart* 2000; 83: 133–40.
• Turner SP, Monaghan MJ. Tissue harmonic imaging for standard left ventricular measurements: fundamentally flawed? *Eur J Echocardiogr* 2006; 7: 9–15.

Prognostic value of pharmacological stress echocardiography in patients with known or suspected coronary artery disease: a prospective, large-scale, multicenter, head-to-head comparison between dipyridamole and dobutamine test

Echo-Persantine International Cooperative (EPIC) and Echo-Dobutamine International Cooperative (EDIC) Study Groups. Pingitore A, Picano E, Varga A, Gigli G, Cortigiani L, Previtali M, Minardi G, Colosso MQ, Lowenstein J, Mathias W, Jr, Landi P. *J Am Coll Cardiol* 1999; 34: 1769–77.

Background

Pharmacological stress echocardiography with either dobutamine or dipyridamole was known to be both effective and useful for the diagnosis of CAD and for the prognostic stratification of patients with known CAD. Overall accuracy of the two tests assessed in a head-to-head fashion was similar (dobutamine 82% vs. dipyridamole 77%)[16]. Whilst there was preliminary data on prognostic value, the purpose of this study was to compare, head-to-head, the prognostic value of dipyridamole and dobutamine stress echocardiography in patients with known or suspected CAD in a large-scale, multicentre, observational, and prospective study design on the basis of evidence collected by 14 different echocardiographic laboratories. All 14 centres passed a rigorous quality control check.

Methods and results

Five hundred and thirty-eight patients who had performed both dipyridamole and dobutamine stress echocardiography were initially selected. Of these, 37 patients were excluded because the two tests were performed within a time interval >15 days, 18 because the two tests were under different therapeutic conditions, and an additional 23 patients were lost to follow-up. Therefore, the final population consisted of 460 patients (379 (82%) men, mean age 60 ± 10 years) with known or suspected CAD. Of these 460 patients: 171 had a recent (<10 days) uncomplicated MI; 108 had a previous (>3 months) MI; 155 had angina pectoris; and 26 complained of atypical chest pain. Each patient performed dipyridamole and dobutamine stress testing on different days, in random order, and within 15 days. A total of 206 patients performed dipyridamole first and 254 patients performed dobutamine first. Three hundred and fifty-eight patients were off therapy at the time of testing, 82 underwent both testing under identical anti-anginal therapy.

Dobutamine was infused in 3-min dose increments, starting from 5 mg/kg/min and increased to 10, 20, 30, and 40 mg/kg/min. When no end point was reached, atropine (in four divided doses of 0.25 mg up to a maximum of 1 mg) was added to the continuing 40 mg/kg/min dobutamine infusion. Dipyridamole was infused intravenously at a dose of 0.56 mg/kg body weight over 4 min, followed by 4 min of no dose and then, if the test was still negative, 0.28 mg/kg over 2 min. When no end point was reached at 3 min after the end of dipyridamole infusion, atropine (in four divided doses of 0.25 mg up to a maximum of 1 mg) was given. Echocardiography at baseline and peak stress were assessed using the Wall-Motion Score Index (WMSI); an average of the interpretable segments was used from the 16-segment model of the LV, each segment ranging from 1 = normal/hyperkinetic to 4 = dyskinetic. A test was deemed positive if there was an increase in score with stress and the change in WMSI was recorded, Delta WMSI. The number of ischaemic segments at peak stress was also recorded. At follow-up events were defined as cardiac-related deaths, non-fatal myocardial infarction, and revascularization procedures.

The dipyridamole test was negative in 253 and positive in 207 patients. The dobutamine test was negative in 242 and positive in 218 patients. The resting WMSI was 1.37 ± 0.38 for the overall population. The WMSI at peak dose increased up to 1.70 ± 0.35 during dipyridamole (p <0.001 vs. rest WMSI) and up to 1.61 ± 0.39 during dobutamine (p <0.005 vs. rest WMSI). Delta WMSI was 0.28 ± 0.16 for dipyridamole and 0.29 ± 0.18 for dobutamine (p = NS). The only serious side effect occurred with sustained ventricular tachycardia in one patient with dobutamine.

Patients were followed up for 38 ± 21 months (range 1–82 months) by review of hospital notes, or contact of the patient or their physician. Eighty-three patients underwent a revascularization procedure within three months of stress testing (PCI n = 50, CABG n = 33) and therefore were censored. During the follow-up period, there were 18 cardiac-related deaths, 22 acute non-fatal myocardial infarctions and 40 revascularization procedures (PCI n = 17; CABG n = 23).

Cardiac events were not significantly different between those with a positive vs. negative test (19% vs. 16%, p = NS) and this was identical with both modalities, and true whether cardiac death, cardiac death/AMI, or cardiac death/AMI/revascularization were end points. There was no significant difference whether the test was positive at low-dose, high-dose, or after atropine.

For all cardiac events, the negative predictive value was 83% for dobutamine and 84% for dipyridamole (p = NS), and the positive predictive value was 17% for dobutamine and 19% for dipyridamole (p = NS).

When the WMSI was examined, both dipyridamole and dobutamine WMSI were univariate predictors of cardiac death (hazard ratio (HR) dipyridamole 7.3, dobutamine 3.3). By stepwise analysis, dipyridamole WMSI was the most important predictor of cardiac death (HR = 7.3), followed by previous PCI.

For cardiac death, the negative predictive value was 96% for dobutamine and 97% for dipyridamole (p = NS), and the positive predictive value was 5% for dobutamine and 6% for dipyridamole (p = NS).

For dipyridamole, survival decreased progressively from negative, down the degrees of positivity (atropine >high-dose >low-dose) and the same was true of dobutamine; other than positive with atropine this was actually associated with better survival than a negative test. However, the only statistically significant worse survival was seen in the dipyridamole low-dose positive group when compared with the dipyridamole-negative group (see Figure 21.2).

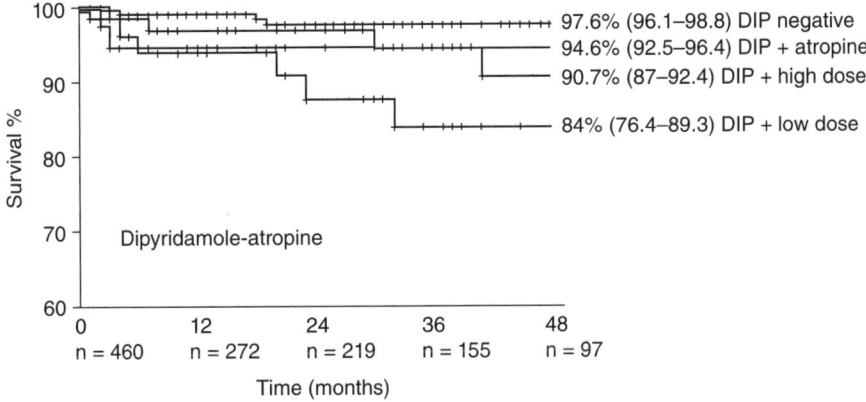

Figure 21.2 Kaplan-Meier survival curves event free of cardiac death in patients with negative and positive dipyridamole tests. Survival is worse in patients with positive tests. Of the positive tests the worst survival is in those positive at low dose, followed by those at high dose, and then finally the best survival of the positive tests occurs if the test was only positive after the use of atropine. Low dose vs. negative, p <0.0001. Cardiac death (n = 18); follow-up 38 ± 21 months.

Reproduced from Pingitore A, *et al.* Prognostic value of pharmacological stress echocardiography in patients with known or suspected coronary artery disease: A prospective, large-scale, multicenter, head-to-head comparison between dipyridamole and dobutamine test. *Journal of the American College of Cardiology* 1999; 34: 9, 1769–77, with permission from Elsevier.

The authors examined survival in the cohort by splitting it with a cutoff of change in WMSI >0.37, determined from ROC curves. The group with larger changes in WMSI with stress had significantly lower survival than the lower group for both techniques.

Strengths and limitations

The strength of this study were the large number of patients involved, a good duration of follow-up, and the rigorous assessment of the multiple centres involved. Despite this, the study was limited by the small number of cardiac deaths, n = 18 (3.9%). This may in part be explained as a significant number of patients (18%) were censored if they had revascularization within three months of the stress test. These revascularization procedures presumably were often ischaemia guided; these patients could have been left in when analysing cardiac death to see real world effects of stress testing on mortality. Additionally, the ability to do two stress tests was required which probably selected a lower risk set of participants. One concern is how applicable these findings are to females given that the vast majority of subjects were male.

Conclusions

This study did confirm that both techniques were feasible and safe. Whether a test was positive or negative had poor positive predictive value for cardiac events or cardiac death. The negative predictive values are better, particularly for predicting cardiac death. It is important to use a more quantitative method to assess ischaemia, the WMSI in this study, as this was more useful for predicting cardiac death. The data also suggest that whilst aggressive protocols with higher doses and atropine may be useful for diagnosis, if the aim of the study is prognostication more conservative protocols are probably warranted, and dipyridamole seems to have a slight advantage. The discussion does, however, highlight that both methods should be widely implemented as in the individual patient one or other technique may be contraindicated, better tolerated, or lead to a diagnostic study.

Learning points

- Stress echocardiography with dobutamine or dipyridamole is feasible and safe.
- Overall a positive test has poor positive predictive value for cardiac events or death.
- Patients with positive tests at lower doses of drug have a worse survival.
- Dipyridamole has a slight advantage at predicting cardiac death.
- Using a quantitative score, the wall motion score index (WMSI), improves prediction of cardiac death.
- Both methodologies should be considered depending on individual patient factors.

Further reading

- Beleslin BD, Ostojic M, Stepanovic J, *et al.* Stress echocardiography in the detection of myocardial ischemia. Head-to-head comparison of exercise, dobutamine, and dipyridamole tests. *Circulation* 1994; 90: 1168–76.
- Picano E, Molinaro S, Pasanisi E. The diagnostic accuracy of pharmacological stress echocardiography for the assessment of coronary artery disease: a meta-analysis *Cardiovasc Ultrasound* 2008; 6: 30.

Clinical utility of Doppler echocardiography and tissue Doppler imaging in the estimation of left ventricular filling pressures: a comparative simultaneous Doppler-catheterization study

Ommen SR, Nishimura RA, Appleton CP, Miller FA, Oh JK, Redfield MM, Tajik AJ. *Circulation* 2000; 102: 1788–94.

Background

Diastolic dysfunction is being increasingly recognized as contributing to the signs and symptoms of heart failure. Doppler echocardiographic assessment of the mitral inflow was the mainstay for assessment of LV filling pressures and diastolic function, but limited by multiple factors that affect mitral flow, particularly ventricular relaxation. Tissue Doppler imaging (TDI) had been proposed to correct for relaxation and was examined in subsets of patients including restrictive[1] and hypertrophic cardiomyopathy[2]. This study sought to critically evaluate TDI by comparison with invasive assessment of LV filling pressures.

Methods and results

One hundred consecutive patients who were referred for cardiac catheterization underwent simultaneous Doppler echocardiography. Micro-manometer tipped catheters in the LV were used to determine mean LV diastolic pressure (M-LVDP) and the time constant of relaxation (T). Conventional pulsed-wave (PW) Doppler included the mitral inflow (early (E) and late (A) diastolic flow, deceleration time (DT) and E/A ratio), and the pulmonary vein (pulmonary vein systolic (PVs) and diastolic (PVd) velocity). Duration of the late diastolic flow was measured at mitral inflow and pulmonary vein. Mitral inflow was also assessed during the Valsalva manoeuvre. Tissue Doppler imaging of the septal and lateral mitral annulus was obtained in the apical four-chamber view for the early (E') and late (A') diastolic velocity. Tissue Doppler imaging intervals were also measured (deceleration time, time to peak velocity, and duration of velocity for E' and A').

Seventy-three patients were referred for evaluation of angina (62 of whom had CAD) with the remaining 27 for heart failure (6 of whom had CAD). Thirty-six patients had EF <50%. 94% of the mitral inflow (61% during Valsalva), 97% of the mitral TDI, and 73% of pulmonary venous signals were adequate.

T was modestly related to E' (r = 0.46), however, with scatter. Examining the standard Doppler variables that correlated with M-LVDP, E/A ratio was strongest (r = 0.59), followed by DT (r = 0.48), although this was mainly due to correlations in those with EF <50%. None of the TDI intervals showed a strong relation to M-LVDP. The best TDI parameter was septal E/E' (r = 0.64) and although this was better when EF <50%, it was reasonable when EF >50% (r = 0.6 and 0.47, respectively), and this was better than lateral E/E' (r = 0.51). The uncorrected E' and A' had weaker correlation.

Previously published criteria for Doppler variables were assessed to see if they predicted M-LVDP >12 mmHg (E/A >2, DT <130 msec, PVd >PVs, pulmonary late diastolic flow ≥30 msec longer than mitral, septal E/E' >10). Septal E/E' was the best, with 71% predictive accuracy for all patients (increasing to 76% if only those with interpretable signals were assessed), area under ROC curve (AUC) 0.82. Looking at M-LVDP >15 mmHg; septal E/E' again had the best AUC of 0.81, with septal E/E' >15 having 64% positive predictive value and E/E' <8 negative

predictive value of 97%. Importantly, this was independent of systolic function.

Some 85% of patients with E/E' <8 had normal M-LVDP and all patients with E/E' >15 had raised M-LVDP (see Figure 21.3). In the intermediate group (E/E' >8 but <15) conventional Doppler was useful; patients with change in E/A >0.5 with Valsalva and/or pulmonary late diastolic flow 30 msec longer than mitral had the highest filling pressures.

Strengths and limitations

As discussed in the study, the presence of RWMA may affect the accuracy of these measures. These patients are representative of those with cardiac disease as they had all been referred for cardiac catheterization. However, they may not be representative of a broader patient group. The fact that echocardiograms were done supine may also have decreased the success rate of some of the conventional techniques, although difficult image acquisition reflects real-world echocardiographic practice. The simultaneous invasive studies, however, are a particular strength, giving real insight into the associations with the echocardiographic measures.

Conclusions

The study confirmed that standard Doppler parameters were useful for assessing filling pressures in the context of systolic dysfunction, but not when systolic function was preserved. Combining the transmitral flow velocity with annular velocity combines the influence of transmitral

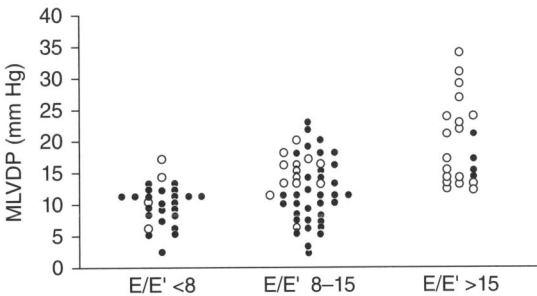

Figure 21.3 M-LVDP versus groups defined by septal E/E'. • indicates patients without conventional Doppler variables suggesting increased filling pressure; □, patients with PVa >30ms MVa; ◊, patients with positive Valsalva manoeuvre; and X, >1 positive variable.

Reproduced from Ommen SR. Clinical Utility of Doppler Echocardiography and Tissue Doppler Imaging in the Estimation of Left Ventricular Filling Pressures: A Comparative Simultaneous Doppler-Catheterization Study. *Circulation* 2000; 102: 15, with permission from Wolters Kluwer Health.

driving pressure with myocardial relaxation when assessing filling pressure. The annular velocity, however, is not a direct measure of relaxation as there was only a modest correlation between the two. Tissue Doppler imaging was easy to obtain and accurate and therefore was proposed as first line for assessment of LV filling pressures. Conventional Doppler measures are helpful when E/E' is between 8 and 15. This study confirmed the promise of TDI with excellent correlations with invasive measure of filling pressure. The importance of this paper is confirmed as TDI remains a central part of current European and American guidelines for assessment of diastolic function.

Learning points

- Tissue Doppler imaging is easy to obtain, with 97% success in this study.

- Septal E/E' is the best predictor of LV filling pressure.
  - <8 strongly predicts normal filling pressure.
  - >15 strongly predicts raised filling pressure.
- Conventional Doppler measures aid assessment when septal E/E' is between 8 and 15.
- E' is not a direct measure of myocardial relaxation.

Further reading

- Mottram PM, Marwick TH. Assessment of diastolic function: what the general cardiologist needs to know. *Heart* 2005; 91: 681–95.

Strain and strain rate imaging: a new clinical approach to quantifying regional myocardial function

Sutherland GR, Di SG, Claus P, D'hooge J, Bijnens B. *J Am Soc Echocardiogr* 2004; 17: 788–802.

Background

This review examined the clinical application of the emergence of strain and strain rate measurements. Strain is a measure of myocardial deformation, the change in length of a myocardial segment over time. Strain rate (SR) is the rate of change of these values. Using TDI a series of velocity curves show a velocity gradient along a length of the myocardial wall. A regression calculation between adjacent tissue velocity data points along this length generates the SR curve, which is then integrated to calculate strain[3]. Strain and SR can then be examined at different points in the cardiac cycle, normally referenced by examining the relationship to aortic valve opening and closure and mitral valve opening. Being a TDI technique it is dependent on alignment with the direction of movement and only strain in this direction can be measured. Strain can be:

1. Radial—directed outwards perpendicular to the epicardium; this can only be measured in the posterior wall on parasternal long or short axis views (difficulties in the septum likely due to the septum being composed of RV and LV myocardium with opposing radial vectors).

2. Longitudinal—parallel with the epicardium in the LV long axis from apex to base; can be measured on all apical long-axis views.

3. Circumferential—perpendicular to radial and longitudinal axis in line with the circumference of the LV short-axis; can be measured in the lateral wall on short-axis views.

There are published normal values in 20–40-year-olds for these measures[4]. Strain and SR are not direct measures of contractility, they are dependent on contraction, but also myocardial stiffness and loading conditions. Mathematical modelling suggest that reduced contractility (such as in ischaemic heart disease or cardiomyopathy) will reduce peak systolic strain, but so would preserved contractility with increased afterload. In contrast, increased preload would increase systolic strain. Strain rate is less dependent on loading conditions. Experimental studies support this, showing that regional SR correlates best with contractility and strain with global haemodynamic measures[5]. Discerning events down to a temporal resolution of about 90 msec is the maximum achievable by visual assessment of wall motion and thickening. Strain and SR analysis can improve this.

The real world clinical application of these measures was examined.

Ischaemic heart disease

There is a progressive reduction in peak systolic strain and SR with increasing severity of ischaemia. It is also possible to detect abnormal thickening of the myocardium after aortic valve closure, post-systolic thickening (PST). Post-systolic thickening can also be detected using M-mode echocardiography, for radial function in basal septum/posterior wall, and for global long axis function, but more detailed regional analysis is not possible.

Using dobutamine stress echo (DSE) these parameters can help distinguish stunned (adequate flow reserve post ischaemia) from actively ischaemic (inadequate flow reserve) myocardium. In stunned myocardium SR/peak strain improve with a decrease in PST, whereas in ischaemic myocardium SR/peak strain does not change or worsen with increasing PST[6]. Additionally, a partial thickness infarct can be distinguished from a transmural one. A partial thickness infarct will show reduced strain at rest, with no change or further reduced strain/SR and increased PST (ischaemic changes) with low-dose dobutamine, whereas a full thickness infarct will show either no strain or abnormal lengthening at rest with no improvement with dobutamine[7]. Clinical studies have replicated these findings, although measuring strain and SR is feasible with pharmacological stress but not with treadmill or bicycle exercise[8]. A practical approach was suggested for DSE: (1) visual inspection—if this looks entirely normal then this is highly predictive of normality. If there is a regional wall motion abnormality then go on to (2) velocity data—if confirms abnormal segmental peak velocity go to (3) strain/SR analysis to define the ischaemic substrate (see Figure 21.4).

Valvular heart disease

In aortic stenosis (AS) afterload related reduction in longitudinal systolic deformation corresponded with aortic valve area and stroke volume and regional deformation profiles could identify those with associated CAD[9]. At this stage there were limited data on the usefulness in regurgitant valve lesions.

Diastolic function

Regional abnormalities in diastolic function may be detectable despite standard measures of global diastolic function (mitral and pulmonary vein velocities) being normal[10]. Strain and SR offer regional diastolic information at high temporal resolution. Regional lengthening usually starts in the mid-inferior septal segment, sometimes before aortic valve closure. This propagates to the apex by the time of mitral valve opening, with the basal segments the last to lengthen, associated with early diastolic flow into the LV. After early filling there is shortening caused by passive recoil, followed by no deformation in diastasis, and finally further lengthening due to filling from atrial contraction. Circumferential shear strain can also be examined to look for abnormalities in twisting and untwisting. Abnormalities in strain and SR can differentiate controls from hypertensives and those with hypertension with and without diastolic dysfunction[11].

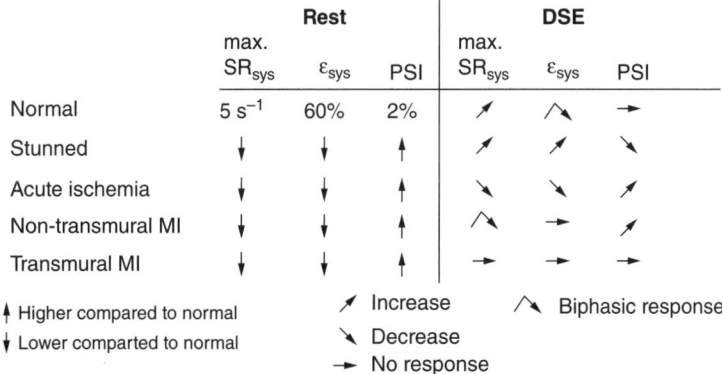

	Rest			**DSE**		
	max. SR$_{sys}$	ε_{sys}	PSI	max. SR$_{sys}$	ε_{sys}	PSI
Normal	5 s^{-1}	60%	2%	↗	⌃↘	→
Stunned	↓	↓	↑	↗	↗	↘
Acute ischemia	↓	↓	↑	↘	↘	↗
Non-transmural MI	↓	↓	↑	⌃↘	→	↗
Transmural MI	↓	↓	↑	→	→	→

↑ Higher compared to normal ↗ Increase ⌃↘ Biphasic response
↓ Lower comparted to normal ↘ Decrease
→ No response

Figure 21.4 Responses to dobutamine stress echocardiography.
PSI=post-systolic index, SR$_{sys}$=systolic strain rate, E$_{sys}$=systolic strain.

Reproduced from Sutherland GR, *et al*. Strain and strain rate imaging: a new clinical approach to quantifying regional myocardial function. *Journal of the American Society of Echocardiography* 2004; 17: 7, 788–802, with permission from Elsevier.

Cardiomyopathies

Strain and SR can discriminate hypertrophic cardiomyopathy (HCM) from physiological hypertrophy better than standard velocity profiles, and better assess response to septal ablation[12]. Dilated cardiomyopathy (DCM) is harder to study with these modalities due to thinner walls and spherical hearts.

Right ventricular function

Only longitudinal RV strain/SR data from the RV free wall can be reliably determined. Peak SR correlates with peak systolic pulmonary artery pressure. In pulmonary stenosis peak systolic strain was related to the systolic pressure increase in the RV[13]. Strain/SR data can also be useful in detecting subtle abnormalities in arrhythmogenic right ventricular dysplasia[14].

Other applications

Using strain/SR for monitoring is potentially more sensitive for detecting changes than standard echo parameters. This may be useful for assessing response to treatments/interventions, or for follow-up, particularly in challenging patients such as those with cardiac transplants or congenital heart disease.

Limitations

The comparison of two velocity data sets to produce the SR curve is susceptible to noise. The TDI technique is inherently angle dependent.

Conclusions

Use of TDI strain and SR imaging brought to the fore the potential of deformation parameters to allow more subtle abnormalities in regional function to be characterized in many disease states. The potential clinical utility in diagnosis and monitoring response to treatment led to rapidly increasing interest in strain assessment. Improvements in

post-processing software have aided analysis of TDI strain data. However, subsequent developments are now moving focus towards newer methods for assessing deformation. Magnetic resonance imaging (MRI) tissue tagging is the subject of much research interest and is subject to the advantages and disadvantages inherent with MRI, but in the field of echocardiography speckle tracking is gaining increasing momentum, primarily due to the removal of problems associated with angle dependence.

Learning points

- Strain is the change in length of a section of myocardium over time.
- Strain rate is a measure of the rate of change of strain.
- These measures of myocardial deformation are more sensitive for detection of abnormalities than standard echocardiographic parameters.
- Tissue Doppler velocity measures were the first to be widely used for this purpose.
- Problems with angle dependence and noise have led to a move towards speckle tracking echocardiography in modern echocardiographic strain assessment.

Further reading

- D'hooge J, Heimdal A, Jamal F, et al. Regional strain and strain rate measurements by cardiac ultrasound: principles, implementation and limitations. *Eur J Echocardiogr* 2000; 1: 154–70 [5].
- Geyer H, Caracciolo G, Abe H, et al. Assessment of myocardial mechanics using speckle tracking echocardiography: fundamentals and clinical applications. *J Am Soc Echocardiogr* 2010; 23: 351–69.

A randomized cross-over study for evaluation of the effect of image optimization with contrast on the diagnostic accuracy of dobutamine echocardiography in coronary artery disease: the OPTIMIZE Trial

Plana JC, Mikati IA, Dokainish H, Lakkis N, Abukhalil J, Davis R, Hetzell BC, Zoghbi WA. *JACC Cardiovasc Imaging* 2008; 1: 145–52.

Background

As reviewed earlier, harmonic imaging had improved image quality, negating the need for contrast studies in

some patients, but the effect of using contrast agents in stress echocardiography was less well characterized. This study examined the impact of contrast use on endocardial visualization, confidence of interpretation, and accuracy of DSE.

Methods and results

Patients with intermediate to high probability of CAD referred for DSE were recruited. They underwent two DSE examinations, one with contrast and one without. The study was a prospective, randomized, cross-over study with a random order of testing at least four hours apart within a 24-hour period. Each patient had the same sonographer for both studies which were performed on one of three machines; it is not clear if the same machine was used in individual patients. For the DSE, dobutamine was infused at 5 mcg/kg/min and increased every 3 minutes to 10, 20, 30, and 40 mcg/kg/min until the target heart rate was achieved. If <85% was achieved atropine in 0.25 mg boluses up to a maximum of 1 mg was given. Images were digitized at baseline, 5 and 10 mcg, and peak dobutamine. In the contrast study at the same time points 0.5 to 1 ml of contrast (Definity, BMS, USA) was given. A single, blinded, experienced observer assessed the images in random order. Regional wall motion was scored for 17-segments at baseline, low dose, and peak dose; normal, ischaemic—development or worsening of wall motion abnormality, scar—wall motion abnormality at rest with no change with stress. This was also done for coronary artery territories; left anterior descending (LAD), non-LAD (also split into circumflex (Cx) and right coronary artery (RCA)). Visualization of the endocardium was scored from 1 = adequate or better, 2 = incomplete endocardial border, 3 = epicardial border only, 4 = not visible, 5 = not obtained, 6 = contrast attenuated (>2 was considered not visualized). If the segment was seen in more than one view the best score was used. Confidence of interpretation for segments and coronary territories was scored 1 = high, 2 = medium, 3 = low. Invasive coronary angiography was carried out within 30 days and a stenosis of ≥70% considered significant.

A group of 108 patients were recruited, 101 had 2 DSE, 92 had coronary angiography, and 87 completed all the studies. Contrast agent increased the visualization of the endocardium at rest (75 ± 24% vs. 95 ± 8% segments) and stress (67 ± 27% vs. 96 ± 7%, p <0.001 for both). At peak stress this was true for all views, with the greatest improvement seen in apical two-chamber >apical four-chamber >short-axis >parasternal long-axis views. The contrast studies were interpreted with a much higher degree of confidence (high confidence 74% vs. 36% for non-contrast, p <0.001). The agreement with presence of CAD was higher with contrast studies, but not quite reaching statistical significance (68% vs. 57%, p = 0.06).

Accurate detection of ischaemia was better with contrast studies (66% vs. 53%, p = 0.02) but this was due to improvement in non-LAD territories (64% vs. 52%, p = 0.016), whereas the LAD territory was better but not significantly so (57% vs. 53%, p = 0.3). If an unenhanced study was interpreted with high confidence the use of contrast did not improve the detection of CAD; however, if the unenhanced study was interpreted with low confidence the accuracy improved from 36% to 68%, p = 0.01 with contrast (see Figure 21.5). This lower confidence of interpretation was associated with lower numbers of visualized segments. If all segments were visualized contrast agent had no effect on accuracy of CAD detection, whereas if >2 segments were not visualized accuracy increased from 28% to 59%, p = 0.005. Overall sensitivity and specificity for detection of CAD was 75% and 51% for unenhanced scans and 80% and 55% for contrast scans, respectively.

Strengths and limitations

The limitations of this study include the use of only luminal stenosis in major epicardial arteries as a predictor of ischaemia. Obviously this does not consider ischaemia due to microvascular dysfunction, but from a practical viewpoint this is an acceptable gold standard. Additionally, anti-ischaemic medications were not stopped prior to stress, perhaps contributing to the low specificity in this study.

Conclusions

As expected and previously shown, this study confirmed that contrast agent improved visualization and added

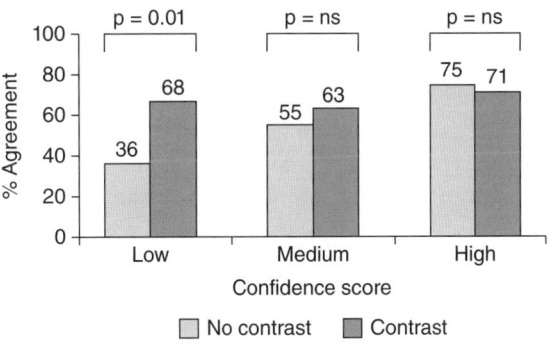

Figure 21.5 Percentage agreement with presence of CAD according to confidence of interpretation.

Reprinted from Plana JC, *et al*. A Randomized Cross-Over Study for Evaluation of the Effect of Image Optimization With Contrast on the Diagnostic Accuracy of Dobutamine Echocardiography in Coronary Artery Disease: The OPTIMIZE Trial. *JACC: Cardiovascular Imaging* 2008; 1: 2, 145–52, with permission from Elsevier.

that this was associated with corresponding improved detection of CAD. This study highlighted that this benefit came from studies where visualization and confidence of interpretation was poor. It also seems that this is less important in LAD disease, presumably due to easier detection of wall motion abnormalities in this larger territory. Difficulties in interpretation are relevant in real-world populations; this study didn't select patients based on image quality and approximately one quarter had >2 segments not visualized or low confidence of interpretation on unenhanced scans. This study would support the use of contrast agent for DSE when resting image quality is suboptimal.

> ## Learning points
>
> ◆ Contrast agent improves endocardial visualization and confidence of interpretation in dobutamine stress echocardiography.
> ◆ This is most helpful for apical views.

◆ Accuracy of detection of coronary disease was only significantly improved in patients with poor visualization or low confidence of interpretation on unenhanced rest scans.
◆ Improvement in detection was mainly due to detection of non-LAD disease.
◆ Contrast use should be planned for suboptimal resting scans.

Further reading

● Abdelmoneim SS, Dhoble A, Bernier M, *et al.* Quantitative myocardial contrast echocardiography during pharmacological stress for diagnosis of coronary artery disease: a systematic review and meta-analysis of diagnostic accuracy studies. *Eur J Echocardiogr* 2009; 10: 813–25.
● Arnold JR, Karamitsos TD, Pegg TJ, *et al.* Adenosine stress myocardial contrast echocardiography for the detection of coronary artery disease: a comparison with coronary angiography and cardiac magnetic resonance. *JACC Cardiovasc Imaging* 2010; 3: 934–43.

Feasibility and clinical decision-making with 3D echocardiography in routine practice

Hare JL, Jenkins C, Nakatani S, Ogawa A, Yu CM, Marwick TH. *Heart* 2008; 94: 440–5.

Background

Accurate assessment of LV function is important for prognosis, determining and monitoring response to therapy in cardiac disease. Quantification by 2D imaging is dependent on image quality and also depends on geometric assumptions regarding the LV. Cardiac MRI needs far less assumptions and is much more reproducible, but is limited by expense, availability, and is less suitable for unstable patients. Real-time 3D echo (RT-3DE) has comparable reproducibility to MRI and this study sought to examine its impact on clinical decision making.

Methods and results

A group of 249 patients referred for routine 2D echo at three centres (in different countries) were recruited; 168 unselected, 81 selected because of congestive heart failure/low EF. The final sample with both 2D and 3D studies was 220 (70% male). The identification of four clinically relevant thresholds was determined (1) LVEF <35% —indication for ICD (2) LVEF <40%—indication for systolic heart failure treatment (3) LV end-systolic volume index (LVESVI) >50 mL/m^2—indication for surgery in regurgitant valve disease (4) LVESVI >30 mL/m^2—prognosis post-MI.

Both 2D and 3D echo were done with respective probes using an ie33 (Philips) machine. Simpson's biplane was used for 2D volumes and EF and Qlab software (Philips) used for semi-automated LV border detection and resulting volume measurements. Real-time 3DE was feasible in 140 patients (83%), failure was mainly due to poor image quality in 24 (14%) with failure of ECG triggering in three, and one unknown reason. On average the RT-3DE took 5.2 minutes longer to acquire and analyse and was less in centres with lower average BMI. On the whole, cohort mean LVEF, LVESVI, and LV end-diastolic volume index (LVEDVI) values were not different with 2D and 3D studies. For LVEF <35%, 19 of 220 (9%) were reallocated, 16 from below to above 35% and 3 from above to below (although the figures in the text are slightly different from those in the table). For LVEF

<40%, 20 of 220 were reclassified (9%), 13 from below to above 40% and seven from above to below. For LVESVI >30 mL/m^2 RT-3DE reclassified 23 of 220 patents (10%), ten moved from below to above the threshold and 13 from above to below. For LVESVI >50 mL/m^2, 8 of 220 (4%) were reclassified, three from below to above the threshold and five from above to below. The presence of a RWMA did not affect re-categorization of LVEF. Twenty-one of 220 patients were visually assessed to have LVEF <40%; 2D echo re-categorized 10 of 220 (4%), five from below to above and five from above to below; RT-RTE re-categorized 10 of 220 (4%), eight from below to above and two from above to below. Visual EF correlated better with 2D than RT-3DE (r = 0.85 vs. r = 0.68).

Strengths and limitations

The reference values used for determining clinical management decisions came from studies using 2D echo; therefore although assessment using RT-3DE might be more accurate (referenced to CMR) it may actually agree less with the classification of these patients had they been in the original research trials. It is also not clear if both studies were performed in the same sitting or at different time intervals.

Conclusions

Real-time 3DE is feasible in >80% of patients with an acceptable increase in time (approximately five minutes). As with 2D, echo patients with increased BMI are more difficult. It is well reported that RT-3DE more accurately correlates with CMR, the gold standard, therefore this study showed that using this method did reclassify 4–10% of patients when examining standard clinical thresholds used to guide management. Real-time 3DE shows much promise. However, whether or not reclassification and subsequent change in clinical management improves outcome in these patients is yet to be proven.

Learning points

- It is established that 3D echo correlates better with the gold standard for cardiac volumes (MRI) than 2D echo.
- Three-dimensional echocardiography is feasible in >80% patients.
- Image acquisition and analysis requires only short increases in time (approx five minutes).
- Real-time 3DE results in reclassification of between 4 and 10% of patients in commonly used clinical thresholds for management decisions when compared with 2D echo.
- Impact of this reclassification on management and outcome is likely but not proven given use of 2D echo in most outcome studies that guide thresholds.

Further reading

- Jenkins C, Moir S, Chan J, Rakhit D, Haluska B, Marwick TH. Left ventricular volume measurement with echocardiography: a comparison of left ventricular opacification, three-dimensional echocardiography, or both with magnetic resonance imaging. *Eur Heart J* 2009; 30: 98–106.
- Pratali L, Molinaro S, Corciu AI, Pasanisi EM, Scalese M, Sicari R. Feasibility of real-time three-dimensional stress echocardiography: pharmacological and semi-supine exercise. *Cardiovasc Ultrasound* 2010; 8: 10.
- Pulerwitz T, Hirata K, Abe Y, *et al.* Feasibility of using a real-time 3-dimensional technique for contrast dobutamine stress echocardiography. *J Am Soc Echocardiogr* 2006; 19: 540–5.

Impact of contrast echocardiography on evaluation of ventricular function and clinical management in a large prospective cohort

Kurt M, Shaikh KA, Peterson L, Kurrelmeyer KM, Shah G, Nagueh SF, Fromm R, Quinones MA, Zoghbi WA. *J Am Coll Cardiol* 2009; 53: 802–10.

Background

It has been estimated that 10–15% of routine echocardiograms have incomplete endocardial resolution, reaching 25–30% in critically ill patients in the intensive care unit. Contrast echocardiography improves image quality and decreases variability of interpretation. The present study was therefore designed to prospectively evaluate the impact of contrast use on cardiac diagnosis and management compared with non-contrast studies in a large cohort of consecutive patients.

Methods and results

Patients who underwent technically difficult echocardiography and subsequent contrast echocardiography were enrolled. A complete echo was performed using either Sonos (Philips) or Vivid 7 (GE) machines optimizing the image and using harmonic imaging. If the echo was deemed technically difficult a contrast agent (Definity®) was used. Offline the non-contrast images were interpreted by one observer and the contrast images and whole study by another observer independently. Analysis was from a pool of six experienced observers. The following were assessed:

1. The number of LV segments visualized (normal vs. abnormal wall motion).
2. Visual estimate of LVEF.
3. The suspicion or presence of an LV thrombus.
4. Image quality (1 = adequate; 2 = technically difficult (>two non-visualized segments); and 3 = uninterpretable (>50% endocardium not visualized and unable to report LVEF)).

After analysis the primary physician was contacted and given the non-contrast findings; he was then asked whether he would order further diagnostic tests (TOE, nuclear, stress test, angiography) or alter the patient's medication. The contrast findings were then given and any changes to the answers to the original plan noted. A cost-benefit analysis was also performed.

A group of 632 patients were consecutively enrolled; this was 14.5 % of the total studies over the time period; 86% were in-patients (around one-third of these on ICU). The first observer deemed 86.7% of studies technically difficult, 11.7% uninterpretable, and 1.6% adequate. After contrast the technically difficult studies dropped from 86.7% to 9.8% and uninterpretable from 11.7% to 0.3%. Therefore adequate studies increased from 1.6% to 89.9% (p <0.0001). The number of visualized segments increased from 11.6 to 16.8 segments per patient (p <0.0001). The total number of abnormal segments visualized increased after contrast from 2.54 ± 4.8 segments to 3.87 ± 6.5 segments (p <0.0001). Interpretation of contrast images produced a significant change in LVEF (≥10%), in a total of 93 (16.7%) patients. The vast majority of these were underestimations of LVEF on the unenhanced contrast images (88 studies (94.5%)). For all the above, results were most marked in the surgical ICU group. The number of suspected thrombi decreased from 35 patients to only 1 patient after contrast utilization (p <0.0001).

Contrast led to avoidance of further diagnostic procedures in 207 patients (32.8%) because of improved assessment of LV function. The avoided procedures were either a TOE (67 patients, 32.4%) or a nuclear imaging study (140 patients, 67.7%). Again, the surgical ICU group had a greater degree of procedures avoided relative to the in-patient ward and outpatient groups (p <0.0001 for both).

From the cohort of 632 patients, 86 patients ultimately underwent coronary angiography, 58 because of the contrast study (22 became interpretable and showed LV dysfunction, 36 showed new wall motion abnormalities). The patients' medical regimen was altered in 67 patients (10.6%) after interpretation of contrast images (p <0.0001). The total impact of contrast (change in drugs, procedures, or both) was seen in 225 patients (35.6%) of suboptimal quality studies. The average savings or diagnostic cost-benefit was $122 per patient. There were no significant complications from contrast administration. Effect on management is summarized in Figure 21.6.

Strengths and limitations

The study was performed with a relatively large group of consecutive patients with no patient drop-out. In addition, each patient served as their own control, as all patients were evaluated both before and after contrast administration. The assessment of impact was obtained immediately before releasing the pre- and post-contrast image results to the primary physician, and then reviewing the medical chart to confirm these findings. One limitation with the design of this study is a bias from the primary physician. It is conceivable that a given physician may alter his or her responses to the question of patient management the more times he or she is contacted. This bias was unavoidable, but was thought to be small given the large number of physicians (n = 65) involved in the cohort over an extended period of time.

Conclusions

Contrast echocardiography in technically difficult patients significantly improves endocardial visualization and impacts cardiac diagnosis, resource utilization, and patient management. The improvement was more pronounced with increasing technical difficulty of the studies, which was more often seen in hospitalized and critically ill patients.

Learning points

◆ Contrast echocardiography:
  ● Decreases uninterpretable scans from approximately 12% to <1%.

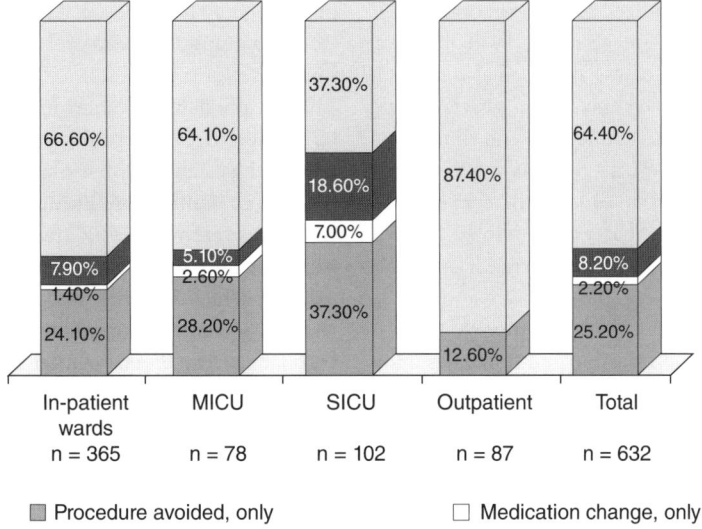

Figure 21.6 Frequency of total impact of contrast use on patient management. The highest impact was observed in inpatients, particularly in the SICU. *p <0.0001 comparing SICU with inpatient ward. †p <0.0001 comparing SICU with outpatients. ‡p <0.0004 comparing SICU and MICU.

Reprinted from Mustafa K, *et al.* Impact of Contrast Echocardiography on Evaluation of Ventricular Function and Clinical Management in a Large Prospective Cohort. *Journal of the American College of Cardiology* 2009; 53: 9, 802–10, with permission from Elsevier.

- Results in a >10% change in EF in approximately one in six patients.
- Is particularly useful to exclude LV thrombus.
- Reduces need for additional procedures (TOE and nuclear studies).
- Has the most benefit in surgical ICU patients.

Further reading

- Mulvagh SL, Rakowski H, Vannan MA, *et al.* American Society of Echocardiography Consensus Statement on the Clinical Applications of Ultrasonic Contrast Agents in Echocardiography. *J Am Soc Echocardiogr* 2008; 21: 1179–201.

Conclusion: the future

Echocardiography is of course only one of several imaging modalities that have evolved over recent years. There are several potential areas of overlap, with several techniques capable of evaluating left ventricular function, valvular heart disease, congenital lesions, and patients with coronary artery disease. What dictates which imaging technique is used on a particular patient in a particular institution depends upon a number of factors and many patients receive more than one type of scan to obtain the same diagnosis. There are some things that echo can do cheaper, quicker, and at the bedside, whereas there are

several conditions where other imaging modalities are clearly superior, albeit at a higher cost. International consensus on the most appropriate applications for echo and other imaging modalities, to avoid unnecessary duplication and keep down healthcare costs, would be our wish for the future. However, given the rate of growth of cardiac imaging over the past decade and the vested interests in the field, we are doubtful that this aspiration will be achieved in the foreseeable future.

Undoubtedly, the technological advances in echo will continue and these will benefit both the low end of the market and the more specialized application of the technique. Three-dimensional image quality will improve, we will see the ability to assess myocardial perfusion in 3D and the use of this technology to provide rapid assessment of left ventricular function. The time taken for an echo examination will decrease as a full-volume cardiac data set acquired in one cardiac cycle will contain all the information that a conventional 2D and Doppler study lasting 40–50 minutes currently contains. Further miniaturization of equipment will also occur so that the current hand-held systems will improve in quality, provide wireless communication and transmission of images, and will contain image recognition software that will provide some degree of automated interpretation/diagnosis. In that way, some forms of echo will be performed by non-specialists in the same way that electrocardiography with automated interpretation is used by all types of medical staff.

These predicted advances in the technique will need to be supported by rigorous, peer-reviewed evaluation of the type highlighted by these landmark papers. For example, a large multi-centre European study (Doppler CIP), which has received EU FP7 funding is currently recruiting to establish which cardiac imaging parameter(s), supplied by which imaging modality, is the most accurate and cost-effective for the follow-up of patients with stable coronary artery disease. Other studies of this type will be needed to help ensure that Echo, alongside its partner imaging modalities continues to evolve in the most appropriate direction in the future.

References

1. Garcia MJ, Rodriguez L, Ares M, et al. Differentiation of constrictive pericarditis from restrictive cardiomyopathy: Assessment of left ventricular diastolic velocities in longitudinal axis by Doppler tissue imaging. *J Am Coll Cardiol* 1996; 27: 108–14.

2. Nagueh SF, Lakkis NM, Middleton KJ, et al. Doppler estimation of left ventricular filling pressures in patients with hypertrophic cardiomyopathy. *Circulation* 1999; 99: 254–61.

3. Marwick TH. Measurement of strain and strain rate by echocardiography: ready for prime time? *J Am Coll Cardiol* 2006; 47: 1313–27.

4. Kowalski M, Kukulski T, Jamal F, et al. Can natural strain and strain rate quantify regional myocardial deformation? A study in healthy subjects. *Ultrasound Med Biol* 2001; 27: 1087–97.

5. Weidemann F, Jamal F, Sutherland GR, et al. Myocardial function defined by strain rate and strain during alterations in inotropic states and heart rate. *Am J Physiol Heart Circ Physiol* 2002; 283: H792–9.

6. Jamal F, Strotmann J, Weidemann F, et al. Noninvasive quantification of the contractile reserve of stunned myocardium by ultrasonic strain rate and strain. *Circulation* 2001; 104: 1059–65.

7. Weidemann F, Dommke C, Bijnens B, et al. Defining the transmurality of a chronic myocardial infarction by ultrasonic strain-rate imaging: implications for identifying intramural viability: an experimental study. *Circulation* 2003; 107: 883–8.

8. Davidavicius G, Kowalski M, Williams RI, et al. Can regional strain and strain rate measurement be performed during both dobutamine and exercise echocardiography, and do regional deformation responses differ with different forms of stress testing? *J Am Soc Echocardiogr* 2003; 16: 299–308.

9. Kowalski M, Herbots L, Weidemann F, et al. One-dimensional ultrasonic strain and strain rate imaging: a new approach to the quantitation of regional myocardial function in patients with aortic stenosis. *Ultrasound Med Biol* 2003; 29: 1085–92.

10. Garcia-Fernandez MA, Azevedo J, Moreno M, Bermejo J, Moreno R. Regional Left Ventricular Diastolic Dysfunction Evaluated by Pulsed-Tissue Doppler Echocardiography. *Echocardiography* 1999; 16: 491–500.

11. Yuda S, Short L, Leano R, Marwick TH. Myocardial abnormalities in hypertensive patients with normal and abnormal left ventricular filling: a study of ultrasound tissue characterization and strain. *Clin Sci* (Lond) 2002; 103: 283–93.

12. Abraham TP, Nishimura RA, Holmes DR, Jr., Belohlavek M, Seward JB. Strain rate imaging for assessment of regional myocardial function: results from a clinical model of septal ablation. *Circulation* 2002; 105: 1403–6.

13. Weidemann F, Eyskens B, Sutherland GR. New ultrasound methods to quantify regional myocardial function in children with heart disease. *Pediatr Cardiol* 2002; 23: 292–306.

14. Herbots L, Kowalski M, Vanhaecke J, Hatle L, Sutherland GR. Characterizing abnormal regional longitudinal function in arrhythmogenic right ventricular dysplasia. The potential clinical role of ultrasonic myocardial deformation imaging. *Eur J Echocardiogr* 2003; 4: 101–7.

Chapter 22

Cardiovascular magnetic resonance

Dr Manish Motwani, Dr Roy Jogiya, and Dr Sven Plein

After the first acquisition with magnetic resonance imaging (MRI) was published in 1973, MRI of the brain and body entered the clinical arena in the early 1980s. Although the potential of MRI to image the heart was recognized early on, the development of cardiovascular magnetic resonance, usually abbreviated to CMR, was initially hampered by the relatively long image acquisition times and the effects of respiratory and cardiac motion. With the advent of more rapid scan techniques and reliable electrocardiographic (ECG) gating, CMR was increasingly used as a research tool in the late 1980s and made its way into clinical practice soon after. Today,

CMR is a highly developed and uniquely versatile imaging modality with multiple clinical applications. The key advantages of CMR compared with other imaging methods are that it does not expose patients to ionizing radiation, that imaging planes can be freely defined, and that many tissue characteristics such as myocardial water, fat, or fibrosis content can be highlighted using an array of CMR methods. The landmark papers highlighted below have each made a particular contribution to the development of CMR as a clinical tool but are ultimately an arbitrary selection from the many outstanding publications in this rapidly expanding field.

Nuclear magnetic resonance tomography of the normal heart

Hawkes RC, Holland GN, Moore WS, Roebuck EJ, Worthington BS. *J Comput Assist Tomogr* 1981; 5: 605–12.

Background

It is difficult to know with certainty when CMR was first performed. The heart and great vessels can be recognized on early MRI images of the chest—but these investigations were not directed at the cardiovascular system. In 1981 Hawkes and colleagues from the University of Nottingham in the UK published a paper that specifically related to cardiac MRI (formerly termed 'nuclear magnetic resonance tomography'), which is widely considered the first landmark paper in the field of CMR.

Methods

Acquisition of a single image took 150 seconds with pixel dimensions of $4 \times 4 \times 10$ mm, interpolated to an in-plane image display of 2×2 mm. The resultant images required corresponding anatomical sections and line drawing for illustration of the anatomy but were of sufficient quality to recognize the future potential of CMR.

Impact on clinical practice

In their introduction, the authors highlighted the major advantage of MRI, which is the lack of ionizing radiation exposure; but also recognized the limitations imposed by cardiac and respiratory motion. They speculated on the potential to overcome image blurring due to cardiac motion by using ECG-triggering. Three years later, Lanzer *et al.*, from the University of California in San Francisco (UCSF) reported ECG-gated CMR in three volunteers, establishing one of the key methods for all future CMR applications.

Conclusions

This was the first published report of CMR, and in the ensuing years the field of CMR has witnessed rapid growth in both clinical and research arenas.

Learning points

- The first CMR images were acquired in the early 1980s.
- Successful CMR requires compensation of cardiac and respiratory motion.

Further reading

- Lanzer P, Botvinick EH, Schiller NB, *et al*. Cardiac imaging using gated magnetic resonance. *Radiology* 1984; 150: 121–7.

Coronary magnetic resonance angiography for the detection of coronary stenoses

Kim WY, Danias PG, Stuber M, Flamm SD, Plein S, Nagel E, Langerak SE, Weber OM, Pedersen EM, Schmidt M, Botnar RM, Manning WJ. *N Engl J Med* 2001; 345(26): 1863–9.

Background

X-ray coronary angiography remains the most widely used test for detecting clinically significant coronary artery disease (CAD). However, it involves exposure to ionizing radiation and a small risk of procedural complications including death. Furthermore, a substantial proportion of patients who undergo coronary angiography are not found to have any significant CAD. An accurate non-invasive technique for the diagnosis of CAD would therefore be an important advance. The first clinical evaluation of coronary magnetic resonance angiography (MRA) was reported in 1993, but wider clinical evaluation was lacking.

Purpose

This was a prospective multi-centre study performed to determine the clinical usefulness of coronary MRA in the diagnosis of native-vessel CAD. The aim was to overcome some of the previous criticisms of single-centre studies, including non-standardized hardware and scanning protocols.

Patients

A group of 109 subjects were recruited to the study at seven institutions in Europe and the USA. All subjects were scheduled to undergo elective X-ray coronary angiography for suspected CAD within 14 days. Exclusion criteria were standard contraindications to magnetic resonance imaging (such as pacemaker or other implantable metallic devices) or sublingual nitrate. In all cases, coronary MRA was performed before X-ray angiography.

Methods

All coronary images were acquired at 1.5-T in mid-diastole using common hardware and standard protocols. A diaphragmatic respiratory navigator was used to compensate for respiratory motion by only accepting end-expiratory data. Images were read by a consensus of two experienced investigators, blinded to clinical and X-ray data. Coronary segments that were not visualized, or that were graded as having poor image quality, were not included in the subsequent analysis. Good quality images were further classified according to disease severity. The diagnostic performance of MRA to detect significant CAD (as determined by X-ray angiography) was determined for each individual vessel and for each patient.

Results

Of the 109 subjects, 759 coronary segments were potentially available for analysis. In 636 (84%) of these, image quality of coronary MRA was sufficient for analysis. The sensitivity, specificity, negative predictive value (NPV), and positive predictive value (PPV) of MRA to detect any significant CAD in a patient were 93% (95% CI: 88–98%), 42% (95% CI: 32–52%), 81% (95% CI: 73–89%), and 70% (95% CI: 61–79%), respectively. The overall diagnostic accuracy (percentage of coronary segments correctly classified) was 72% (95% CI: 63–81%), increasing to 87% (95% CI: 81–93%) for the identification of patients with left main stem (LMS) or three-vessel CAD. Four patients with significant CAD not detected by coronary MRA had isolated single-vessel disease, with two having isolated left circumflex (LCx) artery disease.

Strengths

This was the first prospective multi-centre study of CMR and the first to compare coronary MRA with X-ray angiography. A standardized protocol was applied in all seven centres worldwide. It showed a reasonable diagnostic accuracy and high NPV especially for patients with LMS and three-vessel CAD.

Limitations

This study had several limitations. Coronary MRA was limited to the proximal coronary segments only and even then 16% of coronary segments and 6% of the study patients could not be fully assessed. The LCx artery was less reliably visualized—presumably due to its relatively small calibre and posterior location resulting in a lower signal-to-noise ratio because of the increased distance from the receiver coils. However, isolated LCx disease was found in only 4% of subjects, suggesting that the absence of clinically significant disease in the remaining coronary system makes LCx disease unlikely, but the poor detection of disease in this vessel remains an important limitation. Furthermore, the recruitment was performed over a one-year period and less than 16 patients were recruited from each centre, raising the question of how applicable this select population is to the usual population referred for coronary angiography. Finally, the scan time was on average 70 minutes, substantially longer than a diagnostic X-ray angiogram or cardiac computed tomography (CCT).

Impact on clinical practice

The small size, tortuous course, and rapid motion of coronary arteries make MRA a demanding technique, which requires very high spatial and temporal resolution. This paper suggests that using coronary MRA for CAD detection may be useful in certain subgroups. For example, in patients with severe left ventricular (LV) impairment without a clinical history of myocardial infarction (MI), MRA may be able to reliably discriminate between severe multi-vessel CAD and non-ischaemic cardiomyopathy—thus avoiding referral for X-ray angiography in the latter. However, despite the significant progress with coronary MRA that this study demonstrates, its main application in current clinical practice remains the identification of anomalous coronary artery origins.

Conclusions

This first multi-centre study of coronary MRA demonstrated that the method has reasonable sensitivity, NPV and overall accuracy for detecting CAD, particularly in patients with three-vessel or LMS disease. This is clinically relevant as surgical revascularization in patients with such disease is prognostically beneficial. Widespread uptake of coronary MRA as a clinical tool has, however, been limited by long scan durations, limited coverage of distal coronary segments, the required level of expertise, relatively low specificity, and significant advances in competing imaging modalities, most notably CCT. With ongoing technological advances, coronary MRA continues to improve, and has also recently been used to image the coronary vessel wall.

> ### Learning points
>
> ◆ Coronary MRA may be used to delineate the course of coronary arteries and may detect proximal coronary artery stenosis, especially in multi-vessel disease.

Further reading

● Jahnke C, Paetsch I, Nehrke K, *et al.* Rapid and complete coronary arterial tree visualization with magnetic resonance imaging: feasibility and diagnostic performance. *Eur Heart J* 2005; 26: 2313–9.

The use of contrast-enhanced magnetic resonance imaging to identify reversible myocardial dysfunction

Kim RJ, Wu E, Rafael A, Chen EL, Parker MA, Simonetti O, Klocke FJ, Bonow RO, Judd RM. *N Engl J Med* 2000; 343(20): 1445–53.

Background

In patients with LV dysfunction and CAD, the distinction between viable and non-viable myocardium is important in making revascularization decisions. In the late 1990s, contrast-enhanced CMR had been demonstrated to accurately delineate the transmural extent of scar and to discriminate between reversible and irreversible myocardial injury in animal models and patients. The effect of hyperenhancement of infarcted or fibrotic myocardium was thought to be related to its higher distribution volume compared with viable myocardium. The spatial resolution of this method is in the millimeter range, allowing a highly detailed accurate assessment of the transmural extent of infarction.

Purpose

In this study, contrast-enhanced CMR was used to predict whether regions of myocardial dysfunction improve after revascularization.

Patients

Fifty patients scheduled to undergo coronary revascularization and with regional wall motion abnormalities on either contrast ventriculography or echocardiography were included. Exclusion criteria were unstable angina, NYHA class IV heart failure, and standard contraindications to CMR. All patients underwent baseline cine and contrast enhanced CMR. Forty-one of the patients underwent repeat CMR 79 ± 36 days after revascularization (27 underwent CABG and 14 PCI).

Methods

Cine CMR images were analysed before and after revascularization by two observers blinded to clinical and contrast-enhanced image data. Segmental wall thickening was graded in consensus on a scale of 0–4 (0 = normal, 4 = dyskinetic) and contrast-enhanced images were scored independently on a scale 0–4 (reflecting increments of 25% scar transmurality). A logistic regression model was used to determine the relationship between the transmural extent of hyperenhancement and improvement in contractility on a segmental basis.

Results

At baseline, 2093 myocardial segments were available for analysis—804 (38%) had abnormal contractility and 694 segments (33%) had hyperenhancement. The transmural extent of hyperenhancement in dysfunctional segments at baseline was significantly related to the likelihood of improved contractility after revascularization (p <0.001). Accordingly, in segments with no hyperenhancement, contractility improved in 78% after revascularization, compared to 60% with 1–25% transmural hyperenhancement, 42% with 26–50% transmural hyperenhancement, 10% with 51–75% transmural hyperenhancement, and 2% in those with >75% transmural hyperenhancement.

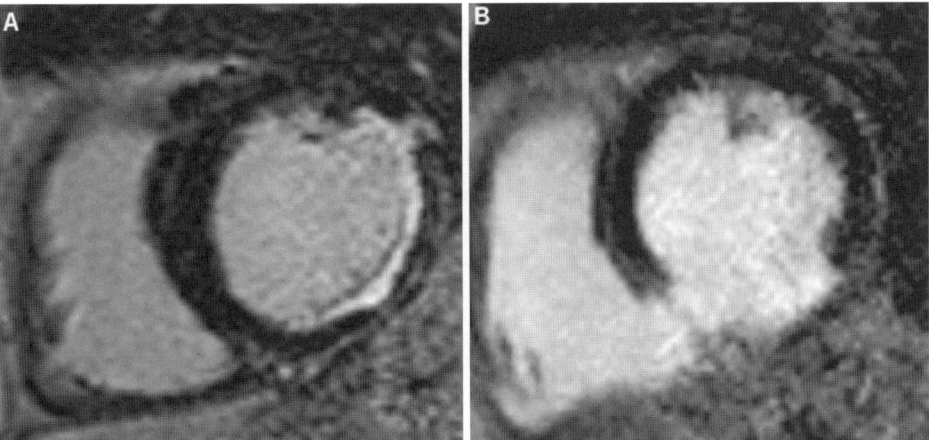

Figure 22.1 Example of LGE images showing myocardial infarction. (A) <25% transmural hyperenhancement in the lateral segments indicates a good chance of functional recovery after revascularization. (B) 100% transmurality in the inferior wall makes recovery unlikely (non-viable).

The association between viability and improvement in global ventricular function was also assessed. An increasing extent of dysfunctional but viable myocardium correlated with greater improvements in both the mean wall-motion score and the ejection fraction (EF) after revascularization (p <0.001).

Strengths

This study was the first to show that the transmural extent of infarction as measured by contrast enhanced CMR is inversely proportional to the likelihood of recovery of function post-revascularization. This landmark paper defined contrast-enhanced CMR as the method of choice for the assessment of myocardial viability and scar (Figure 22.1).

Limitations

The study had some limitations. Analyses of wall motion and the magnitude of hyperenhancement were performed visually rather than by quantitative measurements. Follow-up studies were performed 11 weeks after revascularization, which may be too soon to see the full functional improvement in hibernating myocardium. The mean EF in the group was 43%, therefore raising the question as to how applicable this might be to patients with more severe LV impairment.

Clinical impact

The study demonstrated the clinical value of contrast-enhanced CMR as a powerful tool for the management of

patients considered for coronary revascularization and is widely considered as the study with the largest impact on the clinical use of CMR (Figure 22.1).

Conclusion

Due to its high spatial resolution and tissue contrast, contrast-enhanced CMR can be used to demonstrate the transmural extent of non-viable myocardium and predict recovery of contractile function in patients with chronic ischaemic heart disease. Dysfunctional segments with less than 25% transmural hyperenhancement are likely to recover after revascularization, whilst those with more than 50% transmural hyperenhancement have a very low probability (10%) of recovery.

Learning points

◆ Cardiac magnetic resonance is a powerful test in patients with previous MI and can predict functional recovery after revascularization.

Further reading

● Kim RJ, Fieno DS, Parrish TB, *et al*. Relationship of MRI Delayed Contrast Enhancement to Irreversible Injury, Infarct Age, and Contractile Function. *Circulation* 1999; 100: 1992–2002.

Abnormal subendocardial perfusion in cardiac syndrome X detected by cardiovascular magnetic resonance imaging

Panting JR, Gatehouse PD, Yang GZ, Grothues F, Firmin DN, Collins P, Pennell DJ. *N Engl J Med* 2002; 346(25): 1948–53.

Background

Up to 20% of patients with typical angina have a normal coronary angiogram. The term 'cardiac syndrome X' (CSX) has often been used to describe the constellation of typical angina, positive exercise stress test, and normal coronary angiography. Various mechanisms have been proposed, including microvascular dysfunction and metabolic abnormalities—but the cause of this phenomenon remains poorly understood. Previous studies with SPECT and PET have attempted to investigate the presence of ischaemia, but results have been inconsistent. Some studies have found abnormal perfusion in only a few subjects and others in the majority. At the time of this landmark paper, it was therefore unclear as to whether symptoms in CSX are non-ischaemic in origin or whether the inconsistent results in previous studies reflect a lack of sensitivity in detecting subendocardial ischaemia.

Purpose

Given the higher spatial resolution of CMR over other myocardial perfusion imaging techniques, this study investigated whether CMR would identify subendocardial ischaemia in patients with CSX.

Patients

Myocardial perfusion CMR was performed in 20 patients diagnosed with CSX. They all had a history of exertional angina, abnormal exercise ECG, and a normal coronary angiogram with no inducible spasm on ergonovine provocation testing. They were matched against ten similar age-matched asymptomatic controls.

Methods

Myocardial perfusion CMR scans were performed at 1.5 Tesla at rest and during adenosine hyperaemia, using a gradient-echo sequence with T1 weighting and acquiring two short axis sections. The myocardium was divided into subendocardial and subepicardial regions. Normalized upslope of myocardial signal enhancement was measured to derive the myocardial perfusion index (MPI) and the myocardial-perfusion reserve index (MPRI)—the ratio of MPI at stress to rest. All patients scored the level of pain associated with the infusion from 1 (no pain) to 5 (worst pain ever experienced).

Results

Adenosine provoked chest pain in 95% of patients with CSX and in 40% of controls. In the control group, MPI significantly increased with adenosine in both the subendocardium (0.12 ± 0.03 to 0.16 ± 0.03, $p = 0.02$) and subepicardium (from 0.11 ± 0.02 to 0.17 ± 0.05, $p = 0.002$). In patients with CSX however, MPI did not change significantly in the subendocardium (0.13 ± 0.02 vs. 0.14 ± 0.03, $p = 0.11$), but increased in the subepicardium (from 0.11 ± 0.02 to 0.20 ± 0.04, $p < 0.001$). Consequently, the ratio of subendocardial to subepicardial MPRI was significantly lower in patients with CSX (0.61 ± 0.11 vs. 0.85 ± 0.13, $p = 0.002$). According to ROC curve analysis, the optimal ratio of subendocardial to subepicardial MPRI for distinguishing CSX patients from controls was 0.72, which yielded a diagnostic accuracy of 90%.

Strengths

Making use of the high spatial resolution of myocardial perfusion CMR, this study demonstrated that subendocardial perfusion abnormalities occur in patients with CSX. These results support the view that the chest pain in these patients may be related to myocardial ischaemia, due to global subendocardial hypoperfusion. The study was one of the key publications to prominently demonstrate the advantages of MRI over other imaging modalities for the assessment of myocardial perfusion.

Limitations

The study has been criticized for not including LV function measurements during stress. It has been suggested that the study therefore cannot prove whether the perfusion images obtained after adenosine are accompanied by the development of myocardial dysfunction and represent ischaemia rather than heterogeneity in transmural perfusion. Furthermore, full quantification of myocardial blood flow, although feasible from CMR myocardial perfusion data, was not performed in this study.

Impact on clinical practice

This study suggested that CMR could be used to demonstrate more subtle myocardial perfusion abnormalities in patients with CSX than can be detected with other methods.

Conclusion

Although this was a landmark paper, its results continue to be discussed. A subsequent CMR study by Vermelt-foort *et al.* in 20 patients with angina and normal coronary angiography showed that MPI increased in both the subendocardial and subepicardial layers by a comparable amount during adenosine infusion. However, the latter study was criticized for its selection (95% had positive SPECT, only 25% had a positive exercise test). A subsequent study in patients with CSX by Lanza *et al.* found abnormal perfusion with CMR and a reduced coronary flow response with high-resolution transthoracic echo Doppler in the LAD artery, supporting the hypothesis of coronary microcirculation dysfunction.

In conclusion, after more than 30 years and a number of different studies, the mechanisms of chest pain in patients with CSX remain open to debate. Although in a good prognostic group, the study by Panting *et al.* was important to help in at least identifying patients who suffer from ischaemia and therefore require closer monitoring and suitable therapy.

Learning points

- ◆ Cardiac magnetic resonance is a powerful test for the assessment of myocardial perfusion due to its high spatial resolution.

Further reading

- Lanza GA, Buffon A, Sestito A, *et al.* Relation between stress-induced myocardial perfusion defects on cardiovascular magnetic resonance and coronary microvascular dysfunction in patients with cardiac syndrome X. *J Am Coll Cardiol* 2008; 51: 466–72.
- Vermeltfoort IAC, Bondarenko O, Raijmakers WRP, *et al.* Is subendocardial ischemia present in patients with chest pain and normal coronary angiograms? A cardiovascular MR study. *Eur Heart J* 2007; 28: 1554–8.

Utility of cardiac magnetic resonance imaging in the diagnosis of hypertrophic cardiomyopathy

Rickers C, Norbert M. Wilke, Jerosch-Herold M, Casey SA, Panse P, Panse N, Weil J, Zenovich AG, Maron BJ. *Circulation* 2005; 112: 855–6.

Background

Hypertrophic cardiomyopathy (HCM) is a relatively common form of inherited cardiomyopathy and is the most frequent cause of sudden cardiac death in the young. At the time of this paper, echocardiography was the standard test used to diagnose HCM. However, echocardiography can be limited by acoustic windows and poor visualization of the apex. Cardiac magnetic resonance can overcome these difficulties, with the ability to image in any plane, and offers highly reproducible measures of LV volumes, EF, and LV mass.

Purpose

The purpose of this study was to determine whether CMR has a greater diagnostic performance than echocardiography in detecting HCM and assessing the extent of LVH.

Patients

This prospective study enrolled 48 consecutive patients in whom a diagnosis of HCM was either suspected or established. Patients were aged 8–69 years (mean 34 ± 16 years) and 34 (71%) were male. Exclusions included standard contraindications to CMR.

Methods

Patients were imaged by both 2D-echocardiography and CMR to assess maximum end-diastolic LV wall thickness in eight anatomical segments (total n = 384 segments). Measurements were made independently by two observers, blinded to the imaging data from the other test. Diagnosis of HCM was based on the presence of LVH without cavity dilatation, in the absence of another cardiac or systemic cause. All patients had the echocardiogram performed first, followed by CMR on the same day.

Results

Maximum LV thickness was similar by echocardiography and CMR (21.7 ± 9.1 vs. 22.5 ± 9.6 mm; p = 0.21). However, echocardiography did not detect LVH in 3 (6%), which CMR subsequently identified to have areas of wall thickening in the anterolateral LV free wall (17–20 mm), which resulted in a new diagnosis of HCM. Compared with CMR, echocardiography underestimated the magnitude of LVH in the basal anterolateral free wall (17 ± 8 vs. 13 ± 6 mm; $p = 0.001$); and the presence of extreme LV wall thickness (≥ 30 mm), which was found in six patients ($p < 0.05$).

Strengths

A relatively small (~5%) but important patient subset was confirmed to have HCM solely by the identification of regional LVH (confined to the anterolateral region) by CMR. This had not been clearly delineated in prior comparative CMR and echocardiographic studies in HCM.

Limitations

This was a small observational study, which only looked at a small number of patients with known or suspected HCM. It did not evaluate end points of cardiovascular death, sudden cardiac death, or heart failure death.

Impact on clinical practice

This landmark paper strongly suggests that the approach to the diagnosis of HCM in the contemporary era should involve CMR imaging, particularly when echocardiography images are limited.

Conclusions

Cardiac magnetic resonance is capable of identifying regions of LVH that are sometimes missed by echocardiography—upon which the diagnosis of the HCM can depend. Cardiac magnetic resonance enhances the assessment of LVH, especially in the anterolateral region and offers an important supplemental test with distinct diagnostic advantages for selected HCM patients.

Learning points

- Due to its greater spatial resolution and unlimited imaging planes, CMR can more reliably detect subtle morphological abnormalities of the heart than echocardiography in the diagnosis of cardiomyopathy.

Further reading

- Moon JC, McKenna WJ, McCrohon JA, *et al.* Toward clinical risk assessment in hypertrophic cardiomyopathy with gadolinium cardiovascular magnetic resonance. *J Am Coll Cardiol* 2003; 41: 1561–7.

Cardiovascular magnetic resonance assessment of human myocarditis: a comparison to histology and molecular pathology

Mahrholdt H, Goedecke C, Wagner A, Meinhardt G, Athanasiadis A, Vogelsberg H, Fritz P, Klingel K, Kandolf R, Sechtem U. *Circulation* 2004; 109(10): 1250–8.

Background

Myocarditis has been reported in up to 12% of young adults with sudden cardiac death and up to 10% of cases develop a chronic dilated cardiomyopathy. Myocarditis can be difficult to diagnose clinically and invasive endomyocardial biopsy is limited by the associated risks and the dependency on biopsying an affected area.

Purpose

The aim of this study was to determine whether CMR can visualize areas of active myocarditis as defined by histopathology. The study also investigated whether CMR could be used to follow the progression of the disease.

Patients

Fifty-eight patients were initially identified based on clinical suspicion. Twenty-one patients were excluded on the basis of angiographic findings of CAD or coronary

spasm, or refused to undergo CMR followed by myocardial biopsy (n = 3). Thirty-two patients fulfilled the clinical criteria for myocarditis and underwent CMR.

Methods

The CMR protocol included cine and late-gadolinium enhancement (LGE) imaging. To determine whether CMR visualizes areas of active myocarditis, endomyocardial biopsies were taken from the region of contrast enhancement on LGE images. The samples were sent for histopathological assessment. A follow-up scan was performed three months later.

Results

Of the 32 patients, contrast enhancement was seen in 28 (88%), usually in a patchy distribution most frequently located in the lateral wall. Endomyocardial biopsy was performed in all 32 patients. Of the 28 patients with enhancement on LGE imaging, biopsies were obtained in the enhanced regions in 21. Histopathologic analysis revealed active myocarditis in 19 patients (parvovirus B19, n = 12; human herpes virus type 6 (HHV6), n = 5). In the remaining 11 patients, in whom biopsies could not be taken from the region of contrast enhancement, active myocarditis was found in one case only (HHV6). Four patients without contrast enhancement had myocarditis without evidence of viral infection on histopathology.

Twenty patients with contrast enhancement in the acute setting attended three months later for a repeat CMR study. At the follow-up scan, the area of contrast enhancement decreased from 9 ± 11% to 3 ± 4% of LV mass and the LVEF improved from 47 ± 19% to 60 ± 10% (Figure 22.2).

Strengths

This study was unique in that patients had both LGE imaging and underwent 'CMR-guided' biopsy in the area of contrast enhancement. The study was therefore able to directly correlate CMR findings and histopathological features.

Limitations

The study included a higher than expected number of patients with myocarditis due to HHV.

Clinical impact

This study has shown that CMR can help identify patients with active myocarditis in the setting of suspected myocardial infection or new onset of heart failure. Based on the results of this and other studies, CMR is now a commonly used test in patients presenting with chest pain and normal coronary angiograms. Furthermore, contrast-enhanced CMR provides information on the exact localization of myocarditis that can be used to guide biopsy, enhancing sensitivity and specificity.

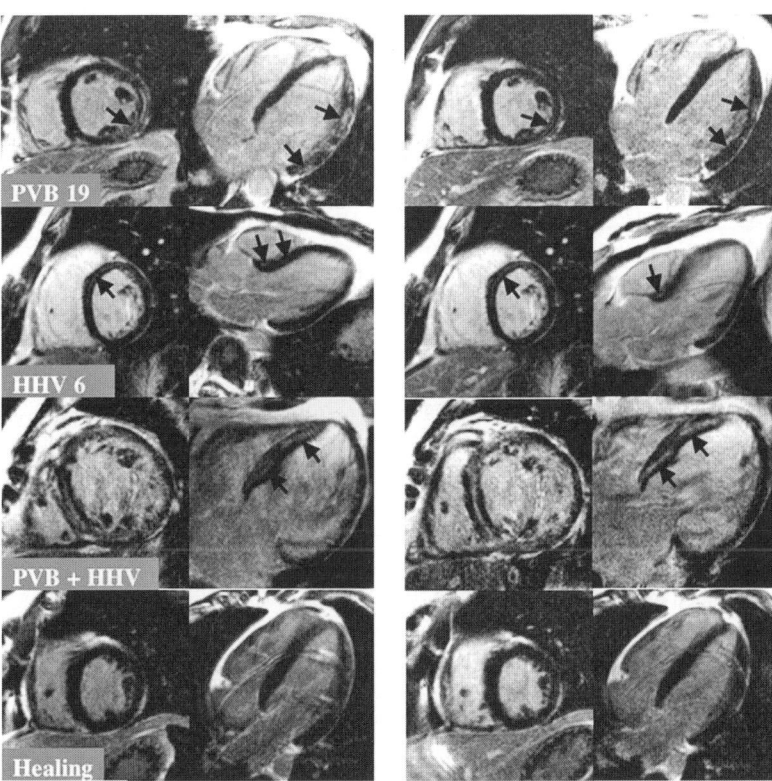

Figure 22.2 Areas of contrast enhancement seen acutely (left) decreased at follow-up (right) as average EF and EDV returned toward normal.

Reproduced from Mahrholdt H. Cardiovascular Magnetic Resonance Assessment of Human Myocarditis: A Comparison to Histology and Molecular Pathology. *Circulation* 2004; 16; 109: 1250–8, with permission from Wolters Kluwer Health.

Conclusions

The authors concluded that contrast enhancement is a frequent finding in the clinical setting of suspected myocarditis and is associated with active inflammation defined by histopathology. Cardiac magnetic resonance findings in myocarditis were most commonly seen in the lateral free wall, consistent with previous post-mortem studies. The areas of contrast enhancement decreased over time as EF and EDV returned toward normal. Incremental diagnostic information can be gained by combining T1 and T2-weighted spin-echo with LGE imaging methods. The role of myocardial damage as measured by contrast CMR as a predictor for long-term outcome warrants further investigation.

Learning points

◆ Cardiac magnetic resonance can significantly aid the diagnosis of myocarditis.

Further reading

● Friedrich MG, Sechtem U, Schulz-Menger J, *et al.* Cardiovascular magnetic resonance in myocarditis: A JACC White Paper. *J Am Coll Cardiol* 2009; 53: 1475–87

MR-IMPACT: comparison of perfusion-cardiac magnetic resonance with single-photon emission computed tomography for the detection of coronary artery disease in a multicentre, multivendor, randomized trial

Schwitter J, Wacker CM, van Rossum AC, Lombardi M, Al-Saadi N, Ahlstrom H, Dill T, Larsson HB, Flamm SD, Marquardt M, Johansson L. *Eur Heart J* 2008; 29: 480–9.

Background

Myocardial perfusion imaging is important in the management of patients with CAD. It helps treatment decisions with regards to optimizing medical therapy and planning revascularization. Cardiac magnetic resonance is emerging as an alternative to nuclear techniques (SPECT and PET) and has several advantages, including higher spatial resolution, better detection of subendocardial ischaemia, shorter scanning times, and, most importantly, the absence of radiation exposure (Figure 22.3).

Purpose

The Magnetic Resonance Imaging for Myocardial Perfusion Assessment in Coronary Artery Disease Trial (MR-IMPACT) was designed to evaluate perfusion CMR in a multi-centre, multi-vendor trial. Aims of the study were to compare the effects of five different contrast doses on image quality and diagnostic accuracy of perfusion CMR. Using the optimum dose of contrast, the diagnostic performance of stress perfusion CMR for the detection of significant coronary stenosis was then compared with SPECT using quantitative angiography as the reference.

Patients

Eligible patients were those scheduled for a coronary angiography (CXA) and/or a SPECT examination for clinical reasons. Before study entry, all patients had to agree to undergo all three tests (CXA, SPECT, and CMR). Exclusion criteria included acute MI within a week before enrolment, unstable angina, previous CABG, decompensated heart failure, and any of the standard contraindications to CMR or adenosine infusion. After exclusions, there were 225 eligible patients with suspected CAD from 18 centres across Europe and the USA. A further 13 studies were excluded (five CMR and eight SPECT) due to inadequate image quality leaving a sample size of 212 for analysis.

Methods

The study had a prospective, double-blind, randomized trial design. All enrolled subjects underwent CXA, SPECT, and perfusion CMR, and were randomly assigned to receive one of five different doses of a gadolinium-based contrast agent (Omniscan) for the CMR study. The SPECT examinations were performed according to current guidelines, using scanners of different vendors, Technetium or Thallium, on one or two-day protocols, and gated or ungated image (~50% studies) acquisition.

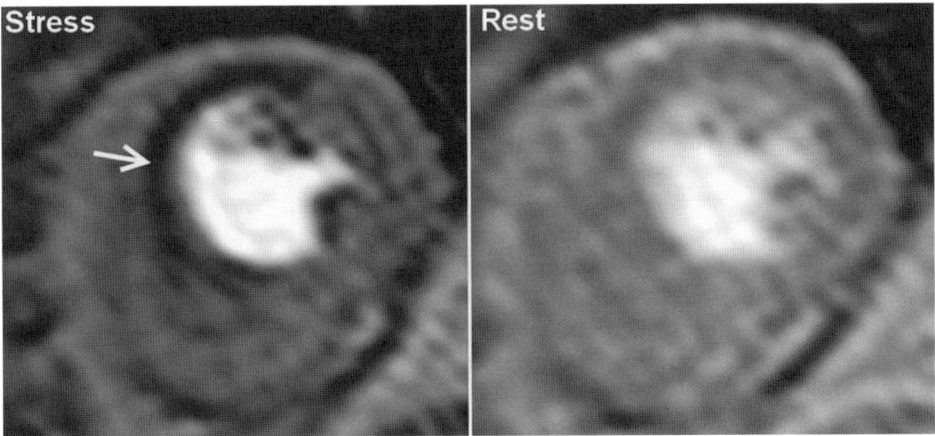

Figure 22.3 Example of perfusion CMR images showing a mid-anterior/anteroseptal stress-induced perfusion defect (white arrow).

Coronary angiography and SPECT had to be performed within four weeks of CMR.

Three experienced readers, blinded to the results of other tests interpreted the data at an independent core laboratory. A semi-quantitative perfusion score was assigned to 16 segments of the left ventricle. The average perfusion score of the three readers for SPECT and CMR were compared using receiver operating characteristic (ROC) curve analysis. Luminal narrowing >50% by quantitative angiography was taken as the reference standard for CAD.

Results

The optimal dosage of gadolinium for perfusion CMR was 0.1 mmol/kg. Using the subgroup of 42 patients randomized to this dose, perfusion CMR was at least as good as SPECT for the detection of CAD on head-to-head analysis (AUC 0.86 ± 0.06 vs. 0.75 ± 0.09; p = 0.12) using angiography as the reference standard. When comparing diagnostic accuracy of perfusion CMR at the optimal contrast dose (n = 42) to the entire SPECT population (n = 212), CMR was found to be superior (AUC: 0.86 ± 0.06 vs. 0.67±0.5, p = 0.013). The differences between perfusion CMR and gated-SPECT did not reach statistical significance. For multi-vessel disease, performance of perfusion CMR was superior vs. the entire multi-vessel disease SPECT population (AUC: 0.89 ± 0.06 vs.0.70 ± 0.5; p = 0.006) (Figure 22.4).

Strengths

This landmark paper had several strengths, including the relatively large number of patients (n = 234), and its multi-centre, randomized design. Previous CMR studies involved smaller patient groups, mostly in single-centre settings and some had produced conflicting results. This study was carried out in a number of different centres with variable experience in CMR perfusion imaging, reflecting real-world practice. Several different CMR machines (Philips, Siemens, and GE) were used in addition to different pulse sequences and image acquisition processes, which is again consistent with routine practice between different institutions. Interestingly, this was also one of the largest multi-centre SPECT studies and the results were reassuring in terms of generating similar values for sensitivity and specificity, which conformed to pre-existing literature.

Limitations

There were a number of limitations in the study design. First, the prevalence of CAD (nearly 80%) was much higher than that seen in general clinical practice and therefore the applicability of the results to lower or intermediate risk groups remains unproven. Second, as this was a dose-finding study, the population was randomized into four different contrast doses and thus the effective sample size at the optimal dose was much smaller (only 42 patients). Third, only stress perfusion images were analysed, but inclusion of rest images in the analysis may have helped in differentiating true perfusion defects from artefacts. Furthermore, no late gadolinium enhanced CMR images were acquired, contrary to routine clinical practice. Finally, the SPECT component of the study has been criticized because gated SPECT was not available in approximately half of the patient cohort, which could have had an influence on the performance of SPECT.

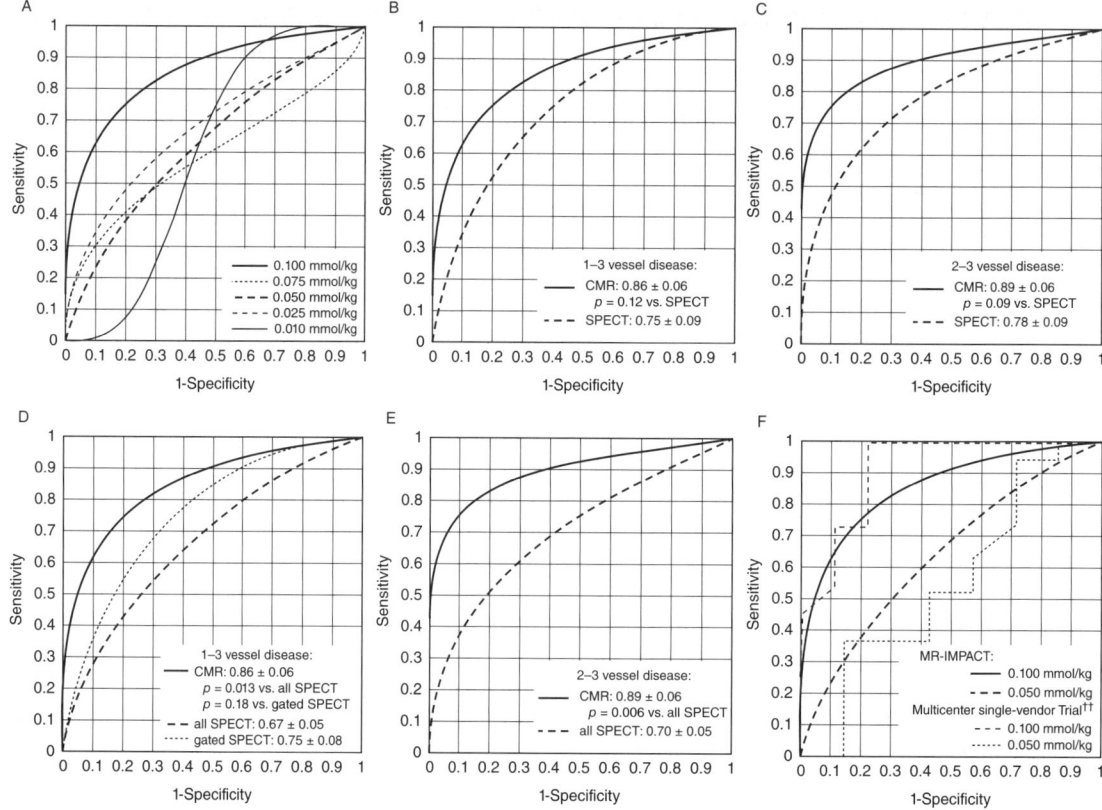

Figure 22.4 The optimal dose of gadolinium was 0.1 mmol/kg (A). There was no significant difference in diagnostic accuracy for CMR vs. SPECT on paired analysis (B, C). At optimal dose, CMR had a significantly higher diagnostic accuracy when compared to the entire SPECT population (D, E). Results were similar to a previous smaller single-vendor trial (F). Numbers indicate mean ± SE of the area under the receiver-operating characteristic curve.

Reproduced from Schwitter J, *et al.* MR-IMPACT: comparison of perfusion-cardiac magnetic resonance with single-photon emission computed tomography for the detection of coronary artery disease in a multicentre, multivendor, randomized trial. *Eur Heart J* 2008; 29: 480–9, with permission from Oxford University Press.

Clinical impact

The MR-IMPACT trial established perfusion CMR as a potential alternative to SPECT in the management of CAD with the advantage of not exposing patients to ionizing radiation.

Conclusion

The MR-IMPACT trial showed that perfusion CMR was at least as good as SPECT in detecting CAD in this first multi-centre and multi-vendor study. A number of limitations in study design led the authors to conclude that although the results were promising, further evaluation in larger trials was required. The subsequent MR-IMPACT II and Clinical Evaluation of MAgnetic Resonance imaging in Coronary heart disease (CE-MARC) trials have studied much larger patient populations and confirmed the high diagnostic accuracy of perfusion CMR.

Learning points

♦ Perfusion CMR is an accurate method of detecting significant CAD, with at least equal performance to nuclear SPECT in single and multi-vessel disease.

Further reading

● Greenwood JP, Maredia N, Younger JF, *et al.* Clinical Evaluation of Magnetic Resonance Imaging in Coronary Heart Disease (The CE-MARC Study): A Prospective Evaluation of 750 Patients. *Circulation* 2010; 122: Abstract A21797.

Cardiovascular magnetic resonance and single-photon emission computed tomography for diagnosis of coronary heart disease (CE-MARC): a prospective trial

Greenwood JP, Maredia N, Younger JF, Brown JM, Nixon J, Everett CC, Bijsterveld P, Ridgway JP, Radjenovic A, Dickinson CJ, Ball SG, Plein S. *Lancet* 2012; 379(9814): 453–60.

Background

The MR-IMPACT study suggested potential superiority of CMR over nuclear perfusion imaging to detect the presence of coronary artery disease (CAD). However, MR-IMPACT was a dose-ranging study and the number of patients in the optimal dose group was small. No large-scale clinical studies had directly compared CMR and nuclear perfusion imaging for the detection of CAD.

Purpose

The CE-MARC study compared the diagnostic accuracy of multi-parametric CMR and single photon emission computed tomography (SPECT) against X-ray coronary angiography as the reference standard in patients with suspected CAD.

Patients

A group of 752 patients with suspected angina pectoris and at least one cardiovascular risk factor were recruited. All patients were scheduled for CMR and SPECT in random order, followed by invasive X-ray coronary angiography.

Methods

This was a prospective study with consecutive patients recruited from two UK hospitals. The CMR protocol included rest and adenosine stress perfusion, cine imaging, late gadolinium enhancement, and MR coronary angiography. Gated SPECT was performed during adenosine stress and at rest using (99 m) Tc tetrofosmin. All angiograms were performed as per usual clinical care. Cardiac magnetic resonance and SPECT studies were visually reported by two experienced observers each, blinded to the results of other tests. A perfusion score was calculated for both methods. Luminal narrowing $\geq 50\%$ in the left main stem and $\geq 70\%$ in any other vessel of more than 2 mm luminal diameter by quantitative angiography was considered to be significant.

Results

Disease prevalence in the 752 recruited patients was 39%. Cardiac magnetic resonance had a sensitivity, specificity, positive, and negative predictive value of 86.5%, 83.4%, 77.2%, and 90.5%, respectively. The same results for SPECT were 66.5%, 82.6%, 71.4%, and 79.1%, respectively. The sensitivity and negative predictive value of CMR and SPECT differed significantly (p <0.0001 for both). Removing coronary MRA from the analysis did not reduce diagnostic performance of CMR. Figure 22.5 compares CMR and SPECT perfusion with ROC curves.

Strengths

This was the largest comparison between CMR and SPECT and the first powered to detect differences between the two methods. All studies were performed with contemporary methodology, including gated SPECT in all patients. Unlike previous studies, there was little referral bias, as all recruited patients underwent CMR, SPECT, and X-ray angiography as part of the study. The disease prevalence was in line with recommendations for referral to an imaging test.

Limitations

The study included only two centres and its applicability to wider practice may be limited.

Clinical impact

Pre-planned future analyses of CE-MARC will also provide critical cost-effectiveness and outcome data for both modalities. The CE-MARC trial may thus have substantial clinical impact as CMR is also safer, not exposing patients to ionizing radiation, and if outcome data suggest equality between CMR and SPECT, CE-MARC may induce a shift towards CMR as the primary diagnostic test in this setting.

Conclusion

The CE-MARC trial showed that multi-parametric CMR is superior to SPECT in detecting CAD in patients with suspected CAD. The coronary MRA component of the multi-parametric CMR study does not add significant diagnostic power.

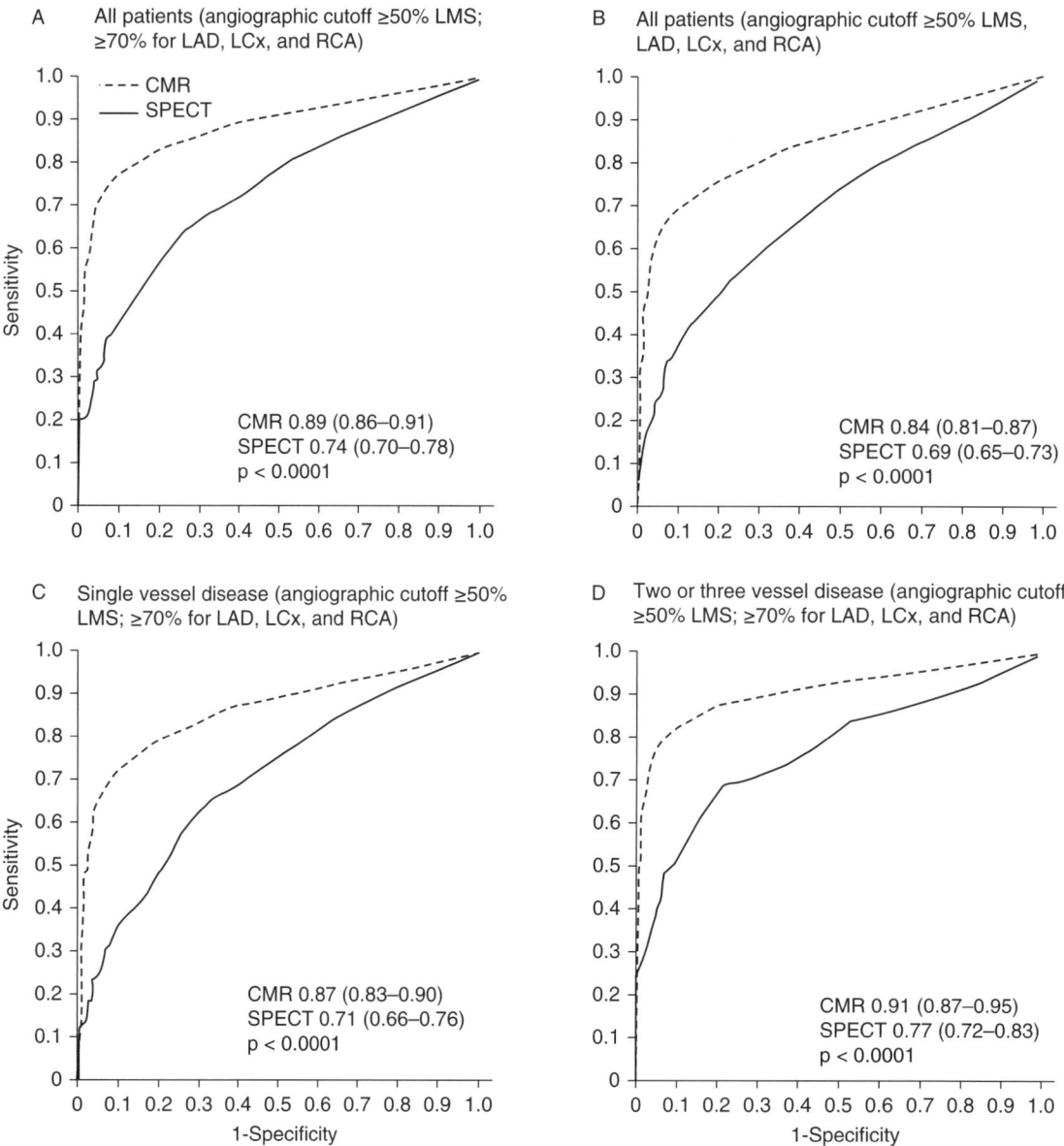

Figure 22.5 Receiver operating characteristic curves generated using summed stress scores with the CMR stress perfusion component and from SPECT (n = 647) for the whole cohort . CMR = cardiovascular magnetic resonance. SPECT = single-photon emission computed tomography. AUC = area under the curve. LMS = left main stem. LAD = left anterior descending. LCx = left circumflex. RCA = right coronary artery.

Reproduced from Greenwood JP, et al. Cardiovascular magnetic resonance and single-photon emission computed tomography for diagnosis of coronary heart disease (CE-MARC): a prospective trial. Lancet 2011; 379: 453–60, with permission of Elsevier.

Learning points

- Cardiac magnetic resonance is more sensitive than SPECT for the detection of significant CAD.

Cardiac T2* magnetic resonance for prediction of cardiac complications in thalassaemia major

Kirk P, Roughton M, Porter JB, Walker JM, Tanner MA, Patel J, Wu D, Taylor J, Westwood MA, Anderson LJ, Pennell DJ. *Circulation* 2009; 120(20): 1961–8.

Background

There are nearly 100 million carriers of β-thalassaemia worldwide and approximately 60,000 homozygotes are born each year. The leading cause of death amongst these patients with β-thalassaemia major is heart failure due to myocardial iron overload from repeated blood transfusions. Death tends to occur at a young age after only a short period of manifested cardiac failure. However, timely introduction of iron chelation therapy has been shown to dramatically improve survival. The potential of T2* mapping to quantify myocardial iron-overload and thus guide chelation therapy has long been recognized but the correlation of T2* measurements and clinical events had not been established prior to this study.

Purpose

The aim of this study was to determine the predictive value of cardiac T2* measurement for heart failure and arrhythmia in β-thalassaemia major patients.

Patients

A group of 652 (319 male: 333 female) patients with thalassaemia major from 21 UK centres participated in this study. Patients were unselectively referred from their local units, but 17 were excluded at the time of their first CMR because of clinical heart failure (n = 11) or arrhythmia (n = 6).

Methods

Heart failure was defined by a clinical diagnosis and CMR derived LVEF <56%. Arrhythmia was diagnosed on the basis of symptoms with objective 12 lead ECG or Holter evidence. T2* CMR images were acquired using a cardiac gated single breath-hold 8 echo sequence (2.6 to 16.7 msec—with 2.02 msec increments) of a single mid-ventricle short-axis slice. When patients had multiple CMR scans, these were analysed as non-independent—so that the unit of analysis was each individual scan and a subsequent one-year of follow up. The ROC analysis compared predictive accuracy for cardiac outcomes across the full range of measured values for cardiac T2*, liver T2* and serum ferritin.

Results

The relative risk for heart failure with cardiac T2* values <10 msec was 160 (95% CI: 39–653). Heart failure occurred in 47% of patients within one year of a cardiac T2* <6 msec with a relative risk of 270 (95% CI, 64–1129). The AUC for predicting heart failure was significantly greater for cardiac T2* (0.948) than for liver T2* (0.589; p <0.001) or serum ferritin (0.629; p <0.001). Cardiac T2* was <10 msec in 98% of scans in patients who developed heart failure (Figure 22.6).

The relative risk for arrhythmia with cardiac T2* values <20 msec was 4.6 (95% CI: 2.66–7.95). Arrhythmia occurred in 14% of patients within one year of a cardiac T2* of <6 msec The AUC for predicting arrhythmia was significantly greater for cardiac T2* (0.747) than for liver T2* (0.514; p <0.001) or serum ferritin (0.518; p <0.001). The cardiac T2* was <20 msec in 83% of scans in patients who developed arrhythmia.

Strengths

This was a large study incorporating >80% of the UK β-thalassaemia major population. Although this study was limited to patients with thalassaemia, the authors speculate that the data would be applicable and relevant in the management of other iron-loading haematological diseases. The study has also given important insight into the biokinetics of iron. Only recently have developments progressed to an understanding of why uptake of iron in the myocardium differs from the liver.

Limitations

The main limitation of this study was that the results were not formally validated in a different cohort. Additionally, ventricular dysfunction was defined using the widely accepted CMR threshold (EF <56%) but single centre data suggested that a slightly higher threshold value may be more relevant to these patients in the absence of cardiac siderosis particularly given their young age.

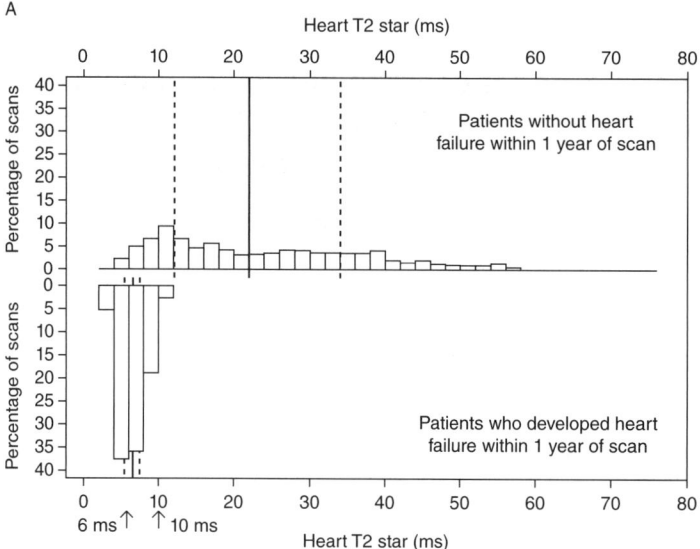

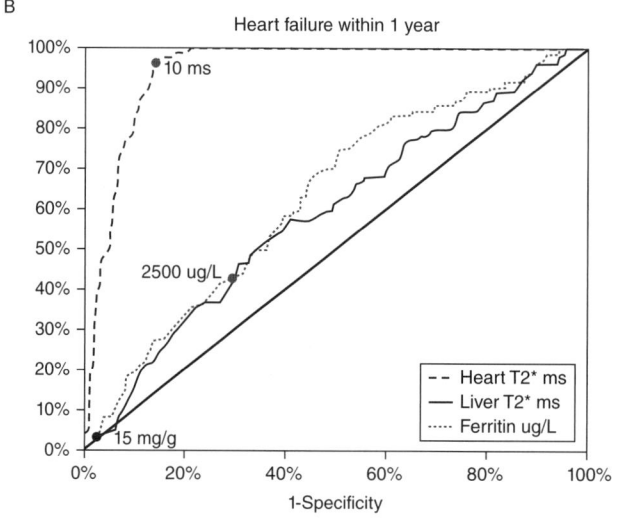

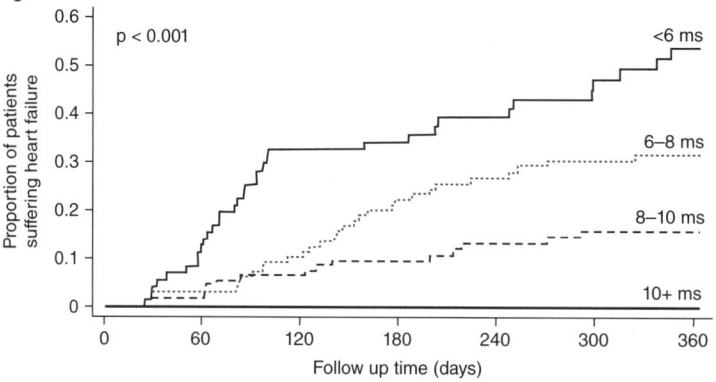

Figure 22.6 (A) Frequency distribution of cardiac T2* values.
(B) Receiver-operating characteristic curve for the prediction of heart failure
within one year of CMR. (C) Kaplan–Meier curves showing the occurrence
of heart failure over one year according to baseline cardiac T2* values.

Reproduced from Kirk P, *et al.* Cardiac T2* Magnetic Resonance for Prediction of Cardiac Complications in
Thalassemia Major. *Circulation* 2009; 17; 120(20): 1961–8, with permission from Wolters Kluwer Health.

Clinical impact

Cardiac T2* measurement by MRI has become a routine test in the management of patients with iron loading and has lead to a dramatic fall in mortality from this condition by timely introduction of chelation therapy and monitoring.

Conclusions

T2*CMR identifies patients at high risk of heart failure and arrhythmia from myocardial siderosis in β-thalassaemia major and is superior to serum ferritin and liver iron parameters.

> ### Learning points
>
> ◆ Cardiac magnetic resonance has the unique ability to quantify cardiac iron concentration and this ability can be used to improve outcome in patients with thalassaemia.

Further reading

- Anderson LJ, Holden S, Davis B, et al. Cardiovascular T2-star (T2*) magnetic resonance for the early diagnosis of myocardial iron overload. Eur Heart J 2001; 22: 2171–9.

Impact of unrecognized myocardial scar detected by cardiac magnetic resonance imaging on event-free survival in patients presenting with signs or symptoms of coronary artery disease

Kwong RY, Chan AK, Brown KA, Chan CW, Reynolds HG, Tsang S, Davis RB. *Circulation* 2006; 113: 2733–43.

Background

Late gadolinium enhancement CMR imaging can detect the extent of myocardial scar resulting from MI. However, the prognostic significance of detected myocardial scar in patients without a clinical history of MI is unknown.

Purpose

The aim of this study was to determine if the presence of myocardial scar on LGE imaging provides additional prognostic data in patients with suspected CAD or known CAD.

Patients

One hundred ninety-five patients with suspected or confirmed CAD undergoing CMR for clinical purposes were studied. Exclusion criteria included suspicion of previous MI, myocarditis, HCM or infiltrative cardiomyopathy; unstable angina; NYHA class IV heart failure; standard CMR contraindications; or normal coronary angiography within the last two weeks.

Methods

A number of baseline demographics including traditional cardiovascular risk factors, results of any prior coronary angiography or non-invasive imaging, and the results of ECG interpretation were recorded. Cardiac magnetic resonance imaging was performed with an LGE pulse sequence starting 15 minutes after a 0.15 mmol/kg dose of gadolinium-DPTA. All images were analysed for quantitative segmental wall motion and presence and extent of hyperenhacement on LGE imaging. Clinical follow-up was performed at a minimum of six months after CMR using standardized telephone interviews, through the patient's physicians, and by hospital records. The primary end point was major adverse cardiac events (MACE) including cardiac death, new acute MI, unstable angina, worsening heart failure requiring in-patient treatment, or ventricular arrhythmias requiring discharge from an ICD.

Results

During a median follow-up of 16 months, 31 patients (18%) experienced MACE, including 17 deaths. Late gadolinium enhancement demonstrated the strongest unadjusted associations with MACE and cardiac mortality (hazard ratios of 8.3 and 10.9, respectively; both $p < 0.0001$) (Figure 22.7). Even patients in the lowest tertile of LGE-involved myocardium (mean LV mass, 1.4%) experienced a >7-fold increased risk for MACE. On multivariate analysis, LGE was independently associated

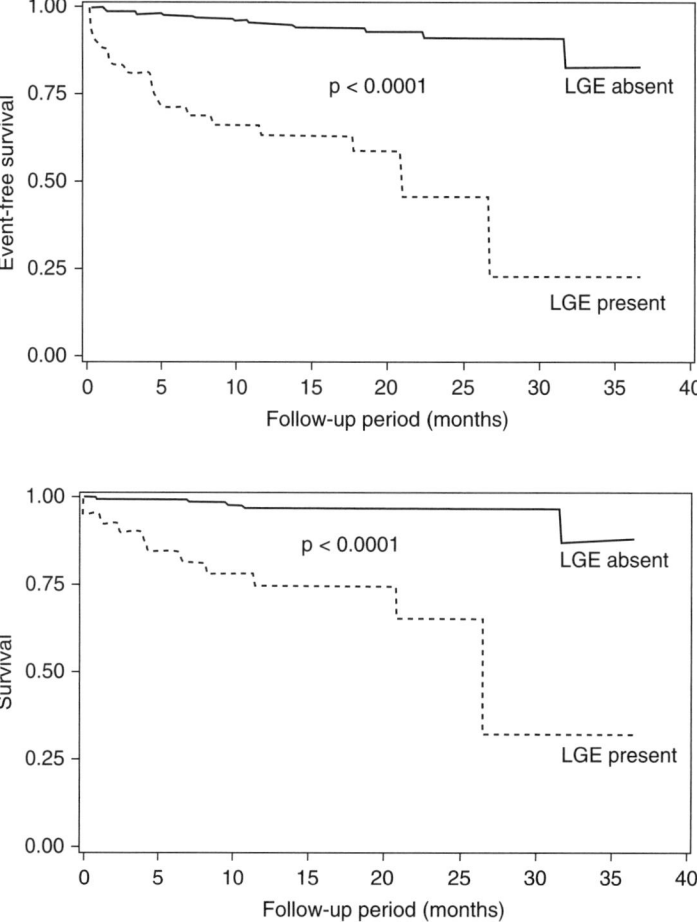

Figure 22.7 Kaplan-Meier curves for MACE (top) and cardiac mortality (bottom).

Reproduced from Kwong RJ, et al. Impact of Unrecognized Myocardial Scar Detected by Cardiac Magnetic Resonance Imaging on Event-Free Survival in Patients Presenting With Signs or Symptoms of Coronary Artery Disease. *Circulation* 2006; 113: 2733–43, with permission from Wolters Kluwer Health.

with MACE beyond the traditional clinical model (p <0.0001) or the clinical model combined with angiographically significant coronary stenosis (p = 0.0007), LVEF (p = 0.001), LV end-systolic volume index (p = 0.0006), or segmental wall motion abnormality (p = 0.002). Late gadolinium enhancement was the strongest predictor in the best overall models for MACE and cardiac mortality.

Strengths

At the time, this paper was the largest and most systematic study to explore the role of LGE in predicting MACE and cardiac mortality. The study also raised intriguing questions as to whether LGE may serve as a new prognostic indicator based on its ability to appreciate myocardial injury and fibrosis. It also highlighted the prevalence and natural course of undetected MI.

Limitations

There was potential for referral bias as this was a single-centre study and all patients were clinically referred for CMR. Second, coronary angiography was not performed in all patients and was at the discretion of the treating clinician. It is therefore unclear whether LGE imaging would maintain its incremental prognostic significance beyond angiographic findings if all patients had undergone coronary angiography. Finally, the results of the CMR studies were made available to the treating clinicians on the same day. As a result, important coronary revascularization decisions may have been influenced by the

CMR report—and the subsequent alteration in prognosis (if any) is not accounted for in this analysis.

Implications for clinical practice

This study highlighted the role of LGE imaging in risk stratification of patients with suspected CAD. Furthermore, as only 7 of the 44 patients with LGE had Q waves on their baseline ECG, it underlined the incremental value of LGE imaging as the reference test for the detection of previous MI, with implications for both clinical purposes and future population-based studies.

Conclusion

Among patients with suspected or confirmed CAD but without a history of MI, LGE even involving a small amount of myocardium carries a high cardiac risk. In addition, LGE imaging provides incremental prognostic

value to MACE and cardiac mortality beyond common clinical, angiographic, and functional predictors.

Learning points

♦ Late gadolinium enhanced CMR is a powerful tool to detect myocardial infarction and this detection determines patient outcome.

Further reading

● Steel K, Broderick R, Gandla V, *et al.* Complementary prognostic values of stress myocardial perfusion and late gadolinium enhancement imaging by cardiac magnetic resonance in patients with known or suspected coronary artery disease. *Circulation* 2009; 120: 1390–400.

Cardiac catheterization guided by MRI in children and adults with congenital heart disease

Razavi R, Hill DL, Keevil SF, Miquel ME, Muthurangu V, Hegde S, Rhode K, Barnett M, van Vaals J, Hawkes DJ, Baker E. *Lancet* 2003; 362: 1877–82.

Background

Congenital heart disease (CHD) has an incidence of 6–8 per 1000 live births. Fluoroscopy remains an important tool in CHD to guide diagnostic cardiac catheterization and percutaneous intervention. Disadvantages of fluoroscopy include poor soft tissue visualization and exposure to radiation. An ideal approach to reduce X-ray exposure would be to combine the versatility and soft tissue detail of CMR with the established techniques of fluoroscopically guided cardiac catheterization.

Purpose

This landmark study investigated the feasibility of cardiac catheterization guided by MRI with radiographic support (XMR).

Patients

The study population consisted of 16 children and adults with CHD referred for cardiac catheterization. Patient selection was made on the basis of those felt to benefit from the additional MRI information and included examples of Alagille syndrome, tricuspid atresia, transverse aortic arch hypoplasia, atrial septal defect (ASD), atrioventricular septal defect (AVSD), and ventricular

septal defect (VSD). Two patients due to have radiofrequency ablation were excluded as the required hardware was not MR compatible. Of the remaining 14 patients, 12 underwent diagnostic cardiac catheterization, two had interventional cardiac catheterizations, and two had radiofrequency ablation for tachyarrhythmias. X-ray doses in patients undergoing X-ray radiography and magnetic resonance (XMR) guided procedures were compared with a retrospectively matched control group undergoing similar procedures with standard fluoroscopy.

Methods

This study took place in a specialized XMR interventional suite comprising a 1.5T MRI scanner, radiography unit, and angiography table in a radiofrequency and X-ray screened room. The MRI tabletop was adapted to enable rapid transfer of the patient between the two. The room was designed so that half the room was outside the 0.5 mT field contour. These facilities enabled the continued use of traditional catheters and devices that are not compatible with MRI. The catheters were made visible to MRI by injection of 1 ml of carbon dioxide. The MRI sequences were a real-time steady state free precession and an interactive mode sequence which allowed 10–14 frames per second to follow catheter manipulation.

Results

In all 14 patients, a substantial proportion or all of the procedure was successfully guided by MRI. In two patients, diagnostic catheterization was completed without the use of any fluoroscopy. In two patients undergoing radiofrequency ablation, catheters were manipulated with fluoroscopic guidance and the outcome was assessed with MRI. All patients received lower amounts of radiation than controls. It was also possible to superimpose fluoroscopic images of electrophysiology electrode catheters on the three dimensional MRI of the cardiac anatomy. The total X-ray dose was consistently lower in patients undergoing XMR-guided procedures than standard fluoroscopy (median values: 5.7 vs. 25.7 Gy/cm^2; $p = 0.006$).

Strengths

Although a small study, this work was the first to demonstrate the use of MRI to guide cardiac catheterization and intervention in patients with CHD. The use of simultaneous invasive pressure measurement and flow data had not been performed before and although there were discrepancies it was suggested that MRI may be more accurate than conventional methods.

Limitations

First, this was only a small feasibility study. Second, additional time was required for preparation and transferring patients between imaging modalities, but this was not examined. However, the authors do report that this improved with increasing experience with the process. Finally, many of the catheters used were designed for use in fluoroscopy and consequently contain ferromagnetic components that could be hazardous with MRI.

Impact on clinical practice

This study showed the feasibility of cardiac catheterization guided by MRI and fluoroscopic images, demonstrating the potential of MRI to replace fluoroscopic based procedures in patients—thus avoiding radiation exposure whilst improving soft tissue imaging. Haemodynamic catheterization data can be combined with anatomical and functional MR imaging to improve management strategies and help evaluate treatment and follow-up. There are many potential developments including the use of robot assistance in MRI guided catheterization.

Conclusion

Cardiac magnetic resonance is an increasingly used test in the management of patients with CHD and adult CHD. In addition to detailed morphological and functional assessment, CMR offers the opportunity to be combined with cardiac catheterization. This study showed that such a combination can be safe and practical in a clinical setting, allows better soft tissue visualization, can provide pertinent physiological information, and results in lower radiation exposure than fluoroscopically guided procedures.

Learning points

- Cardiac magnetic resonance has the potential to replace fluoroscopic guidance and avoid radiation exposure.

Further reading

- Rickers C, Jerosch-Herold M, Hu X, *et al.* Magnetic resonance image-guided transcatheter closure of atrial septal defects. *Circulation* 2003; 107: 132–8.

Overall conclusions

With increasing evidence from clinical trials about the use of CMR, and improving image quality with simpler, faster, and more standardized scanning protocols, the clinical role of CMR will continue to expand. Clearly, with the rapid development of cardiac computed tomography, the role of CMR needs to be redefined. For example, it seems unlikely that CMR is going to be a first-line test for anatomical imaging of the coronary arteries, but as a test that does not expose patients to ionizing radiation, it will play a prominent role in ischaemia and scar detection. Large trials such as the CE-MARC study have begun the task of defining this role more conclusively. Whereas the CE-MARC study compared CMR and SPECT as diagnostic tests for the non-invasive detection of coronary artery disease, outcome studies such as MR Perfusion Imaging to Guide Management of Patients With Stable Coronary Artery Disease (MR-INFORM) will provide much needed prognostic information for CMR in ischaemic heart disease. Other ongoing studies will show the prognostic value of CMR in predicting outcome in non-ischaemic heart disease, such as HCM and arrhythmogenic right ventricular cardiomyopathy, and demonstrate that as in iron-loading, the unique tissue characterization provided by CMR offers clinically relevant information that can guide patient management and save lives. These will be the landmark CMR studies of the future.

Chapter 23

Cardiac computed tomography

Dr Srikanth Iyengar and Professor Carl Roobottom

Introduction

The use of computed tomography (CT) for imaging of the heart has evolved rapidly over the last three decades. The first CT scanner was developed in 1971 by Sir Godfrey Hounsfield. During the 1970s and 1980s, rapid advancements in technology enabled the use of CT scanners for the real-time assessment of stationary organs in the human body. Despite the development of slip-ring technology, allowing rotational gantry movement, it was considered that CT technology would never be capable of imaging the beating heart.

The temporal limitations of mechanical gantry rotation were overcome by the development of electron-beam CT (EBCT) in the 1980s. With its high temporal resolution EBCT ushered in the new era of cross-sectional imaging for cardiac anatomy and cardiac function. The recognition of atherosclerotic calcification in the coronary artery as a surrogate marker for coronary disease, led to the development of calcium scoring and the extensive use of EBCT for coronary artery disease (CAD) assessment in the early 1990s. The late 1990s saw the introduction of the first contrast enhanced EBCT scans for the assessment of coronary disease; however, limitations of EBCT technology prevented its widespread dissemination.

Simultaneously, the increasing availability of spiral and subsequently multi-detector row CT scanners spurred further research into the use of conventional CT systems for cardiac imaging. The scans were initially performed on spiral and 4-slice scanners which had poor spatial resolution and a temporal resolution lower than EBCT. The subsequent development of 16, 32, and 64-slice CT scanners significantly reduced image acquisition times, vastly improved spatial and temporal resolution, and provided clinically useful images of the coronary arteries. Improvements in image reconstruction time (greater computational power), faster gantry rotation speeds (~350 msec), improved spatial resolution of the CT detectors (0.4–0.6 mm), and the utilization of beta-blocker medications to induce transient bradycardia, further enhanced the quality of cardiac CT examinations. This led to the rapid realization of cardiac CT and in particular CT coronary angiography (CTCA) as a viable non-invasive tool in the diagnostic armamentarium for cardiovascular disease.

Most of the landmark papers discussed in this chapter have been selected because they highlight the important advances in the technique and justification for CTCA, which forms the bulk of cardiac CT examinations. Many of the concepts described in these publications are applicable to other cardiac CT indications and have served in firmly establishing CTCA as a valuable technique in the diagnostic pathway for cardiac disease.

Quantification of coronary artery calcium using ultrafast computed tomography

Agatston AS, Janowitz WR, Hildner FJ, Zusmer NR, Viamonte M Jr, Detrano R. *J Am Coll Cardiol* 1990; 15 (4): 827–32.

Background

Coronary artery calcium (CAC) was recognized as a marker for coronary atherosclerotic disease and there was evidence to suggest that CT had greater sensitivity in detecting CAC compared to fluoroscopy. However, there was no evidence regarding the value of CAC quantification. The authors conducted a study to determine the ability of EBCT to detect and quantify CAC.

Methods

Patients who underwent EBCT for proven or suspected CAD and a second group of patients who had undergone coronary angiography were recruited into the study.

High resolution non-contrast enhanced EBCT images were obtained with 3 mm slice thickness, ECG-triggering, and breath-holding. Twenty contiguous images were obtained at 80% of the R-R interval, starting at the lower margin of pulmonary artery bifurcation. In 58 patients, an additional scan was performed to acquire 40 images covering both proximal and distal coronary arteries. Images were assessed for the presence of calcium (density >130 Hounsfield units within four contiguous pixels) and scored using an automated programme. A score was obtained for each lesion by multiplying the area with the density score (1 = 130–199 HU, 2 = 200–299 HU, 3 = 300–399 HU and 4 ≥400 HU). Total score was calculated as the sum of scores obtained from all lesions.

In patients undergoing both coronary angiography and EBCT, fluoroscopy was performed before coronary angiography to look for CAC.

Results

A group of 584 patients underwent only EBCT and 50 patients undergoing coronary angiography were subjected to additional EBCT and fluoroscopy.

Electron-beam CT detected CAC in 96% patients with clinically established CAD. In other patients, prevalence of CAC increased with age. Electron-beam CT was superior to fluoroscopy in demonstrating CAC (96% vs. 57%). The absence of CAC had a high negative predictive value in ruling out clinical CAD (100–98%). The CAC cutoff points for the presence of CAD in patients in their 40/50s and 60s were 50 and 300, respectively. These results, too, were superior to those of fluoroscopy and stress testing. However, CAC demonstrated low specificity for CAD across all ages.

The 20% inter-observer disagreement of CAC score was ascribed to computer hardware error, motion artefacts, and ostial calcifications bordering the aortic wall.

Strengths and limitations

Strengths—this landmark study was the first to develop a scoring system for CAC and elegantly demonstrated the high negative predictive value of the absence of CAC in ruling out CAD.

Limitations—coronary artery imaging was performed on selected patients and the predictive value of CAC in asymptomatic patients was not fully explored. There was a significant degree of inter-observer variability in CAC assessment. Although CAC was shown to be superior to fluoroscopy and stress testing in the prediction of CAD, the overall value was limited by absence of prognostic data.

Conclusion

This was the first of many publications demonstrating the value of CAC assessment in ruling out the presence of coronary disease, providing the basis for the CAC score as a marker of the severity of CAD.

Learning points

◆ Assessment of CAC using EBCT is an excellent tool for detecting CAD.
◆ The absence of CAC has a high negative predictive value in ruling out CAD.

Further reading

● Margolis JR, Chen JT, Kong Y, *et al.* The diagnostic significance of coronary artery calcification. *Radiology* 1980; 137: 609–16.

Detection of coronary artery stenoses by contrast-enhanced, retrospectively electrocardiographically-gated, multi-slice spiral computed tomography

Achenbach S, Giesler T, Ropers D, Ulzheimer S, Derlien H, Schulte C, Wenkel, E Moshage W, Bautz W, Daniel WG, Kalender WA, Baum U. *Circulation* 2001; 103: 2535–8.

Background

Invasive coronary angiography (ICA) was the reference standard for assessment of CAD, despite the risk of complications. The non-invasive alternatives (MRI and EBCT) were limited by unreliable image quality and lack of spatial resolution. A new generation of multi-slice CT scanners (MDCT) were shown to be capable of visualizing coronary arteries. A group at the University of Erlangen studied the accuracy of MDCT technology compared to ICA for detection of significant disease in proximal coronary artery segments.

Methods

A group of 64 consecutive patients with suspected CAD underwent MDCT coronary angiography followed by conventional ICA. Contrast enhanced (160 mL at 4 mL/s) CTCA was performed with spiral acquisition on a four-slice MDCT. Using simultaneously recorded ECG, images were reconstructed using retrospective gating into ten datasets (0–90% of the R-R interval). Three-dimensional and thin slice sliding maximum intensity projections were used for multi-planar evaluation. Vessels larger than 2.0 mm were visually assessed for the presence of high-grade stenosis (>70% diameter reduction).

Following MDCT all patients underwent conventional ICA within 1–3 days. The stenoses seen on ICA were evaluated using quantitative coronary angiography (QCA) software.

Results

The results of the QCA were considered as the reference standard. Some 256 coronary arteries (64 patients) were imaged on MDCT; 82 arteries (32%) could not be evaluated due to reduced image quality from either motion artefacts or atheromatous calcification. Multi-slice CT correctly detected six occlusions and 26/29 high-grade stenoses. The three lesions underestimated by MDCT were within diagonal vessels. However, in 22 arteries, high-grade stenoses were incorrectly detected by MDCT.

Multi-slice CT had 91% sensitivity and 84% specificity for detection of high-grade stenoses in the evaluable segments; however, if the non-evaluable segments were included, sensitivity dropped to 58%. The positive predictive value (PPV) and negative predictive value (NPV) of MDCT for the detection of high-grade stenosis were 59% and 98%, respectively.

Strengths and limitations

Strengths—this was one of the earliest studies demonstrating the feasibility of CTCA using MDCT. It demonstrated a high degree of sensitivity and specificity for the detection of high-grade stenosis, especially emphasizing the high NPV of MDCT. This was also one of the first studies to compare MDCT results with QCA, thus reducing the bias introduced by interpreter variability in the assessment of high-grade stenoses.

Limitations—a large number of coronary artery segments were not considered evaluable, greater than those imaged by EBCT. However, this shortcoming was compensated for by the better spatial resolution of MDCT. Despite the use of a low tube current (150 mA), the estimated radiation exposure was several times higher than EBCT (1.7 mSv compared to 3.9–5.8 mSv).

Conclusion

This study demonstrated the feasibility of CTCA using MDCT and the value of the technique in ruling out significant disease in patients with suspected CAD.

Learning points

♦ Multi-slice CT has a high NPV for the assessment of significant CAD.
♦ The limited temporal resolution of four-slice MDCT results in a large proportion of coronary artery segments that could not be evaluated.

Further reading

● Budoff MJ, Oudiz RJ, Zalace CP, *et al*. Intravenous three-dimensional coronary angiography using contrast-enhanced electron beam computed tomography. *Am J Cardiol* 1999; 83: 840–5.
● Nieman K, Oudkerk M, Rensing BJ, *et al*. Coronary angiography with multi-slice computed tomography. *Lancet* 2001; 357: 599–603.

Detection of coronary artery stenoses with thin-slice multi-detector row spiral computed tomography and multiplanar reconstruction

Ropers D, Baum U, Pohle K, Anders K, Ulzheimer S, Ohnesorge B, Schlundt C, Bautz W, Daniel WG, Achenbach S. *Circulation* 2003; 107: 664–6.

Background

Contrast enhanced MDCT coronary angiography suffered from low reliability in demonstrating arterial stenoses in a large proportion of studies. Previous studies had observed that the image quality was critically influenced by the patient's heart rate; 60 beats per minute being the threshold below which motion artefacts were significantly reduced. Contemporaneously, several new MDCT scanners with higher temporal and spatial resolution were introduced. This was a landmark study assessing the combined use of thin slice spiral scanning (improved spatial resolution) and routine administration of beta blockers to reduce the patient's heart rate (improved temporal resolution).

Methods

A group of 77 consecutive patients, referred for ICA, underwent CTCA following 50 mg of oral atenolol one hour before and sub-lingual isosorbide dinitrate immediately before the scan. A 16-slice MDCT was used to acquire volume data using a spiral scanning technique. Tube current was modulated according to the patient's ECG, with maximum current centred at 55% of the cardiac cycle and 80% reduction during the rest of the cycle. Invasive coronary angiography was performed the next day and the images were assessed using QCA.

Results

The mean ± SD heart rate was 62 ±10 at the time of MDCT. All patients with a heart rate of >60 bpm, were administered oral atenolol for heart rate control. All coronary arteries were evaluable in 57/77 patients; 38 coronary arteries were classified as unevaluable, 26/38 due to motion artefact. In the 36 patients with a heart rate of below 60 bpm, 138 of 144 coronary arteries were classified as evaluable.

Overall there were 16 occlusions and 62 stenoses (>50%), 57/78 lesions were detected by MDCT (per-lesion sensitivity of 73%). However, when the non-evaluable arteries were excluded, 57/62 lesions were correctly identified by MDCT (sensitivity: 92%, specificity: 93% and accuracy: 93%). Multi-slice CT overestimated 14 lesions (false-positive); however, there was no further assessment of the cause of overestimation.

On a per-patient basis, 35/41 patients with significant coronary disease were correctly detected by MDCT (sensitivity of 85% and specificity of 78%).

Strengths and limitations

Strengths—this study addressed two important shortcomings (spatial and temporal resolution) of coronary artery evaluation by MDCT. The significant reduction in the proportion of unevaluable coronary arteries provided proof of concept and safety of beta-blocker administration to improve MDCT image quality. The 16-slice MDCT provided higher spatial resolution and the reduction in scan duration and faster scanner rotation resulted in shorter breath-hold and higher temporal resolution.

Limitation—the analysis was performed on a coronary artery and overall patient level; per-segment level analysis was not attempted. There was no attempt to compare the number of evaluable segments or the anatomical identification of the segments compared to ICA. The MDCT images were analysed by visual assessment, whereas the ICA utilized QCA, possibly resulting in a subjective bias. Finally, only modest heart rate control

was obtained by oral beta blockade (range 43 to 97 bpm) and the effect of heart rate variability was not assessed.

Conclusion

This landmark study demonstrated the feasibility of heart rate control with beta blockade prior to MDCT and the incremental value of using a 16-slice MDCT with shorter gantry rotation time in improving temporal resolution.

Learning points

◆ Use of beta blockers for heart rate control results in an improvement of CTCA image quality.
◆ Higher spatial and temporal resolution can be obtained by using 16-slice MDCT scanners.

Further reading

● Harpreet KP, Alvarez W, Fishman EK. ß-Blockers for Cardiac CT: A Primer for the Radiologist. *AJR* 2006; 186: S341–5.
● Morgan-Hughes GJ, Roobottom CA, Owens PE, Marsahll AJ. Highly accurate coronary angiography with submillimetre, 16 slice computed tomography. *Heart* 2005; 91(3): 308–13.

Electron-beam tomography coronary artery calcium and cardiac events: a 37-month follow-up of 5635 initially asymptomatic low to intermediate-risk adults

Kondos GT, Hoff JA, Sevrukov A, Daviglus ML, Garside DB, Devries SS Chomka EV, Liu K. *Circulation* 2003; 107: 2571–6.

Background

Prospective epidemiological studies had established the association between major risk factors and development of significant CAD; however, they failed to explain a large proportion of morbidity and mortality associated with CAD. According to the Framingham study, nearly 50% of deaths attributable to CAD occurred in asymptomatic individuals with no previous history of CAD. Preventive healthcare strategies were focusing on strategies to predict the magnitude of CAD risk and defining the population at risk of CAD. Coronary artery calcium (CAC) measured by EBCT was proposed as a surrogate marker for atherosclerotic disease in asymptomatic individuals.

The purpose of this study was to assess the association between CAC score and cardiac events in asymptomatic low to intermediate-risk individuals.

Methods

A group of 10,132 individuals (age 30–76 years), self-referred for EBCT CAC-screening, were included in the study. All patients undertook pre-EBCT CAD risk assessment questionnaire. Patients with history of cardiac chest pain or established CAD were excluded from the study. Electron-beam computed tomography was used to calculate Agatston-CAC score for all patients, which was further expressed as age/sex percentiles. Hard events, defined as death or myocardial infarction (MI) and soft cardiac events, defined as percutaneous revascularization or coronary artery bypass grafting, were recorded over a follow-up period of 37 ± 3 months, with only the first event being recorded for each individual.

Results

The study was designed to assess incremental value of CAC score over traditional cardiovascular risk factors in predicting the presence of CAD in asymptomatic low to intermediate-risk individuals. A group of 8,855 patients were included in the study. The response rate to follow-up was 64% (5,635/8,855) and barring minor differences, the responders were a good representation of the overall population. Prevalence figures for cardiovascular risk factors, with the exception of hypercholesterolaemia, were lower in the study population compared to general population, probably due to the selection of low to intermediate-risk individuals. Coronary artery calcium was detected in 74% of men and 51% of women. There were 224 confirmed events: 58 hard events (death and MI) and 166 soft events (CABG and catheter-based interventions).

The CAC score was significantly higher in individuals with all events compared to those without. Individuals with hard events had a higher mean CAC score compared to those with soft events. Coronary artery calcium was independently associated with cardiac events. Controlling for age and risk factors, the presence of CAC was significantly associated with hard, soft, and all events in men. In women, the presence of CAC was significantly associated with soft and all events, although its association with hard events could not be established due to lack of power.

In both genders increasing CAC score was associated with increasing risk of revascularization procedures. Individuals in the highest quartile of age/sex corrected CAC scores were at higher risk of hard and soft events in men and soft events in women. This demonstrated that age/sex corrected CAC scores may provide more accurate assessment of cardiovascular risk in asymptomatic individuals.

Strengths and limitations

Strengths—this was a large cross-sectional study exploring the value of CAC scores in low to intermediate-risk individuals with a reasonably long period of follow-up

and robust assessment of hard and soft outcomes. Although the follow-up rate of 64% was typical of non-incentivised studies, the study population was representative of the overall population.

Limitations—the relative risks from hard events may not be accurate due to the probable inclusion of non-cardiac deaths in 'hard events'. The greater numbers of soft events were probably triggered by positive CAC screening results in asymptomatic individuals. Therefore the associations with soft and all events have limited value. The study population consisted of self-referring individuals with lower overall presence of cardiovascular risk factors compared to the general population. This is likely to dilute the impact of traditional risk factors for prediction of hard and soft events. On the other hand, presence of CAC on EBCT may have motivated a certain number of individuals to modify their lifestyle or commence cholesterol lowering therapy, further influencing the number of cardiac events at follow-up.

Conclusion

This study demonstrated that presence or absence of CAC on EBCT could provide incremental information over the recommended conventional CAD risk assessment scores.

Learning points

- ◆ Detection of coronary artery calcium provides incremental prognostic information when added to cardiovascular risk factor based models of assessment.
- ◆ A CAC score in the highest age/sex corrected quartile is significantly associated with an adverse coronary event in asymptomatic low to intermediate-risk individuals.

Further reading

- Polonsky TS, McClelland RL, Jorgensen NW, *et al.* Coronary artery calcium score and risk classification for coronary heart disease prediction. *JAMA* 2010; 303(16): 1610–6.
- Raggi P, Gongora MC, Gopal A, *et al.* Coronary artery calcium to predict all-cause mortality in elderly men and women. *J Am Coll Cardiol* 2008; 52(1): 17–23.

Coronary artery calcium score combined with Framingham score for risk prediction in asymptomatic individuals

Greenland P, LaBree L, Azen SP, Doherty TM, Detrano RC. *JAMA* 2004; 291(2): 210–5.

Background

Coronary risk stratification was used to estimate an individual's risk of coronary heart disease (CHD) and to identify patients who would benefit form primary preventive treatment. The Framingham risk score (FRS), was a commonly recommended statistical model, but like many other statistical models, was limited in its ability to differentiate individuals who were and those who were not at a significant risk of coronary event. There was increasing evidence that quantification of CAC score improved risk prediction over that provided by office based risk assessment models. The objective of this study was to determine the combined value of the CAC score and FRS for assessment of CHD risk.

Methods

A group of 1,461 asymptomatic individuals from the South Bay Heart Watch study were prospectively enrolled in this study. Individuals with prior history of heart disease or angina and previous revascularization were excluded. Thirty months after enrolment, 1,312 surviving participants underwent a second risk assessment and concurrent CAC score assessment with CT. Patients with diabetes were excluded from further follow-up as diabetes on its own was considered to be a significant risk factor for CHD and was deemed to reduce the prognostic value of the CAC score.

Participants underwent yearly assessment for cardiovascular events for a period of up to 8.5 years (mean = 7 years). Follow-up assessment was performed using clinic appointments or telephonic interview and medical record screening for surviving patients. Follow-up assessment of deceased patients included screening of relevant medical records and conversation with the next of kin. At least one follow-up assessment was completed by 99% of patients, with an overall follow-up rate of 87.5% for the final assessment. The study focused on two hard CHD end points (1) non-fatal MI proven by patients' medical records and (2) death assigned to CHD as assessed by three blinded experts (cardiologists) using the majority rule.

Results

After exclusion of diabetics and participants with established coronary events prior to CT, the study cohort consisted of 1,029 participants. The mean (SD) age at CT scan

was 65.7 (7.8) years and an overwhelming majority of patients were white men. During the follow-up period 84 participants experienced either non-fatal MI (n = 68) or CHD death (n = 16).

The risk of hard CHD end points for participants with CAC of >300 was 3.9 times that of participants with CAC of zero (HR, 3.9; 95% CI, 2.1–7.3; **P** <.001) while the risk for participants in the highest FRS group (>20%) was 14.3 times that of participants in the lowest FRS group (<10%). When both CAC and FRS were considered together, there was no significant increased risk with a CAC of >300 in the lowest FRS group (0–9%). In the 10–15% FRS group a CAC of >300 modified the risk to a level comparable with the >20% FRS group with a CAC of >300.

In this study, both FRS and CAC were able to independently rank participants according to CHD risk in a graded fashion. Coronary artery calcium significantly modified risk in all participants with an FRS of at least 10%, especially when the CAC was >300. However, in participants with CAC of zero, there were 14 coronary events over the period of follow-up, thus establishing that absence of CAC did not preclude the risk of a CHD event.

Strengths and limitations

Strengths—the patient cohort was more representative of the general asymptomatic population than any previous study. Unlike other previous studies, the coronary risk factors were actually measured rather than estimated, providing more accurate risk assessment. This study also benefited from a long follow-up interval and used hard end points rather than a combination of hard and soft end points for follow-up assessment. This reduced the bias introduced by the influence of CAC score on subsequent coronary interventions.

Limitations—the higher proportion of older, predominantly white males in the study cohort may not be representative of the population in other parts of the world. The data may also have limited applicability in women due to the unusually low proportion of females in the study cohort (~10%). As with previous studies with prolonged follow-up intervals, the results of this study may have been influenced by risk-modifying lifestyle changes by patients with high CAC score. However, the impact of such practices on the study result would be difficult to assess in any long cross-sectional study.

Conclusion

This study demonstrates that for patients in the high to intermediate-risk group, CAC score of >300 is associated with a significantly increased risk of CHD related events, compared to that predicted by FRS alone. This is particularly relevant in the intermediate risk group, where clinical decision-making could be altered due to modification in the predicted risk. It also suggests that CAC does not provide significantly incremental improvement in risk prediction over and above FRS in the low risk (<10%) or the high-risk groups (>20%). Finally, a CAC score of zero does not completely exclude future risk of CHD-related events, probably due to the presence of the vulnerable 'soft plaque' in this group of patients.

Learning points

♦ Presence of CAC is significantly associated with a future risk of adverse coronary events in low to intermediate-risk asymptomatic patients.
♦ A CAC score of zero does not completely exclude the risk of future adverse coronary events.

Further reading

- Gottlieb I, Miller J, Arbab-Zadeh A, *et al.* The absence of coronary calcification does not exclude obstructive coronary artery disease or the need for revascularization in patients referred for conventional coronary angiography. *J Am Coll Cardiol* 2010; 55(7): 627–34.
- Wilson SR, Lin FY, Min JK, *et al.* Role of Coronary Artery Calcium Score and Coronary CT Angiography in the Diagnosis and Risk Stratification of Individuals with Suspected Coronary Artery Disease. *Curr Cardiol Rep* 2011; 13(4): 271–9.

Diagnostic accuracy of non-invasive coronary angiography using 64-slice spiral computed tomography

Raff GL, Gallagher MJ, O'Neill WW, Goldstein JA. *J Am Coll Cardiol* 2005; 46: 552–7.

Background

The 16-slice MDCT scanners had high accuracy for the identification of significant CAD in vessels larger than 1.5 mm. However, there was a wide variation in the reported sensitivities and specificities. Advancement of CT technology resulted in the introduction of the 64-slice MDCT scanner (32 detector rows and dual focal spots per detector row) with improved spatial and temporal resolution compared to the 16-slice scanners. This study was designed to assess the accuracy of CTCA using the new 64-slice scanner in patients referred for ICA.

Methods

A group of 70 consecutive patients, who had undergone ICA for assessment of suspected CAD, were subjected to 64-slice CTCA. A combination of oral and intravenous beta blockers were used to achieve acquisition heart rates of <65 bpm. An initial calcium scoring scan was followed by a contrast enhanced spiral scan using retrospective ECG-gating without tube current modulation at 120 kV/750–850 mA. The data was initially reconstructed at 65% and 35% of the R-R cycle, with additional reconstruction windows being used if motion artefacts were present on the initial reconstructions. Lesions with well-defined borders were quantitatively assessed and those with hazy or irregular borders were visually assessed using an ordinal scale. Patients were classified as positive if there was at least a single stenosis of >50%. Invasive angiograms were evaluated by a single observer and lesions were assessed using quantitative coronary analysis software. The accuracy of CTCA for the detection of significant stenosis (>50%) was compared to ICA on per-segment, per-artery, and per-patient levels.

Results

Of the 1,065 coronary artery segments visualized, 935 segments (88%) were analysed either qualitatively or quantitatively and 773 segments were assessed by both MDCT and QCA; 130 segments demonstrated stenoses. On a per-segment basis CTCA had 86% sensitivity and 95% specificity for detecting a significant stenosis. Multidetector CT could analyse 279 of 280 arteries (99%) and the per-artery sensitivity and specificity were 91% and 92% respectively. On a per-patient level MDCT had 95% sensitivity and 93% specificity, accurately demonstrating the status of CAD in 65 of 70 patients (93%).

The presence of high levels of CAC (>400 Agatston U) significantly reduced the specificity of CTCA, although the numbers were extremely small. Multidetector CT had reduced sensitivity (90%) and specificity (86%) in obese patients. Similarly, acquisition heart rate was a major influencing factor, with the sensitivity and specificity deteriorating to 88% and 71% respectively with heart rates >70 bpm. Faster gantry speed enabled diagnostic image acquisition in patients with higher heart rates, although the loss of accuracy proved that heart rate control was still essential.

Strengths and limitations

Strengths—this study was conducted in patients referred for ICA, resulting in a high incidence of significant disease. Despite inclusion of a significant proportion of patients with higher heart rates, obesity, and high calcium scores, 64-slice CTCA demonstrated a high level of accuracy. The number of coronary arteries that could not be assessed was impressively small and no patient was excluded due to poor image quality.

Limitations—the high incidence of CAD may have resulted in the high sensitivity of CTCA. The results were expressed on a per-patient level rather than per-artery or per-segment level, which may have been clinically more relevant. Computed tomography coronary angiography data was assessed using quantitative analysis, probably for ease of comparison to QCA and did not reflect routine practice. The study also suffers from a single high volume expert centre and small sample size bias, which could limit its applicability to other centres with limited experience.

Conclusion

This study demonstrated the incremental accuracy of 64-slice CTCA. The very high negative predictive value suggested that CTCA could be used as an accurate rule-out test in the acute setting, for patients with equivocal stress tests, who would have otherwise required ICA to rule out coronary disease.

Learning points

- Computed tomography coronary angiography performed using 64-slice MDCT demonstrates excellent accuracy, comparable to QCA, in the absence of high levels of CAC.
- A 64-slice MDCT can be used to exclude significant CAD with a high degree of accuracy.

Further reading

- Meijboom WB, Meijs MF, Schuijf JD, *et al.* Diagnostic accuracy of 64-slice computed tomography coronary angiography: a prospective, multicenter, multivendor study. *J Am Coll Cardiol* 2008; 52(25): 2135–44.

Feasibility of low-dose coronary CT angiography: first experience with prospective ECG-gating

Husmann L. Valenta I, Gaemperli O, Adda O, Treyer V, Wyss CA, Veit-Haibach P, Tatsugami F, von Schulthess GK, Kaufmann PA. *Eur Heart J* 2008; 29: 191–7.

Background

Introduction of 64-slice and dual-source CT scanners led to a rapid growth in the use of CTCA for the assessment of patients with low to intermediate pre-test probability of significant CAD. There was increasing recognition of the risk of cancer induction associated with high radiation exposure from CTCA examinations.

Prospective ECG-gating was proposed as the next step in radiation dose reduction for CTCA examination; however, its feasibility and impact on image quality had not been assessed in the clinical setting. This study presented the first experience of CTCA with prospective ECG-gating and its effect on radiation dose reduction.

Methods

A group of 41 consecutive patients, who were scheduled to undergo CTCA for suspected or known CAD, were prospectively recruited. Intravenous beta blockers were used if necessary to achieve a target heart rate of <65 bpm. Computed tomography coronary angiography examinations were performed using a sequential axial scanning protocol using the smallest X-ray window (75% of the R-R interval) and 40 mm z-axis coverage with 5 mm overlap between blocks. Body mass index (BMI) adapted tube voltage (100–120 kV) and tube current (450–650 mA) were used to optimize radiation exposure. The effective radiation dose (ED) was calculated using scanner generated dose-length product (DLP) and chest specific conversion factor (k = 0.017 mSv/mGy cm). Coronary segments >1.5 mm were assessed by two independent readers, using a standardized AHA coronary segment model and images were scored using a five-point visual assessment scale.

Results

One patient was excluded due to atrial fibrillation; 30/40 patients were administered intravenous beta blockers and 10/40 patients were on oral beta blockers as part of their baseline medication, resulting in a mean acquisition heart rate of 57.3 ± 6.2 (range 39–66) bpm. The mean DLP from the CTCA scan was 124.9 + 37.3 mGy.cm (range 65.0–179 mGy.cm) resulting in an estimated ED of 2.1 + 0.6 mSv (range 1.1–3.0 mSv).

Diagnostic quality images were obtained for 95% of segments, with 54.6% of segments rated excellent; 26/519 segments (5%) had non-diagnostic quality images, either due to coronary motion (46%) or step-artefact due to incorrect fusion of the image blocks (46%). The most significant factor influencing image quality was acquisition heart rate, with diagnostic quality being achieved in all segments in 93% of patients with heart rate below 63 bpm. Body mass index adapted scan parameters reduced the impact of high BMI on image quality. Despite sequential acquisition of data at every second heartbeat, contrast opacification was not a problem.

Strengths and limitations

Strengths—this was the first study to demonstrate the feasibility of CTCA with prospective ECG-gating. A high proportion of diagnostic quality images were obtained with very low radiation exposure, especially when the heart rate was below 63 bpm. This study provided an additional step in radiation dose optimization techniques, in addition to those already being employed in clinical practice.

Limitations—the study was conducted on a small homogenous group of patients, reducing its applicability in routine clinical practice with a more heterogeneous patient population. Furthermore, the accuracy of the CTCA examinations was not compared to the accepted gold standard—invasive coronary angiography.

Conclusions

This landmark study demonstrated the feasibility of CTCA using prospective ECG-gating. Diagnostic image quality was achieved in a large proportion of patients despite very low radiation exposure.

Learning points

- Computed tomography coronary angiography using prospective ECG-gating can be used to achieve diagnostic quality images with low-radiation doses.
- Aggressive heart rate reduction (<63 bpm) with the help of beta blockers is essential when using prospective ECG-gating.

Further reading

- Herzog BA, Wyss CA, Husmann L, et al. First head-to-head comparison of effective radiation dose from low-dose 64-slice CT with prospective ECG-triggering versus invasive coronary angiography. 2009; 95(20): 1656–61.
- Lehmkuhl L, de Waha S, Desch S, et al. Diagnostic performance of prospectively ECG triggered versus retrospectively ECG gated 64-slice computed tomography coronary angiography in a heterogeneous patient population. *Eur J Radiol* 2011. (Epub ahead of print).
- Scheffel H, Alkadhi H, Leschka S, et al. Low-dose CT coronary angiography in the step-and-shoot mode: diagnostic performance. *Heart* 2008; 94(9): 1132–7.

Coronary computed tomography angiography for early triage of patients with acute chest pain: the ROMICAT (Rule Out Myocardial Infarction using Computer Assisted Tomography) Trial

Hoffmann U, Bamberg F, Chae CU, Nichols JH, Rogers IS, Seneviratne SK, Truong QA, Cury RC, Abbara S, Shapiro MD, Moloo J, Butler J, Ferencik M, Lee H, Jang IK, Parry BA, Brown DF, Udelson JE, Achenbach S, Brady TJ, Nagurney JT. *J Am Coll Cardiol* 2009; 53: 1642–50.

Background

Patients presenting to the emergency department with suspected ischaemic chest pain, but with equivocal or normal initial ECG and biochemical markers of myocardial necrosis, represent a major diagnostic challenge. The majority of these patients are admitted and undergo further investigations, including stress testing to rule out acute coronary syndrome (ACS). Several small studies had explored the use of CTCA as a triage tool in this group of patients. However, the spectrum of CTCA findings in this group of patients and their association with the diagnosis of ACS was not established. This study was designed to assess the usefulness of CTCA in low to intermediate-risk patients presenting with suspected ischaemic chest pain.

Methods

Patients presenting to the ED with suspected ischaemic chest pain, normal initial troponin, and normal/equivocal initial ECG were recruited in this prospective observational study. Patients with previously established CAD were excluded. All patients underwent CTCA with a 64-slice MDCT, using a standardized retrospective ECG-gated protocol with dose modulation where appropriate, before being admitted to the hospital. Intravenous beta blockers were used for heart rate control where necessary.

The coronary arteries were assessed by two independent investigators using the 17-segment AHA model for the presence of atherosclerotic plaques and significant stenosis (>50% luminal diameter reduction). Segments were considered positive if significant stenosis could not be excluded due to non-diagnostic image quality.

The clinical end points were ACS defined as MI or unstable angina during the index admission and major adverse cardiac events (MACE) defined as death, MI, or coronary revascularization during the six-month follow-up period. The assessment for MACE was conducted via telephone interview or review of medical records by two experienced clinicians blinded to the CTCA result.

Results

The study cohort consisted of 368 eligible patients out of a total of 1869. In this group 31 patients had ACS and the remaining 337 patients had neither ACS nor MACE. At CTCA, 50.3% patients (183/368) were free of CAD, 31.2% (117/368) had coronary plaque, and 18.5% had significant stenosis (34 positive and 34 inconclusive CTCA).

The absence of coronary artery plaque or stenosis had high negative predictive values of 100% and 98% respectively, for ACS. In seven patients with ACS, but no significant stenosis on CTCA, microvascular disease, rupture or thrombosis in a sub-critical plaque or stenosis in distal/small calibre vessels not assessed by CTCA, were considered as possible explanations. Fourteen patients with significant stenosis on CTCA did not have ACS or MACE on subsequent follow-up, suggesting that although significant disease was detected on CTCA, its haemodynamic or clinical significance was unclear in this subset of patients.

Presence of plaque in each additional coronary segment was associated with a 37% incremental risk and presence of stenosis with a 20-fold incremental risk of ACS even after adjustment for age, gender, and TIMI risk score. This suggested that CTCA could independently risk stratify low to intermediate-risk patients.

Strengths and limitations

Strengths—due to the large sample size this study was able to provide robust proof of the negative predictive value of CTCA in suspected ACS. The study provides an unbiased assessment because CTCA was not used as part of standard patient care.

Limitations—the patient recruitment was limited to daytime hours, limiting the applicability and value of CTCA assessment in busy emergency departments during all hours. Patients with renal impairment were excluded from this study, many of whom were elderly and could have benefitted from early non-invasive assessment with CTCA. Lastly, like other studies, this study suffers from a single expert centre bias and the results may be difficult to replicate across departments with varying levels of expertise.

Conclusion

This was a landmark study assessing the applicability of CTCA as a triage tool in patients presenting to the emergency department with suspected ACS. It demonstrated the excellent negative predictive value of coronary CTCA and proved that up to 50% patients (in the low to intermediate-risk category) presenting with suspected ACS are free of CAD.

Learning points

- ◆ A significant number of patients presenting to the emergency department with symptoms of ACS, are free of CAD.

- ◆ The high negative predictive value of CTCA makes it an effective triaging tool in the assessment of suspected ACS; however, its limited availability has prevented its widespread use in the acute setting.

Further reading

- Achenbach S, Daniel WG. Cardiac imaging in the patient with chest pain: coronary CT angiography. *Heart* 2010; 96(15): 1241–6.
- Hollander JE, Chang AM, Shofer FS, McCusker CM, Baxt HI. Coronary computed tomographic angiography for rapid discharge of low-risk patients with potential acute coronary syndromes. *Ann Emerg Med* 2009; 53(3): 295–304.

Diagnostic performance of coronary angiography by 64-row CT

Miller JM, Rochitte CE, Dewey M, Arbab-Zadeh A, Niinuma H, Gottlieb I, Paul N, Clouse ME, Shapiro EP, Hoe J, Lardo AC, Bush DE, de Roos A, Cox C, Brinker J, Lima JA. *N Eng J Med* 2008; 359: 2324–36.

Background

Indirect evaluation of CAD through stress testing has significant limitations and ICA remains the gold standard despite its associated risks. Several small studies had proposed the use of CTCA as a non-invasive alternative; however, published literature highlighted the marked variation in the diagnostic accuracy of CTCA compared to ICA. In addition, the value of CTCA in predicting the need for revascularization in symptomatic patients was not established.

To address these inconsistencies and lack of evidence, the authors of this study conducted a multi-centre, international study using centralized analysis to assess the diagnostic accuracy of 64-slice CTCA in symptomatic patients with a view to identifying the subset of patients who would benefit from referral to ICA or revascularization.

Methods

The CORE-64 study was a prospective study performed at nine hospitals in seven countries on patients who were referred for ICA for assessment of suspected symptomatic CAD. Patients underwent a calcium scoring scan and CTCA before ICA. The CTCA was performed at 120 kV/240–500 mA using retrospective ECG gating to achieve a total study dose of 12–15 mSv capped at 20 mSv. Patients with a resting heart rate >70 bpm were given beta blockers and patient data was excluded from the analysis if the acquisition heart rate was >80 bpm. The data from patients with a calcium score of >600 AU was collected but excluded from the primary analysis. The raw image datasets were analysed in the independent central core laboratory. Stenoses were visually assessed using a six-point ordinal scale by two independent observers and those >30% were quantitatively assessed. Segments were labelled uninterpretable if there was agreement between two observers for visual assessment or three observers for quantitative assessment and considered negative for stenosis in the analysis. Invasive coronary angiography was performed within 30 days of CTCA and images were similarly assessed visually and quantitatively (QCA) using a condensed 19-segment model for comparison with CTCA. The Duke Coronary Artery Disease Index was used for both CTCA and ICA to assess the severity of coronary disease.

Results

Of the 405 patients enrolled for the study, 316 patients had a calcium score of <600 and after exclusions 291 patients were included in the analysis. At QCA 163 patients (56%) had at least one obstructive stenosis (>50%).

The visual and quantitative assessments of stenosis by CTCA were similar and almost all coronary artery segments could be evaluated (~100%). The diagnostic performance of CTCA was comparable to QCA for stenosis >50% (AUC—0.93) and suffered only when the reference standard for stenosis was set at 80–90%. These results indicated that CTCA had a powerful discriminative ability to identify within symptomatic patients, the subset with obstructive CAD, although it could not entirely replace ICA due to its limited PPV (91%) and NPV (83%).

Despite its anatomical accuracy, CTCA misclassified 13% of patients as compared to QCA when the threshold of obstructive stenosis was set at 50%. However, this was not reflected in the modified Duke Coronary Artery Disease Index where there was good correlation between QCA and CTCA, suggesting that both modalities had similar abilities for identifying patients who would benefit from revascularization (0.84 for CTCA and 0.82 for QCA).

The mean effective doses from CTCA for men and women were 14 mSv and 15 mSv respectively. These doses were consistent with other studies using 64-slice CT and indeed comparable to other cardiac imaging modalities using ionizing radiation.

Strengths and limitations

Strengths—this was a large multi-centre study performed across different geographical regions with diverse patient populations, representative of the subset who would require anatomical assessment of coronary arteries. The data obtained from all the sites was analysed in a central core laboratory leading to robustness of analysis.

Limitations—there is a high prevalence of obstructive CAD in this study conducted on symptomatic patients, limiting its applicability to asymptomatic or low-risk patients. Due to exclusion of data from patients with CAC >600, the results cannot be applied to patients with calcified atherosclerotic disease. The study used retrospective-gating, resulting in a very low percentage of uninterpretable segments, although there was a significantly higher radiation exposure. With the increasing use of prospective ECG-gating these results may be difficult to replicate.

Conclusion

This study demonstrated the high diagnostic accuracy of 64-slice CTCA and its ability to characterize disease severity in symptomatic patients with calcium scores of <600.

Learning points

- A 64-slice CTCA yields a robust diagnostic performance in the assessment of symptomatic patients with suspected CAD and calcium scores of <600.
- A 64-slice CTCA cannot be used as a simple replacement for ICA due to its limited PPV and NPV.

Further reading

- Genders TS, Dedic A, Nieman K, Hunink MG. Prognostic value of Cardiac Computed Tomography Angiography. *J Am Coll Cardiol* 2011; 57: 1237–47.
- Hay CS, Morse RJ, Morgan-Hughes GJ, *et al.* Prognostic value of coronary multidetector CT angiography in patients with an intermediate probability of significant coronary heart disease. *Br J Radiol* 2010; 83(988): 327–30.

Prevalence and clinical significance of accidental findings in electron-beam tomographic scans for coronary artery calcification

Hunold P, Schmermund A, Seibel RM, Grönemeyer DH, Erbel R. *Eur Heart J* 2001; 22: 1748–58.

Background

Electron-beam computed tomography was primarily used for non-contrast enhanced CAC scoring scans, to provide prognostic information and for risk stratification. However, the use of EBCT for the assessment of other organ systems, was less common due to inferior spatial resolution compared to spiral CT.

While there was an increasing body of literature describing the value of EBCT in the assessment of the non-coronary cardiac structures, there were a few case reports of accidental extra-cardiac pathology being detected on CAC and little evidence regarding the frequency and importance of these findings in the context of an increasing number of cardiac EBCT examinations. This landmark paper was the first investigation into the frequency and value of accidental cardiac and extra-cardiac findings on cardiac EBCT and paved the way for further debate on this controversial subject.

Methods

A group of 1,812 patients undergoing EBCT based CAC assessment for suspected or proven CAD were recruited. In 32% of patients an additional contrast-enhanced EBCT was performed for assessment of CAD. Electron-beam computed tomography images were obtained as 3 mm contiguous slices from the level of the main pulmonary artery to the diaphragm and CAC score calculated using a validated method. In patients receiving contrast, the EBCT protocol was set to obtain a CT coronary angiogram. The scans were assessed by two experienced assessors for the presence of non-coronary cardiac and extra-cardiac pathologies. The diagnostic and therapeutic consequences of these accidental findings were recorded from the patients' medical records.

Results

Abnormalities of the heart, aorta, and lungs represented a majority of the accidental findings. Accidental findings were identified in 953 (53%) patients, of which non-coronary cardiac findings were observed in 681 (38%) patients. Although the patients with extra-coronary findings were older and had higher calcium scores, there was no difference in the prevalence between those with non-contrast and those with contrast enhanced studies. Not surprisingly, contrast studies demonstrated a greater number of cardiac thrombi, tumours, and lung atelectasis.

In 191 (9.3%) patients, an additional diagnostic test was considered for further evaluation of pathology, the most frequent additional test being transthoracic echocardiography for assessment of valvular abnormalities (317 patients—18%). In a significant number of patients, detection of accidental abdominal findings led to additional assessment of abdominal organs. Incidental malignancy was identified in three patients (0.2%). This would have remained undetected but for the detailed assessment at EBCT. Twenty-two patients (1.2%) underwent therapeutic intervention related to an accidental finding.

Strengths and limitations

Strengths—the study elegantly demonstrates the value of assessment of non-coronary structures on cardiac EBCT images. The importance of detailed assessment even in the non-contrast enhanced studies is underlined by the fact that there was no demonstrable difference in the prevalence of accidental findings between the native and contrast enhanced scans.

Limitations—the scan assessments were exclusively based on limited field of view images on a tissue window setting, possibly resulting in a number of missed pulmonary lesions, some of which may have been malignant. In a large proportion of patients, the accidental findings were not clinically significant, but led to further diagnostic tests.

Conclusion

This landmark study was the first to demonstrate that accidental non-coronary pathology was frequently detected even in non-contrast enhanced EBCT scans acquired for the assessment of CAC, and highlighted the importance of sound knowledge and adequate training for the assessment of non-coronary structures in a cardiac CT study.

Learning points

◆ A significant proportion of patients undergoing cardiac CT reveal non-coronary pathology.
◆ A sound knowledge of thoracic pathology and accurate assessment of non-coronary structures is essential for high quality interpretation of the CT images.

Further reading

● Johnson KM, Dennis JM, Dowe DA. Extracardiac findings on coronary CT angiograms: Limited versus complete image review. *Am J Roentgenol* 2010; 195(1): 143–8.
● Killeen RP, Dodd JD, Cury RC. Noncardiac findings on cardiac CT part I: Pros and cons. *J Cardiovasc Comput Tomogr* 2009; 3(5): 293–9.
● Killeen RP, Cury RC, McErlean A, Dodd JD. Noncardiac findings on cardiac CT. Part II: spectrum of imaging findings. *J Cardiovasc Comput Tomogr* 2009; 3(6): 361–71.

Estimating risk of cancer associated with radiation exposure from 64-slice computed tomography coronary angiography

Einstein AJ, Henzlova MJ, Rajagopalan S. *JAMA* 2007; 298(3): 317–23.

Background

Since its approval in 2004, 64-slice CTCA has provided a viable non-invasive alternative to ICA. While its role is evolving, CTCA is expected to become the test of choice for assessment of patients with low and intermediate pre-test probability of CAD. The volume of CTCA examinations has undergone an exponential increase and the test is being increasingly used in younger patients.

However, CTCA is still considered a radiation intensive examination. The 2006 AHA scientific statement on CTCA estimated a risk of 1 in 2000 of fatal cancer following 10 mSv CT exposure, although the effects of patient and scan specific factors on CTCA associated radiation exposure were not discussed. The authors sought to estimate the lifetime attributable risk (LAR) of cancer incidence associated with radiation exposure from a single CTCA study using the method proposed in BEIR VII report (2006) and assess the influence of age, gender, and scan protocols in the estimated cancer risk.

Methods

Four scan protocols were used for modelling: (1) standard CTCA, (2) CTCA with ECG-gated tube current modulation (ECTCM), (3) extended scan covering the thoracic aorta and the heart for triple rule-out studies and assessment of CABG, and (4) extended scan with ECTCM. The aim was to estimate doses to individual organs by using Monte Carlo simulations and then using the BEIR VII approach to calculate cancer risk.

A 64-slice scanner was modelled using 120 kV/ 170 mA for a slice thickness of 0.6 mm with a pitch of 0.2. A 15 cm scan length was assumed for the standard scan and 25 cm for the extended scan. Simulations were performed using an Impact Dose package for both males and females using all four scan protocols yielding a total of eight estimates.

The lifetime attributable risks (LARs) of cancer incidence for each gender, organ, and age (range of 20–80 years), were determined for a 100 mSv exposure from the BEIR VII report and then scaled linearly using the organ dose estimate from Monte Carlo simulation. Whole body LAR was determined by adding the specific LARs, estimating each component was done using tissue weighting factors specified by the ICRP-60 publication.

Results

There was a marked variation in the cancer risk associated with CTCA, depending on the patient's age, gender, and scan protocol. The LAR for women was greater than men at all ages. From a standard CTCA, the LAR for a 20-year-old woman was as high as 1 in 143 compared to 1 in 686 in a 20-year-old man, while LAR in an 80-year-old woman was 1 in 1,338 compared to 1 in 3,261 in an 80-year-old man. Similarly, the relative risk of attributable cancer incidence compared to an 80-year-old male was 2.4 times in an 80-year-old female and 23 times in a 20-year-old female. This difference was attributed to the risk of breast cancer in females due to exposure of breast tissue within the scan field and greater radiosensitivity of the female lung compared to a male lung at all ages, according to BEIR data. In women, the risk of breast cancer was higher than that of lung cancer until the age of 32 years, after which lung cancer risk was greater.

Tube current modulation of 35% with ECTCM, reduced the cancer risk by 35% across both genders and at all ages. Extended scan protocols increased the cancer risk in men by 43–46% and women by 24–28%.

Strengths and limitations

Strengths—the study presents simplified cancer risk estimates based on the best available data and modelling techniques and provides medical practitioners with objective parameters to assess the risk and benefit of individual CTCA examinations. Second, the method presented in the BEIR VII report is considered extremely robust.

Limitations—the risk estimates are based on mathematical modelling rather than epidemiological data and do not provide estimates of relative uncertainty or error. The BEIR VII risk model is not universally accepted and its applicability across different populations has not been assessed. Finally, the study assessed retrospectively gated CTCA protocols which are subject to higher radiation exposure compared to prospectively gated protocols, limiting their applicability in current practice.

Conclusion

This study confirms that CTCA is a high radiation dose examination associated with significant LAR of cancer induction. However, this risk varies widely with age, gender, and scan protocol. It provides further impetus for physicians to optimize patient selection and employ dose reduction strategies to limit the radiation dose from CTCA examinations.

Learning points

◆ The significant LAR of cancer induction associated with CTCA examinations make it unsuitable for use as a screening tool for young asymptomatic individuals.

◆ Medical personnel involved in performing CTCA must strive to improve scan protocols in order to achieve the lowest possible radiation dose without affecting diagnostic quality.

Further reading

● Herzog BA, Wyss CA, Husmann L, *et al*. First head-to-head comparison of effective radiation dose from low-dose 64-slice CT with prospective ECG-triggering versus invasive coronary angiography. *Heart* 2009; 95(20): 1656–61.
● Nickoloff EL, Alderson PO. A comparative study of thoracic radiation doses from 64-slice cardiac CT. *Br J Radiol* 2007; 80(955): 537–44.

Evaluation of a 'triple rule-out' coronary CT angiography protocol: use of 64-section CT in low-to-moderate risk emergency department patients suspected of having acute coronary syndrome

Takakuwa KM, Halpern EJ. *Radiology* 2008; 248: 438–46.

Background

Evaluating patients presenting with acute chest pain, ACS, or other time-critical intra-thoracic conditions is a difficult challenge for emergency department (ED) physicians. A majority of these patients, who are eventually considered normal, are unnecessarily admitted to the hospital, while a small but significant proportion suffering from ACS are not admitted. While several studies demonstrated the accuracy of CTCA in the exclusion of significant CAD in this group of patients, there was a lack of evidence regarding the incidence and outcome of other important, related causes of chest pain such as pulmonary embolism (PE) and acute aortic syndrome (AAS). A 'triple rule-out' CT protocol (of the above) was the suggested alternative; however, there was no available data regarding the utility of this protocol in an acute setting. This study was conducted to assess the utility of a triple rule-out scan in the acute setting, with a view to identifying the subset of patients who could be confidently discharged without adverse outcome over 30 days.

Methods

Patients presenting to the ED with appropriate clinical symptoms, negative initial ECG, and serum cardiac enzymes were prospectively enrolled in the study. Patients with contraindications to contrast-enhanced CT or previously treated CAD were excluded.

Contrast enhanced CT was performed using 120–140 kV tube voltage with 600–1000 mA tube current and ECG-gated tube current modulation was used where patient's heart rate was ≤65 bpm. Intravenous beta blocker was administered for heart rate control (HR >65 bpm). Bi-phasic contrast injection technique, (80 mL of neat contrast followed by 50 mL of 50% strength contrast) was used to facilitate visualization of pulmonary arteries, aorta, and coronary arteries. Coronary lesions, cardiac motion, and ejection fractions were assessed for all studies using multiphase datasets. Extra-coronary findings were evaluated using a large field of view images reconstructed at 3 mm slice-thickness.

Patients with minimal or no CAD were generally discharged home or underwent stress-testing depending on the level of clinical concern. Patients with mild CAD underwent methoxyisobutylisonitrile (MIBI) scans and were treated accordingly. Patients with moderate to severe CAD were assessed by cardiologists and underwent further assessment with MIBI scan, transthoracic echo, or ICA, before receiving further treatment. Extra-cardiac findings correlating with the presenting symptoms were treated accordingly. In case of a discrepancy between test results, ICA was considered to be the reference standard. Patients were followed up for a period of 30 days for cardiac and related events.

Results

A group of 201 patients were enrolled for the study. Data from 197/201 patients was used for the final analysis; four patients were excluded due to technical problems during scanning. Prospective ECG-gated tube current modulation was used in 30% of the scans. The mean effective dose with dose modulation was 8.7 mSv and without dose modulation was 18 mSv.

Computed tomography demonstrated moderate/severe CAD in 22 patients (10%), most of whom underwent further diagnostic evaluation. Suboptimal coronary visualization was obtained in 19 patients (10%); however, its effect on final patient outcome was not clear. Clinically important extra-coronary diagnoses that explained the patient's symptoms were demonstrated in 22 patients (11%), while those not correlating with the patient's symptoms were found in 27 patients (14%).

Some 133/175 patients with no more than mild CAD were either safely discharged or treated without further tests. The absence of ACS was accurately predicted in 174/175 patients (NPV—99.4%), by CT interpretation of no or mild CAD. One patient with negative CT had a positive stress test and ICA confirmed high-grade stenosis requiring treatment; subsequent review of CT images revealed observational error. No adverse outcomes were reported at 30 days.

The study results demonstrate that in a population of low to moderate-risk patients with suspected ACS, triple rule-out CT is an excellent triage tool and can be used to accurately identify the subgroup of patients who can benefit from early discharge.

Strengths and limitations

Strengths—this was a well conducted study demonstrating the feasibility of a triple rule-out CT triage in the acute setting. It is one of the largest outcome studies using a triple rule-out CT protocol and focused on the short-term clinical outcomes rather than CT accuracy. This study further adds to a growing evidence base that supports the value of 64-slice CTCA as a highly accurate negative rule-out test.

Limitations—this study was conducted on a selected subset of patients, limiting its applicability in routine ED practice. The design precludes any comparative assessment of CT accuracy. In addition, the follow-up period of 30 days is relatively short for the assessment of adverse cardiovascular outcomes. In this context, a negative CT scan is unlikely to completely exclude CAD, further influencing the value of a triple rule-out scan as a definitive test.

Conclusion

The study demonstrates that in patients with a low to moderate risk of ACS, a triple rule-out CT often demonstrates important extra-coronary diagnoses, identifies the subset of patients who will benefit from further assessment of CAD, and facilitates safe and rapid discharge of a majority of patients with a negative scan.

Learning points

- In a significant proportion of patients presenting to the emergency department with symptoms of ACS, the chest pain is a result of potentially lethal but treatable extra-coronary pathology.
- A triple rule-out CT can be used as an accurate triage tool in low-risk patients presenting with acute chest pain in the emergency department.

Further reading

- Halpern EJ. Triple-rule-out CT angiography for evaluation of acute chest pain and possible acute coronary syndrome. *Radiology* 2009; 252(2): 332–45.
- Krissak R, Henzler T, Prechel A, *et al.* Triple-rule-out dual-source CT angiography of patients with acute chest pain: Dose reduction potential of 100 kV scanning. *Eur J Radiol* 2010. (14 Dec 2010, Epub ahead of print).

Estimated radiation dose associated with cardiac CT angiography

Hausleiter J, Meyer T, Hermann F, Hadamitzky M, Krebs M, Gerber TC, McCollough C, Martinoff S, Kastrati A, Schömig A, Achenbach S. *JAMA* 2009; 301(5): 500–7.

Background

A 64-slice CTCA has emerged as a useful diagnostic tool in the assessment of patients with low-to-intermediate pre-test probability of significant CAD and in some settings for the initial triage of patients presenting to the ED with acute chest pain. With increasing acceptance of CTCA as a mainstream tool, an increasing number of CTCA examinations are being performed worldwide. However, CTCA is considered a radiation intensive investigation and its usefulness has to be weighed against the cancer inducing risk from radiation exposure. Due to its rapid evolution, many clinicians were unaware of the magnitude of radiation exposure from CTCA and effects of dose optimization techniques. The Prospective Multicenter Study On Radiation Dose Estimates Of Cardiac CT Angiography In Daily Practice I (PROTECTION-1) study was designed to provide information on: (1) the radiation dose associated with typical CTCA examination, (2) factors contributing to radiation exposure, and (3) the effect of dose optimization strategies on both scan quality and eventual radiation exposure.

Method

The PROTECTION-1 study was a prospective multicentre observational study conducted across 120 sites worldwide, with a view to enrolling at least 20 sites performing a minimum of 20 CTCA studies over one month.

Typical CTCA patients were defined as those with a BMI of 20 to 30 in stable sinus rhythm at the time of image acquisition. Radiation dose parameters from each study included volume CT dose index (CTDIvol) and dose length product (DLP). Estimated effective dose (ED) was calculated using a validated gender averaged chest weighting factor (k = 0.014 mSv/mGy cm). The specific dose reduction strategies included automatic exposure control (AEC), ECG-controlled tube current modulation (ECTCM), BMI adapted tube voltage, and sequential axial scanning (prospective ECG-gated step-and-shoot). All CTCA studies were assessed by an independent blinded core laboratory. A third of randomly selected CTCA studies, were assessed on a binary scale of diagnostic versus non-diagnostic.

Results

There were 50 participating sites contributing data on 1965 CTCA examinations performed in daily practice. There was a mix of sites, with differing workloads, prior experience, scanner manufacturers, and scanner technology.

The majority of scans were performed using 64-slice scanners (96%) for visualization of CAD (82%). Most of the patients were in sinus rhythm (95%) and for approximately half of the studies (46%) beta blockers were administered for heart rate control. Some 1,197/1,546 patients undergoing CTCA for visualization of CAD, had a BMI of between 20 and 30. The median DLP was 885 (IQR, 568–1259) mGy.cm, corresponding to an ED of 12 mSv (IQR, 8–18 mSv). There was a large variability of median DLP between sites (331 to 2146 mGy x cm), illustrating the difference in CTCA protocols and use of dose saving algorithms between individual sites.

In the multivariate regression analysis, absence of sinus rhythm and increasing patient weight were independently associated with higher DLP. The most significant factors in reducing radiation exposure were scan length, sequential axial scanning, use of 100 kV tube potential, and ECTCM. Increase in scan length by 1 cm, was associated with 5% increase in DLP. The use of ECTCM, 100 kV tube-voltage and sequential axial scanning resulted in DLP reduction of 25%, 46%, and 78%, respectively. The use of AEC, ECTCM, or sequential axial scanning did not result in significant deterioration in image quality. The 100 kV tube potential was used in only 82 (5%) patients, but resulted in a higher proportion of diagnostic studies compared to higher tube voltages. The increase in site experience with CTCA resulted in a small reduction of median DLP (1% for 12 months of experience).

Strengths and limitations

Strengths—the study was conducted over multiple sites worldwide and with a large proportion of non-academic sites. This therefore is the most accurate representation of CTCA practice in the present literature. The data represents real-world practice and probably the full spectrum of patients that may be subject to CTCA examinations.

The study demonstrates the applicability of dose saving algorithms in daily practice and their minimal impact on diagnostic quality, further strengthening the rationale for ongoing improvement in CTCA technique for radiation exposure optimization.

Limitations—the data on 100 kV tube potential and sequential axial scanning is subject to selection bias and has limited value. The radiation dose associated with unenhanced calcium scoring scan was not included in the results. Although it results in very small radiation exposure, this is likely to represent a significant proportion of the exposure in low-dose acquisitions using optimal dose-saving algorithms.

Conclusion

This study highlights the significant variation in radiation exposure from CTCA examinations between centres regularly performing these procedures. It proves that radiation reduction strategies can be effectively used to reduce the radiation burden without affecting diagnostic quality; however, the acceptance and use of these techniques is infrequent.

Learning points

- ◆ Radiation dose reduction strategies result in significant reduction of the radiation exposure from CTCA examinations; however, some of these techniques can only be used in carefully selected patients.
- ◆ Due to concerns regarding diagnostic quality, the use of dose saving techniques is infrequent; however, education and training could address this shortcoming.

Further reading

- Feuchtner GM, Jodocy D, Klauser A, *et al*. Radiation dose reduction by using 100-kV tube voltage in cardiac 64-slice computed tomography: a comparative study. *Eur J Radiol* 2010; 75(1): e51–6.
- Hausleiter J, Martinoff S, Hadamitzky M, *et al*. Image quality and radiation exposure with a low tube voltage protocol for coronary CT angiography results of the PROTECTION II Trial. *JACC Cardiovasc Imaging* 2010; 3(11): 1113–23.

Cost-effectiveness of coronary MDCT in the triage of patients with acute chest pain

Ladapo JA, Hoffmann U, Bamberg F, Nagurney JT, Cutler DM, Weinstein MC, Gazelle GS. *AJR* 2008; 191: 455–63.

Background

Patients presenting with acute chest pain form a large proportion of patients presenting to ED and their triage and management has significant cost implications for any hospital or healthcare system. Up to 30% of these patients are hospitalized, with clinical suspicion of ACS; however, a majority of these patients do not have ACS, rendering their hospitalization unnecessary. Computed tomography coronary angiography, which has a very high negative predictive value in the assessment of low-to-intermediate-risk patients presenting with ACS symptoms, is likely to facilitate rapid triage of these patients. To assess the financial impact of using CTCA in the emergency setting, the authors constructed an analytical model comparing 64-slice CTCA to the established standard-of-care (SOC).

Methods

A Monte-Carlo microsimulation model was developed to compare SOC with CTCA based management using estimates for several patient and test variables derived from published literature. For SOC based management, patients were assessed with stress test and admitted for ICA if the results were abnormal. For CTCA based management, patients were either discharged, underwent stress test, or ICA, based on the severity of disease as assessed by CTCA. Following discharge from ED the patients were returned to a baseline health status while accruing costs resulting from their ED/hospitalization period, medications, and interventional treatment. It was assumed that a proportion of patients would progress to various states of CAD. Those that did not progress to CAD would have an annual risk of 20% for ED visits with chest pain, over the next five years. Patients in the low-risk non-ACS group were assumed to be healthy. Bayesian methods were used to calculate disease distribution in patients subsequently visiting ED with chest pain. Patients with missed diagnosis of ACS were assigned higher mortality risk. Data on long-term survival and hospitalization/healthcare costs were derived from published estimates.

A non-diagnostic rate of 4% for CTCA was derived from per-segment based data from previous studies. These patients were further assessed by stress testing. Diagnostic performance data for other tests and risk-benefit data for CTCA and ICA were similarly derived from published literature.

Results

Using CTCA for the triage of patients with chest pain increased hospital cost by $110 and total healthcare cost by $200 for men, while there was reduction in hospital cost of $410 and total healthcare expenditure of $380 for women. In real-world terms, the increase in expenditure for men was due to earlier detection and treatment of CAD and the cost-saving in women a result of a higher discharge rate from ED.

There was a higher detection rate of CAD in both men and women at first ED visit in the CTCA group (97% vs. 85%). Emergency department discharge rates in both men (69% vs. 62%) and women (82% vs. 65%) were higher in the CTCA group, with small incremental improvements in the life expectancy compared to SOC (ten days for men and six days for women). The rate of missed ACS in men remained unchanged (1%), but in women increased to 2% with CTCA compared to 1% with SOC. However, patients discharged wrongfully by CTCA triage were considered to have low risk of mortality due to higher incidence of 'Syndrome X'.

Reducing the negative predictive value of CTCA in healthy patients by 25% increased the cost of CTCA based triage in men, but made little difference in women. Minimizing the positive predictive value of CTCA in patients with CAD only marginally affected its cost effectiveness in men, although it was still cost saving in women. Increasing the CTCA non-diagnostic rate to 10%, which could be expected in centres with less expertise, had an insignificant impact on the results. The model randomly assigned stress testing to stress-SPECT, stress-echo, and exercise tolerance test (ETT). Exclusively using stress-SPECT made CTCA based strategy cost saving in both men and women,

whereas using stress-echo or ETT exclusively increased the overall cost in men and decreased the cost in women.

Strengths and limitations

Strengths—this was one of the first studies to assess the economic impact of using CTCA as a triage tool in low-risk patients presenting with chest pain. Despite being modelled on a selected patient population, the results are applicable in many other patient populations.

Limitations—the study is limited by the use of disease prevalence and severity estimates rather than actual patient based data. It does not account for significant non-cardiac causes of chest pain in discharged patients. It also does not account for incidental CT findings, which may have an impact on patient management and healthcare costs. In the CTCA arm all patients with moderate disease were submitted to stress testing. However, the real world management of these patients is highly variable and could influence the overall healthcare costs.

Conclusion

This landmark study demonstrates the cost effectiveness of 64-slice CTCA in the management of low-risk patients presenting with acute chest pain in the emergency department.

Learning points

- The use of CTCA in the triage of low-risk patients presenting with chest pain is moderately cost effective compared to SOC.
- Computed tomography coronary angiography examinations results in identifying both coronary and extra-coronary and non-coronary pathologies that may result in higher rates of intervention or further investigation.

Further reading

- Cheezum MK, Hulten EA, Taylor AJ, *et al.* Cardiac CT angiography compared with myocardial perfusion stress testing on downstream resource utilization. *J Cardiovasc Comput Tomogr* 2011; 5(2): 101–9.
- Goehler A, Ollendorf DA, Jaeger M, *et al.* A simulation model of clinical and economic outcomes of cardiac CT triage of patients with acute chest pain in the emergency department. *AJR* 2011; 196(4): 853–61.

The future

The last few years have seen a tremendous increase in the application of cardiac CT to the clinical setting. Computed tomography coronary angiography is now the established method of assessment of low-to-intermediate-risk patients with suspected CAD. The advent of new dose reduction strategies has enabled some centres to achieve sub-1mSv scans with excellent diagnostic image quality. While this is still presently only applicable to patients with low BMI, further clinical studies are underway to expand its applicability to more patient groups.

An exciting area of development is the application of iterative reconstruction techniques to CTCA. While iterative reconstruction has resulted in further radiation dose saving, the net improvement in image quality has led to further endeavours in reducing the dose of iodinated contrast, improving the diagnostic accuracy, and expanding the remit of CTCA in patients with calcified atherosclerotic disease.

The rapid development of CT technology has seen the introduction of high end scanners capable of providing high-definition CTCA. Scanners with tubes capable of focal spot toggle, dual energy imaging, and spectral imaging, have rekindled interest in CT assessment of stents, CT myocardial perfusion, and plaque characterization. The development of dual-source and 256/320-slice scanners has enabled several centres to perform CTCA in patients with higher heart rates, without radiation dose penalty. Further evidence regarding value of these developments is awaited.

Establishment of several national and multi-centre CTCA registries has facilitated collation of prognostic data in patients and comparison with established diagnostic tests. As the evidence for the use of CTCA continues to evolve, we are likely to experience an exponential growth in the number and variety of cardiac CT examinations all over the world.

Part VII

Chapter 24

Congenital heart disease

Dr Alexander Opotowsky, Professor Anji T. Yetman, and Professor Gary Webb

Over the last 30 years, we have witnessed a transformation in the care provided to both children and adults with congenital heart disease (CHD). As a result of medical and surgical advances, there has been an exponential growth in the number of patients with increasingly complex CHD surviving into adulthood.

While the sentinel events that have altered the landscape of congenital cardiology over the past 30 years are contained in the literature, a landmark 'event' is often not captured by a single publication. Rather, what we see is a collection of papers, the first of which documents a novel finding, often times the feasibility of a new treatment. This is followed by subsequent corroborative publications which serve to refine and expand upon the initial approach. Finally, publications appear which, on a larger scale, document not only the feasibility but also the therapeutic success of the new treatment. It is this collection of papers which leads to, or perhaps reflects, a gradual paradigm shift in care. In looking back at the congenital cardiac literature since 1980, it is this process of serial publications which depicts the evolutionary tale in this field.

Cardiac catheterization for congenital heart defects

Landmark papers in the field

Rashkind WJ, Mullins CE, Hellenbrand WE, Tait MA. Nonsurgical closure of patent ductus arteriosus: clinical application of the Rashkind PDA Occluder System. *Circulation* 1987; 75(3): 583–92.

Lock JE, Rome JJ, Davis R, Van Praagh S, Perry SB, Van Praagh R, Keane JF. Transcatheter closure of atrial septal defects. Experimental studies. *Circulation* 1989; 79(5): 1091–9.

Lock JE, Bass JL, Amplatz K, Fuhrman BP, Castaneda-Zuniga W. Balloon dilation angioplasty of aortic coarctations in infants and children. *Circulation* 1983; 68(1): 109–16.

Kan JS, White RI, Jr, Mitchell SE, Gardner TJ. Percutaneous balloon valvuloplasty: a new method for treating congenital pulmonary-valve stenosis. *N Engl J Med* 1982; 307(9): 540–2.

Lababidi Z, Wu JR, Walls JT. Percutaneous balloon aortic valvuloplasty: results in 23 patients. *Am J Cardiol* 1984; 53(1): 194–7.

O'Laughlin MP, Perry SB, Lock JE, Mullins CE. Use of endovascular stents in congenital heart disease. *Circulation* 1991; 83(6): 1923–39.

Ebeid MR, Prieto LR, Latson LA. Use of balloon-expandable stents for coarctation of the aorta:

initial results and intermediate-term follow-up. *J Am Coll Cardiol* 1997; 30(7): 1847–52.

Bonhoeffer P, Boudjemline Y, Saliba Z, Merckx J, Aggoun Y, Bonnet D, Acar P, Le Bidois J, Sidi D, Kachaner J. Percutaneous replacement of pulmonary valve in a right-ventricle to pulmonary-artery prosthetic conduit with valve dysfunction. *Lancet* 2000; 356(9239): 1403–5.

Between 1980 and 2010, the treatment of many patients with congenital heart defects moved from the operating room to the cardiac catheterization laboratory. Device closure for various cardiac defects was first described in the 1960s and 1970s. Not until the 1980s, however, were safe and effective devices developed and systematically evaluated for widespread clinical use in CHD. These advances fundamentally changed the clinical approach to the management of atrial septal defects (ASD), patent ductus arteriosus, aortic coarctation, pulmonic stenosis, and other lesions.

Rashkind *et al.* developed and improved, through a long iterative process, an effective and safe device for percutaneous closure of patent ductus arteriosus[1]. This paper describes the process of development from initial studies of the device at a single institution to a multi-centre experimental protocol. The evolution of not only device design but also procedural technique are outlined, providing a reminder that the safety and efficacy of a device is not simply a result of the device itself but also the skill and experience of the operators implanting them.

Lock *et al.* described an elegant and comprehensive series of experiments on the feasibility, safety, and efficacy of device closure of atrial septal defects[2]. The investigators started with a detailed description of the atrial septum in 50 human pathologic specimens with secundum ASD, with assessment of which defects might be closed by the device to be tested. They proceeded to create iatrogenic ASDs in lambs and attempted closure. Based on problems encountered in these experiments, they redesigned the device, which they called a 'clamshell device', and further tested it in the animal laboratory. These studies laid the foundation for the first clinically applicable technology to close atrial septal defects and, with modification, patent foramen ovale and ventricular septal defects (VSDs). Over the next 10–15 years, device closure of secundum ASDs improved and became the standard of care for the majority of patients with uncomplicated defects.

Concomitant with the development of these devices, techniques for balloon angioplasty and valvuloplasty

transformed the approach to congenital aortic and pulmonary valve stenosis as well as coarctation of the aorta and pulmonary artery branch stenoses.

In 1983, Lock and colleagues described balloon dilation of aortic coarctation in eight infants and children, three with unoperated, and five with previously repaired coarctation[3]. Even in this small preliminary report, there was the suggestion that balloon angioplasty may not be as effective in patients with native coarctation as in those with recurrent stenoses. Within the same year, Kan *et al.* described a similar successful experience with balloon angioplasty in seven children with recurrent coarctation following prior surgical repair[4].

Kan *et al.* subsequently presented data on a series of patients who underwent transluminal balloon valvuloplasty for congenital pulmonary valve stenosis[5]. Since then, almost all such cases are managed successfully in the cardiac catheterization laboratory, with excellent long-term results.

Lababidi *et al.* first presented data on the use of balloon valvuloplasty for treatment of congenital aortic stenosis[6]. Subsequent published series ensued, noting this treatment to be safe and feasible for severe neonatal aortic stenosis[7].

The first reported series of the use of endovascular stents in patients with congenital heart disease appeared in *Circulation* in 1991. Forty-five stents were placed in 30 patients ranging from infancy to adulthood[8]. Indications included branch pulmonary stenoses in the majority, Fontan obstruction, superior vena cava obstruction, and recurrent coarctation. The manuscript documented the feasibility of balloon expandable stent placement for a variety of clinical indications. Ebeid, Prieto, and Latson subsequently reported on the favourable initial and intermediate term results of stent placement for recurrent coarctation in a larger series of patients[9]. The use of either balloon angioplasty or stent placement has transformed the management of recurrent aortic coarctation in patients of all ages.

The past decade has witnessed the advent of percutaneously deployable bioprosthetic valves. Bonhoeffer *et al.*[10], after detailed early studies in animals, described the use of a stented bovine jugular venous valve in a 12-year-old boy with right ventricular-to-pulmonary artery conduit stenosis and regurgitation. This group went on to successfully develop the Melody valve, which has been used in over 1000 patients needing conduit repairs. While catheter-delivered valves are still very much a work in progress, there is little question that the availability of such valves will revolutionize clinical management of cardiac valvar dysfunction.

One clear implication of all these successes is that the complexity of cardiac surgical procedures for congenital heart defects will increase as the more straightforward cardiac defects will be amenable to percutaneous intervention.

Surgery for congenital heart disease

Landmark papers in the field

Macartney FJ, Taylor JF, Graham GR, De Leval M, Stark J. The fate of survivors of cardiac surgery in infancy. *Circulation* 1980; 62(1): 80–91.

Bove EL, Behrendt DM. Open-heart surgery in the first week of life. *Ann Thorac Surg* 1980; 29(2): 130–4.

Norwood WI, Lang P, Casteneda AR, Campbell DN. Experience with operations for hypoplastic left heart syndrome. *J Thorac Cardiovasc Surg* 1981; 82(4): 511–9.

Ohye RG, Sleeper LA, Mahony L, Newburger JW, Pearson GD, Lu M, Goldberg CS, Tabbutt S, Frommelt PC, Ghanayem NS, Laussen PC, Rhodes JF, Lewis AB, Mital S, Ravishankar C, Williams IA, Dunbar-Masterson C, Atz AM, Colan S, Minich LL, Pizarro C, Kanter KR, Jaggers J, Jacobs JP, Krawczeski CD, Pike N, McCrindle BW, Virzi L, Gaynor JW; Pediatric Heart Network Investigators. Comparison of shunt types in the Norwood procedure for single-ventricle lesions. *N Engl J Med* 2010; 362(21): 1980–92.

Hoffman TM, Wernovsky G, Atz AM, Bailey JM, Akbary A, Kocsis JF, Nelson DP, Chang AC, Kulik TJ, Spray TL, Wessel DL. Prophylactic intravenous use of milrinone after cardiac operation in pediatrics (PRIMACORP) study. Prophylactic Intravenous Use of Milrinone After Cardiac Operation in Pediatrics. *Am Heart J* 2002; 143(1): 15–21.

Newburger JW, Silbert AR, Buckley LP, Fyler DC. Cognitive function and age at repair of transposition of the great arteries in children. *N Engl J Med* 1984; 310(23): 1495–9.

da Silva JP, Baumgratz JF, da Fonseca L, Franchi SM, Lopes LM, Tavares GM, Soares AM, Moreira LF, Barbero-Marcial M. The cone reconstruction of the tricuspid valve in Ebstein's anomaly. The operation: early and midterm results. *J Thorac Cardiovasc Surg* 2007; 133(1): 215–23.

Flinn CJ, Wolff GS, Dick M, 2nd, Campbell RM, Borkat G, Casta A, Hordof A, Hougen TJ, Kavey RE, Kugler J. Cardiac rhythm after the Mustard operation for complete transposition of the great arteries. *N Engl J Med* 1984; 310(25): 1635–8.

Jatene AD, Fontes VF, Paulista PP, Souza LC, Neger F, Galantier M, Sousa JE. Anatomic correction of transposition of the great vessels. *J Thorac Cardiovasc Surg* 1976; 72(3): 364–70.

Lecompte Y, Zannini L, Hazan E, Jarreau MM, Bex JP, Tu TV, Neveux JY. Anatomic correction of transposition of the great arteries. *J Thorac Cardiovasc Surg* 1981; 82(4): 629–31.

Castaneda AR, Norwood WI, Jonas RA, Colon SD, Sanders SP, Lang P. Transposition of the great arteries and intact ventricular septum: anatomical repair in the neonate. *Ann Thorac Surg* 1984; 38(5): 438–43.

Carvalho JS, Shinebourne EA, Busst C, Rigby ML, Redington AN. Exercise capacity after complete repair of tetralogy of Fallot: deleterious effects of residual pulmonary regurgitation. *Br Heart J* 1992; 67(6): 470–3.

Gatzoulis MA, Till JA, Somerville J, Redington AN. Mechanoelectrical interaction in tetralogy of Fallot. QRS prolongation relates to right ventricular size and predicts malignant ventricular arrhythmias and sudden death. *Circulation* 1995; 92(2): 231–7.

de Leval MR, Kilner P, Gewillig M, Bull C. Total cavopulmonary connection: a logical alternative to atriopulmonary connection for complex Fontan operations. Experimental studies and early clinical experience. *J Thorac Cardiovasc Surg* 1988; 96(5): 682–95.

Mavroudis C, Backer CL, Deal BJ, Labile INRs: time within therapeutic Johnsrude CL. Fontan conversion to cavopulmonary connection and arrhythmia circuit cryoblation. *J Thorac Cardiovasc Surg* 1998; 115(3): 547–56.

Bridges ND, Lock JE, Castaneda AR. Baffle fenestration with subsequent transcatheter closure. Modification of

the Fontan operation for patients at increased risk. *Circulation* 1990; 82(5): 1681–9.

Prior to 1980, definitive cardiovascular surgery, with few exceptions, was not routinely undertaken during infancy. Rather, infants presenting with intractable heart failure underwent palliative surgical procedures to restrict or augment pulmonary blood flow as required. Definitive intracardiac repair was performed in later childhood in those that survived. Macartney and colleagues were the first to look at the long-term outcome of patients with a variety of cardiac lesions surviving cardiac surgery in infancy, and compared the outcome in those undergoing a staged approach versus definitive primary repair[11]. In a group of 600 infant surgeries, they found a marked reduction in long-term mortality in those infants with TGA, isolated VSD, aortic coarctation, or critical pulmonary stenosis who underwent primary, rather than staged, repair in infancy. Numerous lesion-specific publications followed noting both the feasibility and improved outcomes of definitive repair in the first year of life. The question of repair for the neonate requiring urgent surgery, however, remained unanswered. Bove and colleagues reviewed the outcome of 212 neonates undergoing cardiac surgery during the five-year period ending in 1980[12]. In contrast to the current era, cardiac surgery in the neonate at that time accounted for only 11% of all congenital heart surgeries, and 3% of all cardiopulmonary bypass procedures performed in a tertiary paediatric cardiology centre. These authors documented extraordinarily high mortality rates, with 57% of neonates requiring cardiopulmonary bypass dying, and 25% of those undergoing off-bypass procedures dying.

During the period from 1980 to 2010, surgical management of the neonate with congenital cardiac defects evolved. The literature is marked by many 'landmark' publications heralding the success of a wide variety of surgical techniques and the overall move to intervene earlier on in life. It is perhaps the fate of the patient with hypoplastic left heart syndrome (HLHS) that was most markedly altered during this time. Until 1980, all patients with HLHS died unless they received a cardiac transplant. In 1981, Norwood and colleagues[13] reported their initial experience with the Norwood procedure for the management of HLHS. In 1983, the same group reported their expanded experience with this three-phase surgical approach[14]. In 2010, Ohye and colleagues[15] reported the results of a multi-centre randomized trial comparing two

different strategies for the first phase of the Norwood procedure, and determined that a right ventricle to pulmonary artery shunt was superior to a modified Blalock Taussig shunt in reducing early mortality in these patients. The number of HLHS patients surviving to the Fontan procedure has continued to rise.

Despite improvements in surgical treatment, cardiac transplantation continued to be used as a successful treatment modality for patients with complex forms of CHD. Lamour and colleagues reported the outcomes of a series of 488 patients transplanted for congenital heart defects. The predominant diagnoses prior to transplantation included single ventricle, complex forms of d-transposition of the great arteries (d-TGA), right ventricular outflow obstruction, and congenitally-corrected TGA (ccTGA). Five-year survival overall was 80%. Patients having undergone a prior Fontan procedure were noted to have a lower five-year survival rate[16].

Surgical advances were not limited to the operating room. During this period of time, specialized paediatric and congenital intensive care units emerged, with focused expertise in the post-operative care of congenital heart disease. Hoffman and colleagues[17] documented the value of post-operative inotropic therapy in children. They assessed whether prophylactic milrinone therapy was effective in preventing low cardiac output syndrome in high risk paediatric cardiac surgical patients. The study was a double-blind, placebo-controlled trial of three parallel groups. Milrinone significantly reduced the risk in a dose-related fashion compared with placebo with an overall risk reduction of 48%. This therapy was subsequently routinely employed in the post-operative management of patients with CHD.

With the attainment of excellent rates of long-term survival, focus shifted to assessing and improving the quality of life of survivors. In 1984, Newburger and colleagues[18] studied the impact of age at repair on late cognitive function in children with d-TGA and intact ventricular septum. They demonstrated that postponing repair in these cyanotic patients was associated with a progressive impairment of cognitive function. In 1993, Newburger and colleagues compared the perioperative neurologic effects of hypothermic circulatory arrest versus low-flow cardiopulmonary bypass in infant heart surgery, noting circulatory arrest to be associated with greater CNS perturbation in the early post-operative period. This led to a series of studies trying to identify the best surgical and operative strategies for neonatal congenital heart surgery.

Another innovation in cardiothoracic surgery was the availability of video-assisted thoracoscopic techniques. In 1995, Burke and colleagues reported the use of this minimally invasive technique in 46 paediatric patients[19]. The operative procedures included patent ductus arteriosus interruption (n = 31), vascular ring division (n = 8), pericardial drainage and resection (n = 3), arterial and venous collateral interruption (n = 2), thoracic duct ligation (n = 2), epicardial pacemaker lead insertion (n = 1), and diagnostic thoracoscopy (n = 1). Procedural success was achieved in 82% of patients, with thoracotomy required to complete nine procedures. There was no operative mortality and most patients were discharged from hospital within 48 hours of the operation.

Ebstein anomay

Da Silva and colleagues reported a new technique for tricuspid valve repair in Ebstein anomaly, and described early echocardiographic results, as well as early and mid-term clinical outcomes[20]. Of 40 consecutive patients, there was one hospital death and one late death. The overall severity of tricuspid regurgitation was reduced from 3.6 to 1.2. After a mean follow-up of four years, NYHA functional class was substantially improved and the improvement was sustained. While the jury is still out, this 'cone procedure' has the potential to transform the outcomes of Ebstein surgery in many patients.

Transposition of the great arteries

One of the most dramatic shifts in the management of congenital heart disease over the past three decades has been from atrial switch to arterial switch for repair of d-transposition of the great arteries.

Throughout the 1980s, the high long-term incidence of adverse outcomes in patients who had atrial switch repair became apparent. Flinn *et al* reported on 372 patients from eight centres who had undergone a Mustard repair, with a focus on cardiac rhythm[21]. While they reported that the Mustard procedure undoubtedly extended life for those who survived the first three months after repair, there was a significant incidence of complete heart block, tachyarrhythmia, and sudden death. Only 57% of the patients were in sinus rhythm eight years after the operation. In addition, the authors noted that there was no obvious predictor as to which patients would die suddenly. The inability to predict such catastrophic events

was confirmed by others, and remained a major challenge in the care of these patients. Trusler *et al.* reported a similarly large population of patients from Toronto who had undergone the Mustard operation between 1963 and 1985[22]. Their data suggested a real improvement in short-term and long-term outcomes over the study period. Despite this, however, there was still a high incidence of arrhythmia in this population. Based on these and other studies revealing increasing prevalence of right ventricular dysfunction and systemic tricuspid regurgitation, clinicians and investigators recognized the need for improved approaches to repair of TGA.

First described by Jatene in the 1970s[23], it was not until the 1980s that the arterial switch approach to TGA became widespread. Improved understanding of coronary anatomy and refined surgical techniques, especially advances in microsurgical approaches to coronary reimplantation, made neonatal arterial switch a feasible safe approach. Lecompte and colleagues reported a modification of Jatene's approach in 1981, where the pulmonary artery bifurcation was brought anterior to the aorta and the right branch pulmonary artery draped anterior, rather than posterior, to the aorta. This 'Lecompte manoeuvre' lessened tension on the pulmonary arteries[24]. The arterial switch was initially performed on patients with elevated left ventricular pressure, the majority of whom had VSDs. Castenada and colleagues at Children's Hospital Boston pioneered the neonatal arterial switch, which avoided the issue of left ventricular remodeling, allowing the procedure to be performed in patients with or without VSDs. This series represented an enormous advance in the care of this heart defect[25].

Backer *et al.* described an experience with 60 infants who underwent either a Mustard procedure or arterial switch in the first three months of life[26]. They found equivalent early and late (mean follow-up) mortality, but a significantly lower incidence of early and late arrhythmias as well as better systemic ventricular function in the arterial switch group.

A study from Children's Hospital Boston looked at hemodynamic effects and longer term neurological correlates of different approaches to vital organ support during arterial switch repair. They found low-flow bypass and circulatory arrest had little influence on mortality or ICU stay, but that circulatory arrest was associated with more central nervous system abnormalities[27, 28]. After 8 years of follow-up, both groups were noted to have an increased risk of neurodevelopmental abnormalities when compared to the general population[29]. These articles highlight a paradigm shift—no longer are we focused merely on short or long-term mortality, but rather, on assessment and improvement of quality of life.

Tetralogy of Fallot

As late as the 1990s, the topic of primary versus staged repair of tetralogy of Fallot (ToF) remained controversial. In 1993, Freedom and colleagues reported on 237 infants with isolated tetralogy of Fallot who required surgical intervention prior to 18 months of age. They noted an overall ten-year survival rate of 89%, with no difference in mortality between those undergoing primary versus staged repair provided that surgery was not required in the neonatal period.

Patients with ToF were often repaired with use of a transannular patch in order to completely relieve any valvar obstruction. Until 1990, the pulmonary regurgitation created by this surgical approach was considered a harmless outcome of surgery. One of the first strong hints that pulmonary regurgitation was harmful was published by Redington's group[30]. The sudden-death risk associated with repaired tetralogy was publicized initially by the Royal Brompton Hospital. Gatzoulis and Redington described the relationship between extreme QRS prolongation (≥180 msec) and the likelihood of syncope, sustained ventricular tachycardia (VT), or sudden death[31]. They demonstrated that extreme QRS prolongation reflected marked right ventricular dilation, defining a mechano-electric relationship. Gatzoulis *et al.* then published a ten-year study looking at outcomes in 782 patients with tetralogy repair[32]. This highlighted the negative impact of pulmonary regurgitation and the association with sudden death. These observations have altered clinical practice such that pulmonary valve replacement is more frequently performed in patients with pulmonary regurgitation following ToF repair.

Therrien *et al.* queried whether we as cardiologists were waiting too long before referring patients for pulmonary valve replacement[33]. These authors noted that right ventricular systolic function was not improved following pulmonary valve replacement in a cohort of older patients. Vliegen and his colleagues published the first sizable series to demonstrate favourable right ventricular remodeling after pulmonary valve placement[34]. Therrien correlated the normalization of right ventricular volumes post-operatively with preoperative values, and defined a threshold of 170 mL/M^2 for recommending pulmonary valve replacement in patients with moderate or severe pulmonary regurgitation following repair of ToF[35].

Whether or not such remodeling is a true surrogate marker for improved outcomes is unclear and again highlights the real difficulties facing investigators in clinical congenital heart disease.

Khairy and colleagues[36] conducted a multi-centre cohort study in high-risk patients with repaired ToF to determine actuarial rates of ICD discharges, to identify risk factors and to characterize ICD-related complications. They enrolled 121 patients from 11 sites and followed them for a median of 3.7 years. Implantable cardioverter defibrillators were implanted for primary prevention in 68 patients and for secondary prevention in 53 patients. Of the 121 patients, 37 received at least one appropriate and effective ICD discharge. Annual actuarial rates of appropriate ICD shocks were 7.7% and 9.8% in primary and secondary prevention, respectively. Inappropriate shocks were experienced in 5.8% of patients annually. They derived risk factors to help identify patients requiring ICD therapy. Interestingly, the most important predictor variable for shock/ventricular VT was elevated left ventricular end-diastolic pressure.

Khairy and colleagues[37] published the results of a multi-centre study of 52 patients with repaired tetralogy of Fallot who had undergone programmed ventricular stimulation. These patients were then followed for a mean of 6.5 years. The authors demonstrated that both sustained monomorphic VT and polymorphic VT at the time of study were powerful predictors of clinical VT and sudden cardiac death.

The Fontan procedure

The successful application of the concept of a 'Fontan procedure' was first described in 1971. This general approach to management of tricuspid atresia, introduced over the following decade, was subsequently applied more broadly to other single ventricle diagnoses. The surgery carried significant short-term risk, yet held out the first real promise of successful surgical palliation for single ventricle defects.

The development of this extraordinary class of single ventricle surgeries was followed quickly by reports of medium and long-term complications, with important implications for patient outcomes, counselling, and management decisions. This also led to important modifications to the Fontan procedure intended to mitigate adverse outcomes. In a landmark review of 15-year outcomes of patients in 1990, Fontan *et al.* clearly showed that even the results of a 'perfect Fontan' seemed to have a markedly increased risk for adverse outcomes attributable to the single ventricle physiology itself, concluding that 'the premature decline in survival and functional status and the late rise in hazard function are from the Fontan state per se and that the Fontan operation is, therefore, palliative but not curative'[38].

Arrhythmia and thrombosis were well described complications in Fontan patients. The initial approach and early modifications were associated with progressive right atrial dilation and consequently an arrhythmic burden. Investigators introduced new surgical approaches, the 'lateral tunnel Fontan' and 'extracardiac Fontan' procedures, in hopes of reducing the significant long-term morbidity associated with the procedure. These surgical modifications resulted in more laminar flow with less energy loss through the baffle[39] in various models, but did not eliminate the complications of earlier techniques.

The earlier cohort of patients undergoing the classic atriopulmonary Fontan connection developed recurrent arrhythmia resistant to standard medical, and later invasive therapies. Mavroudis and colleagues pioneered and honed a technique to 'convert' older Fontan types to the more streamlined total cavopulmonary anastomosis, often in association with surgical intervention for the arrhythmia. The results, though applicable to a relatively small subset of patients, provided successful improvement in arrhythmia burden, at least over the short term[40].

Another important modification to the Fontan procedure was baffle fenestration to address problematic acute post-operative complications of Fontan surgery, namely low cardiac output and pleural effusions. Bridges *et al.* described placement of a fenestrated baffle during surgery for patients at increased risk for these outcomes, followed by later device closure of the fenestration[41].

Along with the development of the lateral tunnel and extracardiac procedures mentioned above, this modest modification translated into improved perioperative outcomes following the Fontan procedure.

Specific complications associated with the Fontan procedure

A number of non-cardiac complications occurring after the Fontan procedure have been well-described and include protein losing enteropathy, plastic bronchitis, and liver dysfunction. Protein losing enteropathy was first described in this population in a patient with a valveless RA-RV conduit and severe regurgitation[42]. While the conclusion of this manuscript was that a valved conduit might prevent the complication and thus should be preferred, it has become only too clear that protein losing enteropathy is a potential complication of all types of single ventricle Fontan palliation. Lemmer *et al.* described a case of 'cardiac cirrhosis' in a 15-year-old girl who had a valved RA-RV conduit style Fontan for tricuspid atresia at age eight[43]. She had done reasonably well but was noted during cholecystectomy to have severe liver fibrosis/cardiac cirrhosis. Through many subsequent publications, it has become apparent that congestive hepatopathy to fibrosis is almost inevitable as these patients age and can result in clinically significant cirrhosis, with implications for patient outcomes, including ascites, vasodilatory cardiac failure, and hepatocellular carcinoma.

Adult congenital heart disease and other miscellaneous paediatric cardiology

Landmark papers in the field

Anderson RH, Becker AE, Freedom RM, Macartney FJ, Quero-Jimenez M, Shinebourne EA, Wilkinson JL, Tynan M. Sequential segmental analysis of congenital heart disease. *Pediatr Cardiol* 1984; 5(4): 281–7.

Freed MD, Heymann MA, Lewis AB, Roehl SL, Kensey RC. Prostaglandin E1 infants with ductus arteriosus-dependent congenital heart disease. *Circulation* 1981; 64(5): 899–905.

Newburger JW, Takahashi M, Burns JC, Beiser AS, Chung KJ, Duffy CE, Glode MP, Mason WH, Reddy V, Sanders SP, Shulman ST, Wiggins JW, Hicks RV, Fulton DR, Lewis AB, Leung DYM, Colton T, Rosen FS, Melish ME. The treatment of Kawasaki syndrome with intravenous gamma globulin. *N Engl J Med* 1986; 315(6): 341–7.

Morris CD, Menashe VD. 25-year mortality after surgical repair of congenital heart defect in childhood. A population-based cohort study. *JAMA* 1991; 266(24): 3447–52.

Hahn RT, Roman MJ, Mogtader AH, Devereux RB. Association of aortic dilation with regurgitant, stenotic and functionally normal bicuspid aortic valves. *J Am Coll Cardiol* 1992; 19(2): 283–8.

Kleinman CS, Hobbins JC, Jaffe CC, Lynch DC, Talner NS. Echocardiographic studies of the human fetus: prenatal diagnosis of congenital heart disease and cardiac dysrhythmias. *Pediatrics* 1980; 65(6): 1059–67.

Anderson and colleagues[44] fundamentally changed the way we look at congenital heart defects by proposing the sequential segmental analysis of CHD. This had a major impact in clarifying our understanding of CHD, particularly in its complex forms.

Prostaglandin E1 became available in the mid-1970s. In 1981, Freed and colleagues[45] reported the results of a large multi-centre trial of prostaglandin E1 in 492 infants with ductus arteriosus-dependent congenital heart disease. The therapy was highly effective in improving the health of these infants, leading to improved survival and better long-term outcomes.

In 1986, Newburger and colleagues reported the efficacy of intravenous gamma globulin plus aspirin versus aspirin alone in reducing the frequency of coronary artery abnormalities in children with acute Kawasaki syndrome in a multi-centre randomized trial[46]. The IV gamma globulin was safe and effective in reducing the prevalence of coronary artery abnormalities when administered early in the course of the disease. This paper changed the standard of care for this condition.

Long-term outcomes

In 1993 Gersony and colleagues[47] published the Second Natural History Study of congenital heart defects. They looked at quality of life in patients with aortic stenosis, pulmonary stenosis, and VSDs. They concluded that these patients had a quality of life in the mid-1980s similar to that of the general American population.

In 1992, Moller and Anderson[48] reported a 26–37-year follow-up of 1000 consecutive children with cardiac malformations. Of the 1000, 285 had died. Of the remainder, 632 were in excellent or good clinical condition. Morris and Menashe[49] conducted a population-based cohort study of Oregon residents looking at 25-year mortality after surgical repair of eight congenital heart defects in childhood. Age at surgery and operative mortality had decreased significantly during the study: Twenty-five-year mortality was 5% for ToF and isolated VSD; 10% for coarctation; 17% for aortic stenosis; 5% for pulmonic stenosis, less than 1% for patent ductus arteriosus and there were no cardiac deaths after childhood following atrial septal defect repair. Cardiac mortality was 15% at 15 years after the Mustard operation for TGA, and was 2% at ten years after the Senning operation for TGA.

In 1990, Murphy and colleagues[50] reported the 27–32-year outcomes of 123 patients who had surgical repair of a secundum atrial septal defect at the Mayo Clinic between 1956 and 1960. While overall survival was quite good, they demonstrated that surgery at a younger age

(under age 25) was associated with better long-term survival and fewer cardiovascular complications. In 1993, Murphy and colleagues[51] also reported the 32-year actuarial survival of 163 patients who had tetralogy repair at the Mayo Clinic and who survived at least 30 days. They demonstrated excellent long-term survival, albeit not as good as in the general population.

Prevalence and mortality

Marelli and colleagues[52] used administrative databases in the province of Quebec to determine the change in prevalence and age distribution of CHD from 1985 to 2000. The median age for all patients with severe CHD was 11 years in 1985 and 17 years in 2000. The prevalence of severe CHD increased, but the increase in adults was significantly higher than that observed in children. In the year 2000, 49% of those alive with severe CHD were adults. The same group later reported temporal trends in all-cause mortality in patients with CHD in Quebec between 1987 and 2005. They noted that most deaths in patients with CHD had historically occurred in early childhood. Overall mortality decreased by 31% from the beginning to the end of the study. Mortality rates decreased in all age groups below 65 years, with the largest reduction being in infant mortality. Gains in survival were mostly driven by reduced mortality in severe forms of CHD. Deaths in CHD have shifted away from infants and towards adult life, with a steady increase in age at death accompanying a decreasing overall mortality.

In 2000, Oechslin and colleagues[53] provided a profile of 199 deceased patients from a clinic population of 2609. Mortality was highest in patients with cc-TGA, tricuspid atresia, and other forms of single ventricle. Sudden death was the mode of death in 26%, followed by progressive heart failure and perioperative deaths. In 2007, Nienamin and colleagues[54] studied all late deaths of patients operated on for congenital heart disease in Finland during the years 1953–1989. Of the 6000 patients who survived their first operation, 9% died during the 45-year follow-up period. The cause of death was confirmed by post-mortem examination in 81% of cases. Death was CHD-related in two-thirds of the patients. The three most common modes of death were heart failure in 40%, perioperative in 26%, and sudden in 22%.

In 1992, Hahn and colleagues[55] reported a two-dimensional echo study of 83 adults with bicuspid aortic valves. They demonstrated a high prevalence of aortic root enlargement in these patients that was unrelated to the aortic valve haemodynamics or the patient's age. These findings supported the hypothesis that bicuspid aortic valve and a predilection to aortic root dilation may reflect a common genetic or developmental defect. As a result of this and similar publications, it is now recognized that the term 'post-stenotic dilation' is at most only part of the story of bicuspid aortopathy and that patients need to be followed both for valvar dysfunction as well as aortic dilation.

Imaging for congenital heart defects

During the 1980–2010 period, there were many advances made in the imaging of congenital heart defects. One of the most important occurred in 1981, when Kleinman and colleagues[56] reported the first use of foetal echocardiography. This has gone on to transform the diagnosis and management of foetal cardiac problems resulting in improved survival of infants born with congenital cardiac defects.

Magnetic resonance imaging (MRI) was first used in adults with congenital cardiac defects prior to being used in children. In 1991, Kilner and colleagues[57] demonstrated the ability of MR imaging to accurately measure gradients in stenotic native heart valves, conduits, Fontan connections, and aortic coarctation. In 1994, his group reported their experience[58] with the use of MRI and trans-oesophageal echocardiography in the assessment of complex congenital heart patients. This established that TOE was best for intracardiac anatomy; MRI was best for extracardiac anatomy; and that the results were best in both categories when both techniques were used. There have been a multitude of incremental improvements in the techniques used. In 2004 Prakash and colleagues[59] used pulsed MRI to successfully evaluate myocardial perfusion and viability in congenital and acquired paediatric heart disease.

Genetics

Landmark papers in the field

Basson CT, Bachinsky DR, Lin RC, Levi T, Elkins JA, Soults J, Grayzel D, Kroumpouzou E, Traill TA, Leblanc-Straceski J, Renault B, Kucherlapati R, Seidman JG, Seidman CE. Mutations in human TBX5 cause limb and cardiac malformation in Holt-Oram syndrome. *Nat Genet* 1997; 15(1): 30–5.

Li QY, Newbury-Ecob RA, Terrett JA, Wilson DI, Curtis AR, Yi CH, Gebuhr T, Bullen PJ, Robson SC, Strachan T, Bonnet D, Lyonnet S, Young ID, Raeburn JA, Buckler AJ, Law DJ, Brook JD. Holt-Oram syndrome is caused by mutations in TBX5, a member of the Brachyury (T) gene family. *Nat Genet* 1997; 15(1): 21–9.

Ewart AK, Morris CA, Atkinson D, Jin W, Sternes K, Spallone P, Stock AD, Leppert M, Keating MT. Hemizygosity at the elastin locus in a developmental disorder, Williams syndrome. *Nat Genet* 1993; 5(1): 11–6.

Tartaglia M, Mehler EL, Goldberg R, Zampino G, Brunner HG, Kremer H, van der Burgt I, Crosby AH, Ion A, Jeffery S, Kalidas K, Patton MA, Kucherlapati RS, Gelb BD. Mutations in PTPN11, encoding the protein tyrosine phosphatase SHP-2, cause Noonan syndrome. *Nat Genet* 2001; 29(4): 465–8.

de la Chapelle A, Herva R, Koivisto M, Aula P. A deletion in chromosome 22 can cause DiGeorge syndrome. *Human Genetics* 1981; 57(3): 253–6.

Schott JJ, Benson DW, Basson CT, Pease W, Silberbach GM, Moak JP, Maron BJ, Seidman CE, Seidman JG. Congenital heart disease caused by mutations in the transcription factor NKX2-5. *Science* 1998; 281(5373): 108–11.

Gross chromosomal abnormalities, often associated with a clinical syndrome, have long been known to cause congenital heart defects. The complex, likely multifactorial, inheritance of congenital heart defects gives the appearance that the vast majority of defects occur sporadically. In recent years, however, investigators have discovered genetic abnormalities underlying many syndromic and non-syndromic congenital heart defects. This section will highlight papers that epitomize the landmark strides made in defining the important role genetic defects have in the predisposition to congenital heart disease. Progress has been incremental and, perhaps more so than for any other topic of this chapter, it is impossible to specify only a few landmark papers. It is equally important to note that unlike many of the other 'landmarks' described in this chapter, these findings have not directly changed current practice to any great extent. Rather, they have shifted our understanding of the cause of congenital heart defects and hold promise to lead to greatly enhanced prediction and even prevention of CHD.

Identification of the genetic basis of syndromic defects

Two papers, by Basson *et al.* and Li *et al.*, describe the identification of single nucleotide mutations in the *TBX5* gene for multiple patients in several families with Holt-Oram syndrome, which classically presents with upper limb abnormalities and cardiac septal defects[60, 61]. Most of the identified mutations result in early termination of transcription and all cause *TBX5* haploinsufficiency. The mutations all occurred in the *TBX5* gene, but different mutations were described for different families. *TBX5* was shown by Li *et al.* to be expressed in human embryos in the primitive atria, ventricles, endocardial cushions, and forelimbs, supporting the role of the *TBX5* gene product in the development of these structures.

Of note, not all patients with clinical manifestations consistent with Holt-Oram syndrome have a mutation in *TBX5*. Likewise, other syndromes such as Noonan syndrome, which appear to have a relatively consistent phenotypic presentation have been shown to result from an array of different mutations. While there are clearly some phenotypic differences based on genetic defect, the similarities highlight the fact that many genes interact with complex environmental cues during cardiac development, and perturbations along a pathway for diverse reasons can result in a similar outcome.

Genetic defects have been discovered to be associated with a wide array of other syndromes, including congenital heart disease. In 1993, Ewart and colleagues reported the presence of elastin gene mutations in four families and five sporadic cases of Williams syndrome[62]. This was followed by validation of a clinically useful technique (fluorescence in situ hybridization or FISH) for the genetic diagnosis of Williams syndrome[63]. While readily available and highly accurate, the benefit of genetic testing for such syndromes in the clinic is still unclear, especially in cases readily diagnosed by clinical findings or those in which reproduction is highly unlikely or impossible.

While some syndromes, such as Williams syndrome, have been found to be associated almost entirely with mutations in a single gene, it has become clear that for many others mutations in any of several genes may result in similar, though often not identical, phenotypes. *PTPN11* gene mutations are now known to be one cause

of Noonan syndrome, as reported by Tartaglia *et al.*[64]. However, only about half the patients with Noonan syndrome have been found to have such a mutation. About 20% of patients classified as having clinical Noonan syndrome have a mutation in *SOS1*, which encodes a protein in the same pathway (Ras/MAP kinase) as the protein product of *PTPN11*[65]. There are phenotypic differences between Noonan syndrome due to different genetic defects, but it has become clear that mutations at multiple levels of a given developmental pathway may result in a similar genetic syndrome. Further research has confirmed the variable, ascertainment, and time-dependent presentation of other genetic syndromes, including 22q11 mutations[66].

Isolated congenital heart and syndromic defects can result from the same genetic basis

It has long been known that conotruncal abnormalities are common among patients with DiGeorge syndrome and velocardiofacial syndrome. The story of the elucidation of a strong association between deletion of a portion of the 22nd chromosome (22q11) and this syndrome highlights advances in basic genetic techniques. In the early 1980s, investigators reported that deletions of this chromosome seem to be able to cause DiGeorge syndrome using data from a handful of families[67, 68, 69]. Larger studies in the late 1980s, using relatively crude chromosome banding technology and therefore missing a large number of true smaller deletions, suggested a sizeable minority of DiGeorge syndrome patients had 22q11 deletions. Only in the early 1990s, however, with improving techniques of high resolution banding and fluorescence was it confirmed that the vast majority of DiGeorge syndrome was associated with a 22q11 deletion[70, 71, 72]. This begged the question of what proportion of conotruncal defects associated with this syndrome may be related to such a deletion in the absence of other syndromic characteristics. A paper by Goldmuntz, followed by other larger and more comprehensive reports, reported that the 22q11 microdeletion was present in only a significant minority of patients with conotruncal defects without clinical evidence of any congenital syndrome[73].

Identification of the genetic basis of non-syndromic defects

Schott *et al.* studied four families with autosomal dominant inheritance of secundum atrial septal defect and atrioventricular conduction delay, along with sporadic occurrences of other congenital defects, including tetralogy of Fallot, pulmonary atresia, and subvalvar aortic stenosis. They performed genome wide linkage analysis and loci on chromosome 5q35, a region which was thought based on non-human organisms to include a gene involved in cardiac development, NKX2.5. They sequenced this gene in the affected families and found several distinct mutations in NKX2.5[74].

Garg et al. described the presence of mutations in the NOTCH1 gene in two families with clear autosomal dominant inheritance of severe left ventricular outflow tract lesions, mainly bicuspid aortic valve[75]. While this provides insight into aortic valve and outflow tract development, it is notable that research since this publication has found that a small minority of patients with bicuspid aortic valve have such mutations.

McElhinney and colleagues sequenced DNA for 608 subjects with congenital heart disease, including atrial septal defect, ToF, TGA, aortic stenosis, and other conotruncal abnormalities. They found that 3% had a NKX2.5 mutation, the majority of whom had no familial congenital defects or conduction system disease. This report highlights the complexity and heterogeneity of presentation for genetic mutations 'causing' congenital heart disease[76].

Implications

Currently, genetic testing can be useful to determine the risk of other organ involvement, to obtain some prognostic information, to provide reproductive counselling, and to support further familial testing. Although advances in genetics have thus far had modest clinical impact, few doubt that genetic testing will become more commonplace for patients with congenital heart defects in the future.

Cardiac development

Landmark papers in the field

Rudolph AM. Distribution and regulation of blood flow in the fetal and neonatal lamb. *Circ Res* 1985; 57(6): 811–21.

Olley PM, Coceani F, Rowe RD, Swyer PR. Clinical use of prostaglandins and prostaglandin synthetase inhibitors in cardiac problems of the newborn. *Adv Prostaglandin Thromboxane Res* 1980; 7: 913–6.

Kirby ML, Gale TF, Stewart DE. Neural crest cells contribute to normal aorticopulmonary septation. *Science* 1983; 220(4601): 1059–61.

An understanding of cardiac development would seem necessary for a thorough understanding of the causes of congenital heart disease. The fundamental aspects of cardiovascular development were described well before the 1980s. Despite what appeared to be a thorough understanding of the gross aspects of cardiac development, there have been real and significant strides in our understanding over the past three decades, made possible in large part as the result of new scientific techniques.

While the anatomy of the cardiovascular system had been studied extensively for decades, the study of foetal physiology was a more difficult proposition until the 1960s. Abraham Rudolph and colleagues pioneered techniques to study the *in vivo* physiology of foetal lambs, allowing quantitative description of foetal blood flow as well as the response of foetal physiology to various interventions. In a 1985 review, Rudolph presented an astoundingly comprehensive yet succinct summary of two decades of work. Experiments involving radionuclide-labelled microspheres and chronically instrumented foetal sheep resulted in a much more nuanced understanding of the extensive modifications of the foetal circulation, allowing maintenance of well-oxygenated umbilical venous blood to supply the developing brain and myocardium in the face of diverse insults[77].

While the immediate clinical impact of these contributions may have been unclear at first, this is no longer the case. These fundamental physiologic studies led to basic scientific and then clinical investigation into the effects of prostaglandin E1 on the ductus arteriosus, perhaps the greatest medical advance in the care of newborns with congenital heart disease over the past 50 years[45,78]. A more recent development, foetal cardiovascular intervention, has also been facilitated by the physiologic understanding of response to such interventions.

There have also been several landmark advances in our understanding of anatomical and structural cardiovascular development. Kirby et al. described an important contribution of the neural crest to aortopulmonary septation, conferring not only improved understanding of outflow tract and semilunar valve development, but also a mechanism to induce aortopulmonary outflow defects in laboratory animals and thus provide animal models for the study of human disease[79]. More recently, advances in molecular and cellular biology have provided unexpected new insights into cardiac development. Perhaps the most surprising finding is that portions of the right ventricle and right ventricular outflow tract are derived from a previously unknown anterior 'secondary heart field'[80, 81]. This has led to intense interest and further research into how this relates to conotruncal abnormalities and promises to lead to better understanding of clinical congenital heart defects and their aetiology.

Pregnancy and transmission

Landmark papers in the field

Whittemore R, Hobbins JC, Engle MA. Pregnancy and its outcome in women with and without surgical treatment of congenital heart disease. *Am J Cardiol* 1982; 50(3): 641–51.

Nora JJ, Nora AH. Maternal transmission of congenital heart diseases: new recurrence risk figures and the questions of cytoplasmic inheritance and vulnerability to teratogens. *Am J Cardiol* 1987; 59(5): 459–63.

Siu SC, Sermer M, Colman JM, Alvarez AN, Mercier LA, Morton BC, Kells CM, Bergin ML, Kiess MC, Marcotte F, Taylor DA, Gordon EP, Spears JC, Tam JW, Amankwah KS, Smallhorn JF, Farine D, Sorensen S. Prospective multicenter study of pregnancy outcomes in women with heart disease. *Circulation* 2001; 104(5): 515–21.

A major theme in the care of congenital heart disease over the past several decades is a shift of focus from short-term survival to optimizing long-term survival and quality of life. That is, the goal has shifted from living to living well. Having a healthy child is, for many people, a large part of a good life. It is not surprising, therefore, that there has been a focus on describing the risk factors for pregnancy outcomes in the growing population of women with congenital heart defects.

In 1985, Ferencz and colleagues reported the results of the Baltimore-Washington Infant Study of the prevalence of congenital heart disease among live born children. They determined the prevalence to be approximately 3.7 per 1000 live births. In 1982, Whittemore *et al.* published the experience of a single paediatric cardiologist with 482 pregnancies in 233 women with congenital heart disease over 34 years[82]. They reported on the course of pregnancy, infant outcomes, transmission of congenital heart disease from mother to offspring, and maternal cardiovascular and obstetric outcomes. In truth little has been added, despite an extensive and growing literature on the topic, to our general understanding of pregnancy in women with congenital heart disease since this early, largely descriptive study—much of which was based on physical examination in the era before echocardiography was widely available. The authors found that cyanosis predisposed to low birth weight; that the incidence of congenital heart defects in offspring is much higher than that seen in the general population; that most women do well with pregnancy (none of the 482 pregnancies resulted in maternal death or endocarditis), but that impaired functional status and left-sided obstructive lesions predispose to adverse cardiovascular outcomes for mothers. Their experiential recommendations for care of pregnant mothers are almost perfectly in line with what is currently recommended: from maintaining contact with the cardiologist to making 'early joint arrangements' with the obstetric team, to only recommending Caesarean section for obstetric reasons.

Whittemore *et al.* reported a very high rate of offspring with congenital heart disease, 14–16% compared with published estimates of 3–5%. If the mother had a congenital heart defect, the recurrence risk was 14.4%. If the father had a congenital heart defect, the recurrence risk was 9.9%. If one removed, from the total figures, the children whose VSDs closed as well as those with genetic syndromes or strong family history, the incidence of CHD in the progeny of affected mothers or fathers was not statistically different (9.8% and 8.2%, respectively).

These results, however, led Nora and Nora to wonder whether there may be a reason for this surprisingly high figure[83]. They noted that Whittemore's study differed in two ways from prior studies: the offspring were examined multiple times over the first three years of life and, by design, all the parents with congenital heart disease in the study were women. Nora and Nora reviewed eight studies, including 3996 offspring of parents with congenital heart disease. They found that offspring of women with congenital heart disease were much more likely than offspring of men with congenital heart disease to be affected with a heart defect themselves. This was generally consistent across all types of defects, though the effect was heterogeneous with aortic stenosis having the greatest maternal predominance (relative risk of 6.39 for the child to have AS if the mother rather than the father had CHD). These data led to improved counselling for pregnant women, and provided a fascinating insight into the complex aetiology of these clearly heritable disorders.

While clinicians had a general sense of the risks of pregnancy, Siu *et al.* prospectively derived a risk score to facilitate risk stratification for women with heart disease. This multi-centre study of 599 pregnancies resulted in the description of the cardiac disease in pregnancy

(CARPREG) Risk Index to predict the estimated risk for maternal cardiovascular events during pregnancy and in the early postpartum period. The factors themselves may have been expected (and in large part are what one could glean from Whittemore's data):

◆ Prior cardiac events or arrhythmia.
◆ Poor NYHA functional class (III or IV).
◆ Left-sided obstructive lesions or systemic ventricular dysfunction.

Women with none of these risk factors were found to have a cardiac event rate of 3–5%, those with one factor had a risk of 24–31%, and those with more than one risk factor had a maternal cardiac event rate of 53–69%[84]. This landmark paper has been of great help to clinicians in providing specific counsel to their patients and determining the appropriate level of monitoring throughout pregnancy. The results also highlight how difficult it is to predict events during pregnancy—a relatively small minority of all cardiovascular events occurred in women with >1 risk factor (9 of 35 in the validation group).

Pulmonary arterial hypertension and congenital heart disease

Landmark papers in the field

Pepke-Zaba J, Higenbottam TW, Dinh-Xuan AT, Stone D, Wallwork J. Inhaled nitric oxide as a cause of selective pulmonary vasodilatation in pulmonary hypertension. *Lancet* 1991; 338(8776): 1173–4.

Roberts JD, Polaner DM, Lang P, Zapol WM. Inhaled nitric oxide in persistent pulmonary hypertension of the newborn. *Lancet* 1992; 340(8823): 818–9.

Kinsella JP, Neish SR, Shaffer E, Abman SH. Low-dose inhalation nitric oxide in persistent pulmonary hypertension of the newborn. *Lancet* 1992; 340(8823): 819–20.

Journois D, Pouard P, Mauriat P, Malhere T, Vouhe P, Safran D. Inhaled nitric oxide as a therapy for pulmonary hypertension after operations for congenital heart defects. *J Thorac Cardiovasc Surg* 1994; 107(4): 1129–35.

Galie N, Beghetti M, Gatzoulis MA, Granton J, Berger RM, Lauer A, Chiossi E, Landzberg M; Bosentan Randomized Trial of Endothelin Antagonist Therapy-5 (BREATHE-5) Investigators. Bosentan therapy in patients with Eisenmenger syndrome: a multicenter, double-blind, randomized, placebo-controlled study. *Circulation* 2006; 114(1): 48–54.

Unlike many other aspects of congenital heart disease over the past 30 years, the most remarkable advances in the management of pulmonary arterial hypertension have been in medical, rather than surgical or interventional, therapy. There are several distinct populations in paediatric and congenital heart disease where pulmonary arterial hypertension plays a major role in determining outcomes, and major strides have been made in each.

Persistently elevated pulmonary vascular resistance after birth is a relatively rare occurrence, but the natural history includes very high mortality. Abraham Rudolph reviewed this phenomenon, including his truly astounding life's work of investigation, in a 1980 paper on postnatal pulmonary hypertension[85]. Such a deep understanding of the various aspects of the pathophysiology of this disease allowed clinicians to better understand how temporizing measures such as extracorporeal membrane oxygenation (ECMO) and later, nitric oxide, could provide a bridge for the pulmonary vasculature to mature. Two landmark papers on ECMO for persistent pulmonary hypertension of the newborn (PPHN) represent a major advance in both the care of this relatively small group of patients as well as the introduction of a new and controversial study design in paediatric cardiology. Bartlett *et al.* described their experience with ECMO in a study of 12 patients and found mortality without ECMO of 100%, while with ECMO none died. This failed to convince clinicians, however. While this was a randomized controlled trial, the study design was 'play the winner' and only one subject ended up getting conventional therapy[86]. While statistically significant, could clinicians really conclude the superiority based on comparison with outcomes for one subject? This highlights the difficulty of performing rigorous trials for therapies in disease with a high mortality in children. O'Rourke *et al.* performed a study where patients would receive or not receive ECMO depending on which intensive care unit they happened to be transferred to. The study was performed in two phases, and after four deaths in the conventional therapy arm, all remaining patients were treated with ECMO. Survival with ECMO was 97%, with conventional therapy resulting in 60% survival. Once again, important ethical considerations were raised, highlighting the difficulty of assessing new therapies for paediatric disease scientifically[87].

Severe paroxysmal pulmonary arterial hypertension following cardiac surgery, referred to as a pulmonary hypertensive crisis, was a major cause of post-operative morbidity and mortality through the first several decades of congenital heart surgery. Hopkins *et al.* described the phenomenon in detail in a thorough landmark observational study[88]. Of note, none of the five children who died and had autopsies showed any pathologic sign of irreversible pulmonary vascular remodelling seen in 'primary pulmonary hypertension', providing further evidence that these paroxysmal events were related to pulmonary arterial vasoreactivity and thus laying the groundwork for development and study of selective pulmonary vasodilators.

The description of acute therapy with inhaled nitric oxide has entirely shifted the care and prognosis for patients with PPHN as well as for post-operative pulmonary hypertensive crises. Pepke-Zaba described the selective pulmonary vasodilation from inhaled nitric oxide in pulmonary hypertension, without the systemic vasodilation seen with prostacyclin[89]. Landmark studies in PPHN and pulmonary hypertensive crises followed, showing improved haemodynamics, reduced need for ECMO and improved outcomes[90, 91, 92, 93].

There has also been landmark progress in the care for patients with Eisenmenger syndrome, as well as incremental improvement in monitoring multi-organ function and haematologic status. There was question over whether pulmonary vasodilator therapy would be harmful in this population given the potential for systemic vasodilation as well. The BREATHE-5 trial of bosentan in patients with symptomatic Eisenmenger syndrome demonstrated improved haemodynamics and functional capacity over a relatively short follow-up in Eisenmenger syndrome patients without an effect on systemic arterial saturation[94]. While there are no definitive data that such therapy, with bosentan or any other pulmonary vasodilator, prolongs the life of these patients, retrospective analysis suggests improved survival may in fact be expected[95].

Conclusion

The care of children and adults with congenital heart disease has seen remarkable strides forward over the past three decades. Would pioneering congenital cardiologists such as Helen Taussig, Alexander Nadas, Paul Wood, and Maude Abbott recognize a field they essentially founded less than a century earlier? While the answer cannot be known, we can be sure they would without exception be overjoyed by the progress in caring for these patients. From pioneering surgeries for previously universally fatal defects, to understanding the genetic cause of several facets of congenital heart disease, to entirely new imaging modalities to define anatomy and physiology *in vivo*, to the emergence of catheter-based therapy, congenital cardiology has been transformed. As important have been the more incremental steps in refining existing therapies and, finally, an acknowledgement that while survival takes priority, the focus must then turn to optimizing the quality of the lives saved.

The medical literature tells a fascinating tale of this evolution by way of numerous landmark articles which highlight both the shortcomings of existing therapies and the discovery of new ones. No one paper stands alone, but rather builds on the work that has gone before it with this body of literature both reflecting, and generating medical advances.

References

1. Rashkind WJ, Mullins CE, Hellenbrand WE, Tait MA. Nonsurgical closure of patent ductus arteriosus: clinical application of the Rashkind PDA Occluder System. *Circulation* 1987; 75(3): 583–92.

2. Lock JE, Rome JJ, Davis R, *et al.* Transcatheter closure of atrial septal defects. Experimental studies. *Circulation* 1989; 79(5): 1091–9.

3. Lock JE, Bass JL, Amplatz K, Fuhrman BP, Castaneda-Zuniga W. Balloon dilation angioplasty of aortic coarctations in infants and children. *Circulation* 1983; 68(1): 109–16.

4. Kan JS, White RI, Jr., Mitchell SE, Farmlett EJ, Donahoo JS, Gardner TJ. Treatment of restenosis of coarctation by percutaneous transluminal angioplasty. *Circulation* 1983; 68(5): 1087–94.

5. Kan JS, White RI, Jr., Mitchell SE, Gardner TJ. Percutaneous balloon valvuloplasty: a new method for treating congenital pulmonary-valve stenosis. *N Engl J Med* 1982; 307(9): 540–2.

6. Lababidi Z, Wu JR, Walls JT. Percutaneous balloon aortic valvuloplasty: results in 23 patients. *Am J Cardiol* 1984; 53(1): 194–7.

7. Magee AG, Nykanen D, McCrindle BW, Wax D, Freedom RM, Benson LN. Balloon dilation of severe aortic stenosis in the neonate: comparison of anterograde and retrograde catheter approaches. *J Am Coll Cardiol* 1997; 30(4): 1061–6.

8. O'Laughlin MP, Perry SB, Lock JE, Mullins CE. Use of endovascular stents in congenital heart disease. *Circulation* 1991; 83(6): 1923–39.

9. Ebeid MR, Prieto LR, Latson LA. Use of balloon-expandable stents for coarctation of the aorta: initial results and intermediate-term follow-up. *J Am Coll Cardiol* 1997; 30(7): 1847–52.

10. Bonhoeffer P, Boudjemline Y, Saliba Z, *et al.* Percutaneous replacement of pulmonary valve in a right-ventricle to pulmonary-artery prosthetic conduit with valve dysfunction. *Lancet* 2000; 356(9239): 1403–5.

11. Macartney FJ, Taylor JF, Graham GR, De Leval M, Stark J. The fate of survivors of cardiac surgery in infancy. *Circulation* 1980; 62(1): 80–91.

12. Bove EL, Behrendt DM. Open-heart surgery in the first week of life. *Ann Thorac Surg* 1980; 29(2): 130–4.

13. Norwood WI, Lang P, Castaneda AR, Campbell DN. Experience with operations for hypoplastic left heart syndrome. *J Thorac Cardiovasc Surg* 1981; 82(4): 511–9.

14. Norwood WI, Lang P, Hansen DD. Physiologic repair of aortic atresia-hypoplastic left heart syndrome. *N Engl J Med* 1983; 308(1): 23–6.

15. Ohye RG, Sleeper LA, Mahony L, *et al.* Comparison of shunt types in the Norwood procedure for single-ventricle lesions. *N Engl J Med* 2010; 362(21): 1980–92.

16. Lamour JM, Kanter KR, Naftel DC, *et al.* The effect of age, diagnosis, and previous surgery in children and adults undergoing heart transplantation for congenital heart disease. *J Am Coll Cardiol* 2009; 54(2): 160–5.

17. Hoffman TM, Wernovsky G, Atz AM, *et al.* Prophylactic intravenous use of milrinone after cardiac operation in pediatrics (PRIMACORP) study. Prophylactic Intravenous Use of Milrinone After Cardiac Operation in Pediatrics. *Am Heart J* 2002; 143(1): 15–21.

18. Newburger JW, Silbert AR, Buckley LP, Fyler DC. Cognitive function and age at repair of transposition of the great arteries in children. *N Engl J Med* 1984; 310(23): 1495–9.

19. Burke RP, Wernovsky G, van der Velde M, Hansen D, Castaneda AR. Video-assisted thoracoscopic surgery for congenital heart disease. *J Thorac Cardiovasc Surg* 1995; 109(3): 499–507; discussion 8.

20. da Silva JP, Baumgratz JF, da Fonseca L, *et al.* The cone reconstruction of the tricuspid valve in Ebstein's anomaly. The operation: early and midterm results. *J Thorac Cardiovasc Surg* 2007; 133(1): 215–23.

21. Flinn CJ, Wolff GS, Dick M, 2nd, *et al.* Cardiac rhythm after the Mustard operation for complete transposition of the great arteries. *N Engl J Med* 1984; 310(25): 1635–8.

22. Trusler GA, Williams WG, Duncan KF, *et al.* Results with the Mustard operation in simple transposition of the great arteries 1963–1985. *Ann Surg* 1987; 206(3): 251–60.

23. Jatene AD, Fontes VF, Paulista PP, *et al.* Anatomic correction of transposition of the great vessels. *J Thorac Cardiovasc Surg* 1976; 72(3): 364–70.

24. Lecompte Y, Zannini L, Hazan E, *et al.* Anatomic correction of transposition of the great arteries. *J Thorac Cardiovasc Surg* 1981; 82(4): 629–31.

25. Castaneda AR, Norwood WI, Jonas RA, Colon SD, Sanders SP, Lang P. Transposition of the great arteries and intact ventricular septum: anatomical repair in the neonate. *Ann Thorac Surg* 1984; 38(5): 438–43.

26. Backer CL, Ilbawi MN, Ohtake S, *et al.* Transposition of the great arteries: a comparison of results of the mustard procedure versus the arterial switch. *Ann Thorac Surg* 1989; 48(1): 10–4.

27. Wernovsky G, Wypij D, Jonas RA, *et al.* Postoperative course and hemodynamic profile after the arterial switch operation in neonates and infants. A comparison of low-flow cardiopulmonary bypass and circulatory arrest. *Circulation* 1995; 92(8): 2226–35.

28. Newburger JW, Jonas RA, Wernovsky G, *et al.* A comparison of the perioperative neurologic effects of hypothermic circulatory arrest versus low-flow cardiopulmonary bypass in infant heart surgery. *N Engl J Med* 1993; 329(15): 1057–64.

29. Bellinger DC, Wypij D, duPlessis AJ, *et al.* Neurodevelopmental status at eight years in children with dextro-transposition of the great arteries: the Boston

Circulatory Arrest Trial. *J Thorac Cardiovasc Surg* 2003; 126(5): 1385–96.

30. Carvalho JS, Shinebourne EA, Busst C, Rigby ML, Redington AN. Exercise capacity after complete repair of tetralogy of Fallot: deleterious effects of residual pulmonary regurgitation. *Br Heart J* 1992; 67(6): 470–3.

31. Gatzoulis MA, Till JA, Somerville J, Redington AN. Mechanoelectrical interaction in tetralogy of Fallot. QRS prolongation relates to right ventricular size and predicts malignant ventricular arrhythmias and sudden death. *Circulation* 1995; 92(2): 231–7.

32. Gatzoulis MA, Balaji S, Webber SA, *et al*. Risk factors for arrhythmia and sudden cardiac death late after repair of tetralogy of Fallot: a multicentre study. *Lancet* 2000; 356(9234): 975–81.

33. Therrien J, Siu SC, McLaughlin PR, Liu PP, Williams WG, Webb GD. Pulmonary valve replacement in adults late after repair of tetralogy of fallot: are we operating too late? *J Am Coll Cardiol* 2000; 36(5): 1670–5.

34. Vliegen HW, van Straten A, de Roos A, *et al*. Magnetic resonance imaging to assess the hemodynamic effects of pulmonary valve replacement in adults late after repair of tetralogy of Fallot. *Circulation* 2002; 106(13): 1703–7.

35. Therrien J, Provost Y, Merchant N, Williams W, Colman J, Webb G. Optimal timing for pulmonary valve replacement in adults after tetralogy of Fallot repair. *Am J Cardiol* 2005; 95(6): 779–82.

36. Khairy P, Harris L, Landzberg MJ, *et al*. Implantable cardioverter-defibrillators in tetralogy of Fallot. *Circulation* 2008; 117(3): 363–70.

37. Khairy P, Landzberg MJ, Gatzoulis MA, *et al*. Value of programmed ventricular stimulation after tetralogy of Fallot repair: a multicenter study. *Circulation* 2004; 109(16): 1994–2000.

38. Fontan F, Kirklin JW, Fernandez G, *et al*. Outcome after a 'perfect' Fontan operation. *Circulation* 1990; 81(5): 1520–36.

39. de Leval MR, Kilner P, Gewillig M, Bull C. Total cavopulmonary connection: a logical alternative to atriopulmonary connection for complex Fontan operations. Experimental studies and early clinical experience. *J Thorac Cardiovasc Surg* 1988; 96(5): 682–95.

40. Mavroudis C, Backer CL, Deal BJ, Johnsrude CL. Fontan conversion to cavopulmonary connection and arrhythmia circuit cryoablation. *J Thorac Cardiovasc Surg* 1998; 115(3): 547–56.

41. Bridges ND, Lock JE, Castaneda AR. Baffle fenestration with subsequent transcatheter closure. Modification of the Fontan operation for patients at increased risk. *Circulation* 1990; 82(5): 1681–9.

42. Crupi G, Locatelli G, Tiraboschi R, Villani M, De Tommasi M, Parenzan L. Protein-losing enteropathy after Fontan operation for tricuspid atresia (imperforate tricuspid valve). *Thorac Cardiovasc Surg* 1980; 28(5): 359–63.

43. Lemmer JH, Coran AG, Behrendt DM, Heidelberger KP, Stern AM. Liver fibrosis (cardiac cirrhosis) five years after modified Fontan operation for tricuspid atresia. *J Thorac Cardiovasc Surg* 1983; 86(5): 757–60.

44. Anderson RH, Becker AE, Freedom RM, *et al*. Sequential segmental analysis of congenital heart disease. *Pediatr Cardiol* 1984; 5(4): 281–7.

45. Freed MD, Heymann MA, Lewis AB, Roehl SL, Kensey RC. Prostaglandin E1 infants with ductus arteriosus-dependent congenital heart disease. *Circulation* 1981; 64(5): 899–905.

46. Newburger JW, Takahashi M, Burns JC, *et al*. The treatment of Kawasaki syndrome with intravenous gamma globulin. *N Engl J Med* 1986; 315(6): 341–7.

47. Gersony WM, Hayes CJ, Driscoll DJ, *et al*. Second natural history study of congenital heart defects. Quality of life of patients with aortic stenosis, pulmonary stenosis, or ventricular septal defect. *Circulation* 1993; 87(2 Suppl): 152–65.

48. Moller JH, Anderson RC. 1,000 consecutive children with a cardiac malformation with 26 to 37-year follow-up. *Am J Cardiol* 1992; 70(6): 661–7.

49. Morris CD, Menashe VD. 25-year mortality after surgical repair of congenital heart defect in childhood. A population-based cohort study. *JAMA* 1991; 266(24): 3447–52.

50. Murphy JG, Gersh BJ, McGoon MD, *et al*. Long-term outcome after surgical repair of isolated atrial septal defect. Follow-up at 27 to 32 years. *N Engl J Med* 1990; 323(24): 1645–50.

51. Murphy JG, Gersh BJ, Mair DD, *et al*. Long-term outcome in patients undergoing surgical repair of tetralogy of Fallot. *N Engl J Med* 1993; 329(9): 593–9.

52. Marelli AJ, Mackie AS, Ionescu-Ittu R, Rahme E, Pilote L. Congenital heart disease in the general population: changing prevalence and age distribution. *Circulation* 2007; 115(2): 163–72.

53. Oechslin EN, Harrison DA, Connelly MS, Webb GD, Siu SC. Mode of death in adults with congenital heart disease. *Am J Cardiol* 2000; 86(10): 1111–6.

54. Nieminen HP, Jokinen EV, Sairanen HI. Causes of late deaths after pediatric cardiac surgery: a population-based study. *J Am Coll Cardiol* 2007; 50(13): 1263–71.

55. Hahn RT, Roman MJ, Mogtader AH, Devereux RB. Association of aortic dilation with regurgitant, stenotic and functionally normal bicuspid aortic valves. *J Am Coll Cardiol* 1992; 19(2): 283–8.

56. Kleinman CS, Hobbins JC, Jaffe CC, Lynch DC, Talner NS. Echocardiographic studies of the human fetus: prenatal diagnosis of congenital heart disease and cardiac dysrhythmias. *Pediatrics* 1980; 65(6): 1059–67.

57. Kilner PJ, Firmin DN, Rees RS, *et al*. Valve and great vessel stenosis: assessment with MR jet velocity mapping. *Radiology* 1991; 178(1): 229–35.

58. Hirsch R, Kilner PJ, Connelly MS, Redington AN, St John Sutton MG, Somerville J. Diagnosis in adolescents and

adults with congenital heart disease. Prospective assessment of individual and combined roles of magnetic resonance imaging and transesophageal echocardiography. *Circulation* 1994; 90(6): 2937–51.

59. Prakash A, Powell AJ, Krishnamurthy R, Geva T. Magnetic resonance imaging evaluation of myocardial perfusion and viability in congenital and acquired pediatric heart disease. *Am J Cardiol* 2004; 93(5): 657–61.

60. Basson CT, Bachinsky DR, Lin RC, et al. Mutations in human TBX5 cause limb and cardiac malformation in Holt-Oram syndrome. *Nat Genet* 1997; 15(1): 30–5.

61. Li QY, Newbury-Ecob RA, Terrett JA, et al. Holt-Oram syndrome is caused by mutations in TBX5, a member of the Brachyury (T) gene family. *Nat Genet* 1997; 15(1): 21–9.

62. Ewart AK, Morris CA, Atkinson D, et al. Hemizygosity at the elastin locus in a developmental disorder, Williams syndrome. *Nat Genet* 1993; 5(1): 11–6.

63. Lowery MC, Morris CA, Ewart A, et al. Strong correlation of elastin deletions, detected by FISH, with Williams syndrome: evaluation of 235 patients. *Am J Hum Genet* 1995; 57(1): 49–53.

64. Tartaglia M, Mehler EL, Goldberg R, et al. Mutations in PTPN11, encoding the protein tyrosine phosphatase SHP-2, cause Noonan syndrome. *Nat Genet* 2001; 29(4): 465–8.

65. Roberts AE, Araki T, Swanson KD, et al. Germline gain-of-function mutations in SOS1 cause Noonan syndrome. *Nat Genet* 2007; 39(1): 70–4.

66. Bassett AS, Chow EW, Husted J, et al. Clinical features of 78 adults with 22q11 Deletion Syndrome. *Am J Med Genet A* 2005; 138(4): 307–13.

67. de la Chapelle A, Herva R, Koivisto M, Aula P. A deletion in chromosome 22 can cause DiGeorge syndrome. *Human genetics* 1981; 57(3): 253–6.

68. Greenberg F, Crowder WE, Paschall V, Colon-Linares J, Lubianski B, Ledbetter DH. Familial DiGeorge syndrome and associated partial monosomy of chromosome 22. *Human Genetics* 1984; 65(4): 317–9.

69. Kelley RI, Zackai EH, Emanuel BS, Kistenmacher M, Greenberg F, Punnett HH. The association of the DiGeorge anomalad with partial monosomy of chromosome 22. *Journal of Pediatrics* 1982; 101(2): 197–200.

70. Wilson DI, Cross IE, Goodship JA, et al. A prospective cytogenetic study of 36 cases of DiGeorge syndrome. *Am J Hum Genet* 1992; 51(5): 957–63.

71. Carey AH, Kelly D, Halford S, et al. Molecular genetic study of the frequency of monosomy 22q11 in DiGeorge syndrome. *Am J Hum Genet* 1992; 51(5): 964–70.

72. Driscoll DA, Budarf ML, Emanuel BS. A genetic etiology for DiGeorge syndrome: consistent deletions and microdeletions of 22q11. *Am J Hum Genet* 1992; 50(5): 924–33.

73. Goldmuntz E, Driscoll D, Budarf ML, et al. Microdeletions of chromosomal region 22q11 in patients with congenital conotruncal cardiac defects. *J Med Genet* 1993; 30(10): 807–12.

74. Schott JJ, Benson DW, Basson CT, et al. Congenital heart disease caused by mutations in the transcription factor NKX2-5. *Science* 1998; 281(5373): 108–11.

75. Garg V, Muth AN, Ransom JF, et al. Mutations in NOTCH1 cause aortic valve disease. *Nature* 2005; 437(7056): 270–4.

76. McElhinney DB, Geiger E, Blinder J, Benson DW, Goldmuntz E. NKX2.5 mutations in patients with congenital heart disease. *J Am Coll Cardiol* 2003; 42(9): 1650–5.

77. Rudolph AM. Distribution and regulation of blood flow in the fetal and neonatal lamb. *Circ Res.* 1985; 57(6): 811–21.

78. Olley PM, Coceani F, Rowe RD, Swyer PR. Clinical use of prostaglandins and prostaglandin synthetase inhibitors in cardiac problems of the newborn. *Adv Prostaglandin Thromboxane Res* 1980; 7: 913–6.

79. Kirby ML, Gale TF, Stewart DE. Neural crest cells contribute to normal aorticopulmonary septation. *Science* 1983; 220(4601): 1059–61.

80. Mjaatvedt CH, Nakaoka T, Moreno-Rodriguez R, et al. The outflow tract of the heart is recruited from a novel heart-forming field. *Dev Biol* 2001; 238(1): 97–109.

81. Waldo KL, Kumiski DH, Wallis KT, et al. Conotruncal myocardium arises from a secondary heart field. *Development* 2001; 128(16): 3179–88.

82. Whittemore R, Hobbins JC, Engle MA. Pregnancy and its outcome in women with and without surgical treatment of congenital heart disease. *Am J Cardiol* 1982; 50(3): 641–51.

83. Nora JJ, Nora AH. Maternal transmission of congenital heart diseases: new recurrence risk figures and the questions of cytoplasmic inheritance and vulnerability to teratogens. *Am J Cardiol* 1987; 59(5): 459–63.

84. Siu SC, Sermer M, Colman JM, et al. Prospective multicenter study of pregnancy outcomes in women with heart disease. *Circulation* 2001; 104(5): 515–21.

85. Rudolph AM. High pulmonary vascular resistance after birth: I. Pathophysiologic considerations and etiologic classification. *Clin Pediatr (Phila)* 1980; 19(9): 585–90.

86. Bartlett RH, Roloff DW, Cornell RG, Andrews AF, Dillon PW, Zwischenberger JB. Extracorporeal circulation in neonatal respiratory failure: a prospective randomized study. *Pediatrics* 1985; 76(4): 479–87.

87. O'Rourke PP, Crone RK, Vacanti JP, et al. Extracorporeal membrane oxygenation and conventional medical therapy in neonates with persistent pulmonary hypertension of the newborn: a prospective randomized study. *Pediatrics* 1989; 84(6): 957–63.

88. Hopkins RA, Bull C, Haworth SG, de Leval MR, Stark J. Pulmonary hypertensive crises following surgery for congenital heart defects in young children. *Eur J Cardiothorac Surg* 1991; 5(12): 628–34.

89. Pepke-Zaba J, Higenbottam TW, Dinh-Xuan AT, Stone D, Wallwork J. Inhaled nitric oxide as a cause of selective pulmonary vasodilatation in pulmonary hypertension. *Lancet* 1991; 338(8776): 1173–4.

90. Roberts JD, Polaner DM, Lang P, Zapol WM. Inhaled nitric oxide in persistent pulmonary hypertension of the newborn. *Lancet* 1992; 340(8823): 818–9.

91. Kinsella JP, Neish SR, Shaffer E, Abman SH. Low-dose inhalation nitric oxide in persistent pulmonary hypertension of the newborn. *Lancet* 1992; 340(8823): 819–20.

92. Journois D, Pouard P, Mauriat P, Malhere T, Vouhe P, Safran D. Inhaled nitric oxide as a therapy for pulmonary hypertension after operations for congenital heart defects. *J Thorac Cardiovasc Surg* 1994; 107(4): 1129–35.

93. Roberts JD, Jr., Fineman JR, Morin FC, 3rd, *et al.* Inhaled nitric oxide and persistent pulmonary hypertension of the newborn. The Inhaled Nitric Oxide Study Group. *N Engl J Med* 1997; 336(9): 605–10.

94. Galie N, Beghetti M, Gatzoulis MA, *et al.* Bosentan therapy in patients with Eisenmenger syndrome: a multicenter, double-blind, randomized, placebo-controlled study. *Circulation* 2006; 114(1): 48–54.

95. Dimopoulos K, Inuzuka R, Goletto S, *et al.* Improved survival among patients with Eisenmenger syndrome receiving advanced therapy for pulmonary arterial hypertension. *Circulation* 2010; 121(1): 20–5

Part VIII

Chapter 25

Obstetric cardiology

Dr John Fryearson and Dr Dawn Adamson

Introduction

The management of cardiac patients who are or want to become pregnant is a complex and challenging field. Each woman's pregnancy is individual, physicians often have limited experience in this area, and there is a paucity of data to call upon for guidance. It involves a complex multi-disciplinary approach, yet despite huge advances in cardiology over the last few decades, maternal death from cardiac causes continues to rise and is now the UK's leading cause of death in pregnant women.

Clinical trials in pregnant women are few and far between, whilst large randomized trials are virtually non-existent. The literature is therefore predominantly experience in the form of single or multiple case reports, registries, and views of those authors who specialize in this area. There is no doubt that in the field of obstetric cardiology, these papers add value to an area with limited data; however, they are clearly open to serious scientific flaws and prone to selection bias.

The landmark papers selected here have been chosen to reflect each area of cardiovascular disease which affects pregnant women, for example ischaemic heart disease (IHD), valvular heart disease, etc. They have been chosen because they are the papers which have influenced and continue to influence the management of women, whether in giving the most accurate pre-pregnancy counselling or in the actual management of the condition.

The Eighth Report of the Confidential Enquiry into Maternal Deaths in the United Kingdom: Saving Mothers Lives

Centre for Maternal and Child Enquiries. 2006–2008. *BJOG* 2011; 118(Suppl. 1): 1–203.

In this latest triennial report, cardiac disease was the leading cause of death overall (2.37 deaths per 100,000 maternities) and has remained the most common cause of indirect maternal death (deaths as a result of pre-existing or newly developed conditions aggravated by pregnancy, e.g. cardiac disease). Disappointingly, the death rate has not fallen since the last report and in fact has been steadily increasing since 1975. Substandard care was identified in 51% of these cases. See Figure 24.1.

In Chapter 9 of the report, on cardiac disease, the deaths of the 53 women are discussed, along with a further eight women who died late (after six months) and were thus not counted in the statistics detailed above. These women died from either cardiomyopathy or endocarditis.

The leading causes of death in this report were myocardial infarction (MI) and IHD, sudden adult death syndrome (SADS) of which there has been a significant increase, dissection of the thoracic aorta, and cardiomyopathy, predominantly peripartum cardiomyopathy.

Deaths from congenital heart disease and pulmonary hypertension continue to fall. Of the women who died, and had their BMI recorded, 60% were either overweight or obese.

Myocardial infarction and ischaemic heart disease

Six women who died had acute infarcts, whereas five had complications of IHD; that is, heart failure and arrhythmias. Of those who had an MI, three had coronary atheroma, one had extensive coronary dissection, and in two the pathology was unknown. The incidence has reduced, however, by nearly 40% compared to the last triennial report. All women who died had at least one identifiable risk factor, that is, obesity, age >35 years, parity >3, smoker, diabetes, pre-existing hypertension, and a family history of coronary artery disease (CAD). The authors recommend a low threshold for investigation and coronary angiography/intervention in women who may be or are suffering from coronary disease.

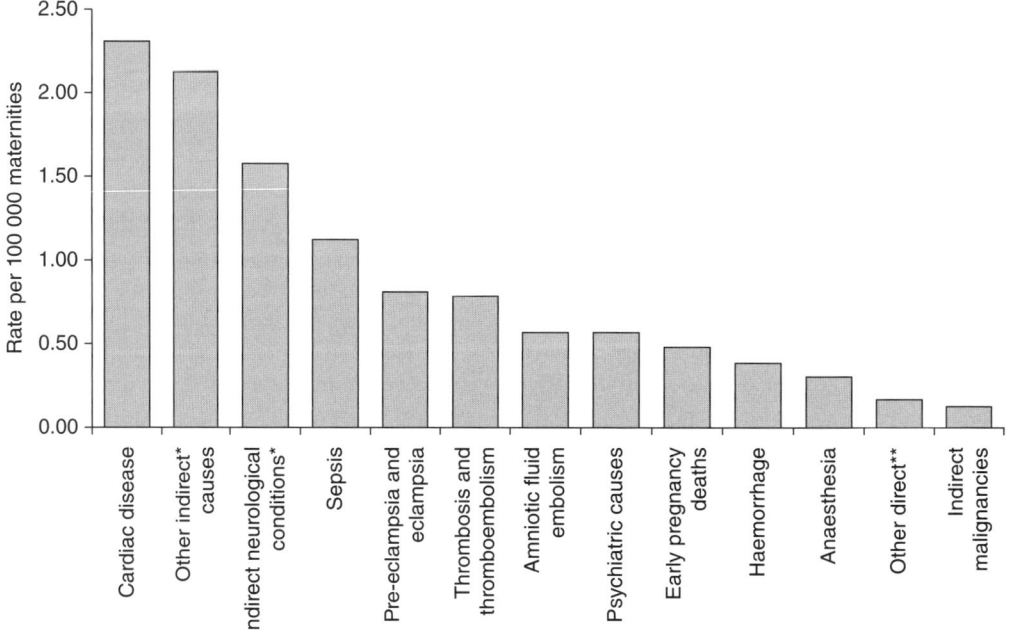

Figure 24.1 Leading causes of maternal death per 100,000 maternities UK; 2006–2008.

Sudden adult death syndrome

Ten women died of SADS this triennia compared to three in the last report. Sudden adult death syndrome is defined as sudden unexpected cardiac death (i.e. presumed fatal arrhythmia) where all other causes of sudden collapse are excluded, including a drug screen for stimulant drugs such as cocaine. These women had an entirely normal morphological heart both on gross examination and histology. It may be that some can be ascribed to known arrhythmic conditions such as channelopathies, though in this report none could be identified from either pre-mortem ECG or family history. This, however, does not exclude such conditions.

Thoracic aortic dissection

Seven women died from aortic dissection, the majority had type A. One had Ehlers-Danlos syndrome, one a bicuspid aortic valve, and the third a family history of dissection. However, the remaining four had no classical risk factors. The majority died within a few days of childbirth. The main concern is that five out of the seven received substandard care because their cause of chest pain was not adequately investigated. Once again the report recommends that all women with pain severe enough to require opiates require a full and senior review with appropriate investigations.

Cardiomyopathy

Thirteen women died from cardiomyopathy of some form, with up to nine being peripartum in aetiology (six definite, three probable). A further six died and are discussed in the late indirect chapter. The mean age was 26 years and the majority had been pregnant before though only two had been previously diagnosed with peripartum cardiomyopathy. Again, 54% of these women received substandard care and the authors recommend that women in late pregnancy or within five months of delivery, with symptoms of breathlessness, orthopnoea, oedema, and who are tachycardic or tachypneoic should be investigated with an echocardiogram. Women diagnosed with cardiomyopthy in pregnancy should be managed in a specialized centre with expertise in the area.

Learning points

- Cardiac disease is the leading cause of maternal death in the UK and continues to rise.
- Substandard care was recorded in 51% of cases.
- Women with chest pain require a low threshold for investigation and coronary angiography if coronary disease is thought to be a cause.
- Any women with pain severe enough to require opiates should have rigorous investigation and senior review—if chest pain is present, consider aortic dissection.
- Women with signs of heart failure at the end of pregnancy or within five months of delivery should have peripartum cardiomyopathy excluded with an echocardiogram.

Prospective Multicenter Study of Pregnancy Outcomes in Women with Heart Disease

Siu S, Sermer M, Colman JM, Alvarez AN, Mercier LA, Morton BC, Kells CM, Bergin ML, Kiess MC, Marcotte F, Taylor DA, Gordon EP, Spears JC, Tam JW, Amankwah KS, Smallhorn JF, Farine D, Sorensen S; Cardiac Disease in Pregnancy (CARPREG) Investigators. *Circulation* 2001; 104: 515–21.

Experience and observational data has shown that maternal and foetal complications during pregnancy are increased in women with cardiovascular disease. The Toronto group (CARPREG investigators) had previously published a risk score (CARPREG score) for assessing adverse events during pregnancy in this patient population based on a study of over 200 patients. They sought to strengthen the validity of the scoring system.

This was a large *prospective* observational study split into two cohorts, with the initial cohort (40%) being used to derive the risk score and the second (60%) to validate it. It was conducted over five years across 13 teaching hospital sites in Canada, with recruitment completed in 1999. After an initial screening of 562 patients, 546 patients encompassing 599 pregnancies were analysed. Clinical variables were recorded at frequent intervals through to six months postpartum. The patient mix was good, with 75% congenital heart disease patients, 20% acquired heart disease, and about 5% of patients having arrhythmia. The initial score index utilized five variables, but this was modified to four without compromising the index's ability to predict future events.

The four factors that were found to be important for maternal outcomes were: a prior event (heart failure, transient ischaemic attack, or cerebrovascular accident) or arrhythmia; NYHA class >II or cyanosis; left heart obstruction (with aortic valve area (AVA) <1.5 cm², mitral valve area (MVA) <2 cm² or left ventricular outflow tract (LVOT) gradient more than 30 mmHg); and left ventricular ejection fraction (LVEF) <40%. For the presence of each factor a score of 1 was given. A total score of 0, 1, and greater than 1 was predictive of a 5%, 27%, and 75% event rate respectively (see Figure 24.2). This was true of either primary (acute pulmonary oedema, symptomatic arrhythmia, stroke, or cardiac arrest) or secondary cardiac events (which included significant deterioration in NYHA class or need for future cardiac intervention). The model held true for subsequent pregnancies and a c-statistic of approximately 0.8 was generated.

The study was also able to identify five factors that predicted neonatal outcomes, without generating a prediction model. These included NYHA class >II or cyanosis, anticoagulation during pregnancy, smoking, multiple gestation, and left heart obstruction. The rate of foetal death doubled to 4% if at least one of these factors was present.

This study was well conducted in a large population, with the use of a derivation and a validation cohort adding to its credibility. It also included patients with a wide range of pathologies, including complex congenital heart disease conditions. The risk model generated is simple to use and easy to calculate. Unfortunately, there is no description of the management of the various patient groups, although the paper states that all the institutions managed patients according to local guidelines.

The generation of this risk index, an extension and modification of previous work, allows us to have a rational and realistic dialogue with these patients to help them understand risk during pregnancy and potential for complications. It allows us to have some confidence in the accuracy of our pre-pregnancy counselling.

Learning points

♦ A simple risk prediction model can be used to identify high-risk patients for future pregnancy, to facilitate pre-pregnancy counselling.

♦ The four factors are NYHA class >II or cyanosis; previous cardiovascular or arrhythmic event; left heart obstruction (see text above); or LVEF <40%.

♦ With none of these present, event risk is 5% but with two or more this increases to 75%.

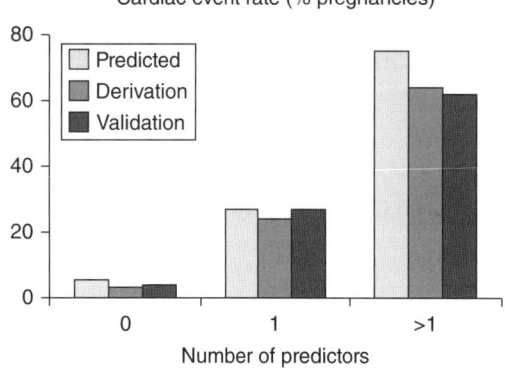

Figure 24.2 Frequency of maternal primary cardiac events, as predicted by the risk index and observed in the derivation and validation groups, expressed as a function of the number of cardiac predictors or points.

Reproduced from Siu SC, *et al*. Prospective multicenter study of pregnancy outcomes in women with heart disease. *Circulation* 2001; 104: 515–21, with permission from Wolters Kluwer Health.

Further reading

● Balint OH, Siu SC, Mason J, *et al*. Cardiac outcomes after pregnancy in women with congenital heart disease. *Heart* 2010; 96(20): 1656 –61. Recent article by the same group looking specifically at pregnancy in patients with congenital heart disease and identifying risk predictors.

● Tanous D, Siu SC, Mason J, *et al*. B-Type Natriuretic Peptide in Pregnant Women with Heart Disease. *J Am Cardiol Coll* 2010; 56(15): 1247–3. Small study demonstrating utility of BNP levels in this population group with a normal value having a 100% negative predictive value.

Acute Myocardial Infarction in Pregnancy and the Puerperium: A Population-Based Study

Ladner HE, Danielsen B, Gilbert WM. *Obstet Gynecol* 2005; 105(3): 480–4.

Acute MI (AMI) in pregnancy is rare. Previous estimates were based on extrapolation from case series and case reports, which had led to widely differing figures. This was the first population-based study to establish systematically the incidence of the condition, and demographic and medical factors associated with risk.

Data was collected over a period of nine years in the state of California from 1991, utilizing birth and death certificates, linking them to hospital databases and discharge summaries. Recorded variables included timing of event, outcome of pregnancy, past medical and obstetric histories. Comparisons were made with the population who did not sustain an event to allow generation of risk factors. A total of 5.4 million deliveries had taken place during this time.

A total of 151 women were identified as having had an AMI. This roughly equated to an incidence of 1 in 35,000 deliveries; but it was noted that the incidence of AMI had tripled in the latter year of the study, in comparison to the first year, to a rate of 1 in 25,000. Maternal age and parity were risk factors, with two-thirds of women being over the age of 30. The classical risk factors of hypertension and diabetes were also predictive. It was thought that the increasing incidence of these factors as well as increasing maternal age contributed to the increased incidence over time, and these were the strongest predictors of AMI. The presence of eclampsia and pre-eclampsia were found to also be associated with AMI. As expected, the overall morbidity and mortality rate was much higher compared to the control population, but an important statistic was that maternal mortality was around 7%—a fifth of previous estimates.

This large study was well conducted and the systematic collection of data allowed for more than 98% of birth records to be matched to hospital records. This allowed exclusion of publication bias and it generated some much needed epidemiological data on this condition. This was a typical western population with a large ethnic contingent.

There was a long lag time between the end of data collection and the study publication, whether this reflects time needed for data collection and analysis by the small group or whether this is an ad hoc retrospective analysis

is not clear. This does have implications, however. There is no comment on how the diagnosis of AMI was reached nor on how it was treated, that is, thrombolysis versus primary angioplasty. The study period was at a time when the recognition of acute coronary syndromes was in its infancy, and in all likelihood AMI in this study represents a combination of ST elevation MI and possibly 'non Q-wave MI'. The contemporary diagnosis of coronary events is more refined and sensitive with increasing recognition of a wider pathophysiology, leading to an increased incidence. This is reflected in the fact that a population-based study published a year later analysing similar information in the years 2000–2002, looked at almost three times as many deliveries and found an incidence just over twice as high as this study.

Nevertheless this was an important seminal work that confirmed that the incidence of AMI in pregnancy was rare but was increasing; and the mortality rate was, somewhat reassuringly, not as high as previously thought. It also confirmed the role of traditional risk factors as well as some maternal ones.

Learning points

- ◆ Acute MI in pregnancy is a rare event, but its incidence is increasing.
- ◆ It is associated with a significant mortality and morbidity rate.
- ◆ Maternal hypertension, diabetes, and age are the strongest risk predictors.

Further reading

- James AH, Jamison MG, Biswas MS, Brancazio LR, Swamy GK, Myers ER. Acute Myocardial Infarction in Pregnancy: A United States Population-Based Study. *Circulation* 2006; 113: 1564–71. Another observational study analysing incidence of AMI in pregnancy.
- Roth A, Elkayam E. Acute Myocardial Infarction Associated with Pregnancy. *J Am Coll Cardiol* 2008; 52: 171–80. Review article of aetiology and management of AMI in pregnancy.

Pregnancy and contraception in heart disease and pulmonary arterial hypertension

Thorne S, Nelson-Piercy C, MacGregor A, Gibbs S, Crowhurst J, Panay N, Rosenthal E, Walker F, Williams D, de Swiet M, Guillebaud J. *J Fam Planning Reprod Health Care* 2006; 32: 74–9.

There is little published information or evidence regarding the use of contraception in patients with heart disease. Whilst pregnancy may be safe in the majority of women, it can be life-threatening in others, and therefore it is important that if a cardiologist advises a woman against a pregnancy, they ensure that contraception is in place. Unfortunately, primary care and gynaecologists who normally specialize in this area, may withhold or prescribe inappropriate contraception due to lack of knowledge of the effects in cardiac patients. As such, some women with heart disease receive inaccurate or incomplete pre-pregnancy counselling. This guideline was developed over two years by a working group of cardiologists, obstetricians, and anaesthetists hoping to generate recommendations to allow appropriate risk stratification and advice to these patients.

The group used the World Health Organization (WHO) (see Table 24.1) classification system for contraceptive use and applied them to specific cardiac lesions as well as types of contraceptive; whereby class I is safe and class IV is contraindicated, with class II and III in between. In this way cardiac lesions were assigned to a status, depending on their risk in pregnancy. A lot of this data has been discussed in previously published articles. Perhaps more importantly, and uniquely to this article, is the classification of the contraceptive methods available. This describes their use in lesions on the basis of safety but also efficacy.

In essence, combined oral contraceptive agents are pro-thrombotic due to oestrogen, which is not necessarily attenuated by concomitant warfarin use. It also has suboptimal efficacy, in comparison to other methods. For most cardiac conditions it is not recommended and receives a class III or IV grouping. Progestogen-only methods, although safer in cardiac conditions, have variable efficacy depending on the preparation. In general, implantable forms are more effective, and Implanon was considered safe for all cardiac lesions with the best efficacy. Sterilization was not a recommended form of contraception due to the haemodynamic demands of the

Table 24.1 WHO risk classifications by medical condition for (A) contraceptive method and (B) pregnancy

WHO Class	(A) Risk for contraceptive method by medical condition	(B) Risk for pregnancy by medical condition
I	Condition with no restriction for the use of the contraceptive method. Always usable	No detectable increased risk of maternal mortality or morbidity.
II	Condition where the advantage of the method generally outweigh the risks. Broadly usable.	Small increased risk of maternal mortality or morbidity.
III	Condition where the advantages of the method usually preferable: Exceptions if: (a) Patient accept risks and rejects alternatives (b) The risk of pregnancy is very high and the only acceptable alternative methods are less effective methods (c) Caution in use	Significantly increased mortality or severe morbidity. Expert counselling required. If pregnancy is decided upon, intensive specialist cardiac and obstetric monitoring needed throughout pregnancy, childbirth, and the puerperium.
IV	Condition where the method represents an unacceptable health risk. Do not use.	Extremely high risk of maternal mortality or severe morbidity: pregnancy contraindicated. If pregnancy occurs termination should be discussed. If pregnancy continues, care as for class III.

Reproduced from the *Medical Eligibility Criteria for Contraceptive Use,* 4th edition, 2009, with permission from the World Health Organization.

Table 24.2 Class of pregnancy according to specific cardiac lesions

Class I pregnancy

Uncomplicated, small or mild:
  pulmonary stenosis
  ventricular septal defect
  patent ductus arteriosus
  mitral valve prolapse with no more than mitral regurgitation
Successfully repaired simple lesions:
  ostium secundum atrial septal defect
  ventricular septal defect
  patent ductus arteriosus
  total anomalous pulmonary venous drainage
Isolated ventricular extrasystoles and atrial ectopic beats

Class II pregnancy (if otherwise well and uncomplicated)

Unoperated atrial septal defect
Repaired tetralogy of Fallot
Arrhythmias

Class 2–3 pregnancy (depending on individual)

Mild LV impairment
Hypertrophic cardiomyopathy
Native or tissue valvular heart disease not considered class 4
Marfan syndrome without aortic dilation (with/without a family history of aortic dissection)
Heart transplantation

Class III pregnancy (unless other risk factors, in which case pregnancy may carry a class IV risk)

Mechanical valve
Systemic right ventricle (congenital heart disease in which the right ventricle supports the systemic circulation)
Post Fontan operation
Cyanotic heart disease
Other complex congenital heart disease

Class IV pregnancy

Pulmonary arterial hypertension of any cause
Severe systemic ventricular dysfunction (NYHA Class III–IV or LVEF <30%)
Previous peripartum cardiomyopathy with any residual impairment of LV function
Severe left heart obstruction
Marfan syndrome with aorta dilated >40 mm

procedure as well as the reduced efficacy in comparison to other methods.

This guideline (see Table 24.2) was predominantly based on expert consensus and extrapolation of information available in healthy patients with regards to contraception use. There was no trial data to guide the decision making. It is an important guideline, however, and filled a large void in the management of contraception in this at-risk patient population. It also reiterated the vital role that counselling plays in these patients about managing their risks during pregnancy.

> **Learning points**
>
> ◆ Female patients with cardiac disease should have access to high quality, accurate, and lesion-specific advice regarding the risks of pregnancy.
> ◆ Thought needs to be given to contraception in these patients, and ideally should be performed by a specialist with prior experience.
> ◆ Not all contraceptive methods are safe or effective and advice needs to be tailored to a woman's individual condition.

Further reading

- Thorne S, MacGregor A, Nelson-Piercy C. Risks of contraception and pregnancy in heart disease. *Heart* 2006; 92(10): 1520–5. An 'Education in Heart' article based on the above paper with associated MCQs.
- Vigl M, Kaemmerer M, Seifert-Klauss V, *et al.* Contraception in women with congenital heart disease. *Am J Cardiol* 2010; 106(9): 1317–21. Study of over 500 patients demonstrating the very poor pre-pregnancy counselling and contraception use in this at-risk group under the care of a tertiary centre.

Managing Palpitations and Arrhythmias during Pregnancy

Adamson DL, Nelson-Piercy C. *Heart* 2007; 93: 1630–6.

Palpitations are a common complaint during pregnancy—with increased heart rate, hormonal influences, sympathetic activity, and reduced venous return all contributing to a reduced threshold for arrhythmia potential. Most palpitations in pregnancy are benign, but significant dysrrhythmias can cause a high level of anxiety as well as being associated with foetal and maternal morbidity and rarely mortality. This review article looked at the incidence of arrhythmias, and how it may be managed in the pregnant patient.

The article reiterates the importance of clinical assessment in these patients, with an emphasis on ensuring that any structural heart disease is identified. It also gives a summary of antiarrhythmic drugs and their safety in pregnancy. Adenosine, digoxin, most beta blockers (including sotalol), and verapamil are relatively safe in pregnancy, but as with all medications in pregnancy should only be used when necessary. The safety of atenolol in pregnancy is addressed and reassurances are given that outside the first trimester the risk of intrauterine growth retardation is minimal, although most experience throughout pregnancy is with metoprolol and propanolol. The management of specific arrhythmias is also discussed, with the importance of their haemodynamic effects and consequent detrimental changes to placental and foetal blood supply being stressed.

This is a trial-naive area, as is the case with a lot of cardiac disorders in pregnancy, and this is reflected in the small number of existing trials the authors had to draw any conclusions from. A lot of the guidance has been gleaned from reviewing all the literature of case reports and case series and adding these to experience.

Despite this, the article is a concise and informative review of the management of this condition in pregnancy and gives the reader more confidence in the management of subsequent patients. This is a commonly encountered condition in the pregnant patient.

Learning points

- Palpitation in pregnancy is a common complaint and usually benign.
- Structural heart disease must be excluded.
- Drug treatment should only be used when necessary with appropriate counselling.
- There are a range of drugs to treat all conditions which have got safety data both in pregnancy and breast feeding.
- Where haemodynamic and potentially foetal compromise may occur, measures must be taken to prevent the arrhythmia and these can include DC cardioversion as well as short use of drugs normally avoided in pregnancy, for example intravenous amiodarone.

Further reading

- Shotan A, Ostrzeqa E, Mehra A, Johnson JV, Elkayam U. Incidence of Arrhythmias in Normal Pregnancy and Relationship to Palpitations, Dizziness, and Syncope. *Am J Cardiol* 1997; 79(8): 1061–4. Article illustrating an increased incidence of supraventricular and ventricular ectopics during pregnancy.
- Silversides CK, Harris L, Haberer K, Sermer M, Colman JM, Siu SC. Recurrence rates of arrhythmias during pregnancy in women with previous tachyarrhythmia and impact on fetal and neonatal outcomes. *Am J Cardiol* 2006; 97(8): 1206–12. Article demonstrating up to 50% occurrence of arrhythmia during pregnancy in patients with known paroxysmal arrhythmias.

Maternal and Fetal outcomes of Subsequent Pregnancies in Women with Peripartum Cardiomyopathy

Elkaym U, Tummala PP, Rao K, Akhter MW, Karaalp IS, Wani OR, Hameed A, Gviazda I, Shotan A. *N Eng J Med* 2009; 344 (21): 1567–71.

Peripartum cardiomyopathy is a rare condition associated with a high maternal morbidity and mortality. Whilst the majority of cases recover at least partially if not completely, around a fifth either die or require cardiac transplantation. The outcome of patients who go on to have a subsequent pregnancy is not well documented; yet it is a common question from women who have had one pregnancy, and want to consider a second. Until this paper, the largest cohort in the literature included only six patients, and so this paper has been pivotal in helping

give more accurate pre- or early pregnancy counselling as to the safety of a subsequent pregnancy.

The group surveyed American College of Cardiology members to ask them about any patients they had cared for, who had had a subsequent pregnancy following a diagnosis of peripartum cardiomyopathy. The case records, including echocardiographic studies, of the identified patients were then analysed to generate data on 60 subsequent pregnancies in 44 patients (six patients having two, and five having three subsequent pregnancies, respectively).

Table 24.3 Outcomes in women undergoing subsequent pregnancy after previous diagnosis of peripartum cardiomyopathy, showing the outcomes of women who were divided depending upon whether or not their LV function had normalized following their previous episode of peripartum cardiomyopthy

	Normal LV pre-pregnancy (%)	Impaired LVEF (%)
Signs of heart failure	21	44
20% decrease in EF	21	25
Persistent LV dysfunction six years later	14	31
Mortality during or after subsequent pregnancy	0	19% total pregnancies, 25% continued pregnancies

Adapted from Elkaym U, *et al*. Maternal and Foetal outcomes of Subsequent Pregnancies in Women with Peripartum Cardiomyopathy. *N Eng J Med* 2009; 344 (21): 1567–71.

They compared two groups of women, those in whom ventricular function had completely normalized prior to subsequent pregnancy (28 women) and those in whom it remained depressed (16 women).

The second group showed a greater reduction in EF during subsequent pregnancy, a greater incidence of heart failure symptoms, and the occurrence of three deaths. There was no perinatal mortality seen in either group, although premature delivery occurred significantly more often in patients in the latter group. The numbers did not achieve statistical significance. However, they also analysed the change in ventricular function in respect to termination of pregnancy and found that those women that continued with pregnancy experienced a statistically significant decrease in EF as compared to those who had an abortion (nine in total, five of which were therapeutic).

The design of this study is open to criticism, with the method being prone to recall and selection bias as noted by the authors themselves. It also uses only EF as the sole determinant of left ventricular function, which will be prone to subjective differences in reporting—echocardiographic images themselves were not analysed. There may well be other markers of ventricular function that are more reliable in predicting future deterioration in function with respect to postpartum cardiomyopathy.

The study did, however, confirm that patients with persistently depressed cardiac function following an episode of postpartum cardiomyopathy remain at high risk for future pregnancies, and that the risk for patients whose function has returned to baseline is unpredictable. See Table 24.3.

Learning points

◆ Subsequent pregnancies in patients with previous peripartum cardiomyopathy incur significant risk to mother and foetus.
◆ Those with persistently depressed cardiac function are at highest risk.
◆ Patients with peripartum cardiomyopathy should be counselled about the risk of future pregnancy and those with impaired LV function should be counselled against future pregnancy as mortality is as high as 25%.

Maternal complications and pregnancy outcomes in women with mechanical prosthetic valves treated with enoxaparin

McClintock C, McCowan L, North R. *BJOG* 2009; 116(12): 1585–92. (Epub 14 Aug 2009).

Warfarin is the most effective anticoagulant for mechanical valves; however, the teratogenicity of warfarin in the first trimester of pregnancy is well documented. Whilst low molecular weight heparin (LMWH) may be a suitable, safe, and effective alternative to warfarin there is limited data to support this. Studies that had been published were exceptionally small, with inconsistent findings; case reports being prone to the usual problems of publication bias. The aim of this group was to publish their local data in terms of actual practice and safety.

It was a retrospective observational study of the management of patients attending their tertiary centre in New Zealand between 1997 and 2008. It included 31 patients with a total of 47 pregnancies. They describe in detail the three alternative regimes available to anticoagulate pregnant patients with metallic heart valves. One is to completely replace warfarin with therapeutic dose enoxaparin for the duration of pregnancy until delivery. Second, to substitute warfarin with enoxaparin during weeks 6–12 and then return to warfarin, until late into the third trimester when enoxaparin is reintroduced again pre/peripartum for planned delivery. Lastly, to continue warfarin through pregnancy, switching to enoxaparin again in preparation for delivery, acknowledging that the increased foetal exposure to warfarin does increase teratogenic risk.

Around 70% of pregnancies were carried out with enoxaparin predominantly for the duration, with almost 30% utilizing warfarin predominantly. No reported pregnancies utilized warfarin throughout. In the enoxaparin group there was a 10% thromboembolic rate, with around 4% in the warfarin groups. However, most events (in both groups) were associated with patients who had poor compliance to treatment or in whom it was difficult to achieve therapeutic levels of enoxaparin, as measured by anti-Xa levels. The study also demonstrated that successful foetal outcomes in patients having enoxaparin treatment throughout pregnancy were much greater, with 96% compared to 75% in the warfarin group. Whilst numbers were small, this was felt to be a significant finding.

This was the largest report of its type looking at the use of enoxaparin in this patient group, with the focus on safety. It had well documented anticoagulation methods which clearly described how the enoxaparin dose was titrated according to anti-Xa levels. It is contemporary and included more modern prosthetic valve types, with just under two-thirds of patients having a tilting disc or bi-leaflet type as opposed to a Starr-Edwards valve. The study, though large for its field, is still a small study, and included a very native population, with 80% being of either Maori or Pacific Islander ethnicity. In their protocols it was stated that all patients should take aspirin as well, although in 20% of pregnancies this was not the case.

The important message of this paper is that women with a metallic valve do have anticoagulation options. The use of enoxaparin (and aspirin) as an alternative to warfarin throughout pregnancy is an effective and safe alternative if utilized appropriately and may indeed lead to improved outcomes for the foetus. No matter which regime is used, compliance is of vital importance. These points should be factored in and offered to patients in the form of pre-pregnancy counselling, so that joint care decisions can be made as soon as possible.

Learning points

- Patients with metallic valves planning to start a family should have counselling, with regard to risks and benefits to both mother and foetus of alternative anticoagulant regimes clarified.
- Enoxaparin in doses titrated according to anti-Xa levels throughout pregnancy in combination with aspirin is a very good alternative.
- Labour/delivery should be planned with adjunct use of unfractionated heparin (UFH) to minimize bleeding risk.
- Compliance with treatment is vital for successful outcomes.

Further reading

- Sbarouni E, Oakley CM. Outcome of pregnancy in women with valve prostheses. *Br Heart J* 1994; 71: 196–201. An article describing outcomes in metallic versus prosthetic valves, noticing an increased risk of bleeding and thromboembolic complication as compared to warfarin, and little in the way of warfarin-induced embryopathy.

Pregnancy in Marfan Syndrome: Maternal and Fetal Risk and Recommendations for Patient Assessment and Management

Goland S, Barakat M, Khatri N, Elkayam U. *Cardiol Rev* 2009; 17(6): 253–62.

Marfan syndrome is recognized to be a cause for concern in the pregnant mother. Not only is there a risk of transmission of this condition, but also there is a serious concern of dissection during pregnancy. This review article helped to identify the level of risk and how to manage these patients and get them as safely as possible through pregnancy.

This article analysed 39 recent case reports and reviews of Marfans in pregnancy from 1995 to 2007. There are several important points with regards to the management of these patients to take from the article. During pregnancy the risk of dissection goes up dramatically compared to outside pregnancy. For patients with an aorta that is larger than 4 cm the risk is 10%, if less than 4 cm then the risk is 1%. Patients who have an aorta that is approaching 5 cm (4.7 cm was suggested as a cutoff) should be considered for early surgery, especially if they are contemplating pregnancy. Aortic dissection during pregnancy can not only be detrimental to maternal health, but it can often have fatal consequences for the foetus. There are some instances of patients with aortas at 4.5 cm that have been taken through pregnancy successfully. Whilst patients with aortas less than 4 cm, in a younger age group (especially under 20) and with slow progression of their aortopathy are at the lowest risk, they still need close follow-up and regular echocardiographic surveillance throughout pregnancy and postpartum.

There are also obstetric complications that Marfans patients are prone to, with an overall 40% higher obstetric complication rate in comparison to the general population. This is mainly due to premature rupture of the membranes.

This paper identified that on the whole pre-pregnancy counselling is done very poorly. Out of the case reports identified only 25% had any form of counselling before conception. As well as the risks of dissection above, patients should be aware that there is a transmission rate of up to 70% for Marfans syndrome to their offspring, and the implications and complications of foetal diagnosis.

This is a clear and concise review article attempting to address a relatively common problem. It is also very recent and utilizes a good wealth of background articles and prior reviews. Unfortunately, there are little in the way of large prospective studies in this area and inferences from case reports and case series are plagued by bias. This review covered some very important points in an area of obstetric cardiology that is frequently seen, both in general as well as specialist clinics.

Learning points

- Pregnancy in Marfans is an added risk factor for aortic dissection.
- Those at highest risk include patients with an aorta/aortic root >4 cm (~10% risk), those with progressive dilatation during pregnancy, and those with previous dissection.
- Obstetric complications are common.
- Pre-pregnancy counselling should be offered to all women with Marfan syndrome.

Further reading

- Immer FF, Bansi AG, Immer-Bansi AS, *et al.* Aortic dissection in pregnancy: analysis of risk factors and outcome. *Ann Thorac Surg* 2003; 76: 309–14. Observational study identifying aortic size of 4 cm indicating a higher risk of dissection in pregnancy in Marfan and bicuspid aortic valve disease.
- Meijboom LJ, Drenthen W, Pieper PG, *et al.* Obstetric complications in Marfan syndrome. *Int J Cardiol* 2006; 110: 53–9. Observational study demonstrating the increased incidence of obstetric complication in Marfan syndrome.

Improved survival in pregnancy and pulmonary hypertension using a multiprofessional approach

Kiely DG, Condliffe R, Webster V, Mills GH, Wrench I, Gandhi SV, Selby K, Armstrong IJ, Martin L, Howarth ES, Bu'lock FA, Stewart P, Elliot CA. *BJOG* 2010; 117: 565–74.

Pulmonary hypertension often affects women of childbearing age and is known to increase maternal mortality. It has been reported that mortality is in excess of 50% in some series and for this reason patients are strongly advised to avoid pregnancy and to consider termination in its event. This group set out to report its contemporary experience in these patients and to challenge some of the prior data.

The group analysed retrospectively ten cases of pregnancy in nine patients with pulmonary hypertension occurring between 2002 and 2009. Their management occurred mostly at a specialist quaternary pulmonary vascular unit. The cause of pulmonary hypertension included idiopathic and familial pulmonary arterial hypertension; secondary to congenital heart disease; secondary to pulmonary venothromboembolic disease, and one case in association with a mixed connective tissue disorder. Lowest systolic pulmonary artery pressure as measured on echocardiography was 45 mmHg and highest 150 mmHg. Four of the patients were diagnosed in the second trimester of the pregnancy, whilst in the other five the diagnosis was already known prior to conception.

All women received 'targeted' therapy, which consisted of daily nebulized iloprost several times a day. Some patients required intravenous or subcutaneous prostaglandin due to deteriorating symptoms and a number were managed on concomitant sildenafil. Most patients received LMWH. All but one delivery was via elective Caesarean section at around 34 weeks with the other being a spontaneous vaginal delivery. No patients had general anaesthesia. Most patients had some form of invasive haemodynamic monitoring with radial arterial and internal jugular venous lines. Cardiac output was also monitored either invasively (early on in the study) or non-invasively.

All pregnancies concluded in a successful live birth of a baby without congenital abnormalities. All patients survived pregnancy. Unfortunately, one patient decided to stop her own targeted treatment four weeks after delivery and died. The remaining eight patients were followed up for a minimum of nine months, with the majority being followed up for over three years.

The study details very well the management of these patients including the assessment, follow-up, and nature of their individual targeted therapies. It is, however, a small series and did not include analysis of two other pregnancies, in the same individual, during the period that both resulted in miscarriage. Whether these sorts of results are attainable outside a specialist pulmonary centre with such intense management is debatable.

This paper demonstrates that for patients with pulmonary hypertension who fall pregnant and wish to continue with the pregnancy despite counselling, management in a specialist centre improves both foetal and maternal outcomes. It suggests that although the mortality rate remains high, it is perhaps not as high as previously documented.

Learning points

- Patients with pulmonary hypertension should receive counselling on contraception and the potential dangers of pregnancy.
- Patients who become pregnant should be given advice with regards to termination of the pregnancy.
- Patients who wish to continue with the pregnancy should be referred early on to experienced centres for targeted therapy and intense management involving a multidisciplinary approach.

Further reading

- Bedard E, Dimopoulos K, Gatzoulis M. Has there been any progress made on pregnancy outcomes among women with pulmonary arterial hypertension? *Eur Heart J* 2009; 30: 256–65. Review article of more contemporary management of patients through pregnancy and associated outcomes.

Hypertension in Pregnancy: the management of hypertensive disorders during pregnancy

NICE Guideline Development Group. London: National Institute for Health and Clinical Excellence. 2010: CG107.

Hypertensive disorders during pregnancy can be life-threatening conditions, associated with increased morbidity and mortality. Pre-eclampsia and related conditions are a real concern for obstetricians and their patients and often require cardiological input. These conditions contribute to around one-third of maternal morbidity, as well as playing a role in neonatal mortality. There have been previous publications outside the NICE guidance regarding the management of pre-eclampsia; however, this guideline will be welcomed by both specialities.

The guideline assesses the evidence base and gives formal definitions on chronic hypertension versus gestational hypertension, pre-eclampsia and severe pre-eclampsia, and significant proteinuria without hypertension. There is advice on patients who are at risk of eclampsia and how they should be managed. There is quite prescriptive advice on the various conditions, how they should be managed, and any medical treatment that should be considered. It also reviews the current antihypertensive agents available for use in pregnancy, whilst acknowledging that few of them have a UK license for their use in pregnancy, and gives guidance on their use in the antenatal and postpartum periods.

The NICE guidelines try to be as robust as possible, but also take into account cost effectiveness when generating guidance. As well as being subject to publication bias when searching for evidence there is often a degree of expert opinion that complements the evidence base when there are gaps, and this can be very subjective. Importantly, the guidelines address conditions that contribute significantly to maternal, and foetal, morbidity and mortality and outline a standard of care that departments can strive towards whilst at the same time auditing shortcomings and improvements over time.

> ### Learning points
>
> - Hypertensive disorders in pregnancy contribute significantly to maternal and foetal outcomes.
> - Not all antihypertensive agents are safe in pregnancy: angiotensin converting enzyme inhibitors and angiotensin receptor blockers are teratogenic and patients of childbearing age on these medications should be counselled appropriately.
> - Aspirin (75 mg) should be considered in patients at high risk of pre-eclampsia from week 12 onwards, which includes those with chronic hypertension.
> - Patients diagnosed with pre-eclampsia should receive an integrated package of care which delineates criteria for escalation of management.

Further reading

- Duckitt K, Harington D. Risk factors for pre-eclampsia at antenatal booking: systematic review of controlled studies. *Br Med J* 2005; 330: 565–7.

Conclusion

Heart disease in pregnancy is the UK's biggest cause of maternal mortality and it is continuing to rise, despite improvements in overall outcome from cardiac conditions outside pregnancy. The reason is multifactorial, but can be partly attributed to a combination of the increased prevalence of risk factors such as diabetes and hypertension in women undergoing a pregnancy, as well as an increase in the age of women becoming pregnant. This is highlighted by data from a study by the UK Obstetric Surveillance System, due to be published in 2012, on the incidence of MI in pregnancy, which demonstrates that for every additional year of maternal age, the odds of MI were increased by 30%.

The management of pregnant women with heart disease remains an area of concern amongst many cardiologists and is reflected in the latest confidential enquiry (detailed above) where substandard care has been identified in 51% of cases. In order to improve outcomes in the future, we need to tackle the lack of expertise amongst cardiologists by improving both education in this area, as well as access of women with heart problems to specialist centres. This does not necessarily mean women having to travel long distances for delivery, which is often a concern for both patient and obstetrician, but a well devised antenatal and delivery plan that may identify areas of potential concern to monitor and allow guidance in the management of such complications for the less experienced team.

The UK has excellent data regarding maternal mortality due to heart disease, for instance from the triennial confidential enquiry reports; however, we have very little data on morbidity or outcomes when pregnancies are terminated or delivered prematurely. The UK-wide prospective population based study into the incidence of MI in pregnancy by the UKOSS, suggests a reduction in the incidence of MI in pregnancy. However, it does rely on information submitted by obstetricians or midwives and one concern is that infarcts occurring in early pregnancy or after delivery may be missed, thus skewing the data. The European Society of Cardiology is also trying to tackle the issue of lack of data in this field with an ongoing EuroHeart survey of 'Pregnancy in patients with structural heart disease'. By combining the experience of cardiologists across Europe, data will be gained on a large variety of cardiac conditions. However, the data will have the usual limitations of a registry. Also, data is mainly being submitted by a few centres from each country which specialize in this area, thus excluding the true outcomes of women who are managed by less experienced teams, particularly if the outcomes are poor. In order to improve the quality of this data, it is important that each country's society encourages all cardiologists to participate, so that the data can be as complete as possible and thus reflect true outcomes with current management. Such data would then allow us to identify not only areas in which we must improve, but also management strategies which have proven to be successful.

Part IX

Chapter 26

Cardiac rehabilitation

Dr Randal J Thomas, Dr Aung Myat, Dr Tushar Kotecha, and Dr Ray W Squires

Introduction

The development of cardiac rehabilitation (CR) over the past 60 years is a fascinating story that is marked by a number of landmark research studies, some evolutionary and others revolutionary. It would be impossible to include all research studies that left a significant mark on the course of CR over the years, but this chapter is an attempt to provide readers with a description of several published papers that are representative of the key advances in the science of CR during its 60-year history.

To identify such landmark studies is no easy feat. While assessment of the impact of a given paper could be attempted by measuring the number of times it is referenced or cited in other articles, this method is not entirely satisfactory since the number of times a paper is cited may vary due to a number of factors, not just the article's soundness and scientific significance. On the other hand, the impact of a given research study could be assessed by asking the opinion of 'experts', but this method is also prone to shortcomings, since those opinions are simply opinions and may be based on non-scientific factors. In the end, we used a combination of the two approaches, combining the subjectivity of expert opinion with the objectivity of the citation index of a given paper.

We first identified the hundred most cited research papers on the topic of 'cardiac rehabilitation' using Scopus. Once those studies were identified, two of the authors (RJT and RWS) each identified from that list (and from other published research studies with which they were familiar) the ten articles that they felt had the biggest impact on the field of CR. This process resulted in 15 articles that were felt to represent landmark papers, either because they introduced important new concepts to CR (i.e. they were 'revolutionary'), or because they expanded previous scientific knowledge that had a lasting impact on the clinical practice of CR (i.e. they were 'evolutionary'). The authors attempted to be as unbiased as possible in this selection process, a fact that may be overlooked by some readers since the authors included (reluctantly) a small number of published papers on which we, ourselves, were contributing authors.

The 15 articles referenced in this chapter, and dozens of others not included, have had a clear impact on the science and practice of CR since its inception in the 1950s.

Particular recognition is warranted for the large number of studies on the physiologic effects of exercise training on cardiovascular health, studies that have helped to establish and explain many of the benefits of CR services. Other studies have identified the important impact of interventional strategies for nutrition, smoking cessation, weight loss, psychological well-being, and long-term treatment adherence. The size limitations of the current article prohibit further descriptions of these important works, but the authors nonetheless pay tribute to the scores of investigators who have collectively contributed to the scientific advancement of CR. While much is already known about CR thanks to these studies, the authors firmly believe that many more important studies are yet to be published, studies that will move the field of CR to even greater heights of impact and will need to be added to a new list of landmark papers in due course.

The 'chair' treatment of acute coronary thrombosis

Levine SA, Lown B. *Trans Assoc Am Physicians* 1951; 64: 317–27.

Background

Until this paper was published, part of the usual treatment for myocardial infarction (MI) included complete bedrest for approximately six weeks. This corresponded to twice the assumed healing time for the damaged myocardium. This period of drastically reduced physical activity unfortunately resulted in a substantial reduction in cardiovascular fitness due to both deconditioning and loss of vasomotor reflexes. In addition, patients perceived that they were invalids who would likely not return to full normal activity. Levine and Lown were aware of some of the deleterious effects of complete bedrest, such as thrombophlebitis, osteoporosis, negative nitrogen balance, atelectasis, etc. They also had observed a critically ill patient with MI improve immediately and dramatically after being sat up in a chair. They hypothesized that sitting in a chair was a better form of rest for the heart than lying in a bed. They reasoned that bedrest facilitated increased venous return and augmented stroke work as well as pooling of blood in the pulmonary circulation. Sitting in a chair, they believed, resulted in venous pooling in the lower extremities and a reduction in venous return and stroke work.

Article summary

Study participants included 58 patients with MI admitted to Peter Bent Brigham Hospital (now the Brigham and Women's Hospital) in Boston. The aim was to have the patients begin sitting in a chair during the first three days of hospitalization, gradually increasing the time, as tolerated. The patients were progressed in 'chair time' until the majority of the day was spent sitting in the chair. Ambulation, of a few steps only, began at the end of the third week. The patients received standard care with the exception of the 'chair treatment'.

Eighty-three per cent of patients began the 'chair treatment' within the first three days in the hospital. No complications were attributed to the new treatment. The authors observed that the patients appeared to have a superior sense of well-being and morale compared to the authors' anecdotal experiences with previous coronary patients who did not receive the 'chair treatment'. They reported that this was especially apparent in the few patients who were hospitalized with their second or third infarct. The authors also wrote that the gradual increase in time spent in the chair provided patients with a clear index of improvement.

Levine and Lown compared hospital mortality in their patients who received the 'chair treatment' (9.0%) to an historical control group of 138 patients treated for MI at Peter Bent Brigham Hospital just before the current study (13.8%). Statistical analysis of these data was not performed and the authors indicated that this comparison was not definitive. They emphasized that their study demonstrated that the 'chair treatment' was not dangerous and that it appeared to have beneficial effects on the 'rehabilitation process'.

Strengths and limitations

This paper startled the medical community by challenging the long-held dogma that any physical activity in the setting of MI was extremely dangerous. The authors made an astute clinical observation—the rapid improvement of one patient who sat up in a chair following acute MI—and designed a study to gather data to determine if this observation was the rule or an aberration. Sixty years after the publication of the data, Dr Bernard Lown wrote of the importance of this early investigation on his stellar career[1]. He noted that in the early 1950s care for MI was largely palliative and patients were confined in bed for weeks, in part because physicians had little to offer these patients. In addition to dealing with the heart attack pain, patients had to cope with the unbearable distress of prolonged bedrest. Physicians believed that complete bedrest was necessary for survival. Dr Lown remarked, 'Visiting Martians, witnessing this travail, might have judged the scene differently, regarding hospitals as prisons where inmates were subjected to a unique form of torture'. He related the difficulty of winning the cooperation of the house staff, who viewed moving critically ill patients from the bed to a chair as 'off-the-wall'. However, when house staff observed even one patient in a chair they became proponents of the treatment. Dr Lown wrote

that, compared with patients confined to bedrest, the chair-treated patients required fewer narcotics, less sedation for anxiety, and expressed a renewed eagerness to resume a normal life. 'Practicing physicians rapidly abandoned the use of strict bedrest . . . Within a few years . . . the period of hospitalization was reduced by half'.

The study was limited by the small number of patients included in the trial, the lack of randomization, and no objective measures of psychosocial or physical function.

Impact on the field

The authors overcame the medical dogma of prolonged, strict bedrest and opened the door to the concept of early mobilization after a cardiac event. The paper inspired other investigators to develop formalized inpatient rehabilitation protocols that formed the basis for the field of CR.

Learning points

- Accepted medical practice not based on sound science may be detrimental for patients.
- An insightful clinical observation can be a powerful tool in formulating hypotheses for clinical research.
- Clinicians can adopt improvements in patient care relatively rapidly if provided with compelling data demonstrating the superiority of a new treatment paradigm.

Further reading

- Irvin WC, Burgess AM. The abuse of bedrest in the treatment of myocardial infarction. *NEJM* 1950; 243: 486.
- Levine SA. Some harmful effects of recumbency in the treatment of heart disease. *JAMA* 1944; 126: 80.

Rehabilitation of the cardiac patient

Hellerstein HK, Ford AB. *JAMA* 1957; 164: 225–31.

Background

In the early 1950s, Dr Herman Hellerstein developed the concept of work classification units for coronary patients. He emphasized the importance of a complete evaluation of the patient, including cardiovascular fitness, emotional status and the ability of the patient to return to the type of occupation they enjoyed prior to the cardiac event.

This paper outlined the process of rehabilitation after a cardiac event. The first sentence of the publication clearly articulated Dr Hellerstein's concept of CR: 'This report describes an orderly plan for the rehabilitation of the patient with heart disease from the initial illness through convalescence to the return to the world of work'. Dr Hellerstein went on to later describe the prescription of exercise after MI and was a powerful advocate for the field of CR. He was a Founding Fellow of the American Association of Cardiopulmonary Rehabilitation in 1985. In 1986, he became the first recipient of that organization's Award of Excellence.

Article summary

The paper's main emphasis was the important role of the physician in the rehabilitation process. In the era in which the paper was published, formal CR programmes did not exist and so, to help address this need, Hellerstein and Ford recommended that physicians assume active leadership for this part of the patients' care. They also emphasized a number of important factors that continue to have an influence on the practice of CR, including the following:

- The importance of rehabilitation for all cardiac patients, not only those with severe impairment.
- The team concept of patient care was proposed and included the attending physician, psychiatrist, social worker, physical and occupational therapists, and vocational counsellor as team members.
- Return to work was a major goal of rehabilitation.
- The frequency of anxiety and depression after a cardiac event was discussed. The term 'emotional disability', later re-named 'cardiac cripple' was defined.
- The role of the physician in either fostering or treating emotional disability was emphasized, and physicians were cautioned against overprotection of the coronary patient.
- Specific recommendations for rehabilitation were included in the paper.
- For example, during the period of hospitalization which lasted three to four weeks in that era, patient education regarding basic pathophysiology and the recovery process was recommended.
- No more than three or four days of inactivity were permitted, and the period of rest should be as short as possible.
- Progressive physical activity, beginning at the bedside and progressing to longer periods of ambulation were to be performed with the supervision of physical and occupational therapists.
- After discharge from the hospital, patients remained at home for several weeks to months before returning to work and normal activity. This phase of rehabilitation was termed 'convalescence'.
- Hellerstein and Ford advocated a gradual return to activities of daily living, including use of stairs, and progressive amounts of walking.

- The authors referred to contemporary animal data demonstrating the development of coronary collateral vessels stimulated by physical activity. Objective evaluation of fitness using the Master two-step test was discussed and recommended.
- Major emphasis was placed on 'work adjustment' and the authors reported their own experience with more than 1000 patients demonstrating that cardiac patients were capable of performing a wide variety of jobs without 'undue physiological stress'.

In the 1950s, coronary risk factors and the pathogenesis of atherosclerosis were not well understood. For example, the authors wrote that:

'Only patients with a demonstrated disturbance of cholesterol balance and fat metabolism should require such stringent diets. The categorical denial of tobacco to all patients must be condemned vigorously. Most patients with heart disease can smoke moderately without apparent harm.'

Today, we read these pronouncements and are amused and amazed at the lack of understanding of practitioners in that era. However, Hellerstein and Ford understood much of the basic concepts of modern CR: the importance of physician involvement, inclusion of all coronary patients in rehabilitation, the usefulness of interdisciplinary teams, the importance of early mobilization and progression of physical activity, the objective measurement of functional capacity, the need to continue the rehabilitation process after hospital discharge, the complex emotional issues surrounding a cardiac event, and the importance of restoring patients to productive, meaningful lives.

Strengths and limitations

This landmark paper provided a template for many of the common processes used in CR programmes today. The authors clearly understood the complexities of the rehabilitation process and provided specific suggestions for both the in-patient and outpatient phases. The paper is limited by the lack of definitive data comparing patients who either did or did not receive rehabilitation. Many years later, randomized, controlled trials were designed and performed that helped address those needs.

Impact on the field

The authors articulated the basic principles of the physical and emotional rehabilitation of patients with coronary disease which are universally applied today.

Further reading

● Hellerstein HK, Goldstein E. Rehabilitation of patients with heart disease. *Postgrad Med* 1954; 15: 265–78.
● Hellerstein HK. Techniques of exercise prescription and evaluation. National workshop: Exercise in the prevention, in the evaluation, and in the treatment of heart disease. *J S C Med Assoc* 1969; (Suppl) 65: 46–56.

Reduction in sudden deaths by a multifactorial intervention progamme after acute myocardial infarction

Kallio V, Hamalainen H, Hakkila J, Luurila OJ. *Lancet* 1979; 2: 1091–4.

Background

The concept of modifying coronary risk factors in patients with documented coronary disease to decrease future events (secondary prevention) was new and largely untested in the 1970s. Some data at that time suggested that smoking cessation and beta blocking drugs might improve prognosis after MI. The World Health Organization (WHO) realized that coronary heart disease was rampant in industrialized countries and devised an international project to test the effects of comprehensive rehabilitation and secondary prevention on outcomes in patients with MI. In the 1960s, Finland had the highest death rate from coronary heart disease in the world, related to a high prevalence of elevated cholesterol, hypertension, and cigarette smoking in the population. Finnish public health officials began a campaign to improve risk factors in the population. They readily agreed to become involved in the WHO rehabilitation and secondary prevention project. The present paper constituted the combined results from the two Finnish sites, Turku and Helsinki.

Article summary

The study randomized consecutive patients (301 men, 74 women), under 65 years of age with MI, to either an intervention programme including exercise training, dietary and smoking cessation advice, or to a control group with three years of follow-up.

Patients in the control group were treated by their own physicians and were seen by the study team once per year. Control patients were in contact with their physicians approximately half as often as intervention patients.

The intervention programme began two weeks after hospital discharge with physician/intervention team visits at least monthly for the first six months, then at least every three months. Team members included a social worker, psychologist, dietitian, and physical therapist. Health education included smoking cessation and diet advice, and discussion of psychosocial issues. An individualized exercise programme was designed for each patient based on the results of a graded exercise test. The exercise programme was supervised for most patients.

At baseline, the two groups of patients were similar in terms of body weight, smoking prevalence, total cholesterol, triglycerides, and blood pressure. The intervention group achieved lower blood lipids and blood pressure at one, two, and three years into the study. Both groups reduced smoking by approximately 50%. Beta blocker usage was similar for both groups at year one, but higher in the intervention group at years two and three. There were no differences in physical fitness for the groups at one, two, or three years.

The three-year cumulative mortality was lower in the intervention patients than in the control group (18.6% vs. 29.4%, p = 0.02). The mortality difference was primarily due to a lower incidence of sudden cardiac death in the intervention group (5.8% vs. 14.4%, p <0.01). The rates of non-fatal reinfarction and angina pectoris were similar for the two groups of patients.

Strengths and limitations

This was the first randomized, controlled trial to demonstrate the efficacy of comprehensive CR and secondary prevention in reducing mortality in patients with coronary heart disease. In fact, Finland was the only WHO trial participant to report such favourable results. The authors demonstrated that the improvement in blood lipids and blood pressure persisted for three years with the intervention. The clinical utility of an interdisciplinary team approach in secondary prevention was demonstrated. The authors subsequently reported favourable ten-year follow-up data in 1989 (see Further reading below). As with other early trials, this study was plagued by a relatively small numbers of participants, a relative lack of women in the cohort, and the exclusion of older coronary patients.

Impact on the field

This study stimulated a proliferation of CR and secondary prevention programmes throughout the western world. While this study showed the importance of using a model of long-term management of coronary risk factors by rehabilitation staff employed, this model was not universally included in most CR programmes of that era.

> ### Learning points
>
> ◆ The team approach to CR and multi-factorial secondary prevention is effective in improving coronary risk factors and in reducing cardiovascular mortality.
> ◆ Long-term coronary disease management is possible and is effective at lowering death rates.

Further reading

● Hamalainen H, Luurila OJ, Kallio V, *et al.* Long-term reduction in sudden deaths after a multifactorial intervention programme in patients with myocardial infarction. *Eur Heart J* 1989; 10: 55–62.

An overview of randomized trials of rehabilitation with exercise after myocardial infarction

O'Connor GT, Buring JE, Yusuf S, Goldhaber SZ, Olmstead EM, Paffenbarger RS Jr, Hennekens CH. *Circulation* 1989; 80: 234–44.

Background

Prior to the publication of this seminal meta-analysis (and an earlier, slightly smaller meta-analysis, see Oldridge *et al.* in the Further reading at the end of this section), there remained a modicum of doubt within the cardiovascular fraternity as to whether the putative medical, physical, psychological, and socio-economic benefits of CR were clinically significant and cost effective. The prevailing issue at the time had been the relatively small size of many of the individual randomized trials of CR, which precluded the establishment of statistically significant study end points. For CR to be fully embraced as an effective clinical tool, it would need to be supported by firm evidence of its benefits, not only improving the functional capacity and quality of life of those individuals having suffered a cardiac event but also reducing morbidity and mortality rates. The randomized trials that had been conducted in CR up to the late 1980s had not been able to provide that level of evidence to a convincing degree.

Article summary

O'Connor and colleagues reviewed all previously published randomized trials of post-MI CR that included a structured exercise component. In general, patients had been randomized to either a structured regimen of physical exercise or to normal activities of daily living. Practically all the trials also included a formal or informal non-exercise component ranging from advice on lifestyle modification through to a fully integrated multidisciplinary intervention that included input from social workers, psychologists, and dieticians. As such, trials selected for the final analysis were classified as either 'exercise only' or 'exercise plus other interventions'.

In all, 36 randomized trials of CR that included a structured exercise component were identified, all having been published between 1960 and 1988. The WHO study of CR had coordinated 24 of these trials, but each one was recognized individually since they differed in their method of randomization. Of the initial 36, 22 were ultimately included in the final analysis. The remainder were excluded as a consequence of significant limitations in study design, including truncation of the study follow-up period, lack of individual patient randomization, and in the case of some WHO sites, lack of contribution of data to the final report.

Study end points included: total mortality, cardiovascular mortality, sudden death, fatal and non-fatal MI. Importantly, definitions of the various end points used by the original investigators of each trial were retained.

Where possible, each end point was assessed with respect to the time from randomization and the effects of rehabilitation were analysed at one, two, and three or more years. Statistical manipulation of the data was based on an 'intention to treat' analysis and, therefore, trial participants were not excluded as a consequence of non-adherence to study protocols.

Overall, 4,554 patients qualified for the meta-analysis and were randomized to CR (n = 2,310) or comparison groups (n = 2,244). With regard to the pre-specified end points, there were 502 deaths in total, 412 designated as cardiovascular-related, and 202 as sudden deaths. There were 701 recurrent MIs and of these, 312 were fatal. Typical odds ratios between the 'exercise only' and 'exercise plus other interventions' groups were reasonably similar in terms of total mortality and recurrent fatal MI; showed a non-significant trend towards favouring the 'exercise plus other interventions' group for cardiovascular death and sudden death; and favoured the 'exercise only' group for non-fatal re-infarction.

O'Connor and colleagues demonstrated from their analysis a statistically significant 20% reduction in total and cardiovascular mortality with exercise-based CR one year after randomization, a finding which persisted throughout the follow-up period. The reduction in overall mortality corresponded to an attenuated risk of cardiovascular mortality and fatal re-infarction out to three years and a reduction in sudden death during the first year and possibly for 1–2 years thereafter. For non-fatal re-infarction there were no significant differences between CR and those randomized to activities of daily living.

Strengths and limitations

By employing the obvious advantages of a wide-ranging meta-analysis, the authors had the statistical power to produce a more robust and convincing estimate of the effect of CR on mortality as compared to previously published smaller, individual studies. They did not attempt to make direct comparisons between individual trials, but tests of heterogeneity were calculated for each end point and for each follow-up period, with generally good agreement for the studies included in the analysis. The authors made every effort to ensure as complete an ascertainment of trial events as possible. For instance, at three years after randomization ascertainment of all-cause mortality, cardiovascular mortality, fatal and non-fatal MI were 100%, 92.5%, 86%, and 90.1% of participants, respectively. The fact that most of the studies included in this analysis were not, by themselves, significant, makes it much less likely that the overall findings of the meta-analysis were confounded by publication bias.

One limitation of this analysis is the lack of reliable data on sudden death. Ascertainment of this end-point was complete in only 68% of participants. This was predominantly due to the fact that the studies included in the analysis commonly had differing definitions of what constituted a 'sudden death'. Another limitation of this study is that the number of women included in the study was relatively small (only 3% of study participants), precluding the accurate assessment of outcomes in women. In addition, insufficient numbers of participants from racial and ethnic minority groups were included in the study. Furthermore, elderly participants were also under-represented, since patients aged over 70 years of age were not included in most of the trials included in the study. The result of these limitations was that the study's findings could only be reliably applied to middle-aged, Caucasian men.

Impact on the field

While a slightly smaller study, with similar findings, published a year earlier by Oldridge and colleagues also deserves recognition as a landmark study, the study by O'Connor was included in our list of landmark papers because it was the largest study of that time period to analyse the clinical benefits of CR. Additional meta-analyses were carried out by other researchers more than a decade later (see Further reading), but clearly, the message of the O'Connor study, on the heels of the Oldridge study, provided a significant 'one-two punch' in major medical journals, that had an immediate and significant impact on the recognition of the benefits of CR on morbidity and mortality rates, and helped push the science and the practice of CR to new levels of acceptance.

Learning points

◆ Exercise-based CR, in randomized controlled trials, reduced all-cause and cardiovascular mortality rates by 20%.
◆ Cardiac rehabilitation may not have an impact on reducing the risk of recurrent, non-fatal MI.
◆ Truly definitive conclusions about the impact of individual components of CR are not possible. This is due to the fact that only a small number of 'exercise only' studies was included, and the fact that sufficient detail on non-exercise components of CR, such as smoking cessation therapy and dietary counselling, was not provided in the individual studies included in this meta-analysis.

Further reading

- Clark AM, Hartling L, Vandemeer B, McAlister FA. Meta-analysis: secondary prevention of programs for patients with coronary artery disease. *Ann Intern Med* 2005; 143: 659–72.
- Joliffe JA, Rees K, Taylor RS, Thompson D, Oldridge NB, Ebrahim S. Exercise-based rehabilitation for coronary heart disease. *Cochrane Database Syst Rev* 2000; (4): CD001800.
- Oldridge NB, Guyatt GH, Fischer MS, Rimm AA. Cardiac rehabilitation after myocardial infarction: Combined experience of randomized clinical trials. *JAMA* 1988; 260: 945–50.
- Taylor RS, Brown A, Ebrahim S, *et al.* Exercise-based rehabilitation for patients with coronary heart disease: systematic review and meta-analysis of randomized controlled trials. *Am J Med* 2004; 116: 682–92.

Regular physical exercise and low-fat diet: effects on progression of coronary artery disease

Schuler G, Hambrecht R, Schlierf G, Niebauer J, Hauer K, Neumann J, Hoberg E, Drinkmann A, Bacher F, Grunze M. *Circulation* 1992; 86: 1–11.

Background

Aggressive lipid-lowering therapy has been shown to attenuate the progression of atherosclerotic coronary lesions and may even stimulate regression of plaques in some patients. Lipid modification has also been shown to result in fewer clinical events and reduced mortality from coronary artery disease. The mainstay of treatment for lipid reduction is HMG-CoA reductase inhibition. Studies carried out in selected, highly motivated patient groups have also shown that regular exercise and elimination of high fat content foods can result in normalization of serum lipid levels. However, benefits in the general population seem less impressive predominantly due to a lack of compliance.

Article summary

This single-centre randomized controlled trial aimed to assess the effects of intensive physical exercise and a low-fat, low-cholesterol diet on progression of coronary atherosclerosis and changes in overall myocardial perfusion in non-selected patients with stable angina, both of which were primary outcome measures. Patients were recruited after routine coronary angiography for stable angina and randomized to intervention (n = 56) or 'usual care' (n = 57). Only males with stable symptoms, previously documented coronary artery stenoses, and motivation to participate for a period of at least 12 months were included. Exclusion criteria included unstable symptoms, left main stem disease, left ventricular ejection fraction <35%, significant valvular disease, insulin-dependent diabetes mellitus, primary hypercholesterolaemia, and an inability to participate in regular exercise. Importantly, all patients satisfying the criteria above were offered trial participation, so that no one was rejected on the basis of possible future non-compliance. The intervention involved intensive physical exercise with group training sessions (minimum two hours per week), daily home exercise (30 minutes a day on a cycle ergometer maintaining pre-determined target heart rates), and a low-fat, low cholesterol diet. Patients randomized to intervention spent the first three weeks on a metabolic ward during which time they were taught how to appropriately lower the fat content of their daily food intake. Those in the 'usual care' cohort spent one week on the same ward but adherence to the guidelines laid out by the trial team was left completely to their own initiative. No lipid lowering therapy was prescribed to either patient group. Repeat coronary angiography was performed at 12 months measuring relative and minimal diameter reductions of the known coronary lesions. In addition, myocardial perfusion was assessed at baseline and 12 months using exercise stress ^{201}Tl scintigraphy. Secondary outcome measures included serum lipid profile, physical work capacity, and erythrocyte sedimentation rate (ESR).

With respect to the minimal diameter reduction of lesions at coronary angiography, 32% of the intervention group showed regression, with 23% showing progression. In the control group 17% showed regression and 48% progression. This difference was statistically significant. In effect, 12 months of an intensive exercise programme and low-fat diet did not promote a net regression of coronary lesions in the overall intervention cohort. On the other hand, there was no progression of disease. Those patients on usual care, however, witnessed a considerable progression of disease.

In terms of ^{201}Tl scintigraphy, the intervention group showed a significant improvement in myocardial perfusion at 12 months. No significant change was demonstrated in the control group. The intervention group also demonstrated a 5% reduction in body weight (p <0.010), 10% reduction in cholesterol (p <0.001), 8% reduction in LDL (p <0.002), and 24% reduction in triglycerides (p <0.001). No change was seen in the control group. Impressively, the number of positive stress tests in the intervention group was significantly lower at 12 months when compared with the control group (p <0.05) and fewer patients were forced to stop the stress test consequent to progressive angina symptoms (p = 0.06).

Strengths and limitations

As this small randomized controlled trial was restricted to men, the results cannot be extrapolated to the female population. There was no explanation as to why this gender restriction was instituted. Following drop-outs and adverse clinical events, complete angiographic data at 12 months was available for 40 out of 56 patients randomized to intervention and 52 out of 57 patients in the control group. Despite this, the trial was sufficiently powered to allow statistically significant inferences to be made. Meticulous attention was also paid to the angiographic analysis of changes in pre-existing coronary lesions which no doubt helped to produce a robust set of results.

Importantly, and as the authors attest to, the patient cohort enrolled in this study were not endowed with exceptional motivation and compliance. Despite this, significantly beneficial haemodynamic and metabolic results were gained from the prescribed interventions. Clearly, with both an exercise programme and dietary restrictions working in tandem, it is difficult to determine which intervention stimulated which improvements.

Impact on the field

This study highlights that regular physical exercise and a low-fat diet can have a significant beneficial impact on the rate of progression of coronary disease in terms of prognostic measures. The same group (Neibaner *et al.*) completed a six-year follow-up on the same cohort and found that the intervention group showed a 28% increase in physical work capacity and showed a significantly slower rate of progression of coronary stenosis (p <0.001), suggesting that benefits of the intervention extend beyond the short term. Subsequently, Hambrecht *et al.* have completed a randomized controlled trial comparing

percutaneous coronary intervention with a 12-month exercise training programme in males under 70 years old with stable angina. They found that the exercise group had a significantly improved event-free survival and exercise capacity. It has also been shown that physical training following PCI in patients with stable angina improves maximal exercise capacity (Astengo *et al.*).

As a result of this landmark study and subsequent work, physical exercise and low-fat diet are recommended in both American and European guidance as part of the management of patients with coronary artery disease.

Learning points

◆ Regular physical exercise and low-fat diet have a positive impact on coronary artery disease in those with stable angina and should be recommended as part of the cardiac rehabilitation programme.

◆ These measures are associated with a beneficial impact on lipid profile which in turn has been shown to improve cardiovascular risk.

Further reading

● Astengo M, Dahl A, Karlsson T *et al.* Physical training after percutaneous coronary intervention in patients with stable angina: effects on working capacity, metabolism and markers of inflammation. *Eur J Cardiovasc Prev Rehabil* 2010; 17(3): 349–54.

● Hambrecht R, Waltner C, Mobius-Winkler S *et al.* Percutaneous coronary angioplasty compared with exercise training in patients with stable coronary artery disease. *Circulation* 2004; 109: 1371–8.

● Lavie CJ, Church TS, Milani RV, Earnest CP. Impact of physical activity, cardiorespiratory fitness, and exercise training on markers of inflammation. *J Cardiopulm Rehabil Prev.* 2011 May-Jun; 31(3): 137–45.

● Neibauer J, Hambrecht R, Velich T *et al.* Attenuated progression of coronary artery disease after 6 years of multifactorial risk intervention. Role of physical exercise. *Circulation* 1997; 96: 2534–41.

● Nikkila EA, Viikinkoski P, Valle M, Frick MH. Prevention of progression of coronary atherosclerosis by treatment of hyperlipidaemia: A seven year prospective angiographic study. *BMJ* 1984; 289: 220–3.

● Ornish D, Brown SE, Scherwitz LW *et al.* Can lifestyle changes reverse coronary heart disease? *Lancet* 1990; 2: 129–33.

Long-term disease management of patients with coronary disease by cardiac rehabilitation program staff

Squires RW, Montero-Gomez A, Allison TG, Thomas RJ. *J Cardiopulm Rehabil Prev* 2008; 28: 180–6.

Background

In the United States, traditional CR programmes include up to 36 sessions of supervised exercise, risk factor education, and counseling generally over a three-month period of time. However, long-term adherence to medications and healthy lifestyle changes remain problematic even for patients who participate in CR. In 1987 Squires *et al.* described their experience with a programme to continue with secondary prevention therapy long-term in patients who had completed an outpatient CR programme (see Further reading). Subsequent randomized controlled clinical trials demonstrated that coronary risk factor control, using nurses as disease case managers, resulted in decreased events over 3–4 years, compared to usual care (see Further reading). An ongoing concern regarding randomized trials is the potential problem of recruitment bias. Patients who agree to be randomized and to participate in a trial may be inherently different from the typical patient encountered in routine clinical practice. The results from randomized trials, therefore, may not be directly applicable to the general population of patients. An additional concern about the applicability of randomized controlled trials is the feasibility of applying, in routine clinical practice, the well-developed disease-management systems used in such trials.

Article summary

The purpose of this study was to determine the feasibility and clinical benefits of a long-term (three-year) disease management of coronary patients in routine clinical practice using CR programme staff. A retrospective analysis of 503 consecutive patients (375 men, 128 women, 54% ≥65 years of age) who participated in outpatient CR and who were available for three years of follow-up (83% of all referred patients) was performed. Face-to-face meetings with disease managers occurred every 3–6 months after completion of outpatient CR. Physicians were readily available for medical decision-making purposes. The following outcome measures were assessed: appropriate use of cardioprotective medications, coronary risk factors, amount of habitual exercise training, and all-cause mortality. After three years, use of appropriate medications was high. With the exception of body mass index, which increased slightly over the three years, coronary risk factors were well-controlled: total cholesterol 164 ± 29 mg/dL, high-density lipoprotein cholesterol 46 ± 11 mg/dL, low-density lipoprotein cholesterol 90 ± 23 mg/dL, systolic blood pressure 126 ± 19 mmHg, diastolic blood pressure 70 ± 11 mmHg. At three years, 95% of patients were tobacco free. Habitual exercise training averaged 139 ± 123 minutes per week. Over the three years of the intervention, there were 29 deaths, yielding an annual all-cause mortality of 1.9%. This compared favourably with the Centers for Disease Control and Prevention's expected annual mortality of 1.6% for average Americans, in the general population without a history coronary disease, of similar ages to these patients.

Strengths and limitations

This paper, for the first time, demonstrated that up to three years of coronary artery disease management intervention using CR staff in routine clinical practice was feasible and generally effective in secondary prevention. The disease-management intervention was part of the routine clinical work of the staff. The amount of time required of physicians was minimal. Limitations of the study were its single-centre retrospective design, use of self-report data (medication usage, exercise, smoking), the lack of data regarding recurrent hospitalizations or overall healthcare costs, and no comparable control group. The authors' institution was a large group practice that facilitates a high enrolment of eligible patients and facilitates follow-up.

Impact on the field

It remains to be seen if this paper (and other studies of long-term secondary prevention) will stimulate the evolution of CR programmes into long-term coronary disease-management programmes.

Learning points

- Optimal secondary prevention of coronary artery disease is achieved by long-term patient adherence to cardioprotective medications and healthy lifestyle habits. This is a difficult task for patients, even those who have participated in outpatient CR.

◆ Previous randomized controlled trials have demonstrated that coronary risk control and medication compliance, using registered nurses as disease managers for 3–4 years, resulted in reduced coronary events compared with usual care.

◆ This paper demonstrated that coronary disease management of patients in routine clinical practice, by non-physicians, was effective in providing effective long-term, secondary prevention treatments and to have similar mortality benefits as have been shown in systems used in previously published clinical trials.

◆ Cardiac rehabilitation programmes are uniquely positioned to provide long-term coronary disease management.

● Giannuzzi P, Temporelli PL, Marchioli R, *et al.*; GOSPEL Investigators. Global secondary prevention strategies to limit event recurrence after myocardial infarction: results of the GOSPEL study, a multicenter, randomized controlled trial from the Italian Cardiac Rehabilitation Network. *Arch Intern Med* 2008; 168(20): 2194–204.

● Haskell WL, Alderman EL, Fair JM, *et al.* Effects of intensive multiple risk factor reduction on coronary atherosclerosis and clinical cardiac events in men and women with coronary artery disease: the Stanford Coronary Risk Intervention Project (SCRIP). *Circulation* 1994; 89: 975–90.

● Squires RW, Gau GT: Cardiac rehabilitation and cardiovascular health enhancement. In: Brandenburg RO, Fuster V, Giuliani ER, McGoon DC (eds). *Cardiology: Fundamentals and Practice*. Chicago: Yearbook Medical Publishers, 1987, pp. 1944–60.

Further reading

● Boden WE, O'Rourke RA, Teo KK, *et al.* Optimal medical therapy with or without PCI for stable coronary disease. *N Engl J Med* 2007; 356: 1503–16.

Cardiac rehabilitation and survival in older coronary patients

Suaya JA, Stason WB, Ades PA, Normand ST, Shepard DS. *J Am Coll Cardiol* 2009; 54: 25–33.

Background

Previous meta-analyses of randomized controlled trials of CR have demonstrated a 15–28% reduction in all-cause mortality. However, these trials included very few patients over the age of 65, women, those from ethnic minorities, or high-risk patients with congestive heart failure. In the USA, more than 55% of acute MIs and 86% of deaths from coronary heart disease occur in those aged over 65 years (Arias *et al.* 2003). This study aimed to assess the effects of CR on survival in a large cohort of older patients with coronary heart disease.

Article summary

This retrospective study utilized Medicare records of patients 65 years or older who were hospitalized in 1997 for coronary disease or revascularization procedures, and had follow-up through to 2002. A total of 601,099 patients were initially identified. The primary outcome measure was all-cause mortality within five years of the index hospitalization. Highly refined statistical methods were used to analyse the data: propensity-based matching that paired CR users with non-users by using all observable risk factors, regression modelling to estimate the impact of CR on mortality of the entire cohort of Medicare beneficiaries included in the analysis, and instrumental variables which were used to enhance regression modelling by protecting against confounding by unobserved variables. Overall, 12.2% of the cohort received one or more CR outpatient sessions. The CR users received a mean of 24 sessions. Users of CR were more likely to be male, white, and younger.

Propensity based matching resulted in 70,040 matched pairs of CR users and non-users. At one year, mortality rates were 2.2% in CR users versus 5.3% in non-users, whilst at five years they were 16.3% versus 24.6%. This represents a relative risk reduction of 58% at one year and 24% at five years (p <0.001). High-dose CR users (>25 sessions) had a lower mortality than low-dose users (1.1% vs. 2.6% at one year and 14.0% vs. 17.2% at five years; p <0.001). Multivariate analysis of the matched pairs demonstrated greater benefit from CR amongst older age groups (>75 years) and in women compared to men.

The greatest difference in five-year mortality was demonstrated in patients with acute MI who also had congestive heart failure (32.5% in CR users vs. 52.0% in non-users).

Regression modelling and instrumental variable analysis of the entire cohort also demonstrated reduced mortality in the CR user group compared to non-users (regression modelling: 4.8% vs. 10.9% at one year, 28.1% vs. 38% at five years; instrumental variables: 6% vs. 10.6% at one year, 29.8% vs. 37.8% at five years). Overall, these results indicated that for every 12 patients treated with CR, one death would be averted over a five-year period.

Strengths and limitations

This was a large study using a representative population in terms of age and socio-demographics. The sample size and five-year follow-up enabled the collection of nearly three million person-years of data. The population received 'real world' treatment rather than 'study treatment'. Furthermore those patients enrolled in randomized controlled trials are often pre-selected, younger, and less severely ill. The authors here use three analytic approaches in an effort to eliminate confounding factors, and all three demonstrated a significant benefit of CR in terms of mortality reduction at all time points to five years.

The predominant limitation of this study was its retrospective construction and reliance on Medicare claims data, the main data source, which has limited patient data. Important potentially confounding variables that were not available to investigators included left ventricular ejection fraction, smoking history, obesity, and medication regimens. The propensity adjusted matched-pair analysis was able to adjust for bias potentially introduced by various patient characteristics, but since the Medicare database did not include many potentially confounding variables, the accuracy of the results may be limited as a result.

Impact on the field

While previous studies have demonstrated the mortality benefits of CR in pre-selected patients in controlled environments, this study confirms, using 'real-world' data, the benefit of CR in a large cohort of older patients, involving both men and women, and individuals from minority and non-minority subgroups. This study also provides strong evidence of the benefits of CR in patients with heart failure.

Learning points

♦ Mortality rates at five years were 21–34% lower in users of CR compared to non-users in patients with coronary artery disease.

♦ Older patients derive significant mortality benefit from CR.

♦ Mortality benefits were noted for men and women, for minority and non-minority groups, and for all diagnostic groups studied (MI, PCI, and CABG, with or without heart failure).

♦ This study provided preliminary evidence of a dose-response relationship between the number of CR sessions and consequent survival benefit.

Further reading

- Bethell H. Cardiac rehabilitation: from Hellerstein to the millennium. *Int J Clin Pract* 2000; 54: 92–7.
- Bongard V, Grenier O, Ferrières J, *et al*. Drug prescriptions and referral to cardiac rehabilitation after coronary events: comparison between men and women in the French PREVENIR survey. *Int J Cardiol* 2004; 93: 217–23.
- Clark A, Hartling L, Vandermeer B, *et al*. Meta-analysis: secondary prevention programs for patients with coronary artery disease. *Ann Intern Med* 2005; 143: 659–72.
- Goel K, Lennon RJ, Tilbury RT, *et al*. Impact of cardiac rehabilitation on mortality and cardiovascular events after percutaneous coronary intervention in the community. *Circulation* 2011; 123: 2344–52.
- Hammill BG, Curtis LH, Schulman KA, Whellan DJ. Relationship between cardiac rehabilitation and long-term risks of death and myocardial infarction among elderly Medicare Beneficiaries. *Circulation* 2010; 121: 63–70.
- Taylor RS, Brown A, Ebrahim S, *et al*. Evidence-based rehabilitation for patients with coronary heart disease: systematic review and meta-analysis of randomised controlled trials. *Am J Med* 2004; 116: 682–92.

Relationship between cardiac rehabilitation and long-term risks of death and myocardial infarction among elderly Medicare Beneficiaries

Hammill BG, Curtis LH, Schulman KA, Whellan DJ. *Circulation* 2010; 121: 63–70.

Background

Exercise-based CR has been shown to improve both survival and the risk of adverse sequelae associated with coronary artery disease (Taylor *et al.*, 2004). However, the optimal dose of CR is unclear. A previous meta-analysis of 14 randomized controlled trials failed to show a dose-response relationship, although most of these trials were prior to 2000 (Taylor *et al.*, 2004). A more recent study of older patients by Suaya *et al.* in 2009 (see previous landmark paper) did show a mortality benefit for patients participating in more than 25 sessions compared to those participating in less than 25 sessions. The investigators set out to determine whether there was an optimal 'dose' of CR that could be prescribed following a cardiac event, and, furthermore, whether or not there was indeed a threshold of sessions above which no extra outcomes benefit could be gained.

Article summary

This retrospective study aimed to characterize the dose-response relationship between the number of CR sessions attended and the long-term risk of death and MI in patients aged over 65 years. The primary outcome was all-cause mortality. A 5% national sample of Medicare beneficiaries was used to provide the sample cohort. The study population was limited to those over 65 years living in the United States and who participated in their first CR session between 1 January 2000 and 31 December 2005 (the index date). Data were collated regarding number of sessions attended, indication for rehabilitation, comorbidities, subsequent hospitalization with MI, and mortality over a follow-up period of four years after the index date.

There were 30,161 patients within the 5% sample who commenced CR within the specified timeframe. Of these, 60.8% were post-coronary artery bypass graft (CABG) surgery, 20.5% post-MI, and 14.9% had had stable angina; 40% also had a diagnosis of heart failure. The median number of sessions attended was 25, with more than 40% of patients attending more than 30 sessions and 13% attending less than 6.

Patients attending 36 sessions were found to have a 14% lower mortality than those attending 24 sessions (HR 0.86, 95% CI 0.77–0.97), a 22% lower risk than those

attending 12 sessions (HR 0.78, 95% CI 0.71–0.86) and a massive 47% lower risk than those attending just one session (HR 0.53, 95% CI 0.47–0.59). The same was true of the incidence of MI: 36 vs. 24 sessions HR 0.88 (95% CI 0.83–0.93), 36 vs. 12 sessions HR 0.77 (95% CI 0.69–0.86), 36 vs. 1 session HR 0.68 (95% CI 0.58–0.81). The results were also analysed by indication for CR. For patients who underwent CABG, there appeared to be a plateau at 24 sessions after which there was no improved outcome in terms of mortality. For those referred with stable angina, there was a similar plateau at 18 sessions. For those referred post-MI, no plateau was noted out to 36 sessions. In terms of risk of MI, attending for 36 sessions was associated with a lower risk than any lower number of sessions, regardless of indication for rehabilitation.

Strengths and limitations

This study included a large number of patients from a national cohort of men and women, from minority and non-minority groups, over 65 years of age. The data analysis was adjusted for demographics, comorbidities and subsequent hospitalization. Outcomes were calculated for a cumulative number of sessions allowing for a more detailed analysis of the dose-response relationship between number of sessions and mortality.

The population selected was limited to Medicare fee-for-service beneficiaries so the results may not be applicable to those on other programmes, those in other countries with different healthcare systems, and younger patients. The analysis was limited to a maximum of 36 CR sessions, since Medicare carriers will not reimburse for additional treatment. Could the positive impact of increasing CR sessions be extrapolated over and above the putative 36-session limit? Furthermore, a direct cause-and-effect relationship that would suggest CR was the sole reason for the improved outcomes could not be established. For instance, attendance in CR may simply be a proxy for other factors, not included in the analysis, such as improved general activity, medication adherence, healthier eating, and smoking cessation. Finally, there may be a potential bias secondary to unmeasured underlying health status, that is, those with poor underlying health may attend fewer CR sessions than those with better health status, and therefore may have worse outcomes.

Impact on the field

This study clearly demonstrates the existence of a dose-response relationship between the number of CR sessions attended and long-term outcomes in terms of mortality and subsequent MI. These results provide important evidence for CR patients, professionals, and other stakeholders, that 'more is better', with regards to CR.

Learning points

- There is a dose-response relationship between the number of cardiac rehabilitation sessions attended and long-term outcomes.
- Attending 36 sessions of CR is associated with a greater reduction in the risk of mortality and subsequent MI when compared with any lesser number of sessions.
- Uptake of CR remains low, with only 18% of patients attending 36 sessions in this particular analysis.

- Patients who are eligible for CR should be encouraged to attend as many sessions as possible to achieve maximal benefits from CR.

Further reading

- Goel K, Lennon RJ, Tilbury RT, *et al*. Impact of cardiac rehabilitation on mortality and cardiovascular events after percutaneous coronary intervention in the community. *Circulation* 2011; 123: 2344–52.
- Suaya JA, Stason WB, Ades PA, *et al*. Cardiac rehabilitation and survival in older coronary patients. *J Am Coll Cardiol* 2009; 54: 25–33.
- Taylor RS, Brown A, Ebrahim S, *et al*. Evidence-based rehabilitation for patients with coronary heart disease: systematic review and meta-analysis of randomised controlled trials. *Am J Med* 2004; 116: 682–92.

Predictors of cardiac rehabilitation participation in older coronary patients

Ades PA, Waldmann ML, McCann WL, Weaver SO. *Arch Intern Med* 1992; 152: 1033–5.

Background

Early studies of CR identified first the safety, and later the benefits of CR services for patients with recent cardiac events. This led to the gradual acceptance of CR services in both research and clinical circles, and gradually led to a significant growth in the number of CR programmes in the United States in the 1980s and 1990s. Despite that growth, however, studies in the 1990s suggested that only a minority of eligible patients were receiving CR following a cardiac event. If CR services had been shown to be beneficial for patients, why were they not participating?

While it was becoming clear that there was a problem with under-utilization of CR, even as early as 1990, the reasons for this problem, and its potential solutions, were largely unclear and unexplored. Particularly perplexing was the finding in some studies that CR was particularly under-utilized in persons who were older than 65 years of age, a group that would seem to have the most to gain from a comprehensive and coordinated approach to their recuperation and rehabilitation. Clearly, starting in the 1990s, under-utilization of CR emerged as a growing concern in the field of CR.

While some clinical investigators help to identify important clinical problems, others work to identify solutions. Philip Ades and colleagues set about to do both in their landmark study from 1992. In this study, Ades sought to identify barriers and potential solutions to the perplexing problem of under-utilization of CR.

Article summary

Research nurses carried out in-hospital interviews with 226 hospitalized patients, 62 years of age or older, who had been hospitalized with MI (47%) or post-CABG surgery (53%). They collected and analysed a variety of demographic, psychosocial, and medical factors to identify predictors of CR participation. Important univariate predictors of CR participation included younger age, shorter commute time, higher education, absence of chronic comorbid medical conditions, being male, having a white collar job, being depressed before the index hospitalization, denial of the severity of his/her cardiac disease, and the strength of the physician recommendation for CR. In the multivariate analysis, the strength of the physician recommendation for CR was the strongest predictor of subsequent CR participation. When the physician's recommendation was considered to be strong by the patient, 66% of the time the patient ended up participating in CR, while only 2% participated when they considered the physician's recommendation for CR to be weak. Other predictors of CR participation in the multivariate model included commute time, patient denial of the severity of his/her cardiac illness, and the presence of depression before hospitalization.

Strengths and limitations

Two important strengths of this study should be noted. First, the investigators collected both objective and subjective data from patients at the time of hospitalization in a prospective manner. Second, patient participation in CR was verified directly by the study's investigators. One limitation of the study is that the study included a group of patients, 62 years of age or older, from one medical centre in the north-eastern United States. Results of the study, therefore, may not be directly applicable to other patient groups in other parts of the world.

Impact on the field

This study has had a lasting impact on the field of CR for a number of reasons. First of all, this paper was one of the first studies of 'outcomes research' in CR. It helped form a basis for future efforts to identify important components and processes of patient care that affect the treatment delivered to patients and, by extension, the outcomes of that treatment. Second, this study was important because it helped identify a somewhat surprising but key factor that greatly affected the enrolment of patients into a CR programme—the strength of the physician's recommendation for CR enrolment. The stronger the endorsement, the more likely it was that patients would actually enrol in a programme. This finding made it clear that the referring physician was an important potential solution to the problem of under-utilization of CR.

Furthermore, this study helped to identify other patient, medical, and healthcare system factors that were potential barriers to CR participation. Subsequent to the

publication of this landmark paper, a number of quality improvement projects have been carried out that have tested various process interventions aimed at overcoming barriers to CR participation. While it is an overstatement to suggest that this paper by Ades and colleagues was the main reason for the application of quality improvement efforts in the field of CR, it is safe to say that this fairly brief paper had an enormous and lasting impact on the subsequent development of quality improvement initiatives in CR.

Learning points

- Various patient, medical, and healthcare system factors influence the likelihood that a patient will participate in CR following a cardiac event.
- The strength of a physician's recommendation for a patient to participate in CR was found to be the strongest predictor of subsequent CR participation.
- The systematic identification of barriers to and predictors of CR participation helped lay the groundwork for the systematic approaches to improving CR participation.

Further reading

- Daly J, Sindone AP, Thompson DR, *et al.* Barriers to participation in and adherence to cardiac rehabilitation programs: a critical literature review. *Prog Cardiovasc Nurs* 2002; 17: 8–17.
- Dunlay SM, Witt BJ, Allison TG, *et al.* Barriers to participation in cardiac rehabilitation. *Am Heart J* 2009; 158(5): 852–9.
- Grace SL, Chessex C, Arthur H, *et al.* Systematizing Inpatient Referral to Cardiac Rehabilitation 2010: Canadian Association of Cardiac Rehabilitation and Canadian Cardiovascular Society joint position paper. *J Cardiopulm Rehabil Prev* 2011; 31(3): E1–8.
- Witt BJ, Thomas RJ, Roger VL. Cardiac rehabilitation after myocardial infarction: a review to understand barriers to participation and potential solutions. *Eura Medicophys* 2005; 41(1): 27–34.

National survey on gender difference in cardiac rehabilitation program: patient characteristics and enrollment patterns

Thomas RJ, Miller NH, Lamendola C, Berra K, Hedback B, Durstine L, Haskell W. *J Cardiopulm Rehabil* 1996; 16: 402–12.

Background

While research over the past 2–3 decades has shown that CR services provide significant health benefits to participating patients, another line of research during that same time has suggested that the true impact of CR is limited by its under-utilization by eligible patients. While the problem of under-utilization was suspected by many CR programmes in the 1980s, large-scale national studies on this issue were lacking. Early studies by Neil Oldridge and others helped to raise awareness of this increasingly recognized gap in CR care in the early 1990s. However, new and important light was shed on this topic by this landmark paper by William Haskell, Nancy Miller, Kathy Berra, and other researchers at Stanford University. They were among the first to report detailed, national enrolment patterns in CR for men, women, and minorities.

Article summary

The authors surveyed 500 randomly chosen CR programmes operating in the United States in 1990, to collect information about the number and characteristics of patients who enrolled in their programmes that year. Responses were received from 163 programmes (33% response rate), including data on 1322 women and 1418 men. Results from these surveys were used to estimate the total number of patients who participated in a CR programme in the United States in 1990 (i.e. the 'numerator'). To estimate the number of patients who were eligible for CR in 1990 (i.e. the 'denominator'), the authors also analysed data from the 1990 National Hospital Discharge Survey to identify the number of patients discharged alive from the hospital in 1990 after MI, percutaneous coronary intervention, or CABG surgery.

Cardiac rehabilitation enrolment rates were found to be low for all patients, from 10.8% of post-MI patients to 23.4% of post-CABG patients. Participation rates were particularly low for women, non-whites, and those older than 65 years of age. In post-MI patients, for example, 13.3% of men enrolled in CR compared to only 6.9% of women (p <0001). While 16.5% of those younger than age 65 enrolled in CR, only 7.0% of those 65 years of age or older enrolled (p <0.001). Participation rates were generally higher following CABG surgery, 24.6% of men and 20.2% of women enrolled in CR. With regards to enrolment in CR by racial group, 11.6% of whites enrolled in CR following MI, while only 5.1% of non-whites enrolled (p <0.001). Following CABG surgery, 24.0% of whites enrolled in CR, with only 16.9% of non-whites enrolling (p <0.001). The gender gap in enrollment in CR was similar in whites and non-whites following MI, but was larger following CABG surgery (i.e. the percentage of women enrolling in CR following CABG surgery was even lower in non-white than in white women). The gender gap remained consistent with increasing age for post-MI patients, but was larger following CABG surgery (i.e. older women were less likely than younger women to enroll in CR).

Strengths and limitations

The strengths of this study include its national scope and sampling of CR programmes, and its use of the National Hospital Discharge Survey to assess the number of patients who were eligible for CR, in general, by gender and racial/ethnic group, and by diagnostic group.

The weaknesses of this study include the fact that the investigators used data from a relatively small sample of CR programmes to estimate the number and characteristics of patients who enrolled in CR. However, since the sample of CR programmes included programmes from various parts of the United States, the estimates appear to be accurate, and are consistent with subsequent studies that have assessed the percentage and characteristics of patients who participate in CR programmes.

Impact on the field

This study, along with others that helped to verify the findings, helped to raise awareness of the low utilization rates for CR among those patients eligible for such services. The identification of this gap in delivery of secondary prevention services helped encourage others in the field to further clarify the barriers to CR participation and explore their potential solutions.

Learning points

- Only a small percentage of eligible patients actually receive CR services in the United States.
- The low CR utilization rates are particularly low for women, older patients, and patients from racial/ethnic minority groups.
- Cardiac rehabilitation participation is higher among patients who have undergone CABG surgery as compared to those who have had an MI.
- Participation rates for CR vary by geographical regions, suggesting that certain barriers to participation may be potentially overcome.

Further reading

- Bittner V, Sanderson B, Breland J, Green D. Referral patterns to a University-based cardiac rehabilitation program. *Am J Cardiol* 1999; 83(2): 252–5, A5.
- Oldridge NB, Streiner DL. The health belief model: predicting compliance and dropout in cardiac rehabilitation. *Med Sci Sports Exerc* 1990; 22(5): 678–83.
- Sharp J, Freeman C. Patterns and predictors of uptake and adherence to cardiac rehabilitation. *J Cardiopulm Rehabil Prev* 2009; 29(4): 241–7.
- Suaya JA, Shepard DS, Normand SL, Ades PA, Prottas J, Stason WB. Use of cardiac rehabilitation by Medicare beneficiaries after myocardial infarction or coronary bypass surgery. *Circulation* 2007; 116(15): 1653–62. (Epub 24 Sep 2007).

Economic evaluation of cardiac rehabilitation soon after acute myocardial infarction

Oldridge N, Furlong W, Feeny D, Torrance G, Guyatt G, Crowe J et al. *Am J Cardiol* 1993; 72(2): 154–61.

Background

Cardiac rehabilitation is considered a standard of care for patients experiencing a qualifying cardiac event. It provides a structured programme of exercise training, patient education, and counselling, and has been shown to accelerate improvement in cardiovascular risk factors, increase exercise tolerance, and improve some aspects of psychological status. Meta-analyses have also shown an approximate 25% reduction in mortality over three years post-acute MI associated with CR.

Economic evaluation of healthcare programmes is defined as the comparative analysis of alternative courses of action in regard to both costs and consequences. One method is cost-utility analysis, in which therapeutic interventions are compared in terms of cost per quality adjusted life year (QALY) gained. One QALY is one year of life in full health. It is calculated by adjusting life expectancy for the quality of those remaining years.

Article summary

Oldridge *et al.* present this randomized controlled trial of CR initiated soon after acute MI for patients with mild to moderate levels of anxiety and depression. The economic evaluation in terms of cost per QALY gained was the primary outcome measure. The intervention involved an eight-week CR programme consisting of supervised exercise, together with group behavioural and risk factor management counselling, initiated within six weeks of MI, and was compared to standard post-MI care. Data were collected at baseline, following the eight-week intervention, and at 4, 8, and 12 months post-index event. The authors hypothesized that patients with mild to moderate depression while in hospital would have the greatest potential for improvement in quality of life with the intervention. A group of 201 eligible patients were randomized, 102 to usual care and 99 to intervention. The cohorts were comparable in terms of age, gender, degree of myocardial damage, and employment status.

The same authors had previously published a detailed analysis of improvement in QALYs related to CR. They selected time trade off as a measure of QALY. This provides a measure based on the maximum number of years a subject would be willing to trade off to live in full health rather than their present health state. Based on this method, the CR programme resulted in 0.052 QALYs gained attributable to the programme at one year (95% CI 0.100 and 0.007). Costs were calculated in terms of costs of the programme, costs to the patient, and savings as a result of reduced healthcare service utilization. At one year, there was no significant difference in utilization of physician services, emergency room visits, hospital in-patient days, allied healthcare visits, or medication use, so these costs were assumed to be the same in each cohort. There was, however, a significant reduction in utilization of community CR visits. After accounting for these costs and savings, the authors estimated an incremental cost of $480 per patient associated with the intervention (95% CI $230–180). The authors calculated a cost of $9,200 per QALY gained (at 1991 US$ rates). A cost-effectiveness analysis was also performed utilizing three-year mortality data from a previous meta-analysis providing a cost of $35,900 per life year gained.

Strengths and limitations

The authors used a randomized controlled trial to collate their data prospectively. In particular, the cost analysis is very thorough, accounting for the costs to the patient as well as the costs of the programme. The time trade off measure of QALYs gained is a tool specifically developed for use in healthcare settings. A full sensitivity analysis was also performed utilizing minimum and maximum estimates for each of the costs.

The data presented only provide a measure based on one-year follow-up. The longer-term benefits for this intervention are therefore unknown. The generalizability of these results to the population at large is unknown, as only those with mild to moderate anxiety and depression were included. In addition, there is no information on the comorbidities of the cohorts. The significance of the cost-effectiveness analysis is debatable given that the meta-analysis used to perform the calculation included studies with differing rehabilitation programmes. In addition, any mortality benefit beyond the three years of study was not considered.

Impact on the field

This study shows that brief CR provided soon after MI in patients with mild to moderate anxiety and depression is an efficient use of resources and can be economically justified. When compared to other interventions, CR seems an economically sound use of resources. For example, CABG surgery for single vessel disease in patients with mild angina costs $68,200/QALY (Goel et al., 1989), lovastatin treatment for hypercholesterolemia costs $17,000/QALY (Goldman et al., 1991), and captopril for hypertension

$106,900/QALY (Edelson et al., 1990). More economic interventions include CABG for left main disease (£7900/QALY), aspirin post-acute MI ($3100/QALY) and beta blockers for high-risk males ($5300/QALY). However, these data are based on costs in the late 1980s, with many drugs cheaper now, and do not include data on percutaneous coronary intervention. Cardiac rehabilitation has previously been demonstrated to be safe and clinically useful and this data support its ongoing use in the management of patients following acute MI.

Learning points

♦ The cost-utility of a relatively brief period of CR post-acute MI in patients with mild-moderate anxiety and depression is $9200 per QALY gained (1991 US$).

♦ Over a one-year period, a gain of 0.052 QALY/patient can be attributed to CR.

♦ Cardiac rehabilitation is an economically justifiable use of resources for patients following an acute MI.

Further reading

● Edelson JT, Weinstein MC, Tosteson ANA, et al. Long-term cost-effectiveness of various initial monotherapies for mild to moderate hypertension. JAMA 1990; 263: 408–13.
● Goel V, Deber RB, Detsky AS. Nonionic contrast media: economic analysis and health policy development. Can Med Assoc J 1989; 140: 389–95.
● Goldman L, Weinstein MC, Goldman PA, Williams LW. Cost-effectiveness of HMG-CoA reductase inhibition for primary and secondary prevention of coronary heart disease. JAMA 1991; 265: 1145–51.
● Oldridge NB, Guyatt G, Jones N, et al. Effects on quality of life with comprehensive rehabilitation after acute myocardial infarction. Am J Cardiol 1991; 67: 1084–9.
● Siegel D, Grady D, Browner WS, Hulley SB. Risk factor modification after myocardial infarction. Ann Intern Med 1988; 109: 213–8.

Cost-effectiveness of cardiac rehabilitation after myocardial infarction

Ades P, Pashkow F, Nestor J. *J Cardiopulm Rehabil* 1997; 17(4): 222–31.

Background

Cardiac rehabilitation often forms part of a secondary prevention strategy aimed at reducing mortality and subsequent coronary events. Cost effectiveness is an indicator of the cost of an intervention per year of survival gained, usually quoted as unit price per year of life saved.

It provides a means of direct comparison between otherwise difficult to compare interventions, for example invasive versus non-invasive interventions for coronary artery disease. Such an analysis is aimed at assisting clinical decision making and the setting of healthcare finance policy. Both the medical benefits and cost effectiveness of standard acute and secondary preventive interventions including invasive revascularization, reperfusion, anticoagulation, blood pressure, and lipid reduction have previously been documented. In this paper, Ades *et al.* provide a cost-effectiveness analysis of CR as compared to standard care for the post-acute MI patient.

Article summary

The authors here utilized three different sources to calculate the cost effectiveness of CR in the post-acute MI population: published results from randomized controlled trials of effect of CR on mortality rates, epidemiological studies of long-term survival in the overall post-MI population, and studies of patient charges for rehabilitation programmes and averted medical expenses for hospitalization after rehabilitation. The primary measure of effectiveness was incremental life expectancy (YLS— years of life saved) attributable to CR for survivors of acute MI. The measure of cost included explicit payments made, or averted, for direct medical services including hospitalization, physician services, other non-physician services, drugs, and diagnostic tests. It did not include indirect or non-medical costs such as travel costs to attend rehabilitation or change in income as a result of rehabilitation. The final calculation of cost-effectiveness was calculated as:

$$\frac{\text{Lifetime total expenditure on intervention} - \text{Lifetime direct saving for averted medical care}}{\text{Incremental life expectancy}}$$

Rates of mortality in the intervention group versus control were adapted from a meta-analysis by O'Connor and colleagues in 1989 of 22 randomized controlled trials of CR. The populations studied were predominantly males below the age of 65 years post-acute MI. The cumulative all-cause mortality in the rehabilitation group was reduced by 16.9% at three years (OR 0.80; 95% CI 0.66–0.96). Beyond follow-up, it was assumed that mortality in both groups follows a natural and predictable course. The Duke University Cardiovascular Disease Database of 4379 post-acute MI patients was used to obtain an average life expectancy of 15.4 years in this group. This resulted in the authors obtaining a value of 0.202 YLS for CR versus standard treatment.

The cost of rehabilitation for the index period, defined by the authors as 1985 to 1986 was $1280, and was obtained from a survey of 626 centres in the USA. The monetary saving from averted hospitalization was obtained from a US-based study by the same author and was calculated at $850.

The primary finding was a cost effectiveness of $2130/ YLS during the index period, equating to $4,950/YLS in 1995, after accounting for inflation and changes in post-acute MI mortality.

Strengths and limitations

This study provides an analysis of the cost-effectiveness of CR following MI. It included estimates and other data that allowed for sensitivity analyses as well as a comparison to other interventions.

The main limitation was that different populations were used for each component of the analysis. For instance, the early mortality data were taken from a group of predominantly younger males and from studies from various countries. The late mortality calculation and the cost calculations were based on a 1995 population from the US only.

Impact on the field

This study was the first to allow direct comparison of the cost effectiveness of CR with other secondary prevention measures post-MI. It showed that the cost effectiveness of CR was acceptably lower than the cost-effectiveness threshold that was typically used at the time the paper was published (less than $20,000/YLS). In fact, the study found that CR was more cost-effective than CABG graft surgery ($8500/YLS for left main stem, $18,700/YLS for three vessels, Wong, 1990), coronary angioplasty ($8700/ YLS one vessel and severe angina, Wong, 1990), and lipid lowering therapy ($9360/YLS for simvastatin, Goldman, 1991) but less cost-effective than smoking-cessation measures ($220/YLS, Krumholz, 1993). Overall, this study proved that CR was an economically viable part of post-acute MI care.

Learning points

- At 1995 rates, the cost effectiveness of CR in post-acute MI patients is $4950/YLS.
- Cardiac rehabilitation is more cost-effective than CABG surgery, coronary angioplasty, and cholesterol lowering drugs according to this calculation but less cost-effective than smoking cessation.

Further reading

- Ades PA, Huang D, Weaver SO. Cardiac rehabilitation participation predicts lower rehospitalization cost. *Am Heart J* 1992; 123: 916–21.
- Balady GJ, Fletcher BJ, Froelicher ES, *et al.* Cardiac rehabilitation programs. A statement for healthcare professionals from the American Heart Association. *Circulation* 1994; 90: 1602–10.
- Goldman L, Weinstein MC, Goldman PA, Williams LW. Cost-effectiveness of HMG-CoA reductase inhibition for primary and secondary prevention of coronary heart disease. *JAMA* 1991; 265: 1145–51.
- Krumholz HM, Cohen BJ, Tsevat J, *et al.* Cost effectiveness of a smoking cessation program after myocardial infarction. *J Am Coll Cardiol* 1993; 22: 1697–1702.
- Kupersmith J, Holmes-Rovner M, Hogan A, *et al.* Cost-effectiveness analysis in heart disease. *Prog Cardiovasc Dis* 1995; 37: 243–71.
- O'Connor GT, Buring JE, Yusuf S, *et al.* An overview of randomized trials of rehabilitation with exercise after myocardial infarction. *Circulation* 1989; 80: 234–44.
- Wong JB, Sonnenberg FA, Salem DN, Pauker SG. Myocardial revascularization for chronic stable angina. *Ann Intern Med* 1990; 113: 852–71.

A case-management system for coronary risk factor modification after acute myocardial infarction

DeBusk RF, Miller NH, Superko HR, Dennis CA, Thomas RJ, Lew HT, Berger WE 3rd, Heller RS, Rompf J, Gee D, Kraemer HC, Bandura A, Ghandour G, Clark M, Shah RV, Fisher L, Taylor CB. *Ann Intern Med* 1994; 120(9): 721–9.

Background

The evolution of CR over the past three decades has been marked by several advances that have been truly innovative. One particular advance was published by Robert DeBusk, lead researcher of the MULTIFIT study, who has been a long-time leader in innovation in cardiovascular disease prevention. Prior to the MULTIFIT study, referenced here, it was thought unsafe and ineffective to have patients carry out their rehabilitation in any location other than a supervised CR setting. DeBusk and colleagues designed a study to challenge that line of thinking, by assessing the potential impact of a physician-directed, nurse-managed, home-based system for patients recuperating from MI. This study has had a lasting impact on the field of CR.

Article summary

Patients (n = 585) were randomized to usual care or the nurse-case management system following MI. The intervention started in the hospital, with the nurse meeting with each intervention patient to initiate exercise training, lipid lowering diet-drug therapy, and smoking cessation therapy (where indicated). Following hospital discharge, intervention patients were contacted periodically by their nurse case manager to follow up on their progress in their treatment plans. Outcomes were assessed at two months and six months following hospital discharge.

Smoking cessation, documented by cotinine levels, was confirmed in 70% of smokers in the intervention group (vs. 53% in usual care, p = 0.03). Low-density lipoprotein cholesterol levels were significantly lower in the intervention group (107 mg/dl vs. 132 mg/dl in the usual care group, p = 0.001), and exercise capacity was significantly higher in the intervention group (9.3 METs vs. 8.43 METs in the usual care group, p = 0.001). Patients with severe medical limitations (22%) were not encouraged to exercise (severe chronic obstructive pulmonary disease, severe peripheral artery disease, musculoskeletal limitations, etc.). No significant exercise-related adverse events occurred in the intervention group. Only 5% of the usual care group participated in group-based exercise training.

Strengths and limitations

The strengths of this study by DeBusk *et al.* include the following:

- All patients in the intervention group were enrolled in a system that provided optimal secondary prevention therapy following MI. This model of care is particularly appealing in view of the low percentage of eligible patients who are referred to CR centres as part of their plan for secondary prevention therapy.
- Although a cost effective analysis was not reported, the nurse-managed system of secondary prevention

appears to be a safe and relatively low cost alternative, and produces outcomes that are superior to those seen in usual care.

The study is limited, however, by the fact that the study was performed in the era when statin therapy was just emerging, and reflected the ability of the nurse-managed care team to manage lipids with the therapeutic tools available to them at the time (principally niacin, fibrates, and resins). In today's 'statin era', it is unclear if a nurse-managed system would be superior to usual care. A major limitation to the study is in the area of generalizability, given that insurance carriers generally did not (and still do not) cover services that are carried out by telephone, such as occurred with the MULTIFIT intervention. One final limitation of the study is that it did not compare the impact of the intervention with the 'gold standard' of programme-based CR, making it hard to assess how the MULTIFIT model compares with the 'traditional' model of secondary prevention following MI.

Impact on the field

This study by DeBusk *et al.* had a significant impact on the field of preventive cardiology by introducing a novel approach to secondary prevention—a nurse-managed, home-based approach to care. Unfortunately, the fact that insurance carriers have generally chosen not to cover such services has limited its full implementation in the United States, but such a model still holds great promise as the US, and other countries search for safe, effective, and lower cost options for high quality secondary prevention care.

Learning points

◆ A physician supervised, nurse-managed system that started in the hospital and continued at home primarily through telephone contacts, was effective and safe in delivering lifestyle and medication therapy for hyperlipidaemia, exercise training, and smoking cessation.

◆ As healthcare systems look to safe, effective, and lower cost options for secondary prevention following MI, the MULTIFIT system approach will be a likely alternative for their consideration.

Further reading

● Allison TG, Farkouh ME, Smars PA, *et al.* Management of coronary risk factors by registered nurses versus usual care in patients with unstable angina pectoris (a chest pain evaluation in the emergency room (CHEER) substudy). *Am J Cardiol* 2000; 86(2): 133–8.
● Berra K, Miller NH, Jennings C. Nurse-based models for cardiovascular disease prevention: from research to clinical practice. *Eur J Cardiovasc Nurs* 2011; 10 Suppl 2: S42–50.
● Gordon NF, English CD, Contractor AS, Salmon RD, Leighton RF, Franklin BA, Haskell WL. Effectiveness of three models for comprehensive cardiovascular disease risk reduction. *Am J Cardiol.* 2002 Jun 1; 89(11):1263–8.
● Miller NH, Haskell WL, Berra K, DeBusk RF. Home versus group exercise training for increasing functional capacity after myocardial infarction. *Circulation* 1984; 70: 645–9.
● Taylor CB, Houston-Miller N, Killen JD, DeBusk RF. Smoking cessation after acute myocardial infarction: effects of a nurse-managed intervention. *Ann Intern Med* 1990; 113: 118–23.

Safety of medically supervised outpatient cardiac rehabilitation exercise therapy: a 16-year follow-up

Franklin BA, Bonzheim K, Gordon S, Timmis GC. *Chest* 1998; 114(3): 902–6.

Background

The safety of CR in the form of physical training was initially demonstrated in two large retrospective surveys. The first by Haskell in 1978 reported one non-fatal event for every 34,673 participant-hours and one fatal event per 116,402 patient-hours over a study period of 17 years. The second by Van Camp and Peterson in 1986 reported 29 cardiovascular complications over 2,351,916 participant-hours. However, these surveys pre-dated the increasing use of revascularization and newer pharmacological therapies.

Article summary

This study by Franklin *et al.* examines the safety of medically supervised outpatient CR therapy at a single centre over a 16-year-period between 1982 and 1998. The primary outcome was major cardiovascular events including cardiac arrest and acute MI. A total of 3,335 patients referred following acute MI or revascularization surgery were included, with an average age of 61.6 years. Patients had a range of cardiac comorbidities, including compensated heart failure, previous heart valve surgery, and device insertion (pacemaker or implantable cardioverter-defibrillator). Approximately 70% of the study population was male.

The exercise programme studied comprised two levels of intervention. Phase 2 involved 50-minute sessions three times a week with continuous ECG telemetry and blood pressure measurements during exercise. The programme duration was four, six, and eight weeks for low, moderate, and high-risk patients respectively. Phase 3 followed a similar format without continuous monitoring; instead ECG was available if required and blood pressure monitored weekly. Patients were encouraged to enter phase 3 following completion of phase 2. An exercise prescription was created for each patient with target heart rate and metabolic equivalents set. The supervising team included nurses, exercise physiologists, and exercise technicians trained in basic or advanced life support.

Overall, 292,254 patient-hours were recorded (45,679 in phase 2 and 246,575 in phase 3). There were five major cardiovascular complications, including three non-fatal MIs and two cardiac arrests. Both patients with cardiac arrest were successfully resuscitated, although one later died in hospital. Each of these patients was deemed moderate to high risk. The overall cardiovascular complication rate was 1 event per 58,451 patient-hours (1 per 146,127 for cardiac arrest and 1 per 97,418 for acute MI). Further analysis showed that cardiovascular complications appear unrelated to the duration of the programme or time following cardiac event.

Strengths and limitations

This study examines a large number of patient hours over 16 years at a single centre, with clear outcome measures. The five patients with complications were examined further in terms of their cardiac history, risk factor profile, and rehabilitation programme. Although all of these patients were deemed moderate or high risk, the statistical significance is unclear because of the low numbers. The population included was diverse in terms of cardiac co-morbidities making it difficult to relate the results to specific cardiac sub-populations.

Impact on the field

This study supports previous studies in the field showing that supervised outpatient CR programmes are safe.

A more recent study by Pavy et al. confirmed these findings with an adverse event rate of 1 per 49,565 patient-hours. Traditional risk factor stratification appears to identify those at risk of developing complications. In addition, the presence of a physician at the sessions does not seem to be necessary as long as staff are trained in advanced life support. The fact this study was performed in the age of cardiac revascularization and aggressive pharmacotherapy supports its continuing use in practice.

Learning points

- Supervised out-patient CR is a safe intervention, with a low frequency of major cardiovascular complications.
- Contemporary risk factor stratification criteria seems to identify patients at risk of complications.
- Direct physician presence does not appear necessary for safety as long as staff are trained in life support.

Further reading

- Balady GJ, Williams MA, Ades PA, et al. Core components of cardiac rehabilitation/secondary prevention programs: 2007 update. *Circulation* 2007; 115: 2675–82.
- Dinnes J, Kleijnen J, Leitner M, Thompson D. Cardiac rehabilitation. *Qual Health Care* 1999; 8: 65–71.
- Haskell WL. Cardiovascular complications during exercise training of cardiac patients. *Circulation* 1978; 57: 920–4.
- Pavy B, Iliou MC, Meurin P, et al. Safety of exercise training for cardiac patients. Results of the French registry of complications during cardiac rehabilitation. *Arch Int Med* 2006; 166: 2329–34.
- Van Camp SP, Paterson SA. Cardiovascular complications of outpatient cardiac rehabilitation programs. *JAMA* 1986; 256: 1160–3.
- Witt BJ, Jacobson SJ, Weston SA, et al. Cardiac rehabilitation after myocardial infarction in the community. *J Am Coll Cardiol* 2004; 44: 988–96.

Effect of cardiac rehabilitation referral strategies on utilization rates: a prospective, controlled study

Grace SL, Russell KL, Reid RD, Oh P, Anand S, Rush J, Williamson K, Gupta M, Alter DA, Stewart DE; for the Cardiac Rehabilitation Care Continuity Through Automatic Referral Evaluation (CRCARE) Investigators. *Arch Intern Med* 2011; 171(3): 235–41.

Background

An important step in the progression of CR has been the development of methods to overcome its underutilization by improving methods of its delivery to eligible patients. A number of important studies have taken place over the years that have attempted to solve the important barriers to CR utilization. While none of these studies have found a perfect solution, several have led to key improvements in the CR referral and enrolment process. Many of these articles are worthy of mention, and are listed in the reference list at the end of this section. The landmark article by Grace *et al.* is important because it developed and tested four different CR referral strategies in an innovative, timely, and rigorous fashion to identify method(s) associated with improved uptake of CR.

Article summary

Patients hospitalized with coronary artery disease (n = 2,635) from 11 hospitals in Ontario, Canada, were prospectively enrolled into this study, and were referred to CR using one of four referral strategies—usual referral, liaison referral (a healthcare professional acting as a referral counsellor or 'coach'), automatic referral (automatic ordering and referral system), and liaison plus automatic referral. One year later, 1,809 of the patients returned surveys that assessed their CR participation following the index hospitalization. Adjusted analyses found that the combined liaison plus automatic referral method produced the highest CR referral and enrolment rates (85% referral, 74% enrolment), followed by the automatic referral method (70% referral, 60% enrolment), the liaison only method (59% referral, 51% enrolment), and the usual referral method (32% referral, 29% enrolment).

Strengths and limitations

The main strength of the study was that it tested four clinically meaningful referral strategies in a prospective and controlled fashion. A weakness of the study is the potential for bias in the results, since the study was not a randomized study and its results could have been affected by differing patient characteristics in each of the 11 study sites. The investigators attempted to overcome this limitation by performing statistical adjustment of the results, correcting for the major differences between sites. Another limitation to the study was that it relied on patient self-report for CR participation. The study may have been underpowered, as reflected by the relatively small number of sites per intervention strategy, and by relatively wide confidence intervals. Still, the findings are timely, important, and clinically relevant to the current practice of CR.

Impact on the field

This study has given new insights into specific methods that can help reduce the gap in CR utilization that has been noted worldwide for the past two decades. It has already helped move the field of CR forward with approaches for improving the uptake of CR that are both feasible and evidence-based.

Learning points

- Among four intervention strategies that were tested, CR referral and enrolment were enhanced most by using a strategy that combined an automatic CR referral process with a clinical liaison (counsellor/coach).
- Use of such a strategy produced a very high rate of CR referral (85%) and enrolment (74%).

Further reading

- Gravely-Witte S, Leung YW, Nariani R, *et al.* Effects of cardiac rehabilitation referral strategies on referral and enrollment rates. *Nat Rev Cardiol* 2010; 7(2): 87–96.
- Mueller E, Savage PD, Schneider DJ, Howland LL, Ades PA. Effect of a computerized referral at hospital discharge on cardiac rehabilitation participation rates. *J Cardiopulm Rehabil Prev* 2009; 29(6): 365–9.

Conclusion

Since its origins in the 1950s, CR has evolved into a multidisciplinary and evidence-based lifesaving service for patients with cardiovascular disease. A rich tapestry of research findings have shown CR to improve both the quality and the quantity of life for patients who receive its services. Cardiac rehabilitation is recommended by national healthcare organizations in their clinical practice guidelines and is covered widely by healthcare plans. Unfortunately, despite the evidence and support for CR services, only a minority of eligible patients participate in CR and receive its numerous benefits.

Researchers have uncovered important CR referral and enrolment tools to improve the utilization of CR services by eligible patients. Likewise, emerging healthcare policy work is helping to increase CR delivery by increasing the level of accountability for healthcare providers in assuring that they provide CR services to all eligible patients, and not just to the minority of patients who receive CR currently.

These recent advances in the science and the application of CR services are likely to continue to expand and bear fruit.

Ongoing and future studies will help clarify several important questions that remain about CR:

- What is the role of CR in patients with heart failure?
- How best can CR programmes assist patients in treating obesity?
- Are new delivery models of care for CR as beneficial and cost effective as centre-based CR?
- Do performance measures for CR help improve the percentage of patients who participate in CR?
- What is the most cost-effective long-term model of follow-up care for patients who have completed early outpatient CR?

The future of CR looks bright, particularly as researchers continue to uncover new and innovative ways to improve CR delivery, and as healthcare policy-makers recognize and cover those new and innovative delivery methods.

This overview of landmark studies in CR includes only a small number of the many important CR studies that have been published in the past. It is very likely that as the field of CR continues to evolve and advance, additional landmark CR studies will appear in the months and years ahead.

Reference

1. http://bernardlown.wordpress.com/2011/02/03/a-chair-to-the-rescue/ Accessed 25 April 2011.

Index